Studies in Classification, Data Analysis, and Knowledge Organisation

Springer
Berlin
Heidelberg
New York
Hong Kong
London
Milan
Paris
Tokyo

Titles in the Series

H.-H. Bock and P. Ihm (Eds.)
Classification, Data Analysis, and Knowledge Organization. 1991 (out of print)

M. Schader (Ed.)
Analyzing and Modeling Data and Knowledge. 1992

O. Opitz, B. Lausen, and R. Klar (Eds.)
Information and Classification. 1993 (out of print)

H.-H. Bock, W. Lenski, and M. M. Richter (Eds.)
Information Systems and Data Analysis. 1994 (out of print)

E. Diday, Y. Lechevallier, M. Schader, P. Bertrand, and B. Burtschy (Eds.)
New Approaches in Classification and Data Analysis. 1994 (out of print)

W. Gaul and D. Pfeifer (Eds.)
From Data to Knowledge. 1995

H.-H. Bock and W. Polasek (Eds.)
Data Analysis and Information Systems. 1996

E. Diday, Y. Lechevallier, and O. Opitz (Eds.)
Ordinal and Symbolic Data Analysis. 1996

R. Klar and O. Opitz (Eds.)
Classification and Knowledge Organization. 1997

C. Hayashi, N. Ohsumi, K. Yajima, Y. Tanaka, H.-H. Bock, and Y. Baba (Eds.)
Data Science, Classification, and Related Methods. 1998

I. Balderjahn, R. Mathar, and M. Schader (Eds.)
Classification, Data Analysis, and Data Highways. 1998

A. Rizzi, M. Vichi, and H.-H. Bock (Eds.)
Advances in Data Science and Classification. 1998

M. Vichi and O. Opitz (Eds.)
Classification and Data Analysis. 1999

W. Gaul and H. Locarek-Junge (Eds.)
Classification in the Information Age. 1999

H.-H. Bock and E. Diday (Eds.)
Analysis of Symbolic Data. 2000

H. A. L. Kiers, J.-P. Rasson, P. J. F. Groenen, and M. Schader (Eds.)
Data Analysis, Classification, and Related Methods. 2000

W. Gaul, O. Opitz, and M. Schader (Eds.)
Data Analysis. 2000

R. Decker and W. Gaul
Classification and Information Processing at the Turn of the Millenium. 2000

S. Borra, R. Rocci, M. Vichi, and M. Schader (Eds.)
Advances in Classification and Data Analysis. 2001

W. Gaul and G. Ritter (Eds.)
Classification, Automation, and New Media. 2002

K. Jajuga, A. Sokolowski, and H.-H. Bock (Eds.)
Classification, Clustering and Data Analysis. 2002

M. Schwaiger, O. Opitz (Eds.)
Exploratory Data Analysis in Empirical Research. 2003

M. Schader, W. Gaul, and M. Vichi (Eds.)
Between Data Science and Applied Data Analysis. 2003

H.-H. Bock, M. Chiodi, and A. Mineo (Eds.)
Advances in Multivariate Data Analysis. 2004

David Banks · Leanna House ·
Frederick R. McMorris · Phipps Arabie ·
Wolfgang Gaul
Editors

Classification, Clustering, and Data Mining Applications

Proceedings of the Meeting of the International Federation of Classification Societies (IFCS),
Illinois Institute of Technology, Chicago, 15–18 July 2004

With 156 Figures and 86 Tables

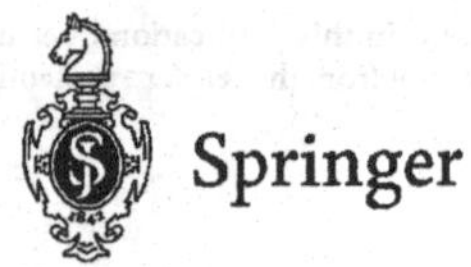

Dr. David Banks
Leanna House
Institute of Statistics and Decision Sciences
Duke University
27708 Durham, NC
U.S.A.
banks@stat.duke.edu
house@stat.duke.edu

Dr. Frederick R. McMorris
Illinois Institute of Technology
Department of Mathematics
10 West 32nd Street
60616-3793 Chicago, IL
U.S.A.
mcmorris@iit.edu

Dr. Phipps Arabie
Faculty of Management
Rutgers University
180 University Avenue
07102-1895 Newark, NJ
U.S.A.
arabie@andromeda.rutgers.edu

Prof. Dr. Wolfgang Gaul
Institute of Decision Theory
University of Karlsruhe
Kaiserstr. 12
76128 Karlsruhe
Germany
wolfgang.gaul@wiwi.uni-karlsruhe.de

ISSN 1431-8814
ISBN 3-540-22014-3 Springer-Verlag Berlin Heidelberg New York

Library of Congress Control Number: 2004106890

Springer-Verlag is a part of Springer Science+Business Media

springeronline.com

Printed in Germany

Softcover design: Erich Kirchner, Heidelberg

SPIN 11008729 88/3130-5 4 3 2 1 0 – Printed on acid-free paper

This book is dedicated to the memory of

Professor Chikio Hayashi

who served as president of the International Federation of Classification Societies from 1998 until 2000. His leadership, his scholarship, and his humanity are an example to us all.

Preface

This book presents some of the key research undertaken by the members of the International Federation of Classification Societies during the two years since our last symposium. If the past is a guide to the future, these papers contain the seeds of new ideas that will invigorate our field.

The editors are grateful to the community of classification scientists. Even those whose work does not appear here have contributed through previous research, teaching, and mentoring. It is a great joy to participate in this kind global academy, which is only possible because its members work to cultivate courtesy along with creativity, and friendship together with scholarship.

The editors particularly thank the referees who reviewed these papers:

Simona Balbi	Lynne Billard	Hans Bock	Paul De Boeck
Jaap Brand	Peter Bryant	Doug Carroll	Edwin Diday
Adrian Dobra	Vincenzo Esposito	Anuska Ferligoj	Ernest Fokoue
John Gower	Andre Hardy	Stephen Hirtle	Krzysztof Jajuga
Bart Jan van Os	Mel Janowitz	Henk Kiers	Mike Larsen
Carlo Lauro	Michael Lavine	Ludovic Lebart	Bruno Leclerc
Herbie Lee	Taerim Lee	Scotland Leman	Walter Liggett
Masahiro Mizuta	Clive Moncrieff	Fionn Murtagh	Noboru Ohsumi
Jennifer Pittman	Alfredo Rizzi	Pascale Rousseau	Ashish Sanil
Bill Shannon	Javier Trejos	Mark Vangel	Rosanna Verde
Kert Viele	Kiri Wagstaff	Stan Wasserman	Stan Young

Durham, North Carolina	*David Banks*
Durham, North Carolina	*Leanna House*
New Brunswick, New Jersey	*Phipps Arabie*
Chicago, Illinois	*F. R. McMorris*
Karlsruhe, Germany	*Wolfgang Gaul*
	March, 2004

Contents

Part I

New Methods in Cluster Analysis

Thinking Ultrametrically

Fionn Murtagh

Queen's University Belfast, Northern Ireland, UK
f.murtagh@qub.ac.uk

Abstract: The triangular inequality is a defining property of a metric space, while the stronger ultrametric inequality is a defining property of an ultrametric space. Ultrametric distance is defined from p-adic valuation. It is known that ultrametricity is a natural property of spaces that are sparse. Here we look at the quantification of ultrametricity. We also look at data compression based on a new ultrametric wavelet transform. We conclude with computational implications of prevalent and perhaps ubiquitous ultrametricity.

1 Introduction

The triangular inequality holds for a metric space: $d(x, z) \leq d(x, y) + d(y, z)$ for any triplet of points x, y, z. In addition the properties of symmetry and positive definiteness are respected. The "strong triangular inequality" or ultrametric inequality is: $d(x, z) \leq \max \{d(x, y), d(y, z)\}$ for any triplet x, y, z. An ultrametric space implies respect for a range of stringent properties. For example, the triangle formed by any triplet is necessarily isosceles, with the two large sides equal. Ultrametricity is a natural property of high-dimensional spaces (Rammal et al., 1986, p. 786); and ultrametricity emerges as a consequence of randomness and of the law of large numbers (Rammal et al., 1986; Ogielski and Stein, 1985).

An ultrametric topology is associated with the p-adic numbers (Mahler, 1981; Gouvêa, 2003). Furthermore, the ultrametric inequality implies non-respect of a relation between a triplet of positive valuations termed the Archimedean inequality. Consequently, ultrametric spaces, p-adic numbers, non-Archimedean numbers, and isosceles spaces all express the same thing.

P-adic numbers were introduced by Kurt Hensel in 1898. The ultrametric topology was introduced by Marc Krasner (Krasner, 1944), the ultrametric inequality having been formulated by Hausdorff in 1934. Important references on ultrametrics in the clustering and classification area are those of Benzécri (1979) representing work going back to 1963, and Johnson (1967).

Watson (2003) attributes to Mézard et al. (1984) the basis for take-off in interest in ultrametrics in statistical mechanics and optimization theory. Mézard et al. (1984) developed a mean-field theory of spin glasses, showing that the distribution of pure states in a configuration space is ultrametric. "Frustrated optimization problems" are ultrametric, and have been shown as such for spin glass and related special cases. Parisi and Ricci-Tersenghi (2000), considering the spin glass model that has become a basic model for complex systems, state that "ultrametricity implies that the distance between the different states is such that they can be put in a taxonomic or genealogical tree such that the distance among two states is consistent with their position on the tree". An optimization process can be modeled using random walks so if local ultrametricity exists then random walks in ultrametric spaces are important (Ogielski and Stein, 1985). Further historical insight into the recent history of use of ultrametric spaces is provided by Rammal et al. (1985) and for linguistic research by Roberts (2001).

P-adic numbers, which provide an analytic version of ultrametric topologies, have a crucially important property resulting from Ostrowski's theorem: Each non-trivial valuation on the field of the rational numbers is equivalent either to the absolute value function or to some p-adic valuation (Schikhof, 1984, p. 22). Essentially this theorem states that the rationals can be expressed in terms of (continuous) reals, or (discrete) p-adic numbers, and no other alternative system.

In this article we will describe a new ultrametric wavelet transform. Our motivation for doing this is to provide analysis capability for situations where our data tends to be ultrametric (e.g., sparse, high-dimensional data). Secondly, in this article, we will present results of Lerman's proposed quantification of ultrametricity in a data set.

2 P-adic Coding From Dendrograms

Dendrograms used in data analysis are usually labeled and ranked: see Figures 2 and 3.

For the ranked dendrogram shown in Figure 2 we develop the following p-adic encoding of terminal nodes, by traversing a path from the root: $x_1 = 0 \cdot 2^7 + 0 \cdot 2^5 + 0 \cdot 2^2 + 0 \cdot 2^1$; $x_2 = 0 \cdot 2^7 + 0 \cdot 2^5 + 0 \cdot 2^2 + 1 \cdot 2^1$; $x_4 = 0 \cdot 2^7 + 1 \cdot 2^5 + 0 \cdot 2^4 + 0 \cdot 2^3$; $x_6 = 0 \cdot 2^7 + 1 \cdot 2^5 + 1 \cdot 2^4$. The decimal equivalents of this p-adic representation of terminal nodes work out as $x_1, x_2, \ldots x_8 = 0, 2, 4, 32, 40, 48, 128, 192$.

Distance and norm are defined as follows. $d_p(x, x') = d_p|x - x'| = 2^{-r+1}$ or $2 \cdot 2^{-r}$ where $x = \sum_k a_k 2^k$, $x' = \sum_k a'_k 2^k$, $r = \text{argmin}_k \{a_k = a'_k\}$. The norm is defined as $d_p(x, 0) = 2^{-1+1} = 1$.

To find the p-adic distance, we therefore look for the smallest level, r (if ordered from terminal to root as in Figure 2) which is identical in the pair of power series, which yields the result of 2^{-r+1}. We find $|x_1 - x_2|_2 = 2^{-2+1} =$

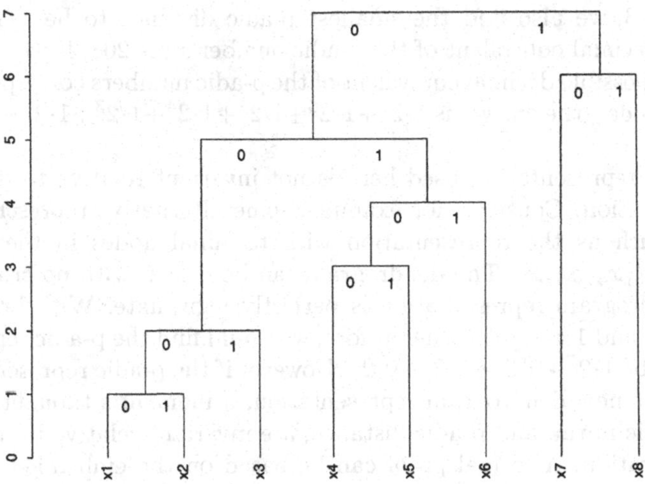

Fig. 1. Labeled, ranked dendrogram on 8 terminal nodes. Branches labeled 0 and 1.

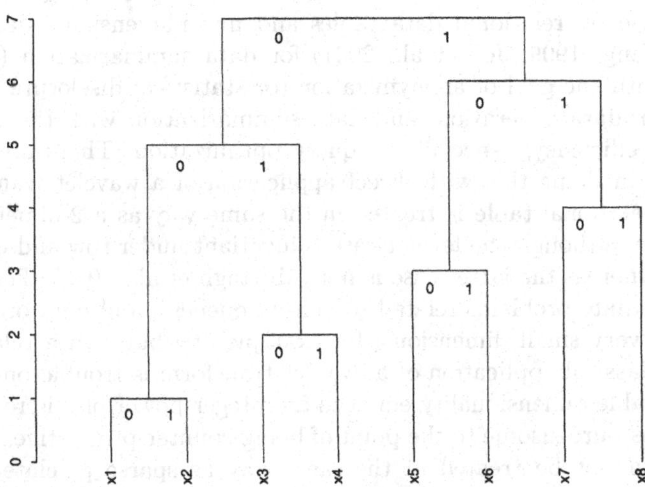

Fig. 2. A structurally balanced, labeled, ranked dendrogram on 8 terminal nodes. Branches labeled 0 and 1.

$1/2; |x_1 - x_4|_2 = 2^{-6+1} = 1/32; |x_1 - x_6|_2 = 2^{-6+1} = 1/32$. The smallest p-adic distance between terminals in Figure 2 is seen to be 1/128.

For Figure 3, we also find the smallest p-adic distance to be 1/128. In Figure 3, the decimal equivalent of the p-adic number x_8 is 208. If we look for the maximum possible decimal equivalent of the p-adic numbers corresponding to 8 terminal nodes, the answer is $1 \cdot 2^7 + 1 \cdot 2^6 + 1 \cdot 2^5 + 1 \cdot 2^4 + 1 \cdot 2^3 + 1 \cdot 2^2 + 1 \cdot 2^1 = 254$.

The p-adic representation used here is not invariant relative to dendrogram representation. Consider, for example, some alternative representation of Figure 2 such as the representation with terminal nodes in the order: $x_7, x_8, x_1, x_2, x_3, x_4, x_5, x_6$. The dendrogram can be drawn with no crossings, so such a dendrogram representation is perfectly legitimate. With branches labeled 0 = left and 1 = right, as heretofore, we would find the p-adic representation of x_1 to be $1 \cdot 2^7 + 0 \cdot 2^5 + 0 \cdot 2^2 + 0 \cdot 2^1$. However if the p-adic representation differs with this new dendrogram representation, a moment's thought shows that both p-adic norm, and p-adic distance, are invariant relative to dendrogram representation. A formal proof can be based on the embedded classes represented by dendrogram nodes.

3 Regression Based on Ultrametric Haar Wavelet Transform

The wavelet transform, developed for signal and image processing, has been extended for use on relational data tables and multidimensional data sets (Vitter and Wang, 1999; Joe et al., 2001) for data summarization (microaggregation) with the goal of anonymization (or statistical disclosure limitation) and macrodata generation; and data summarization with the goal of computational efficiency, especially in query optimization. There are problems, however, in doing this with direct application of a wavelet transform. Essentially, a relational table is treated in the same way as a 2-dimensional pixelated image, although the former case is invariant under row and column permutation, whereas the latter case is not (Murtagh et al., 2000). Therefore there are immediate problems related to non-uniqueness, and data order dependence. For very small dimensions, for example attributes in a relational data table, a classical application of a wavelet transform is troublesome, and in addition if table dimensionality equal to an integer power of 2 is required, the procedure is burdensome to the point of being counter-productive. Sparse tabular data cannot be treated in the same way as sparse pixelated data (e.g. Sun and Zhou, 2000) if only because row/column permutation invariance causes the outcome to be dominated by sparsity-induced effects. In this article we will develop a different way to wavelet transform tabular data. A range of other input data types are also capable of being treated in this way.

Our motivation for the development of wavelet transforms in ultrametric or hierarchical data structures is to cater for "naturally" or enforced ultrametric data. An example of the former case is questionnaire results with embedded question sets. An example of the latter case is that of data with already strong ultrametric tendency such as sparsely coded data in speech analysis, genomics and proteomics, and other fields, and complete disjunctive form in correspondence analysis.

The Haar wavelet transform is usually applied to 1D signals, 2D images, and 3D data cubes (see Starck et al. 1998; Starck and Murtagh, 2002). Sweldens (1997) extended the wavelet transform to spherical structures, still in Hilbert space. We extend the wavelet transform to other topological structures, in particular hierarchies which have a natural representation as trees. In regard to the wavelet transform, we focus in particular on the Haar wavelet transform, in its redundant (Soltani et al., 2000; Zheng et al., 1999) and non-redundant versions (e.g., Frazier, 1999).

The Morlet-Grossmann definition of the continuous wavelet transform (Grossmann et al. 1989; Starck and Murtagh 2002) holds for a signal $f(x) \in L^2(\mathbb{R})$, the Hilbert space of all square integrable functions. Hilbert space $L^2(\mathbb{R})$ is isomorphic and isometric relative to its integer analog $l^2(\mathbb{Z})$. The discrete wavelet transform, derived from the continuous wavelet transform, holds for a discrete function $f(x) \in l^2(\mathbb{Z})$.

Our input data is decomposed into a set of band-pass filtered components, the wavelet coefficients, plus a low-pass filtered version of our data, the continuum (or background or residual). We consider a signal, $\{c_{0,l}\}$, defined as the scalar product at samples i of the real function $f(x)$, our input data, with a scaling function $\phi(x)$ which corresponds to a low-pass filter: $c_0(k) = \langle f(x), \phi(x-k) \rangle$.

The wavelet transform is defined as a series expansion of the original signal, c_0, in terms of the wavelet coefficients. The final smoothed signal is added to all the differences: $c_{0,i} = c_{J,i} + \sum_{j=1}^{J} w_{j,i}$. This equation provides a reconstruction formula for the original signal. At each scale j, we obtain a set, which we call a wavelet scale. The wavelet scale has the same number of samples as the signal, i.e. it is redundant, and decimation is not used.

Now consider any hierarchical clustering, H, represented as a binary rooted tree. For each cluster q'' with offspring nodes q and q', we define $s(q'')$ through application of the low-pass filter $\begin{pmatrix} 0.5 \\ 0.5 \end{pmatrix}$:

$$s(q'') = \frac{1}{2}(s(q) + s(q')) = \begin{pmatrix} 0.5 \\ 0.5 \end{pmatrix}^t \begin{pmatrix} s(q) \\ s(q') \end{pmatrix} \tag{1}$$

Next for each cluster q'' with offspring nodes q and q', we define detail coefficients $d(q'')$ through application of the band-pass filter $\begin{pmatrix} 0.5 \\ -0.5 \end{pmatrix}$:

$$d(q'') = \frac{1}{2}(d(q) - d(q')) = \begin{pmatrix} 0.5 \\ -0.5 \end{pmatrix}^t \begin{pmatrix} d(q) \\ d(q') \end{pmatrix} \tag{2}$$

The scheme followed is illustrated in Figure 3, which shows the hierarchy constructed by the median method, using the first 8 observation vectors in Fisher's iris data (Fisher, 1936).

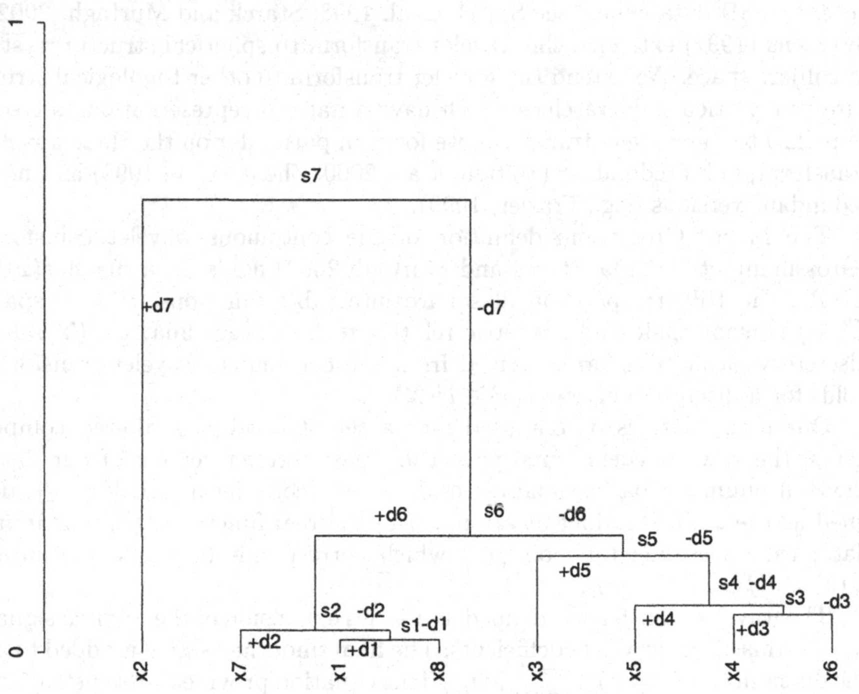

Fig. 3. Dendrogram on 8 terminal nodes constructed from first 8 values of Fisher's iris data. Median method used in this case.

For any $d(q_j)$ we have: $\sum_k d(q_j)_k = 0$, i.e. the detail coefficient vectors are each of zero mean. The inverse transform allows exact reconstruction of the input data. If an observation vector is denoted by x_i, then the ultrametric wavelet transform defines the p-adic encoding for x_i given by $\sum_1^{n-1} a_k p_k$ where $a_k \in \{0, 1\}$ and $p_k = 2^k$. The wavelet transform is defined by $x_i = s_{n-1} + \sum_1^{n-1} a_k d_k$ where s_{n-1} is the final smooth component, and d_k are the detail or wavelet signals (or vectors).

Setting wavelet coefficients to zero and then reconstructing the data is referred to as hard thresholding (in wavelet space) and this is also termed wavelet smoothing or regression. Table 1 shows the excellent results that can be obtained for Fisher's iris data. Further results on the energy compacting or compression properties of this new ultrametric Haar transform are given in Murtagh (2003b), together with R code for this new transform and its inverse.

Filtering threshold	% coefficients set to zero	mean square error
0	16.95	0
0.1	70.13	0.0098
0.2	91.95	0.0487
0.3	97.15	0.0837
0.4	97.82	0.1040

Table 1. Ultrametric Haar filtering results for Fisher's 150 × 4 iris data. Filtering is carried out by setting small (less than the threshold) wavelet coefficient values to zero. The data is then reconstructed. The quality of reconstruction between the input data matrix, and the reconstructed data matrix, is measured using mean square error.

4 Lerman's H-Classifiability

The work of Rammal et al. (1986) used the discrepancy between the subdominant ultrametric (provided by single link hierarchical clustering) and input metric values as a measure of how ultrametric the given data set was. Their work is further discussed below, in this section. We distrust the single link method in view of its known chaining and other disadvantages. We will now review an alternative measure of ultrametricity in a data set, due to Lerman (1981).

On a set E, a binary relation is a *preorder* if it is reflexive and transitive. Let F denote the set of pairs of distinct units, where a unit is from E. A distance defines a total preorder on F:

$$\forall\{(x,y),(z,t)\} \in F : (x,y) \leq (z,t) \Longleftrightarrow d(x,y) \leq d(z,t)$$

This preorder will be denoted ω_d. Two distances are equivalent on a given set E iff the preordonnances associated with each on E are identical. A total preorder is equivalent to the definition of a partition (defining an equivalence relation on F), and to a total order on the set of classes. A preorder $\bar{\omega}$ is called ultrametric if:

$$\forall x,y,z \in E : \rho(x,y) \leq r \text{ and } \rho(y,z) \leq r \Longrightarrow \rho(x,z) \leq r$$

where r is a given integer and $\rho(x,y)$ denotes the rank of pair (x,y) for $\bar{\omega}$, defined by non-decreasing values of the distance used. A necessary and sufficient condition for a distance on F to be ultrametric is that the associated preorder (on $E \times E$, or alternatively preordonnance on E) is ultrametric.

Looking again at the link between a preorder and classes defining a partition, $\forall x, y, z \in E$ s.t. $(x, y) \leq (y, z) \leq (x, z)$ we must have: $(x, z) \leq (y, z)$, i.e. (x, z) and (y, z) are in the same class of a preorder $\bar{\omega}$.

We move on now to define Lerman's H-classifiability index (Lerman, 1981), which measures how ultrametric a given metric is. Let $M(x, y, z)$ be the median pair among $\{(x, y), (y, z), (x, z)\}$ and let $S(x, y, z)$ be the highest ranked pair among this triplet. J is the set of all such triplets of E. We consider the mapping τ of all triplets J into the open interval of all pairs F for the given preorder ω defined as:

$$\tau : J \longrightarrow]M(x, y, z), S(x, y, z)[$$

A measure of the discrepancy between preorder ω and an ultrametric preorder will be defined from a measure on all pairs F that is dependent on ω.

Given a triplet $\{x, y, z\}$ for which $(x, y) \leq (y, z) \leq (x, z)$, for preorder ω, the interval $]M(x, y, z), S(x, y, z)[$ is empty if ω is ultrametric. Relative to such a triplet, the preorder ω is "less ultrametric" to the extent that the cardinal of $]M(x, y, z), S(x, y, z)[$, defined on ω, is large. In practice we ensure that ties in the ranks, due to identically-valued distances, are taken into account, by counting ranks that are strictly between M and S.

We take J into account in order to define discrepancy between the structure of ω and the structure of an ultrametric preordonnance where $|\cdot|$ denotes cardinality:

$$H(\omega) = \sum_J |]M(x, y, z), S(x, y, z)[|/(|F| - 3)|J|$$

If ω is ultrametric then $H(\omega) = 0$. As shown in simple cases by Lerman (1981, p. 218), data sets that are "more classifiable" in an intuitive way, i.e. they contain "sporadic islands" of more dense regions of points – a prime example is Fisher's iris data contrasted with 150 uniformly distributed values in $\mathbb{R}^4$ – such data sets have a smaller value of $H(\omega)$. For Fisher's data we find $H(\omega) = 0.0899$, whereas for 150 uniformly distributed points in a 4-dimensional hypercube, we find $H(\omega) = 0.1835$.

Generating all unique triplets is computationally intensive: for n points, $n(n-1)(n-2)/6$ triplets have to be considered. Hence, in practice, we must draw triangles randomly from the given point set. For integer indices i, j, k, we draw $i \sim [1 \ldots n-2], j \sim [i+1 \ldots n-1], k \sim [\max\,(i, j) + 1 \ldots n]$ where sampling is uniform.

Rammal et al. (1985, 1986) quantify ultrametricity as follows. The Rammal ultrametricity index is given by $\sum_{x,y}(d(x, y) - d_c(x, y)) / \sum_{x,y} d(x, y)$ where d is the metric distance being assessed, and d_c is the subdominant ultrametric. The Rammal index is bounded by 0 (= ultrametric) and 1. As pointed out in Rammal (1985, 1986), this index suffers from "the chaining effect and from sensitivity to fluctuations". The single link method, yielding the subdominant ultrametric, is subject to potential pathologies. For this reason the Lerman index is to be preferred. The latter is unbounded and, given the definition used above, we have found maximum values (i.e. greatest non-ultrametricity) in the region of 0.25.

Rammal et al. (1985, 1986) discuss a range of important cases: a set of n binary words, randomly defined among the 2^k possible words of k bits; and n words of k letters extracted from an alphabet of size K. For binary words, $K = 2$; for nucleic acids, four nucleotids give $K = 4$; for proteins, twenty amino acids give $K = 20$; and for spoken words, around 40 phonemes give $K = 40$. Using the Rammal ultrametricity index, experimental findings demonstrate that random data, in the sparse limit (i.e., with increasing dimensionality and with increasing sparseness), are increasingly ultrametric.

Our experimental findings are different, given the very different way we assess ultrametricity, and we contribute some important clarifications in the light of Lerman's H-classifiability to the Rammal et al. discovery that ultrametricity is "a natural property of large spaces".

We use uniformly distributed data and also uniformly distributed hypercube vertex positions. The latter is used to simulate the multivalued words considered by Rammal et al. Random values are converted to hypercube vertex locations by use of complete disjunctive data coding (Benzécri, 1992). For example, for $K = 4$ we use four fixed intervals. A value of x falling in the first interval receives a 4-valued set: $1, 0, 0, 0$; a value of x falling in the second interval receives the 4-valued set: $0, 1, 0, 0$; and so on. Such complete disjunctive coding is widely used in correspondence analysis. It is easily verified that the row marginals are constant. In this important case, Lerman (1981) develops an analytic probability density function for the H-classifiability index.

In our experiments (see Murtagh, 2003a), we found that there is no increase in H-classifiability, i.e. departure from ultrametricity, for increasing numbers of points, n, at least for the range used here: $n = 1000, 2000, 3000, 4000, 5000$. In the results shown in Figure 4 we note the following additional findings:

- There is increase in H-classifiability, i.e. departure from ultrametricity, for increasing dimensionality. Again this holds for the dimensionalities examined here: $m = 50, 100, 250, 500$.
- Random hypercube vertex data are "more classifiable", i.e. such data has smaller H-classifiability and is more ultrametric, compared to uniformly distributed data.

In our experimentation we chose data sets with no a priori clustering. These data sets were random, being either

- uniformly distributed, or
- sparsely coded as hypercube vertices.

We see that the latter is consistently more ultrametric than the former.

Our results point to the importance of the "type" of data used or, better expressed, how the data are coded. Binary data representing any categori-

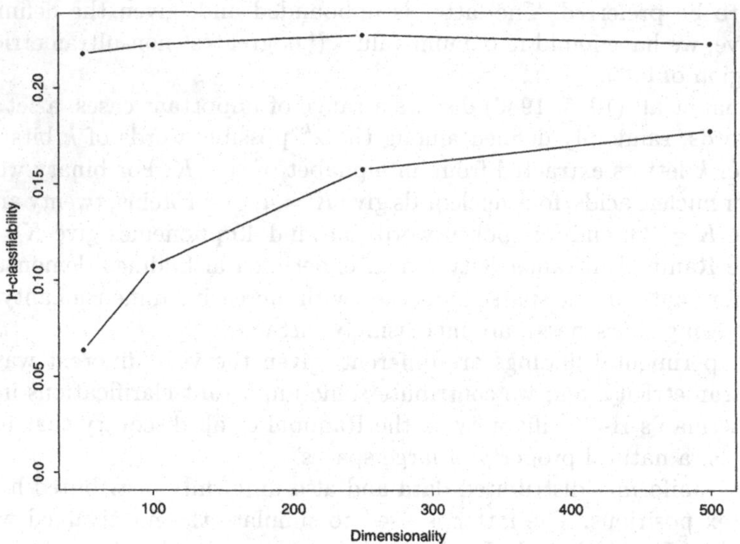

Fig. 4. Upper curve: uniformly distributed values. Lower curve: random hypercube vertex points. A low value of H-classifiability is related to near-ultrametricity. Each point shows an average of different experiments corresponding to numbers of points $n = 1000, 2000, 3000, 4000, 5000$.

cal (qualitative) variables are consistently more ultrametric than uniformly distributed data. Further experiments on quantifying ultrametricity are in Murtagh (2004).

Given that sparse forms of coding are considered for how complex stimuli are represented in the cortex (see Young and Yamane, 1992), the ultrametricity of such spaces becomes important because of this sparseness of coding. This suggests the possibility that semantic pattern matching is best accomplished through ultrametric computation. Our justification in indicating this is that once we have a dendrogram data structure nearest neighbor computation has constant computational complexity, i.e. it is of $\mathcal{O}(1)$ computational cost. Other operations also enjoy good computational properties once we have a binary rooted tree data structure that defines interrelationships.

5 Conclusion

We have shown that sparse coding tends to be ultrametric. This is an interesting result in its own right. However a far more important result is that certain computational operations can be carried out very efficiently indeed in space endowed with an ultrametric. Chief among these computational results is that nearest neighbor finding can be carried out in (worst case) constant computational time. We have noted how forms of sparse coding are considered to be used in the human or animal cortex. We raise the interesting question as to whether human or animal thinking can be computationally efficient precisely because such computation is carried out in an ultrametric space.

We have developed a new form of the Haar wavelet transform for topologies associated with hierarchically structured data sets. We have demonstrated the effectiveness of this transform for data filtering and for data compression.

References

1. Benzécri, J. P. (1979). *La Taxinomie*, 2nd ed., Paris:Dunod.
2. Benzécri, J. P. (1992). Transl. T.K. Gopalan. *Correspondence Analysis Handbook*, Basel:Marcel Dekker.
3. Fisher, R. A. (1936). "The Use of Multiple Measurements in Taxonomic Problems," *The Annals of Eugenics*, **7**, 179–188.
4. Frazier, M. W. (1999). *An Introduction to Wavelets through Linear Algebra*, Springer-Verlag, New York.
5. Gouvêa, F. Q. (2003). *P-Adic Numbers*, Springer-Verlag, New York, 2nd edn., 3rd printing.
6. Grossmann, A., Kronland-Martinet, R., and Morlet, J. (1989). "Reading and Understanding the Continuous Wavelet Transform," in *Wavelets: Time-Frequency Methods and Phase-Space*, eds. J. Combes, A. Grossmann, and P. Tchamitchian, New York:Springer-Verlag, pp. 2–20.
7. Joe, M. J., Whang, K.-Y., and Kim, S.-W. (2001). "Wavelet Transformation-Based Management of Integrated Summary Data for Distributed Query Processing," *Data and Knowledge Engineering*, **39**, 293–312.
8. Johnson, S. C. (1967). "Hierarchical Clustering Schemes," *Psychometrika*, **32**, 241-254.
9. Krasner, M. (1944). "Nombres Semi-Réels et Espaces Ultramétriques," *Comptes-Rendus de l'Académie des Sciences, Tome II*, **219**, 433.
10. Lerman, I. C. (1981). *Classification et Analyse Ordinale des Données*, Dunod, Paris.
11. Mahler, M. (1981). *P-adic Numbers and Their Functions*, 2nd edn., Cambridge:Cambridge University Press.
12. Mézard, M., Parisi, G., Sourlas, N., Toulouse, G., and Virasoro, M. A. (1984). "Nature of the Spin-Glass Phase," *Physical Review Letters*, **52**, 1156–1159.
13. Murtagh, F., Starck, J.-L., and Berry, M. (2000). "Overcoming the Curse of Dimensionality in Clustering by Means of the Wavelet Transform," *The Computer Journal*, **43**, 107–120.
14. Murtagh, F. (2003a). "On Ultrametricity, Sparse Coding and Computation," submitted.
15. Murtagh, F. (2003b). "Hierarchical or Ultrametric Haar Wavelet Transform in Multivariate Data Analysis and Data Mining," submitted.
16. Murtagh, F. (2004). "Quantifying Ultrametricity," *COMPSTAT 2004*, submitted.

17. Ogielski, A. T. and Stein, D. L. (1985). "Dynamics of Ultrametric Spaces," *Physical Review Letters*, **55**, 1634–1637.
18. Parisi, G. and Ricci-Tersenghi, F. (2000). "On the Origin of Ultrametricity," *Journal of Physics A: Mathematical and General*, **33**, 113–129.
19. Rammal, R., Angles d'Auriac, J. C., and Doucot, B. (1985). "On the Degree of Ultrametricity," *Le Journal de Physique–Lettres*, **46**, L-945–L-952.
20. Rammal, R., Toulouse, G., and Virasoro, M.A. (1986). "Ultrametricity for Physicists," *Reviews of Modern Physics*, **58**, 765-788.
21. Roberts, M. D. (2001). "Ultrametric Distance in Syntax," at Internet URL http://arXiv.org/abs/cs.CL/9810012.
22. Schikhof, W. H. (1984). *Ultrametric Calculus*, Cambridge:Cambridge University Press.
23. Soltani, S., Boichu, D., Simard, P., and Canu, S. (2000). "The Long-Term Memory Prediction by Multiscale Decomposition," *Signal Processing*, **80**, 2195–2205.
24. Starck, J.-L., Murtagh, F., and Bijaoui, A. (1998). *Image and Data Analysis: The Multiscale Approach*, Cambridge University Press, Cambridge.
25. Starck, J.-L., and Murtagh, F. (2002). *Astronomical Image and Data Analysis*, Springer-Verlag, New York.
26. Sun, W., and Zhou, X. (2000). "Sampling Theorem for Wavelet Subspaces: Error Estimate and Irregular Sampling Theorem," *IEEE Transactions on Signal Processing*, **48**, 223–226.
27. Sweldens, W. (1997). "The Lifting Scheme: A Construction of Second Generation Wavelets," *SIAM Journal on Mathematical Analysis*, **29**, 511–546.
28. Vitter, J. S., and Wang, M. (1999). "Approximate Computation of Multidimensional Aggregates of Sparse Data Using Wavelets," in *Proceedings of the ACM SIGMOD International Conference on Management of Data*, pp. 193–204.
29. Watson, S. (2003). "The Classification of Metrics and Multivariate Statistical Analysis," preprint, York University, 27 pp.
30. Young, M. P. and Yamane, S. (1992). "Sparse Population Coding of Faces in the Inferotemporal Cortex," *Science*, **256**, 1327–1331.
31. Zheng, G., Starck, J.-L., Campbell, J. G., and Murtagh, F. (1999). "Multiscale Transforms for Filtering Financial Data Streams," *Journal of Computational Intelligence in Finance*, **7**, 18-35.

Clustering by Vertex Density in a Graph

Alain Guénoche

Institute de Mathématiques de Luminy - CNRS, France
guenoche@iml.univ-mrs.fr

Abstract: In this paper we introduce a new principle for two classical problems in clustering: obtaining a set of partial classes and a partition on a set X of n elements. These structures are built from a distance D and a threshold value σ giving a threshold graph on X with maximum degree δ. The method is based on a density function $De : X \to \mathbb{R}$ which is computed first from D. Then, the number of classes, the classes, and the partitions are established using only this density function and the graph edges, with a computational complexity of $\mathcal{O}(n\delta)$. Monte Carlo simulations, from random Euclidian distances, validate the method.

1 Introduction

Given a distance matrix on X, extracting partial classes (in which not all the elements are clustered) or establishing partitions (all the elements are clustered in disjoint classes) is generally made by optimizing a criterion over the set of all partitions with a given number of classes. For most of the criteria, the optimization problem is NP-Hard and so heuristics are applied (too many authors deserve to be cited to just select a few of them, so these references are omitted).

In this paper, we investigate a different approach. First, we select a threshold σ and, considering only pairs having a distance value lower than or equal to σ, we build the corresponding graph. Thus we are lead to the clustering problem in valued graphs, well known in Combinatorial Data Analysis.

The method we propose is based on the evaluation of a density function in each vertex. Then we search for connected parts having a high density value, as has been proposed in the percolation methods (Trémolières, 1994). The algorithm differs from similar approaches (Bader and Hogue, 2003; Rougemont and Hingamp, 2003) in many ways; e.g., we use the valuation of the edges to measure a density and we perform progressive clustering, adding the elements in three steps:

- we first realize a *kernel* which is a connected part of the vertices for which the density is locally maximum and greater than the average;
- then, these classes are extended, adding vertices that are connected to only one kernel ;
- finally the unclassified elements are assigned to one of the previous classes.

This method can be applied to any data in a metric space—quantitative, qualitative or binary, sequences—using an appropriate distance. We emphasize that the number of classes in not given a priori. It is defined as the number of local maxima of the density function and, with simulations, we prove that the correct number can very often be recovered, when classes do not intersect.

Given a distance matrix, $D : X \times X \to \mathbb{R}$, the first step is to select a threshold σ to build a graph. Its edge set E is the set of pairs having a distance value less than or equal to σ. Let $n = |X|$, $m = |E|$, and let $\Gamma_\sigma = (X, E)$ be the corresponding graph. When there is no ambiguity on the threshold value, it will simply be denoted Γ. For any part Y of X, let $\Gamma(Y)$ be the set of vertices adjacent to Y which do not belong to Y. Thus, the neighborhood of x is denoted by $\Gamma(x)$, the degree of a vertex x is $Dg(x) = |\Gamma(x)|$, and let δ be the maximum degree in Γ.

The paper is organized as follows. In Section 2 we define three density functions that will be compared in Section 4. In Section 3 we detail the algorithm for building partial classes and partitions, giving its complexity. In Section 4 we evaluate classes and partitions using Monte Carlo simulations; several criteria estimate partition quality.

2 Threshold Value and Density Functions

The nested family of threshold graphs is obtained from a distance matrix by making σ vary from 0 to $Dmax$, the largest distance value. Let σ_c be the *connectivity threshold* value, i.e., the largest edge length of a minimum spanning tree of D. A value larger than or equal to σ_c, gives a connected graph and a lower value always yields several connected components. For $\sigma = Dmax$ the graph is complete.

Choosing a threshold value is a delicate problem. It has an influence on the number of classes since they are the connected part of X and thus necessarily included in the connected components of the graph. Hence we replace this problem by choosing a percentage of the number of edges of the complete graph. Indicating the percent α will define a threshold distance value σ, and the graph will contain $\alpha \times \frac{n(n-1)}{2}$ edges.

For each vertex x, we define a density value denoted $De(x)$ which is high when the elements of $\Gamma(x)$ are close to x. We propose three functions:

- The first only depends on the minimum distance value from x, and is

$$De_1(x) = \frac{\sigma - \min_{y \in \Gamma(x)} D(x,y)}{\sigma}.$$

- The second is computed from the average length of the edges from x and is

$$De_2(x) = \frac{\sigma - \frac{1}{Dg(x)} \sum_{y \in \Gamma(x)} D(x,y)}{\sigma}.$$

- The third corresponds to the maximum distance value in $\Gamma(x)$, and is

$$De_3(x) = \frac{\sigma - \max_{y \in \Gamma(x)} D(x,y)}{\sigma}.$$

The computation of the threshold graph from D is of order $\mathcal{O}(n^2)$. To evaluate these functions it is sufficient to test the edges in the neighborhood of x which contains at most δ vertices. So the computation of the density function is thus $\mathcal{O}(n^2)$.

3 Classes and Partitions

The dense classes are by definition connected parts in Γ that share high density values. Our initial idea was to search for a density threshold and to consider the partial subgraph whose vertices have a density greater than this threshold. Classes would be the connected components. This strategy does not give the expected results. Enumerating all the possible threshold values, we observed that often none was satisfying. By decreasing the threshold, we often obtain only a single growing class, and many singletons. Since there is no straightforward way to fix a threshold, the *local maximum values* of the density function need to be considered.

3.1 Classes at Three Levels

We successively compute the *kernels* of the classes, the *extended classes* that do not cover X, and the *complete classes* that make a partition. For these three levels, the classes are nested.

Kernels

A kernel, denoted K, is a connected part of Γ obtained by the following algorithm: we first search for the local maximum values of the density function and we consider the partial subgraph of Γ reduced to these vertices:

$$\forall x \in K,\ \forall y \in \Gamma(x) \text{ we have } De(x) \geq De(y).$$

The initial kernels are the connected components of this graph. More precisely, if several vertices with the maximum value are in the same kernel, they necessarily have the same density value; otherwise the initial kernels are singletons. Then, we assign recursively to each kernel K the vertices (i) having a density greater than or equal to the average density value over X, and (ii) that are adjacent to only one kernel. By doing so, we avoid any ambiguity in the assignment, reserving the decision when several are possible.

The number of kernels is the number of classes and it will remain unchanged in the following. Hence it is not required to indicate this number, as is needed for all the alternative methods that optimize a criterion. We shall see that it performs well when there are a small number of classes, each having at least 30 to 50 elements.

Extended Classes

At the second level, we simply assign elements that are connected to a unique kernel, whatever their density is. If an element not in a kernel is connected to several ones, the decision is again postponed.

Complete Classes

Finally, to get partitions, we assign the remaining elements to one class. For x and any extended class C to which it is connected, we compute the number of edges between x and C, and also its average distance to C. Finally there are two alternative choices, the majority connected class C_m and the closest one C_d. If they are identical, then x is connected to it; if they differ we apply the following empirical rule: if $\frac{|C_m|}{|C_d|} > 1.5$, class C_m is joined, because the number of links to C_m is clearly larger than to C_d; otherwise C_d is joinned.

3.2 Complexity

Kernel computation is of order $\mathcal{O}(n\delta)$ to find the local maximum vertices, and $\mathcal{O}(m) \leq \mathcal{O}(n\delta)$ to determine the kernel elements. During the extension steps, for any x we count its connections to the kernels, and then to the extended classes. Both are also $\mathcal{O}(n\delta)$, so that is the complexity of the whole algorithm.

With this very low computation time, the method enables us to treat large distance matrices ($n \gg 1000$) more efficiently than other optimization procedures on distance matrices which are, in the best case, order $\mathcal{O}(n^2)$. It permits to test several threshold values to find an interval in which the number of classes remains the same. For disjoint classes, the corresponding threshold value always exists and the expected number of classes can easily be recovered.

More interesting is the fact that to build the threshold graph, it is not necessary to memorize the whole distance matrix ; it is sufficient to read it row after row and to keep in memory the adjacency lists or an adjacency matrix. This is very important for biological applications that are increasingly common; in one year, starting with sixty entirely sequenced genomes, we get more than one hundred, each one possessing several thousands of genes. And DNA chips quantify the expression of several thousands of genes simultaneously.

4 Experimental Validation

In order to show that this method allows to recover existing classes, we have tested it, comparing the efficiency of the density functions. First, we have developed a random generator of Euclidian distances in which there is a given number of classes denoted by p; and n points are generated in an Euclidian space having dimension $m \geq p$; the coordinates of each point are selected uniformly at random between 0 and 1 except for one coordinate, corresponding to its class number, which is selected in [1,2]. So the "squares" of any two groups share a common border providing many small inter-class distance values, and the split of the initial partition is much smaller than its diameter. The Euclidian distance is then computed. So, the generator of random distances depends on three parameters:

- n: the number of elements,
- p: the number of initial classes,
- $m > p$: the dimension of the Euclidian space.

The initial partition is denoted $P = \{C_1, ..C_p\}$.

4.1 Quality of the Classes Compared to the Initial Partition

For the three levels, we would like to estimate the quality of the resulting classes, and thus the efficacy of the clustering process. Let n'_c be the number of classified vertices at each level. They are distributed in p' classes denoted by $C'_1, \ldots, C'_{p'}$ that realize a partition P' over a subset of X for the kernels and the extended classes.

We first aim to map the classes of P' onto those of P by evaluating $n_{ij} = |C_i \bigcap C'_j|$. We define the *corresponding* class of C'_j, denoted by $\Theta(C'_j)$, as the one in P that contains the greatest number of elements of C'_j. So $\Theta(C'_j) = C_k$ if and only if $n_{kj} \geq n_{ij}$ for all i from 1 to p.

In order to measure the accuracy of the classes, we evaluate three criteria:

- τ_c, the percentage of clustered elements in P' ($\tau_c = \frac{n'_c}{n}$).
- τ_e, the percentage of elements in one of the p' classes which belong to its corresponding class in P;

$$\tau_e = \frac{\sum_i |\Theta(C'_i) \bigcap C'_i|}{n'_c}.$$

- τ_p, the percentage of pairs in the same class in P' which are also joined together in P.

The first criterion measures the efficiency of the clustering process at each level; if very few elements are clustered, the method is inefficient. For the second criterion, we must compute, for each class in P', the distribution of the elements of any initial class to define its corresponding class in P. Thus it

can be interpreted as a percentage of "well classified" elements. The third one estimates the probability that a pair in one class of P' to belong to a single class in P.
Remark: The last two criteria may reach their maximum value (1.0) even when partitions P and P' are not identical. When a class in P is subdivided in two parts, they will have the same corresponding class in P; all their elements will be considered as well classified, and the rate of pairs will also be equal to 1. Consequently, we indicate in Table 3 the percentage of trials for which the correct number of classes has been found.

4.2 Results

We first evaluate the number of recovered classes according to the percentage of edges in the threshold graph. We have generated 300 distances on 200 points distributed in 5 classes, and we have computed the number of local maxima, using the De_2 density function. In a first series, the dimension of the Euclidian space is equal to the number of classes ($m = 5$). For the second series, this dimension is doubled ($m = 10$), the new coordinates being selected uniformly at random in [0,1]. These new variables do not provide any information for partitioning; they just add noise.

We study the average number of classes corresponding to increasing values of α and the dimension m of the Euclidian space. The results in Table 1 prove that the correct number is predictable from taking α to be 20% to 45%. These computations can be made for a single distance matrix and the number of classes is then the one remaining the same along a large interval for α. Table 2 indicates the percentage of trials giving each computed number of classes.

Table 1. Average number of classes determined with a threshold graph having $\alpha \cdot n(n-1)/2$ edges.

α	.10	.15	.20	.25	.30	.35	.40	.45	.50	.55	.60	.65	.70
$m = 5$	10.4	6.0	5.0	5.0	4.9	4.9	4.9	4.8	4.7	4.2	3.0	1.6	1.1
$m = 10$	9.8	6.0	5.0	4.7	4.6	4.5	4.2	3.8	3.0	2.1	1.3	1.1	1.0

One can see that for 25% of edges, 5 classes have been determined in more than 95% of the trials when the dimension is equal to the number of classes, and in practically 75% of the trials when it is double. In the other cases, the number of classes is very close to 5. These results remain good when the number of elements increases up to 1000. They are weakened when the number of elements per class goes below 30. The results are equivalent if there are only 3 classes in a 3 dimensional space, but the best results (100% of exact prediction) are obtained with 30 to 40 percent of edges. This can be generalized; the larger the expected number of classes is, the smaller the α should be.

Table 2. Distribution of the number of classes according to the percentage of edges.

	m = 5					m = 10						
Nb. of classes	3	4	5	6	7	1	2	3	4	5	6	7
20%	0.0	.03	.86	.10	.01	0.0	0.0	.01	.14	.70	.14	.02
25%	0.0	.03	.96	.01	0.0	0.0	0.0	.03	.21	.74	.01	0.0
30%	0.0	.06	.94	0.0	0.0	0.0	0.0	.04	.33	.62	.01	0.0
35%	0.0	.10	.90	0.0	0.0	0.0	.01	.08	.37	.54	0.0	0.0
40%	.01	.13	.86	0.0	0.0	0.0	.03	.15	.41	.41	0.0	0.0
45%	.01	.19	.80	0.0	0.0	.01	.08	.27	.41	.23	0.0	0.0

Now we compare the density functions using the same protocol for distances ($n = 200$, $p = 5$, $m = 5, 10$), keeping 25% of the edges in the threshold graph to evaluate the density. The results are shone in Table 3.

Table 3. Average results of the quality criteria on the 3 types of classes for the 3 density functions. The row labelled K indicates the kernels, the row labelled C indicates the classes, the row labelled P indicates the partitions, and the row labelled % is the percentage of trials that found 5 classes.

	$m = 5$									$m = 10$								
	De_1			De_2			De_3			De_1			De_2			De_3		
	τ_c	τ_e	τ_p	τ_c	τ_e	τ_p	τ_c	τ_e	τ_p	τ_c	τ_e	τ_p	τ_c	τ_e	τ_p	τ_c	τ_e	τ_p
K	.30	.82	.72	.36	1.0	.99	.23	.99	.99	.26	.75	.62	.29	.97	.94	.19	.97	.95
C	.54	.78	.68	.54	.99	.99	.50	.99	.99	.49	.71	.60	.46	.95	.91	.39	.97	.95
P	1.0	.72	.59	1.0	.96	.93	1.0	.93	.88	1.0	.60	.45	1.0	.89	.80	1.	.83	70
%	.30			.94			.67			.21			.73			.31		

The superiority of functions De_2 is evident. Function De_1 is not satisfying, at any level, because it recovers the correct number of classes too rarely. In fact, every pair of mutual nearest neighbors constitutes a kernel. It seems to be better for function De_3 but it predicts too many classes and the criteria encourage this bias. For function De_2, 1/3 of the elements belong to the kernels and 1/2 are in the extended classes. More than 90% of the joined pairs of elements come from the same initial class.

4.3 Evaluating Final Partitions

In the preceding IFCS conference, Guénoche and Garreta (2002) proposed several criteria to evaluate whether a partition P fits with a distance D. We review some of these which are based on the principle that the large distance values should be between-class, or external links, and the small distance values should be within-class, or internal links. A partition P on X induces a bipartition on the pair set. Let $(L_e|L_i)$ be this bipartition, and let N_e and N_i be the number of elements in each part.

These quantities induce another bipartition of the $n(n-1)/2$ pairs in X. After ranking the distance values in decreasing order, we can distinguish the N_e greatest values, on the left side, and the N_i smallest values, on the right side. This bipartition is denoted by $(G_d|S_d)$. A perfect partition on X would lead to identical bipartitions on pairs. To compare these two bipartitions, we compute:

- *The rate of agreement on pairs.* This rate, denoted by τ_a, is the percentage of pairs belonging to L_e and G_d (external links and large distances) or to L_i and S_d (internal links and small distances).
- *The rate of weight.* This is computed from the sums of distances in each of the four classes, respectively denoted by $\sum(L_e)$, $\sum(L_i)$, $\sum(G_d)$, and $\sum(S_d)$:
$$\tau_w = \frac{\sum(L_e)}{\sum(G_d)} \times \frac{\sum(S_d)}{\sum(L_i)}.$$
These two ratios correspond to the weight of external links divided by the maximum that could be realized with N_e distance values and to the minimal weight of N_i edges divided by the weight of the internal links. Both are less than or equal to 1 and so is τ_w. A rate close to 1 means that the between-class links belong to the longest distance set and the intra-class links have been taken from the smallest ones.
- *The ratio of well designed triples.* We only consider triples made of two elements x_1 and x_2 belonging to the same class in P and a third external element y. We say that such a triple is *well designed* if and only if $D(x_1,x_2) \leq \inf\{D(x_1,y), D(x_2,y)\}$. The criterion τ_t is just the percentage of well designed triples.

After 200 trials, we have computed the average of these three criteria, first for the initial partitions P (they do not reach the theoretical maximum of 1 because there are many small distance values between elements in different squares) and for the final partitions P'. The results in Table 4 prove that the latter practically have the same quality when compared to the distances.

Table 4. Comparison of three fitting criteria between initial partitions and final partitions as recovered by the density clustering method.

	$m=5$			$m=10$		
	τ_a	τ_w	τ_t	τ_a	τ_w	τ_t
Initial partitions	.90	.91	.92	.88	.91	.88
Final partitions	.89	.90	.90	.84	.88	.82

The method has also been tested with other types of distances, such as Boolean distances (symmetrical difference distance on binary vectors) or graph distance (Sczekanovski-Dice distance on graphs). The existence of classes is always guaranteed by using generating procedures that cannot be detailed here. The partition quality remains the same, as $\tau_e = .96$ and $\tau_p = .93$ for graphs on 300 vertices distributed in 5 classes.

5 Conclusion

The density clustering method has many advantages over classical partitioning ones.

- It allows one to both extract classes that do not cover the complete set of elements and to build a partition. The first problem becomes very important with DNA microarray data for which not all the genes have to be clustered.
- It provides, according to a threshold distance value or a percentage of edges in the threshold graph, the number of classes, and this number is very often the correct one and always very close if classes have a few tens of elements.
- It has an average complexity proportional to the number of elements and to the average degree in the graph. This makes it very efficient to treat large problems with distance matrices that cannot be completely memorized, as for complete genome comparisons.

Also, it is a one parameter method (the threshold distance value or the percentage of edges in the threshold graph) that can be used for large clustering problems with biological data.

Acknowledgements

This work is supported by the program inter-EPST "BioInformatique."

References

1. G. D. Bader and C. W. Hogue (2003). "An Automated Method for Finding Molecular Complexes in Large Protein Interaction Networks," *BMC Bioinformatics*, **4**.
2. Guénoche, A., and Garreta, H. (2002). "Representation and Evaluation of Partitions," in *Classification, Clustering and Data Analysis*, ed. K. Jajuga et al., Berlin:Springer-Verlag, pp. 131–138.
3. Matsuda, H., Ishihara, T., and Hashimoto, A. (1999). "Classifying Molecular Sequences Using a Linkage Graph with Their Pairwise Similarities," *Theoretical Computer Science*, **210**, 305–325.
4. Rougemont, J., and Hingamp, P. (2003). "DNA Microarray Data and Contextual Analysis of Correlation Graphs," *BMC Bioinformatics*, **4**.
5. Trémolières, R. C. (1994). "Percolation and Multimodal Data Structuring," in *New Approaches in Classification and Data Analysis*, ed. E. Diday et al., Berlin:Springer-Verlag, pp. 263–268.

Clustering by Ant Colony Optimization

Javier Trejos, Alex Murillo, and Eduardo Piza

University of Costa Rica, Costa Rica
{jtrejos,murillo,epiza}@cariari.ucr.ac.cr

Abstract: We use the heuristic known as ant colony optimization in the partitioning problem for improving solutions of k-means method (McQueen (1967)). Each ant in the algorithm is associated with a partition, which is modified by the principles of the heuristic; that is, by the random selection of an element, and the assignment of another element which is chosen according to a probability that depends on the pheromone trail (related to the overall criterion: the maximization of the between-classes variance), and a local criterion (the distance between objects). The pheromone trail is reinforced for those objects that belong to the same class. We present some preliminary results, compared to results of other techniques, such as simulated annealing, genetic algorithms, tabu search, and k-means. Our results are as good as the best of the above methods.

1 Introduction

The partitioning problem is well known for its problems with local minima. Indeed, most of the methods for clustering with a fixed number of classes find local optima of the criterion to be optimized, such as k-means or its variants (dynamical clusters, transfers, Isodata (Diday et al. (1982), Bock (1974)). This is the reason why the implementation of modern combinatorial optimization heuristics has been studied, such as simulated annealing (Aarts & Korst (1988)), tabu seach (Glover et al. (1993)) and genetic algorithms (Goldberg (1989)), which have shown to have good features when implemented in different problems. These heuristics have been widely studied by the authors in clustering (Trejos et al. (1998), Trejos & Castillo (2000), Trejos & Piza (2001), Castillo & Trejos (2002)), with good results.

In this article we study a recent optimization heuristic, the *ant colony optimization* (ACO) (Bonabeau et al. (1999)), which has shown to have good performances in some well known problems of operations research. Section 2 reminds us of the partitioning problem that is considered here: a data table with numerical data and criterion to be optimized. Section 3 presents the technique and takes a closer look at ACO with the help of two problems where it has found good results: the traveling salesman problem and the quadratic assignment problem. In Section 4 we present the algorithm using ACO for the minimization of the intra-classes variance: an algorithm for the modification of partitions by the transfer of objects according to a probabilistic rule based on a pheromone trail of reinforcement and a local criterion of closeness of objects. Finally, in Section 5 we report the obtained results on some empirical data tables.

2 Partitioning

We are in the presence of a data set $\Omega = \{\mathbf{x}_1, \ldots, \mathbf{x}_n\}$ of objects in $\mathbb{R}^p$, and we look for a partition $P = (C_1, \ldots, C_K)$ of Ω that minimizes the intra-classes variance

$$W(P) = \sum_{k=1}^{K} \sum_{\mathbf{x}_i \in C_k} \omega_i \, \|\mathbf{x}_i - \mathbf{g}_k\|^2, \tag{1}$$

where $\mathbf{g}_k$ is the gravity center or mean vector of class C_k and ω_i is the weight of object $\mathbf{x}_i$; in the simplest case, $\omega_i = 1/n$. It is well known that the minimization of $W(P)$ is equivalent to the maximization of the inter-classes variance

$$B(P) = \sum_{k=1}^{K} \mu_k \, \|\mathbf{g}_k - \mathbf{g}\|^2, \tag{2}$$

where $\mu_k = \sum_{\mathbf{x}_i \in C_k} \omega_i$ is the class weight of C_k, and $\mathbf{g} = \sum_{i=1}^{n} \omega_i \, \mathbf{x}_i$ is the overall gravity center, since $I = W(P) + B(P)$, $I = \sum_{i=1}^{n} \omega_i \, \|\mathbf{x}_i - \mathbf{g}\|^2$ is the total variance of Ω.

The most widely known method of partitioning is k-means, which is a local seach method; the final solution depends deterministically on the initial partition. The application of modern optimization heuristics (Trejos et al. (1998), Piza & Trejos (1995), Murillo (2000)) —such as simulated annealing, tabu search and genetic algorithms— is based on the transfer of objects between classes. In the case of **simulated annealing** we use the Metropolis rule (cf. Aarts & Korst (1988)) for deciding whether a transfer of an object from a class to another one —both selected at random— is accepted. In **tabu search**, we construct a set of partitions (the neighborhood of a given partition) by the transfer of a single object and the best neighbor is chosen accordingly to the rules of this technique. Finally, we apply a **genetic algorithm** with a chromosomic representation of n allele in an alphabet of K letters that represent a partition, and we use a roulette-wheel selection proportional to $B(P)$, mutations (that correspond to transfers), and a special crossover operator called "forced crossover" (a good father imposes membership in a class —chosen at random— to another father). In all three cases, the use of the heuristics showed a clearly better performance than k-means or Ward hierarchical clustering (Bock (1974), Diday et al. (1982)). We have also adapted these heuristics to binary data, making the corresponding changes to the dissimilarities, distances and aggregation indexes in that context, since usually there is no "centroid" for binary data (except for the L_1 distance).

3 Ant Colony Optimization

The underlying metaphor of ant colony optimization (ACO) is the way that some insects living in collaborative colonies look for food. Indeed, if an ant nest feels a food source, then some expeditions of ants go —by different paths— to search for this food, leaving a pheromone trail, a chemical substance that animals usually have, but very important for insects. This pheromone trail is an olfactory signal for other ants, that will recognize the way followed by its predecessors. Between all expeditions of ants, there will be some that arrive first to the food source because they took the shortest path, and then they will go back to the nest first than the other expeditions. Then, the shortest path has been reinforced in its pheromone trail; therefore, new expeditions will probably take that path more than others will, unless new better paths (or parts of paths) are found by some expeditions. It is expected that the pheromone trail of the shortest path is more and more intense, and the one of the other paths will evaporate.

When applying this principle to combinatorial optimization problems, we look for an implementation that uses the principle of *reinforcement of good solutions*, or parts of solutions, by the intensification of a value of "pheromone" that controls the probability of taking this solution or its part of solution. Now, this probability will depend not only on the pheromone value, but also on a value of a "local heuristic" or "short term vision", that suggests a solution or part of solution by a local optimization criterion, for example as greedy algorithms do.

An optimization method that uses ACO has at least the following components:

- A *representation*, that enables the construction or modification of solutions by means of a probabilistic transition rule, that depends on the pheromone trail and the local heuristic.
- A *local heuristic* or *visibility*, noted η.
- An *update rule* for the pheromone, noted τ.
- A *probabilistic transition rule*, that depends on η and τ.

One of the principles of ACO is that it handles in parallel a set of M agents or ants, and each one constructs or modifies a solution of the optimization problem.

The general algorithm of ACO, in the case that states are vertices $i, j, \dots$ on a graph of n nodes, is the following:

```
Algorithm ACO
Initialize τ_ij = τ_0
Put each ant (from 1 to M) in a vertex
for t = 1 to t_max do:
   for m = 1 to M do:
      Construct a solution S^m(t) applying n − 1 times a rule
      of construction or modification, choosing
      a pheromone trail τ and a local heuristics η
      Calculate the cost W^m(t) of S^m(t)
   end-for
   for each arc (i, j) do:
      Update τ
   end-for
end-for.
```

We briefly explain how ACO has been implement in the travelling salesman problem (TSP) and the quadratic assignment problem (QAP).

In the TSP, each ant constructs a permutation; at each step, the m-th ant is on a city i and selects the next city j with probability $p_{ij}^m = [\tau_{ij}(t)]^\alpha [\eta_{ij}]^\beta / \sum_{h \in J_i^m(t)} [\tau_{ih}(t)]^\alpha [\eta_{ih}]^\beta$, where $J_i^m(t)$ is the set of cities that can be visited by m when it is on i, and t is the current iteration; α and β are weighting parameters fixed by the user. The local heuristics is the inverse of the distance: $\eta_{ij} = 1/d_{ij}$. Many variants have been proposed (Bonabeau et al. (1999)), for example the use of elite states for updating the pheromone value. Here $\tau_{ij}(t+1) = (1-\rho)\tau_{ij}(t) + \rho \sum_{m=1}^M \Delta^m \tau_{ij}(t+1)$ where $i, j \in \{1, \ldots, n\}$, $\rho \in (0, 1]$, and

$$\Delta^m \tau_{ij}(t+1) = \begin{cases} Q/L_k & \text{if ant } m \text{ uses arc } (i,j) \text{ in its permutation} \\ 0 & \text{otherwise,} \end{cases}$$

is the amount of pheromone left by ant m, Q being a constant and L_k the length of the cycle constructed by m.

For the QAP, there is also a constructive algorithm very similar to the TSP one, with a local heuristic $\eta_{ih} = d_i f_h$, where $d_i = \sum_{j=1}^n d_{ij}$ and $f_h = \sum_{k=1}^n f_{hk}$ is the sum of activities flux. There is also a modifying algorithm for QAP (Gambardella et al. (1999)), where each ant is associated to a permutation π^m (initialized at random and improved by a local search method). The ant modifies π^m by means of R swaps, $\pi^m(i) \leftrightarrow \pi^m(j)$. With probability $q \in (0, 1)$, j is chosen such that $\tau_{i\pi^m(j)} + \tau_{j\pi^m(i)}$ is maximized, and with probability $1-q$ it is chosen j with probability $p_{ij}^m = \tau_{i\pi^m(j)} + \tau_{j\pi^m(i)} / \sum_{\substack{l=1 \\ l \neq i}}^n \tau_{i\pi^m(l)} + \tau_{l\pi^m(i)}$. The pheromone trail $\tau_{i\pi(i)}$ is updated by $\Delta\tau_{ij}(t) = 1/C(\pi^+)$ if (i, j) belongs to the best state π^+ found so far; that is, there is an elite of one element. There are some other aspects, such as intensification and diversification that can be consulted in Gambardella et al. (1999).

4 Application of ACO in Partitioning

We propose an iterative algorithm such that in each iteration the behavior of every ant is examined. At the beginning, an ant m is associated to a partition P^m randomly generated, the k-means method is applied and converges to a local minimum of W. During the iterations, the ant will modify P^m in the following way: an object i is selected at random, and another object j is selected at random using a roulette-wheel with probability p_{ij}, where p_{ij} depends on the pheromone trail and a local heuristic. We can say that the ant decides whether to assign j to the same class as i.

The value of the pheromone trail is modified according to the rule

$$\tau_{ij}(t+1) = (1-\rho)\tau_{ij}(t) + \rho\,\Delta\tau_{ij}(t+1), \tag{3}$$

where the values τ_{ij} associate two objects i, j in Ω, and $\rho \in (0,1]$ is an *evaporation parameter*. We put

$$\Delta\tau_{ij}(t+1) = \sum_{m=1}^{M} \Delta^m\tau_{ij}(t+1), \tag{4}$$

$\Delta^m\tau_{ij}(t+1)$ being the quantity of pheromone by agent in the association of objects i, j to the same class, defined by

$$\Delta^m\tau_{ij}(t+1) = \begin{cases} B(P^m)/I & \text{if } i,j \text{ belong to the same class of } P^m \\ 0 & \text{otherwise.} \end{cases} \tag{5}$$

$B(P^m)$ being the inter-classes variance of partition P^m. That way, two objects classified into the same class leave a pheromone trail.

The local heuristic or short-term visibility is defined as

$$\eta_{ij} = \frac{1}{\|\mathbf{x}_i - \mathbf{x}_j\|}, \tag{6}$$

in such a way that two near elements give a big value in order to influence in the probability of assigning them to the same class.

If ant m is at object i, object j is chosen with probability

$$p_{ij} = \frac{[\tau_{ij}]^\alpha[\eta_{ij}]^\beta}{\sum_{l=1}^{n}[\tau_{il}]^\alpha[\eta_{il}]^\beta}. \tag{7}$$

Then, j is assigned to the same class as i. This random choice is similar to the so called roulette-wheel of genetic algorithms: the rows of matrix $(p_{ij})_{n\times n}$ sum 1; given i, the value p_{ij} is the probability of choosing j, which is modeled using the cumulative probabilities and generating uniformly random numbers.

With the above elements, the algorithm is as follows:

Algorithm Acoclus
Initialize $\tau_{ij} = \tau_0$
Calculate η according to (6)
Initialize the probabilities p
Initialize at random partitions $P^1, \ldots, P^M$ associated to each ant
Run k-means on each P^m in order to converge to a local minimum of W
for $t = 1$ to $t_{\max}$ do:
  for $m = 1$ to M, do S times:
    Choose at random an object i
    Choose an object j according to (7)
    Assign j to the class of i
  end-for
  Calculate $B(P^1), \ldots, B(P^M)$ and keep the best value
  Update τ according to (3), (4) and (5)
end-for.

Notice that the algorithm has the following parameters: the number M of ants, the initial value of pheromone τ_0, the maximum number of iterations $t_{\max}$, weight α of the pheromone in (7), weight β of the local heuristic in (7), the evaporation coefficient ρ in (3), and the number S of transfers for each ant.

5 Results and Perspectives

As with other metaheuristics, in ant colony optimization there is a problem with the tuning of the parameters. In ACO this problem is more complicated, because it has more parameters than the other heuristics. In ACO we have 7 parameters to be fixed, instead of 4 in simulated annealing and 2 in tabu search.

We also tried another rule for choosing j when i has been selected: with probability $q \in (0,1)$ choose j that maximizes τ_{ij}: $j = \text{argmax}_h\{\tau_{ih}\}$, and with probability $1-q$ choose j according to (7). However, this change did not give better results.

A significant improvement was obtained when k-means was run before starting the iterations, since at the beginning of our experimentation initial partitions were purely at random and ants improved them only during the iterations. So, we can see our method as a method for improving k-means solutions in partitioning.

With all the above considerations, the following results were obtained by the application of AcoClus with: a population size $M = 20$, a maximum number of 30 iterations, 25 runs, a number of transfers $S = 2 \times n$, $\alpha = 0.7$, $\beta = 0.8$, $\rho = 0.5$, and $\tau_0 = 0.001$.

The method is applied several times with the same parameters, and the attraction rate of the best minimum of W is examined. Table 1 shows the results of applying the methods based on combinatorial optimization heuristics and AcoClus (applied 25 times), on four data tables described by the literature (Trejos et al. (1998)). Tabu search was applied 150 times, while simulated annealing was applied 1,000 times on the first table, 200 times on the second and third, and 25 on the fourth; the genetic algorithm was applied 100 times on the first three tables, and 50 times on the fourth. The dimension $n \times p$ of each table appears close to the table's name. Only the best value of W is reported, and for each method we report the percentage of times this value was found. We also report the results for k-means (applied 10,000 times) and Ward hierarchical clustering (applied only once since it is deterministic).

Results on table 1 show that ACO performs well, as good as simulated annealing and tabu search. However, some experimentation has yet to be done for deciding some features of the method. For example, we have to decide whether to use elite agents, to "kill" the ants before restarting a new iteration or not, and the use of another rule for selecting j from i. A complete Monte Carlo comparison is being performed at the present time, controlling four factors: the data table size, the number of clusters, the cardinality and the variance of each class. The results should compare ant colony optimization, simulated annealing, tabu search, genetic algorithms, particle swarm optimization, k-means and Ward's hierarchical clustering.

Table 1. Best value of the intra-classes variance W^* and percentage of times this value is obtained when each method is applied several times: ant colony optimization (ACO), tabu search (TS), simulated annealing (SA), genetic algorithm (GA), k-means (kM), and Ward's hierarchical clustering.

K	W^*	ACO	TS	SA	GA	KM	Ward
	French Scholar Notes (9×5)						
2	28.2	100%	100%	100%	100%	12%	0%
3	16.8	100%	100%	100%	95%	12%	0%
4	10.5	100%	100%	100%	97%	5%	100%
5	4.9	100%	100%	100%	100%	8%	100%
	Amiard's Fishes (23×16)						
3	32213	100%	100%	100%	87%	8%	0%
4	18281	100%	100%	100%	0%	9%	0%
5	14497	68%	97%	100%	0%	1%	100%
	Thomas' Sociomatrix (24×24)						
3	271.8	100%	100%	100%	85%	2%	0%
4	235.0	96%	100%	100%	24%	0.15%	0%
5	202.6	84%	98%	100%	0%	0.02%	0%
	Fisher's Iris (150×4)						
2	0.999	100%	100%	100%	100%	100%	0%
3	0.521	100%	76%	100%	100%	4%	0%
4	0.378	100%	60%	55%	82%	1%	0%
5	0.312	100%	32%	0%	6%	0.24%	0%

References

1. Aarts, E. M., Korst, J. (1988). *Simulated Annealing and Boltzmann Machines*, Wiley, Chichester.
2. Bock, H.-H. (1974). *Automatische Klassifikation*, Vandenhoeck & Ruprecht, Göttingen.
3. Bonabeau, E., Dorigo, M., and Therauluz, G. (1999). *Swarm Intelligence. From Natural to Artificial Systems*, Oxford University Press, New York.
4. Castillo, W., and Trejos, J. (2002). "Two-Mode Partitioning: Review of Methods and Application of Tabu Search," in *Classification, Clustering, and Data Analysis*, eds. K. Jajuga, et al., Berlin:Springer, pp. 43–51.
5. Diday, E., Lemaire, J., Pouget, J., and Testu, F. (1982). *Eléments d'Analyse des Données*, Dunod, Paris.
6. Gambardella, L. M., Taillard, E. D., and Dorigo, M. (1999). "Ant Colonies for the QAP," *Journal of Operations Research Society*, **50**, 167–176.
7. Glover, F., et al. (1993). "Tabu Search: An Introduction," *Annals of Operations Research*, **41**, 1–28.
8. Goldberg, D. E. (1989). *Genetic Algorithms in Search, Optimization and Machine Learning*, Addison-Wesley, Reading MA.
9. McQueen, J.B. (1967). "Some Methods for Classification and Analysis of Multivariate Observations," *Proceedings of the 5th Berkeley Symposium on Mathematical Statistics and Probability*, Vol. 1, Berkeley:University of California Press.
10. Murillo, A. (2000). "Aplicación de la Búsqueda Tabú en la Clasificación por Particiones," *Investigación Operacional*, **21**, 183–194.
11. Piza, E., and Trejos, J. (1995). "Particionamiento Usando Sobrecalentamiento Simulado y Algoritmos Genéticos," in *IX SIMMAC*, ed. J. Trejos, Universidad de Costa Rica, Turrialba, pp. 121–132.
12. Trejos, J., Murillo, A., and Piza, E. (1998). "Global Stochastic Optimization for Partitioning," in *Advances in Data Science and Classification*, eds. A. Rizzi et al., Berlin:Springer, pp. 185–190.
13. Trejos, J., and Castillo, W. (2000). "Simulated Annealing Optimization for Two-Mode Partitioning," in *Classification and Information Processing at the Turn of the Millenium*, eds. W. Gaul and R. Decker, Berlin:Springer, pp. 133-142.
14. Trejos, J., and Piza, E. (2001). "Critères et Heuristiques d'Optimisation pour la Classification de Données Binaires," in *Journées de la Société Francophone de Classification*, Guadeloupe, pp. 331–338.

A Dynamic Cluster Algorithm Based on L_r Distances for Quantitative Data

Francisco de A. T. de Carvalho[1], Yves Lechevallier[2], and Renata M.C.R. de Souza[1]

[1] Cidade Universitaria, Brazil
{fatc,rmcrs}@cin.ufpe.br
[2] INRIA - Rocquencourt, France
Yves.Lechevallier@inria.fr

Abstract: Dynamic clustering methods aim to obtain both a single partition of the input data into a fixed number of clusters and the identification of a suitable representation of each cluster simultaneously. In its adaptive version, at each iteration of these algorithms there is a different distance for the comparison of each cluster with its representation. In this paper, we present a dynamic cluster method based on L_r distances for quantitative data.

1 Introduction

Clustering (Bock, 1993; Jain, et al., 1999) is an exploratory data analysis method that aims to group a set of items into clusters such that items within a given cluster have a high degree of similarity, while items belonging to different clusters have a high degree of dissimilarity. The most popular cluster analysis techniques are hierarchical and partitioning methods (Spaeth, 1980; Gordon, 1999; Everitt, 2001).

Hierarchical methods yield complete hierarchy, i.e., a nested sequence of partitions of the input data. Hierarchical methods can be either agglomerative or divisive. Agglomerative methods start with trivial clustering, where each item is in a unique cluster, and end with the trivial clustering, where all items are in the same cluster. A divisive method starts with all items in the same cluster and performs divisions until a stopping criterion is met.

Partition methods try to obtain a single division of the input data into a fixed number of clusters. Often, these methods look for a partition that optimizes (usually locally) a criterion function. To improve the cluster quality, the algorithm is run multiple times with different starting points, and the best configuration obtained from all the runs is used as the output clustering.

Dynamic cluster algorithms (Diday and Simon, 1976) are iterative two-step relocation algorithms involving, at each iteration, the construction of the clusters and the identification of a suitable representative or exemplar (means, axes, probability laws, groups of elements, etc.) of each cluster by locally optimizing an adequacy criterion between the clusters and their corresponding representatives. The k-means algorithm, with class representatives updated after all objects have been considered for relocation, is a particular case of dynamical clustering with the adequacy criterion being a variance criterion such that the class exemplar equals the center of gravity for the cluster.

In these algorithms, the optimization problem can be stated as follow. Let Ω be a set of n objects indexed by $i = 1, \ldots, n$ and described by p quantitative variables. Then each object i is described by a vector $\mathbf{x}_i = (x_i^1, \ldots, x_i^p) \in \Re^p$. The problem is to find the partition $P = (C_1, ..., C_K)$ of Ω into K clusters and the system $Y = (\mathbf{y}_1, ..., \mathbf{y}_K)$ of class exemplars that minimize a partitioning criterion $g(P, Y)$ which measures the fit between the clusters and their representatives.

This optimization process starts from a set of representatives or an initial partition and interactively applies an "allocation" step (the exemplars are fixed) in order to assign the individuals to the classes according to their proximity to the exemplars. This is followed by a "representation" step (the partition is fixed) where the exemplars are updated according to the assignment of the individuals in the allocation step, and these steps alternate until the algorithm converges, i.e., until until the adequacy criterion reaches a stationary value.

The algorithm converges and the partitioning criterion decreases at each iteration if the class exemplars are properly defined at each representation step. Indeed, the problem is to find the exemplar $\mathbf{y}_k = (y_k^1, \ldots, y_k^p) \in \Re^p$ of each cluster C_k, $k = 1, \ldots, K$, which minimizes an adequacy criterion $f(\mathbf{y}_k)$ measuring the dissimilarity between the exemplar $\mathbf{y}_k$ and the cluster C_k.

The adaptive dynamic clusters algorithms (Diday and Govaert, 1977) also optimize a criterion based on a measure of fit between the clusters and their representation, but at each iteration there is a different distance for the comparison of each cluster with its representative. The idea is to associate each cluster with a distance which is defined according to the intra-class structure of the cluster. These distances are not determined once and for all, and they are different from one class to another. The advantage of these adaptive distances is that the clustering algorithm is able to recognize clusters of different shapes and sizes.

In these algorithms, the optimization problem is now to find the partition $P = (C_1, \ldots, C_K)$ of Ω into K clusters, its corresponding set of K exemplars $Y = (\mathbf{y}_1, \ldots, \mathbf{y}_K)$, and a set of K distances $d = \{d^1, \ldots, d^k\}$, each one associated with a cluster, which minimizes a partitioning criterion $g(P, Y, d)$ that measures the fit between the clusters and their representatives.

The initialization, the allocation step and the stopping criterion are nearly the same in the adaptive and non-adaptive dynamic cluster algorithm. The main difference between these algorithms occurs in the representation step which has two stages: the first stage, where the partition and the distances are fixed and the exemplars are updated, is followed by the second one, where the partition and its corresponding representatives are fixed and the distances are updated. The adaptive dynamic cluster algorithm converges and the partitioning criterion decreases at each iteration if the class exemplars and the distances are properly defined at each representation step.

The aim of this paper is to present a dynamic cluster method based on L_r distances for quantitative data. Sections 2 and 3 present, respectively, the non-adaptive and the adaptive version of this method. An example concerning adaptive and non-adaptive dynamic clustering based on L_2 distance is given in Section 4 and the concluding remarks are given in Section 5.

2 Dynamic Clusters Based on a Non-Adaptive L_r Distance

Let $\mathbf{x}_i = (x_i^1, \ldots, x_i^p)$ and $\mathbf{x}_{i'} = (x_{i'}^1, \ldots, x_{i'}^p)$ be two quantitative feature vectors representing objects i and i' belonging to class C_k. We use the L_r distance function to measure the dissimilarity between $\mathbf{x}_i$ and $\mathbf{x}_{i'}$:

$$d_r(\mathbf{x}_i, \mathbf{x}_{i'}) = \sum_{j=1}^{p} (|x_i^j - x_{i'}^j|)^r, \quad r \geq 1 \tag{1}$$

In equation (1), $r = 1$ and $r = 2$ give, respectively, the L_1 and L_2 distances.

2.1 The Optimization Problem for Class Exemplars

As presented in the introduction, the exemplar $\mathbf{y}_k$ of a cluster C_k is defined in the framework of the dynamic cluster algorithm by optimizing an adequacy criterion f that measures the dissimilarity between the cluster and its representative. Here, we search for the vector $\mathbf{y}_k = (y_k^1, \ldots, y_k^p)$ that minimizes the following adequacy criterion:

$$f(\mathbf{y}_k) = \sum_{i \in C_k} d_r(\mathbf{x}_i, \mathbf{y}_k) = \sum_{i \in C_k} \sum_{j=1}^{p} (|x_i^j - y_k^j|)^r, \quad r \geq 1, \tag{2}$$

where d_r is the distance between two vectors of quantitative data as given by equation (1).

The criterion (2) can also be written:

$$f(\mathbf{y}_k) = \sum_{j=1}^{p} \overbrace{\sum_{i \in C_k} (|x_i^j - y_k^j|)^r}^{\tilde{f}(y_k^j)} \tag{3}$$

and we search, for $j = 1, \ldots, p$, for the quantity y_k^j which minimizes:

$$\tilde{f}(y_k^j) = \sum_{i \in C_k} (|x_i^j - y_k^j|)^r. \tag{4}$$

When $r \in \{1, 2\}$ the minimum of the equation (4) has an analytical solution. For $r = 1$, y_k^j is the median of $\{x_i^j, i \in C_k\}$; for $r = 2$, y_k^j is the average of $\{x_i^j, i \in C_k\}$.

For $r > 2$, let $\{x_i^j \,|\, i \in C_k\}$ and $X_{C_k}^j = \{x_{(1)}^j, \ldots, x_{(\#C_k)}^j\}$ be the sets of increasing ordered values of $\{x_i^j \,|\, i \in C_k\}$; i.e., $\forall\, l \in \{1, \ldots, \#C_k\}$, $x_{(l)}^j \in \{x_i^j \,|\, i \in C_k\}$ and $\forall\, l \in \{1, \ldots, \#C_k - 1\}$, $x_{(l)}^j \leq x_{(l+1)}^j$.

Let the functions $\tilde{f}_t, t = 0, \ldots, \#C_k$, be defined by

$$\tilde{f}_t(y_k^j) = \sum_{l=1}^{\#C_k} (|x_{(l)}^j - y_k^j|)^r, \; y_k^j \in \mathcal{B}_t \tag{5}$$

where $\mathcal{B}_0 = (-\infty, x_{(1)}^j]$, $\mathcal{B}_t = [x_{(l)}^j, x_{(l+1)}^j]$, for $t, l = 1, \ldots, \#C_k - 1$, and $\mathcal{B}_{\#C_k} = [x_{(\#C_k)}^j, \infty)$.

In this case, the quantity y_k^j which minimizes (4) belongs to the union of two sets: the set $\{x_i^j \,|\, i \in C_k\}$ and the set of roots of the derivatives, for $y_k^j \in \mathcal{B}_t$, of the functions $\tilde{f}_t$ for $t = 0, \ldots, \#C_k)$.

2.2 The Dynamic Cluster Algorithm

The dynamic cluster algorithm searches for the partition $P = (C_1, \ldots, C_K)$ of Ω and the system $Y = (\mathbf{y}_1, ..., \mathbf{y}_K)$ of class exemplars that locally minimizes the following partitioning criterion based on the distance d_r defined in (1):

$$g(P, Y) = \sum_{k=1}^{K} \sum_{i \in C_k} d_r(\mathbf{x}_i, \mathbf{y}_k) = \sum_{k=1}^{K} \sum_{i \in C_k} \sum_{j=1}^{p} (|x_i^j - y_k^j|)^r. \tag{6}$$

This algorithm proceeds by iteratively repeating an "allocation" step and a "representation" step. During the "representation" step, the partition is fixed and the algorithm computes for each cluster C_k its representative $\mathbf{y}_k$ that minimizes the adequacy criterion given in (2). During the "allocation step," the exemplars are fixed and the algorithm performs a new partition by reassigning each object i to the closest class exemplar $\mathbf{y}_{k*}$ where $k* = \text{argmin}_{k=1,...,K}\, d(\mathbf{x}_i, \mathbf{y}_k)$.

Thus the algorithm can be written as follows:

(a) Initialization.
Choose a partition $(C_1, \ldots, C_K)$ of the data set Ω or choose K distinct objects $\mathbf{y}_1, ..., \mathbf{y}_K$ among Ω and assign each object i to the closest exemplar $\mathbf{y}_{k*}$ for $k* = \text{argmin}_{k=l,...,K}\, d(\mathbf{x}_i, \mathbf{y}_k))$ to construct the initial partition $(C_1, \ldots, C_K)$.

(b) The "representation" step (the partition is fixed).
For k in 1 to K compute the exemplar $\mathbf{y}_k = (y_k^1, \ldots, y_k^p)$.
(c) The "allocation" step (the exemplars are fixed).
$test \leftarrow 0$.
For i in 1 to n do:
Define the cluster C_{k*} such that $k* = \text{argmin}_{k=l,\ldots,K}\, d(\mathbf{x}_i, \mathbf{y}_k)$.
If $i \in C_k$ and $k* \neq k$
$test \leftarrow 1$
$C_{k*} \leftarrow C_{k*} \cup \{i\}$
$C_k \leftarrow C_k \backslash \{i\}$.
(d) If $test = 0$ then END, else go to (b).

3 Dynamic Clusters Based on Adaptive L_r Distance

As before, let $\mathbf{x}_i = (x_i^1, ..., x_i^p)$ and $\mathbf{x}_{i'} = (x_{i'}^1, , ..., x_{i'}^p)$ be two quantitative feature vectors, representating objects i and i' belonging to class C_k, respectively. We consider the following adaptive L_r distance function, which is parameterized by the weight vector $\boldsymbol{\lambda}_k = (\lambda_k^1, \ldots, \lambda_k^p))$, to measure the dissimilarity between $\mathbf{x}_i$ and $\mathbf{x}_{i'}$:

$$d_r^k(\mathbf{x}_i, \mathbf{x}_{i'}) = \sum_{j=1}^{p} \lambda_k^j (|x_i^j - x_{i'}^j|)^r, \quad r \geq 1. \tag{7}$$

In equation (7), $r = 1$ and $r = 2$ give, respectively, adaptive L_1 (Diday and Govaert, 1977) and adaptive L_2 distances.

3.1 The Optimization Problem for Class Exemplars

We search for the vectors $\mathbf{y}_k = (y_k^1, ..., y_k^p)$ and $\boldsymbol{\lambda}_k = (\lambda_k^1, \ldots, \lambda_k^p)$ that minimize the following adequacy criterion:

$$f(\mathbf{y}_k, \lambda_k) = \sum_{i \in C_k} d_r^k(\mathbf{x}_i, \mathbf{y}_k) = \sum_{i \in C_k} \sum_{j=1}^{p} \lambda_k^j (|x_i^j - y_k^j|)^r, \quad r \geq 1, \tag{8}$$

where d_r^k is the adaptive distance between two vectors of quantitative data given in (7).

The criterion (8) can also be written:

$$f(\mathbf{y}_k, \lambda_k) = \sum_{j=1}^{p} \lambda_k^j \overbrace{\sum_{i \in C_k} (|x_i^j - y_k^j|)^r}^{\tilde{f}(y_k^j)} \tag{9}$$

and the optimization problem will be solved in two stages.

In the first step the vector $\boldsymbol{\lambda}_k = (\lambda_k^1, \ldots, \lambda_k^p)$ is fixed and we search, for $j = 1, \ldots, p$, for the quantity y_k^j that minimizes:

$$\tilde{f}(y_k^j) = \sum_{i \in C_k} (|x_i^j - y_k^j|)^r. \tag{10}$$

The solution is the same as the one pointed out in Section 2.1.

In the second step, the vector $\mathbf{y}_k = (y_k^1, ..., y_k^p)$ is fixed and we search for the $\boldsymbol{\lambda}_k = (\lambda_k^1, \ldots, \lambda_k^p)$ that minimizes the adequacy criterion $f(\mathbf{y}_k, \boldsymbol{\lambda}_k)$. According to the standard adaptive method (Diday and Govaert, 1977), we look for the coordinates λ_k^j $(j = 1, \ldots, p)$ of the vector $\boldsymbol{\lambda}_k$ that satisfies the following restrictions:

$$\lambda_k^j > 0 \ (j = 1, \ldots, p) \text{ and } \prod_{j=1}^{p} \lambda_k^j = 1. \tag{11}$$

These coordinates, which are calculated according to the Lagrange multiplier method (Govaert, 1975), are:

$$\lambda_k^j = \frac{\left[\prod_{h=1}^{p} \left(\sum_{i \in C_k} (|x_i^h - y_k^h|)^r\right)\right]^{1/p}}{\sum_{i \in C_k} (|x_i^j - y_k^j|)^r}, \quad j = 1, \ldots, p. \tag{12}$$

3.2 The Adaptive Dynamic Cluster Algorithm

The dynamic cluster algorithm searches for the partition $P = (C_1, ..., C_K)$ of Ω into K clusters, its corresponding set of K exemplars $Y = (\mathbf{y}_1, ..., \mathbf{y}_K)$, and a set of K distances $d = \{d_r^1, \ldots, d_r^k\}$, each one associated with a cluster, which locally minimizes the following partitioning criterion based on the distance d_r^k defined in (7):

$$g(P, Y, d) = \sum_{k=1}^{K} \sum_{i \in C_k} d_r^k(\mathbf{x}_i, \mathbf{y}_k) = \sum_{k=1}^{K} \sum_{i \in C_k} \sum_{j=1}^{p} \lambda_k^j (|x_i^j - y_k^j|)^r. \tag{13}$$

As in the standard dynamic cluster algorithm, this method performs an "allocation" step (the partition and the exemplars are fixed) in order to assign the individuals to the classes according to their proximity to the class representative, followed by a two-stage "representation" step where, according to the assignment of the individuals in the allocation step, in the first stage the partition and the distances are fixed and the class exemplars are updated, and in the second stage the partition and the exemplars are fixed and the distances are updated. The algorithm iterates these steps until convergence, when the partitioning criterion reaches a stationary value. The algorithm schema is the following:

(a) Initialization.
Choose a partition $(C_1, \ldots, C_K)$ of the data set Ω or choose K distinct objects $\mathbf{y}_1, \ldots, \mathbf{y}_K$ among Ω and assign each object i to the closest exemplar $\mathbf{y}_{k*}$ ($k* = \text{argmin}_{k=l,\ldots,K}\ d_r^k(\mathbf{x}_i, \mathbf{y}_k)$) to construct the initial partition $(C_1, \ldots, C_K)$.
(b) The "representation" step.
a) (The partition P and the distances d_r^k are fixed.)
For $k = 1$ to K compute the exemplar $\mathbf{y}_k$.
b) (The partition P and the exemplars $\mathbf{y}_k$ are fixed.)
For $j = 1, \ldots, p$ and $k = 1, \ldots, K$, compute λ_k^j.
(c) The "allocation" step.
test $\leftarrow 0$.
For i in 1 to n do:
Define the cluster C_{k*} such that $k* = \text{argmin}_{k=l,\ldots,K}\ d_r^k(\mathbf{x}_i, \mathbf{y}_k)$.
Ff $i \in C_k$ and $k* \neq k$
test $\leftarrow 1$
$C_{k*} \leftarrow C_{k*} \cup \{i\}$
$C_k \leftarrow C_k \backslash \{i\}$.
(d) If *test* $= 0$ the END, else go to (b).

4 Experimental Evaluation with Artificial Data

The adaptive dynamic cluster method based on L_1 distance has been studied by Diday and Govaert (1977). As an example of adaptive and non-adaptive dynamic clusters based on L_r distances, we consider here the comparison between the adaptive and the non-adaptive methods for the case of L_2 distance. To accomplish this comparison we cluster quantitative data sets scattered in $\Re^2$ using both methods and we evaluate the clustering results based on a Monte Carlo experiment.

The basic data set considered here is described in Diday and Govaert (1977). It has 150 points scattered among three clusters of size 50 and unequal shapes: two clusters with elliptical shapes and one cluster with spherical shape. Figure 1 shows an example of this data set. The data points in each cluster were drawn according to a bivariate normal distribution with correlated components according to the following parameters:

a) Class 1: $\mu_1 = 0$, $\mu_2 = 0$, $\sigma_1^2 = 4$, $\sigma_{12} = 1.7$, $\sigma_2^2 = 1$ and $\rho_{12} = 0.85$;
b) Class 2: $\mu_1 = 0$, $\mu_2 = 3$, $\sigma_1^2 = 0.25$, $\sigma_{12} = 0.0$, $\sigma_2^2 = 0.25$ and $\rho_{12} = 0.0$;
c) Class 3: $\mu_1 = 4$, $\mu_2 = 3$, $\sigma_1^2 = 4$, $\sigma_{12} = -1.7$, $\sigma_2^2 = 1$ and $\rho_{12} = -0.85$.

The clustering results are evaluated based on a external index in the framework of a Monte Carlo experiment with 100 replications. In each replication an L_2 clustering method (non-adaptive or adaptive) is run (until the convergence to a stationary value of the partitioning criterion) 50 times and the best result, according to the partitioning criterion, is selected.

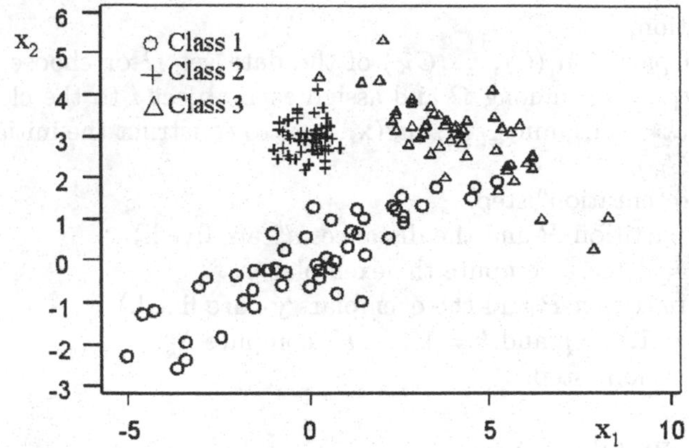

Fig. 1. Quantitative data set showing three clusters.

The average of the corrected Rand (CR) index (Hubert and Arabie, 1985) among these 100 replications is calculated. The CR index assesses the degree of agreement (similarity) between an a priori partition and a partition furnished by the clustering algorithm. The CR index takes values in the interval [-1,1], where the value 1 indicates perfect agreement between the partitions and values near 0 (or negative values) correspond to cluster agreements found by chance (Milligan, 1996).

The CR indices for the clustering results are 0.64 and 0.61 for the methods with adaptive and non-adaptive L_2 distances, respectively. The comparison between these results is achieved by a paired Students' t-tests at a 5% significance level. The observed value of the test statistic, which follows a t-distribution with 99 degrees of freedom under the null, was 3.3. From this observed value, we reject the hypothesis that the average performance of the adaptive L_2 method is inferior to the non-adaptive L_2 method. The results of this experiment show that the performance of the adaptive methods is superior to the non-adaptive method, at least for this data set.

5 Conclusion

Our approach proposes a framework which permits one to generalize easily the dynamic cluster method for the case of the adaptive and non-adaptive L_r distances. If r is equal to 1 and 2 we recover the usual exemplars (median and mean, respectively) of the clusters but now the difficulty is to find a realistic interpretation for the cluster representatives when $r > 2$. Moreover, the adaptive dynamic cluster method based on L_1 distance has been studied by Diday and Govaert (1977). In this work we accomplished a similar study concerning the adaptive dynamic cluster method based on L_2 distance. In this study, the accuracy of the results furnished by the adaptive and non-adaptive methods for the L_2 distance have been assessed by an external index in the framework of a Monte Carlo experiment. These results clearly show that the adaptive method outperforms the non-adaptive one concerning the quality of the clusters as measured by the corrected Rand index.

Acknowledgments

The authors would like to thank CNPq (a Brazilian agency) for its financial support.

References

1. Bock, H. H. (1993). "Classification and Clustering: Problems for the Future," in *New Approaches in Classification and Data Analysis*, eds. E. Diday, et al., Berlin:Springer, pp. 3–24.
2. Diday, E., and Govaert, G. (1977). "Classification Automatique avec Distances Adaptatives," *R.A.I.R.O. Informatique Computer Science*, **11**, 329–349.
3. Diday, E., and Simon, J. J. (1976). "Clustering Analysis," in *Digital Pattern Recognition*, ed. K. S. Fu, Berlin:Springer, pp. 47–94.
4. Everitt, B. (2001). *Cluster Analysis*, Halsted, New York.
5. Gordon, A. D. (1999). *Classification*, Chapman and Hall/CRC, Boca Raton, Florida.
6. Govaert, G. (1975). *Classification Automatique et Distances Adaptatives*, Thèse de 3ème cycle, Mathématique appliquée, Université Paris VI.
7. Hubert, L., and Arabie, P. (1985). "Comparing Partitions," *Journal of Classification*, **2**, 193–218.
8. Jain, A. K., Murty, M. N., and Flynn, P. J. (1999). "Data Clustering: A Review," *ACM Computing Surveys*, **31**, 264–323.
9. Milligan, G. W. (1996). "Clustering Validation: Results and Implications for Applied Analysis," in *Clustering and Classification*, eds. P. Arabie et al., Singapore:Word Scientific, pp. 341–375.
10. Spaeth, H. (1980). *Cluster Analysis Algorithms*, Wiley, New York.

The Last Step of a New Divisive Monothetic Clustering Method: the Gluing-Back Criterion

Jean-Yves Pirçon and Jean-Paul Rasson

University of Namur, Belgium
{jean-yves.pircon,Jean-Paul.Rasson}@fundp.ac.be

Abstract: Pirçon and Rasson (2003) propose a divisive monothetic clustering method. In that work, the selection of relevant variables is performed simultaneously with the formation of clusters. The method treats only one variable at each stage; a single variable is chosen to split a cluster into two sub-clusters. Then the sub-clusters are successively split until a stopping criterion is satisfied. The original splitting criterion is the solution of a maximum likelihood problem conditional on the fact that data are generated by a nonhomogeneous Poisson process on two disjoint intervals. The criterion splits at the place of the maximum integrated intensity between two consecutive points.

This paper extends Pirçon and Rasson (2003) by developing a "gluing-back" criterion. The previous work explained the new method for combining trees and nonhomogeneous Poisson processes and the splitting criterion. It was shown that the maximum likelihood criterion reduces to minimization of the integrated intensity on the domain containing all of the points. This method of clustering is indexed, divisive and monothetic hierarchical, but its performance can be improved through a gluing-back criterion. That criterion is developed in this paper, after a brief review of the main ideas.

1 Introduction

Clustering is a significant tool for data analysis. It aims at finding the intrinsic structure of the data by organizing the data into distinct and homogeneous groups, called *clusters*. The objects in the same cluster must be similar to each other and different from objects in other clusters.

Generally, very little attention has been paid to the correspondence between statistical models and data structures; interpretation takes a lot of time. But for monothetic methods, interpretaion is easy.

Monothetic methods were first proposed by Williams and Lambert (1959) and recent ideas are reviewed in Chavent (1998). With these methods, each node can be clearly expressed according to the variables used in its construction, which makes it an attractive strategy for cluster analysis. Our original contribution lies in the way of splitting a node. Each cut is based on the assumption that the distribution of points at that node can be modelled by nonhomogeneous Poisson processes whose intensity can be estimated by histograms. The cut is made in order to maximize the likelihood function. Indeed, to find a partition, we must optimize an objective function that measures the homogeneity within clusters and/or the separation between clusters; in our case, this function is related to the likelihood.

In the next section, we recall the main results of the first steps of the method. Then we describe the gluing-back criterion and finish with several applications.

2 First Steps

The method developed in Pirçon and Rasson (2003) builds a tree of clusters. We successively split clusters into two sub-clusters on the basis of a single variable. Therefore, finding the cutting criterion is a one-dimensional problem. Afterwards we simplify the structure of the tree by pruning. For the cutting criterion and the pruning methods, this paper just gives the main results. For the development, we refer thc reader to the previous article.

Consider the problem of clustering points that are generated by a nonhomogeneous Poisson process with intensity $q(\cdot)$. Since we work variable by variable, we can write univariate formulas. The likelihood function for observations $\boldsymbol{x} = (x_1, x_2, \ldots, x_n)$ with $x_i \in I\!R, i = 1, \ldots, n$, is:

$$F_D(\boldsymbol{x}) = \frac{1}{(\rho(D))^n} \prod_{i=1}^{n} 1_D(x_i).q(x_i)$$

where $\rho(D) = \int_D q(x)\,dx$ is the integrated intensity of the process and $1_D(\cdot)$ is the indicator function.

Consequently, if the intensity of the process is known and D is the union of g disjoint and convex domains $D_1, \ldots, D_g \subset I\!R$, the domains which maximise the likelihood will correspond to g disjoint convex domains containing all the points and for which the sum of their integrated intensities is minimal:

$$\max_{D_1,\ldots,D_g} F_{\cup D_k}(\boldsymbol{x}) \iff \min_{D_1,\ldots,D_g} \sum_{k=1}^{g} \rho(D_k).$$

When the intensity is unknown, it must be estimated for all x in D. Our approach to estimation uses histograms with equal frequencies in each of the windows. Since we work variable by variable, the histograms are one-dimensional. Their construction depends on the type of variable—we don't treat qualitative and quantitative information in the same way.

For ordinal variables (i.e., qualitative variables where the categories have an order relation), the number of bins in the histogram equals the number of modalities of the variable. And the length of the windows is automatically given by the levels.

For quantitative variables, we must choose the number of bins and their widths. Jobson (1991, p. 35-36) gives a theoretical argument for choosing the number of bins n_h to satisfy $2^{n_h} < n < 2^{n_h+1}$ where n is the number of points. To choose the borders of these n_h bins, we build them in such way that the number of points each bin contains is approximately constant. For this, we calculate the theoretical number of points which each class should contain: $n_{pt} = \left[\frac{n}{n_h}\right] + 1$. Then we determine widths of bins so that each bin contains, as nearly as possible, n_{pt} points. In this manner, we avoid empty bins.

Basically, ignoring the possibility of tied values, the histogram is defined by the order statistics $x_{(1)}, \ldots, x_{(n)} \in I\!R$ of the observations $x_1, \ldots, x_n \in I\!R$ with $x_{(1)} \leq \cdots \leq x_{(n)}$ according to:

$$\begin{aligned} \text{class } k &= (x_{(kn_{pt})}, x_{((k+1)n_{pt})}], \\ f_k &= n_k(x_{((k+1)n_{pt})} - x_{(kn_{pt})}) \quad k = 1, \ldots, n_h - 1 \end{aligned}$$

where n_k is the number of points in class k. The value of the intensity is then $q(x) = f_k$ if $x \in$ class k.

2.1 Cutting Criterion

To split a node, we assume there are two convex disjoint sets whose observed points are generated by a nonhomogeneous Poisson process on $I\!R$. Since we treat one variable at a time, we need only work with the real line. By maximum likelihood, an optimal cut is the one that generates convex disjoint domains D_1 and D_2 ($D_1, D_2 \subset I\!R$) where $\rho(D_1) + \rho(D_2)$ is minimized:

$$\min_{D_1, D_2} \rho(D_1) + \rho(D_2) \iff \max_{\Delta} \rho(\Delta)$$

where Δ is a gap between two consecutive observations. So, our cutting procedure is the following: at each node, we start by using histograms to estimate the intensity of the points that lie in the node. Once the intensity is estimated, we find the two convex disjoint domains for which the integrated estimated surface is as small as possible. When we proceed in this way, variable by variable, we are able to select the variable which generates the largest value of the likelihood—it is the variable with the smallest integrated estimated surface on the two domains.

Moreover, in order to find the two disjoint convex domains for which the integrated surface is the smallest, we measure this surface for each pair of consecutive points. In order to avoid cutting between outliers, we compute Tukey's barrier, given by the following interval (Jobson, 1991, p. 56-59): $[Q_1 - (1.5)Q, Q_3 + (1.5)Q]$, where Q_1 and Q_3 are the first and third quartiles, respectively, and Q is the interquartile range. Consequently, we calculate the integrated surface for all pairs of consecutive points inside Tukey's barrier and we take, for the variable under consideration, the cut between the two consecutive points whose gap has the maximum integrated intensity.

Thanks to this cutting criterion, we have a divisive hierarchical method for clustering. The procedure stops only if:

- it meets a node whose points have all the same value;
- the removed surface (the surface of the "hole") is lower than a threshold (fixed at 0.00001);
- it meets a node which contains less than 10% of the sample.

For the remainder, we don't use a test in order to decide whether a cut is significant or not. Indeed, during the various numerical experiments, we often found that a bad cut was followed by a good cut. Consequently, we build the tree all the way to the end before testing whether a cut is significant. That decision is the role of the pruning procedure.

2.2 Pruning Criteria

To prune the tree, we introduce two different criteria :

- *"Elbow" Pruning*: First, we compute the intraclass inertia $I(\cdot)$ for all possible numbers of classes: Let $\mathcal{P}_k = \{D_1, \ldots, D_k\}$ be a partition into k classes, and for all $k = 1, \ldots, n$ set

  $$W(\mathcal{P}_k) = \sum_{i=1}^{k} I(D_i), \quad \text{for} \quad I(D) = \frac{1}{n} \sum_{i=1}^{n} d(x_i, c)$$

  where c is the center of gravity center and $d(\cdot, \cdot)$ is the Euclidian distance or the Manhattan distance for quantitative or qualitative variables, respectively. Then we trace the graph associated with intraclass inertia according to k, the number of classes. The presence of an "elbow" in this curve indicates the number of classes to be used.
  We have created an algorithm that finds the largest elbow in such a graph. Thus, this method of pruning chooses the number of classes by the elbow method and prunes superfluous cuts. We must pay attention to the graph of the elbow to make sure it does not decrease too smoothly; in such a case, that indicates an absence of structure.
- *Gap Test Pruning*: This procedure is based on an hypothesis test called the *gap test* (Rasson and Kubushishi, 1994 and Kubushishi, 1996). Suppose that we have n observations in $D \subset \mathbb{R}$, separated into two classes $D_1 \subset \mathbb{R}$ (with n_1 points) and $D_2 \subset \mathbb{R}$ (with n_2 points). The gap test compares the null and alternative hypotheses:
  H_0: there is $n = n_1 + n_2$ points in $D_1 \cup D_2$
  H_1: there are n_1 points in D_1 and n_2 points in D_2 with $D_1 \cap D_2 = \emptyset$.

This pruning method crosses the tree branch by branch from its root to its end in order to index the good cuts (gap test rejects the null) and the bad cuts (gap test fails to reject). The ends of the branches in which there are only bad cuts are pruned.

Given that the statistic of the gap test is only valid for data following a homogeneous Poisson process, we make a change of variables (Kubushishi, 1996, p. 105) of the type $\tau = \int_{x_{(1)}}^{t} q(x)dx$ where $q(x)$ is the intensity of the Poisson process. We denote the maximum distance between two consecutive values in $\tau_{(1)}, \ldots, \tau_{(n)}$ by Δ^*. Consequently, as shown in Pirçon and Rasson (2003), the critical region is

$$\{m' | m' = \frac{n\Delta^*}{\tau_{(n)}} - \ln \Delta^* \geq K_\alpha = -\ln(-\ln(1-\alpha)\}.$$

3 Gluing-Back Criteria

The pruning method tests if two clusters with the same parent node should be considered as one group or two. The gluing-back criterion can join two clusters that have been separated by a previous cut. For example, examine Ruspini's data in Fig. 1. In this scatterplot, we see that after pruning there are five classes. But Ruspini's data should have only four classes. In fact, both groups with an asterisk should form only one class.

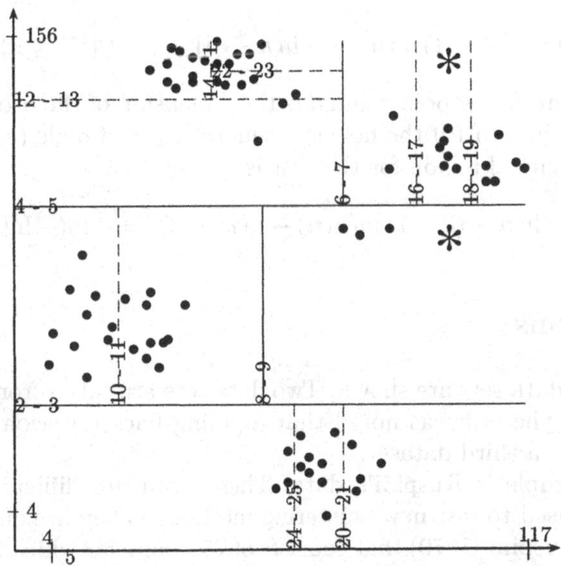

Fig. 1. Ruspini's data: An example in which gluing-back is needed.

As there are two different pruning methods, we have two associated gluing back criteria.

3.1 The Elbow Gluing-Back Criterion

This criterion is easy. We first compute the intraclass inertia for k classes where k decreases from the number of groups after pruning to 1. For each k, we choose the best gluing to have the maximum intraclass inertia after joining two groups. Then, as previously for pruning, we examine the graph that plots the best intraclass inertia against k. The presence of an elbow in this curve indicates the number of classes that should be retained and we glue the corresponding groups.

3.2 The Gap Test Gluing-Back Criterion

Suppose we want to test whether to glue back groups on D_1 and on D_2. The test statistic is the same as for the gap test pruning method. But this time, after the change of variables, we work in multidimensional space with $D_1, D_2 \subset \mathbb{R}^d$.

First, using a square 4-connexity frame (Schmitt and Mattioli, 1993), the weak convex envelopes of D_1 and D_2 ($\overline{D_1}$, $\overline{D_2}$) are estimated. Then we compute the weak convex envelope of the gluing group ($\overline{D_1 \cup D_2}$). The asymptotic distribution of the statistic of the largest hole $\Delta = \overline{D_1 \cup D_2} \backslash (\overline{D_1} \cup \overline{D_2})$ was found by Kubushishi (1996):

$$n\, m(\Delta) - \ln n - (d-1)\ln(\ln n) - \ln \kappa \xrightarrow{\mathcal{L}} W \quad , \quad P(W \leq x) = e^{-e^{-x}}$$

where n is the number of points and d is the dimension of the problem. Here κ is a parameter equal to 1 if the hole is a square or a rectangle (Janson, 1986). Therefore, the critical region for the test is

$$\{\Delta | n\, m(\Delta) - \ln n - (d-1)\ln(\ln n) - \ln \kappa \geq K_\alpha = -\ln(-\ln(1-\alpha))\} .$$

4 Applications

Three different data sets are shown. Two data sets are taken from Pirçon and Rasson (2003), where it was noted that a gluing-back criterion was needed. We also consider a third dataset.

The first sample is Ruspini's data. These data are difficult to classify; they are often used to test new clustering methods. They are an artificial set introduced by Ruspini (1970) that consists of 75 points for which two measures were calculated. The data are divided into four rather distinct groups but most of methods only find three, and wrongly combine two of the groups into one.

This error happens because there is a "bridge" of 8 points between the two groups.

The second dataset shows how our method works when there are classes which cannot be completely separated by cuts that are perpendicular to the axes. This "Triangle" dataset is artificial with 85 points and 2 variables. These observations cluster in three elliptical groups laid out to form a triangle.

The third dataset requires, by the structure of its clusters, several gluings. This "Sourire" dataset is artificial and consists of 100 points and 2 variables.

In Fig. 2, we can see the results from the elbow and gap test pruning and gluing-back criteria. The dotted lines are pruned cuts and the dashed lines represent the groups that are glued. For Ruspini's data, the results are perfect. But this is not the case for the other two datasets. For the Triangle data, results are not very good. Regarding the gap test pruning and gluing-back criteria, this is due to the fact that some points in different clusters are very close. Regarding the elbow method, there is no gluing-back because the inertia tends to make spherical groups. For the Sourire data, the elbow method fails for the same reason. But in this case, there are some gluing-backs to make more spherical groups.

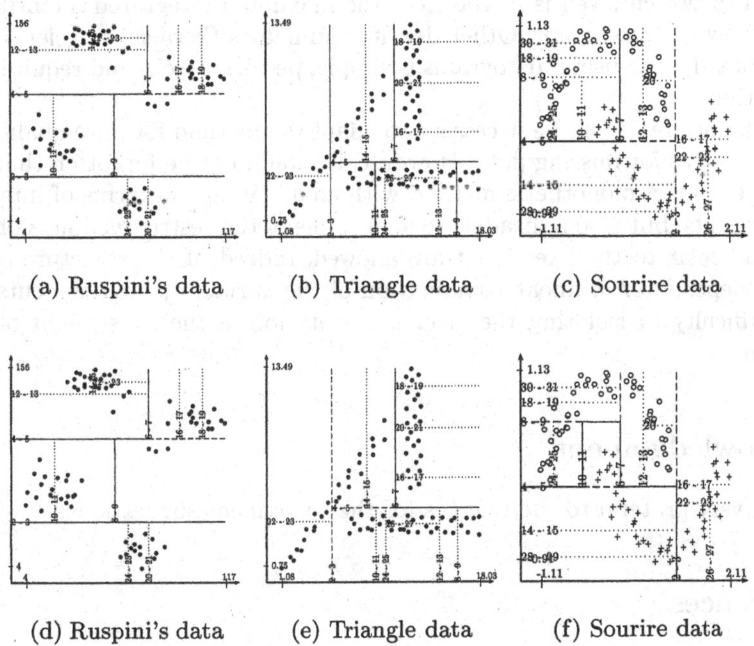

(a) Ruspini's data (b) Triangle data (c) Sourire data

(d) Ruspini's data (e) Triangle data (f) Sourire data

Fig. 2. Results with elbow pruning and gluing ((a),(b),(c)) and with gap test pruning and gluing ((d),(e),(f)).

5 Conclusion

The last step of a proposed new method is described in this article. With the gluing-back criterion, we partially resolve the disadvantages of the method. Since our method is monothetic, the cuts are necessarily perpendicular to axes. But with the gluing back criterion, we can glue together some clusters that do not the same parent node in the tree.

The elbow pruning and gluing-back criteria have the drawback that they tend to form spherical groups. With the gap test, the results are better for elliptical groups. For spherical groups, results are good with both kinds of pruning and gluing. Indeed, we have the good classes for Ruspini's data and for Sourire data. But, for the Triangle data, the problem is the proximity between two clusters. The gap test rejects the hypothesis of two different groups for any value of α up to 0.75. Other standard methods (single, average, or complete linkage, k-means, etc.) do not correctly find the three classes.

With this last criterion, our method is complete. The method is indexed, divisive, and monothetic hierarchical. Our principal contributions in this method are the cutting criterion, the pruning methods, and the gluing-back criteria which make only the assumption that points are distributed according to a nonhomogeneous Poisson process. A new measure for separating one group into two children is introduced: the maximum integrated intensity estimated by the histogram. Other density estimators (kernels, wavelets) were tested but the one using histograms is simple, performs well, and requires less calculation.

In the future, it will be necessary to adapt the method for pure qualitative data as well as for missing data. However, it should not be forgotten that this new method is a monothetic method with an advantage in terms of interpreting results, but also a disadvantage in terms of the restrictive kinds of cuts (perpendicular to the axes) that are allowed. Indeed, if the structure of the groups depends on a linear combination of the variables, then the cuts will have difficulty in isolating the groups. A rotation of the axes might offer a solution.

Acknowledgement

We are very grateful to the referees for their pertinent suggestions.

References

1. Chavent, M. (1998). "A Monothetic Clustering Method," *Pattern Recognition Letters*, **19**, 989–996.
2. Everitt, B. S. (1993). *Cluster Analysis*, third edition, Edward Arnold, London.
3. Gordon, A. D. (1998). "Cluster Validation," in *Data Sciences, Classification, and Related Methods*, eds. C. Hayashi et. al., Berlin:Springer, pp. 22–39.

4. Janson, S. (1986). "Random Coverings in Several Dimensions," *Acta Mathematica*, **156**, 83–118.
5. Jobson, J. (1991). *Applied Multivariate Data Analysis. Volume I: Regression and Experimental Design.* Springer-Verlag, New York.
6. Kubushishi, T. (1996). *On Some Applications of the Point Process Theory in Cluster Analysis and Pattern Recognition.* PhD thesis, Facultés Universitaires Notre-Dame de la Paix.
7. Pirçon, J.-Y. and Rasson, J.-P. (2003). "A New Monothetic Method of Clustering Based on Density Estimation by Histograms," submitted to the *Journal of Classification.*
8. Rasson, J.-P. and Kubushishi, T. (1994). "The Gap Test: An Optimal Method for Determining the Number of Natural Classes in Cluster Analysis," in *New Approaches in Classification and Data Analysis*, eds. E. Diday, Y. Lechevallier, M. Schader, P. Bertrand, and B. Burtschy, Berlin:Springer, pp. 186-193.
9. Ruspini, E. M. (1970). "Numerical Methods for Fuzzy Clustering," *Information Sciences*, **2**, 319–350.
10. Schmitt, M. and Mattioli, J. (1993). *Morphologie Mathématique.* Masson, Paris.
11. Williams, W. T. and Lambert, J. M. (1959). "Multivariate Methods in Plant Ecology: 1. Association Analysis in Plant Communities," *Journal of Ecology*, **47**, 83–101.

Standardizing Variables in K-means Clustering

Douglas Steinley

University of Illinois Urbana-Champaign, USA
steinley@cyrus.psych.uiuc.edu

Abstract: Several standardization methods are investigated in conjunction with the K-means algorithm under various conditions. We find that traditional standardization methods (i.e., z-scores) are inferior to alternative standardization methods. Future suggestions concerning the combination of standardization and variable selection are considered.

1 Introduction

There is some current debate in the literature about the "proper" way to standardize variables when performing a K-means clustering. To date, the only comprehensive study examining variable standardization was conducted by Milligan and Cooper (1988) who investigated eight different methods of standardization under several error conditions. Milligan and Cooper (1988) concluded that standardizing by the range (instead of relying on the usual z-score) was the most effective method; Dillon, Mulani, and Frederick (1989) indicate variable standardization (z-scores specifically) can result in misleading conclusions when true group structure is present; Späth (1985) notes that a z-score is as arbitrary as any other type of scaling. In contrast, Vesanto (2001) argues that z-scores are more interpretable and should be chosen in lieu of standardizing by the range, subsequently creating a measure of "variable quality" based on the z-score. Vesanto (2001), however, fails to carry out a comprehensive study, and his assertion is not as strongly supported as Milligan and Cooper's (1988) results, who unfortunately only investigated agglomerative hierarchical techniques.

Schaffer and Green (1996) studied the effects of variable standardization on K-means clustering across ten empirical datasets and found results that were not commensurate with those of Milligan and Cooper (1988), supporting Stoddard's (1979) conjecture that standardization based on the entire sample variance is likely to eliminate valuable between-cluster variation. Schaffer and Green (1996) note that part of the discrepancy between the two studies could be due to the different clustering algorithms employed (K-means vs. hierarchical methods). To the author's knowledge, a comprehensive analysis of the effects of variable standardization has not been conducted on the K-means method when the cluster structure is known.

1.1 K-means Clustering

The K-means method (MacQueen, 1967) is designed to partition two-way, two-mode data (that is, N objects each having measurements on P variables) into K classes $(C_1, C_2, \ldots, C_K)$, where C_k is the set of n_k objects in cluster k, and K is given. If $\mathbf{X}_{N\times P} = \{x_{ij}\}_{N\times P}$ denotes the $N \times P$ data matrix, the K-means method constructs these partitions so that the squared Euclidean distance between the row vector for any object and the centroid vector of its respective cluster is at least as small as the distances to the centroids of the remaining clusters. The centroid of cluster C_k, $\bar{\mathbf{x}}^{(k)}$, is a point in P–dimensional space found by averaging the values on each variable over the objects within the cluster. A typical algorithm used for this purpose is:

1. K initial seeds are defined by P-dimensional vectors $(s_1^{(k)}, \ldots, s_P^{(k)})$, for $1 \leq k \leq K)$.
2. Based on the initial seeds, the squared Euclidean distance, $d^2(i,k)$, between the ith object and the kth seed vector is obtained:
$$d^2(i,k) = \sum_{j=1}^{P} (x_{ij} - s_j^{(k)})^2. \tag{1}$$
Objects are allocated to clusters with the minimum squared Euclidean distance to its defining seed.
3. Once all objects have been initially allocated, cluster centroids are computed and the initial seeds, $s_j^{(k)}$, are replaced with $\bar{x}_j^{(k)}$.
4. Objects are compared to each centroid (using $d^2(i,k)$) and allocated to the cluster whose centroid is closest.
5. New centroids are calculated with the updated cluster membership (by calculating the centroids after all objects have been assigned).
6. Steps 4 and 5 are repeated until no objects can be reallocated to different clusters.

A common problem in K-means clustering is convergence to a local optimum (Steinley, 2003a). To combat this problem, Steinley (2003a) suggests performing K-means several thousand times and on each implementation, randomly choosing different seed vectors to begin the algorithm; the solution is chosen as the partitioning of the data that minimizes the overall within cluster variance (i.e., the solution with the most compact clusters). This procedure was shown to outperform several other commonly implemented initialization procedures.

1.2 Methods of Standardization

This section introduces the five standardization methods studied in this experiment (Milligan & Cooper (1988) studied seven methods, but two of them are redundant when using squared Euclidean distance). The following notation first needs to be defined:

$\bar{\mathbf{x}}' = (\bar{x}_1, \ldots, \bar{x}_P)$, the $1 \times P$ grand centroid row vector ($1 \leq p \leq P$);
$\mathbf{s}' = (s_1, \ldots, s_P)$, the $1 \times P$ vector of variable standard deviations;
$(\mathbf{x}^m)' = (\max(x_1), \ldots, \max(x_P))$, the $1 \times P$ vector of maxima for each variable;
$(\mathbf{x}_m)' = (\min(x_1), \ldots, \min(x_P))$, the $1 \times P$ vector of minima for each variable;
$\mathbf{j}$ = an $N \times 1$ vector of ones;
$\mathbf{Z}$ = an $N \times P$ matrix of standardized values;
Rank($\mathbf{X}$) = within column ranking of observations of the data matrix, $\mathbf{X}$.
$\mathbf{A}./\mathbf{B}$ = the element by element division of $\mathbf{A}$ by $\mathbf{B}$.

The original data and the five standardizations are:

$$\mathbf{Z}_0 = \mathbf{X} \;, \tag{2}$$

$$\mathbf{Z}_1 = (\mathbf{X} - \mathbf{j}\bar{\mathbf{x}}')./\mathbf{j}\mathbf{s}' \;, \tag{3}$$

$$\mathbf{Z}_2 = \mathbf{X}./\mathbf{j}(\mathbf{x}^m)' \;, \tag{4}$$

$$\mathbf{Z}_3 = \mathbf{X}./(\mathbf{j}(\mathbf{x}^m)' - \mathbf{j}(\mathbf{x}_m)') \;, \tag{5}$$

$$\mathbf{Z}_4 = \mathbf{X}./(N\mathbf{j}\bar{\mathbf{x}}') \;, \tag{6}$$

and

$$\mathbf{Z}_5 = \text{Rank}(\mathbf{X}) \;. \tag{7}$$

Noting that all of the methods perform within column (variable) standardization, they can be conceptualized as: $\mathbf{Z}_0$ represents the original data; $\mathbf{Z}_1$ is the common z-score standardization method for each variable; $\mathbf{Z}_2$ divides each variable by its maximum; $\mathbf{Z}_3$ divides each variable by its range; $\mathbf{Z}_4$ divides each variable by its sum; and $\mathbf{Z}_5$ transforms the data matrix into ranks.

2 Experimental Design

The design of the simulation study follows that presented in Steinley (2003a) with some modifications based on Milligan and Cooper (1988) and some extensions in general. For the general data generation procedure, Milligan (1985) requires the first dimension of the clusters to be non-overlapping (subsequently, all other dimensions are allowed to overlap or not). Furthermore, all of the dimensions are generated using a slightly truncated multivariate normal distribution. Using this method allows for the manipulation of four factors: the number of clusters, the number of variables, relative scale of variables, and probability of overlap on the first dimension. The fifth factor alters the original data generation procedure (1985) by following the method in Steinley (2003a), generating clusters that may overlap. Generally, simulated data sets reported in the clustering literature have contained anywhere from 50 to 300 objects (Brusco & Cradit, 2001; Milligan & Cooper, 1988). The present study includes datasets with 300 objects.

The first factor, the number of clusters present in the datasets, was examined at three levels, $K = 3, 4$, and 5. The second factor, the number of variables, had values $P = 4, 6, \text{and } 8$. The third factor, relative scale of variables, has two different levels. The first level assumes that the variables are each sampled from the same type of scale (i.e., each variable has a comparable range). The second multiplies a random subset of $P/2$ variables by a random constant between 5 and 10 (thus increasing the variance of a variable between 25 and 100 times its original value). This factor (relative scale of variables) is extremely important because of the additive nature of (1), and is designed to address one of the common criticisms that K-means gives too much priority to variables with large variances. Milligan and Cooper (1988) examined a similar factor that manipulated the within cluster variance; however, they found it did not significantly impact the results of their study. The fourth factor, probability of overlap on the first dimension, had ten different levels ranging from 0 to .45 in increments of .05. The fifth and final factor was the type of standardization procedure used and had six different levels, $\mathbf{Z}_0$–$\mathbf{Z}_5$. This design results in $3 \times 3 \times 2 \times 10 \times 6 = 1080$ conditions. Commensurate with other studies, three datasets were generated for each condition (Milligan, 1980; Milligan & Cooper, 1988; Brusco & Cradit, 2001), resulting in a total of 3,240 datasets.

2.1 Recovery Measure

To examine the appropriateness of the standardization procedures, the ability to reproduce the generated data is considered the most important quality. The adjusted Rand index (Hubert & Arabie, 1985) was used as the recovery measure and the dependent variable in the study. This index is frequently used and has been shown to possess several desirable properties Steinley (2003b). The adjusted Rand index (ARI) assumes a value of unity when there is perfect agreement between the recovered structure and the known, "true" structure; the ARI assumes a value of zero when there is only chance agreement between the recovered partition and the "true" partition.

3 Results

Because five datasets were sampled for each separate condition, the ARI can be treated as the response variable and analyzed as a fixed effects ANOVA where the class variables are the factors included in the simulation (consistent with other simulation studies, see Brusco & Cradit, 2001). To conserve space, only main effects are reported here; however, significant interactions are discussed where relevant. The factors are discussed in the order presented in the ANOVA table (all effects in the ANOVA table were significant, $p < .0001$).

Table 1. ANOVA Results for Simulation Factors

Effect	DF	SS	MS	F
K	2	24.19	12.09	489.41
P	2	10.18	5.09	205.95
Scale	1	1.65	1.65	66.58
Overlap	9	0.90	0.10	4.05
Standardization	5	5.12	1.02	41.45

The first factor is the number of clusters in the dataset. The means for the three conditions ($K = 3, 4, 5$) are 0.74, 0.90, and 0.95, respectively. This general increase is attributable to the inherent property of the ARI that, if all other factors are held constant, the ARI increases as the number of groups increases (cf. Steinley, 2003b). So the effects of this factor are a direct result of the recovery measure instead of the clustering technique.

The second factor is the number of variables per cluster. The means for the three conditions ($P = 4, 6, 8$) are 0.79, 0.88, and 0.93. The increase in recovery as the number of dimensions increases is consistent with several other simulation studies (Milligan, 1980; Steinley, 2003a) and is attributable to an increase of information due to the inclusion of several variables with the same underlying cluster structure.

The third factor, relative scale, shows an ARI of 0.89 when all of the variables are from the same relative scale; if the variables have disproportionate amounts of relative variance, the average ARI decreases to 0.84. The effect of the scale factor will be discussed in more depth in the context of the interaction with the type of standardization performed.

The overlap factor mirrored the results of Steinley (2003), indicating a gradual decrease in cluster recovery as the probability of overlap increases. The decrease follows the same steady trend indicated in the previous study and moves from an ARI of 0.89 when probability of overlap on the first dimension is zero to an ARI of 0.84 when probability of overlap increases to 0.45.

The final factor, the type of standardization, plays an important role in understanding these results. The means of different conditions ($\mathbf{Z}_0$–$\mathbf{Z}_5$) were 0.78, 0.88, 0.89, 0.90, 0.86, and 0.88, respectively. The similarity in results may be in part attributed to the method of using several thousand random restarts proposed by Steinley (2003a), making it easier for the unstandardized and standardized data to arrive at the same final partitioning of the dataset. However, a greater difference is noticed if the means for the standardization methods are examined by the relative scale factor (the interaction, scale × type is significant: p-value $< .0001$; see Table 2 for cell means). Furthermore, $\mathbf{Z}_0$ is the only variable that exhibited significantly different recovery capabilities between the two types of scale ($p < .0001$). To determine which standardization methods performed best, the Ryan-Einot-Gabriel-Welsch multiple range test was conducted and the final group of top-performing methods (indicated by a * in Table 2) consisted of $\mathbf{Z}_2$ and $\mathbf{Z}_3$.

Table 2. Standardization Recovery Results by Relative Scale Condition

Condition	$\mathbf{Z}_0$	$\mathbf{Z}_1$	$\mathbf{Z}_2$	$\mathbf{Z}_3$	$\mathbf{Z}_4$	$\mathbf{Z}_5$
Scale Equal	0.91	0.89	0.89	0.90	0.86	0.88
Scale Not Equal	0.65	0.87	0.89	0.90	0.86	0.88
Overall	0.78	0.88	0.89*	0.90*	0.86	0.88

The standardization of variables was additionally helpful in making K-means more robust with respect to overlap on the first dimension of the clusters. Figure 1 plots the performance of the unstandardized data as probability of overlap increases (the bottom line), and the average performance of the top performing standardization methods ($\mathbf{Z}_2$ and $\mathbf{Z}_3$) as probability of overlap increases. Two important differences can be gleaned from this graph: (a) the standardization methods consistently perform better in the presence of a given level of overlap, and (b) the decrease in performance of the standardization methods is not as great, indicating that standardized data are not as dramatically affected by changes in overlap as unstandardized data.

4 Conclusion

Under the studied conditions, standardization of the data before clustering never has a detrimental effect on the recovery method, and when the variances of the variables are disparate, standardization can actually increase the general recovery of the K-means clustering method. Second, the overall results presented here support the conclusions of Milligan and Cooper (1988) that standardizing variables by their range is the most effective standardization method. Additionally, for K-means clustering, it is shown that the standardization of variables by their maximum is also an effective method of standardization. Contrary to arguments made by Vesanto (2001), standardization by the z-score is not the most effective method for standardization, giving more weight to the remark by Späth (1985) that z-scores are an arbitrary transformation of scale. Compared to $\mathbf{Z}_2$ and $\mathbf{Z}_3$, $\mathbf{Z}_1$ may perform worse because it is too much of an "equalizer". Specifically, $\mathbf{Z}_1$ fixes the variances of all variables to unity; $\mathbf{Z}_2$ and $\mathbf{Z}_3$ make the variables more compatible while allowing differences based on their original compositions to remain (in the form

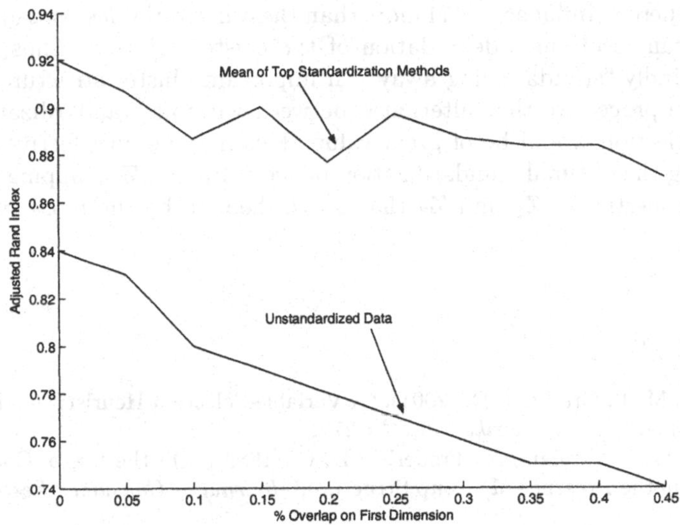

Fig. 1. Resilience to Overlap: Unstandardized data vs. Standardized data

of variances of different magnitude)—creating a transformed variable that lies somewhere between $\mathbf{Z}_0$ and $\mathbf{Z}_1$ in terms of impact on (1).

These results also contradict the findings of Schaffer and Green (1996); however, since they were analyzing empirical datasets, other factors could have complicated their results (for example, incorrectly specifying the correct number of clusters). An added benefit of variable standardization in K-means clustering is the general resilience of cluster overlap, the problem Steinley (2003a) indicated as the most hindering when trying to recover the correct clusters underlying the observed data.

4.1 Future Directions

Although interesting results were provided, there are several extensions of this study that might be pursued. First, it would be of interest to determine how different the variances of the variables have to be before standardization becomes effective. Also, how many variables must have larger variances before standardization becomes necessary. A cluster generation procedure that controls for different types of overlap on all dimensions would prove invaluable in pinpointing the optimal performance for different methods (a method is currently under development, see Steinley & Henson, 2003), leading to a standardization method that helps combat the interference of several overlapping dimensions and noisy cluster structure.

Possibly of greater interest is the notion of combining standardization methods with variable selection procedures. Specifically, if the variable that defines the cluster structure the most is also the variable with the greatest variance (thereby influencing (1) more than the other variables), standardizing the data can result in a degradation of the cluster solution. Thus, to help prevent blindly "standardizing away" an important cluster structure, a type of iterative procedure that alternates between variable standardization and variable selection would be of great value. This may be an effective method for locating the optimal standardization between $\mathbf{Z}_0$ and $\mathbf{Z}_1$, tapping into the implicit properties of $\mathbf{Z}_2$ and $\mathbf{Z}_3$ that cause them to be the more successful methods.

References

1. Brusco, M. J., Cradit, J. D. (2001). "A Variable-Selection Heuristic for K-means Clustering," *Psychometrika*, **66**, 249–270.
2. Dillon, W. R., Mulani, N., Frederick, D. G. (1989). "On the Use of Component Scores in the Presence of Group Structure," *Journal of Consumer Research*, **16**, 106–112.
3. Hubert, L., Arabie, P. (1985). "Comparing partitions," *Journal of Classification*, **2**, 193–218.
4. MacQueen, J. (1967). "Some Methods of Classification and Analysis of Multivariate Observations," in *Proceedings of the 5th Berkeley Symposium on Statistics and Probability*, eds. L. Le Cam and J. Neyman, Berkeley, CA: University of California Press, pp. 281–297.
5. Milligan, G. W. (1980). "An Examination of the Effect of Six Types of Error Perturbation on Fifteen Clustering Algorithms," *Psychometrika*, **45**, 325–342.
6. Milligan, G. W. (1985). "An Algorithm for Generating Artificial Test Clusters," *Psychometrika*, **50**, 123–127.
7. Milligan, G. W., Cooper, M. C. (1988). "A Study of Standardization of Variables in Cluster Analysis," *Journal of Classification*, **5**, 181–204.
8. Schaffer, C. M., Green, P. E. (1996). "An Empirical Comparison of Variable Standardization Methods in Cluster Analysis," *Multivariate Behavioral Research*, **31**, 149–167.
9. Späth, H. (1985). *Cluster Dissection and Analysis–Theory, FORTRAN Programs, Examples.* Wiley, New York.
10. Steinley, D. (2003a). "K-means Clustering: What You Don't Know May Hurt You," *Psychometric Methods*, **8**, 294–304.
11. Steinley, D. (2003b). "Properties of the Hubert-Arabie Adjusted Rand Index," Manuscript submitted for publication.
12. Steinley, D., Henson, R. (2003). "OCLUS–An Analytic Method to Generate Clusters with Known Overlap," Manuscript submitted for publication.
13. Stoddard, A. M. (1979). "Standardization of Measures Prior to Cluster Analysis," *Biometrics*, **35**, 765–773.
14. Vesanto, J. (2001). "Importance of Individual Variables in the K-means Algorithm," in *Proceedings of the Pacific–Asia Conference in Knowledge Discovery and Data Mining*, eds. D. Cheung, G. J. Willimas, and J. Li, New York: Springer, pp. 513–518.

A Self-Organizing Map for Dissimilarity Data

Aïcha El Golli[1,2], Brieuc Conan-Guez[1,2], and Fabrice Rossi[1,2]

[1] INRIA-Rocquencourt, France
aicha.el_golli,brieuc.conan-guez@inria.fr
[2] Université Paris Dauphine, France
rossi@ufrmd.dauphine.fr

Abstract: Treatment of complex data (for example symbolic data, semi-structured data, or functional data) cannot be easily done by clustering methods that are based on calculating the center of gravity. We present in this paper an extension of self-organizing maps to dissimilarity data. This extension allows to apply this algorithm to numerous types of data in a convenient way.

1 Introduction

The Kohonen Self-Organizing Map (SOM) introduced by Kohonen (1997) is an unsupervised neural network method which has both clustering and visualization properties. It can be considered as an algorithm that maps a high dimensional data space, $\mathbb{R}^p$, to a lattice space which usually has a lower dimension, generally 2, and is called a Map. This projection enables a partition of the inputs into "similar" clusters while preserving their topology. Its most similar predecessors are the k-means algorithm (MacQueen, 1967) and the dynamic clustering method (Diday et al., 1989), which operate as a SOM without topology preservation and thus without easy visualization.

In data analysis, new forms of complex data have to be considered, most notably structured data (data with an internal structure such as intervals data, distributions, functional data, etc) and semi-structured data (trees, XML documents, SQL queries, etc.). In this context, classical data analysis based on calculating the center of gravity cannot be used because inputs are not $\mathbb{R}^p$ vectors. In order to solve this problem, several methods can be considered according to the type of data (for example, recoding techniques for symbolic data (de Reyniès, 2003) or projection operators for functional data (Ramsay and Silverman, 1997). However, those methods are not fully general and an adaptation of every data analysis algorithm to the resulting data is needed.

We propose in this article an adaptation of the SOM to dissimilarity data as an alternative solution. Kohonen's SOM is based on the notion of center of gravity and, unfortunately, this concept is not applicable to many kind of complex data, especially semi-structured data. Our goal is to modify the SOM algorithm to allow its implementation on dissimilarity measures rather than on raw data. With this alternative only the definition of a dissimilarity for each type of data is necessary to apply the method and so treat complex data.

The paper is organized as follows: we first recall the SOM algorithm in its batch version. Then we describe our adaptation. We conclude the paper by experiments on simulated and real world data.

2 Self-Organizing Map (SOM)

Kohonen's SOM is used nowadays across many domains and has been successfully applied in numerous applications. It is a very popular tool for visualizing high dimensional data spaces. SOMs can be considered as doing vector quantization and/or clustering while preserving the spatial ordering of the input data reflected by implementing an ordering of the codebook vectors (also called prototype vectors, cluster centroids or *referent vectors*) in a one- or two-dimensional output space. The SOM consists of neurons organized on a regular low-dimensional grid, called the map. More formally, the map is described by a graph (C, Γ). The C is a set of m interconnected neurons having a discrete topology defined by Γ. For each pair of neurons (c, r) on the map, the distance $\delta(c, r)$ is defined as the shortest path between c and r on the graph. This distance imposes a neighborhood relation between neurons (see figure 1 for an example). Each neuron c is represented by a p-dimensional referent vector $w_c = \{w_c^1, ..., w_c^p\}$, where p is equal to the dimension of the input vectors. The number of neurons may vary from a few dozen to several thousand depending on the application.

The SOM training algorithm resembles k-means clustering (MacQueen, 1967). The important distinction is that in addition to the best-matching referent vector, its neighbors on the map are updated: the region around the best-matching vector is stretched towards the training sample presented. The end result is that the neurons on the grid become ordered: neighboring neurons have similar referent vectors.

The SOM takes as its input a set of labeled sample vectors and gives as output an array of neurons with the input vectors labels attached to these neurons. Let n be the number of sample vectors $z_i \in \mathbb{R}^p$, $i = 1, 2, ..., n$, where each sample vector z_i is identified by a label.

2.1 Batch Training Algorithm

The batch training algorithm is an iterative algorithm in which the whole data set (denoted by Ω) is presented to the map before any adjustments are made. In each training step, the data set is partitioned according to the Voronoi regions of the map referent vectors. More formally, we define an affectation function f from $\mathbb{R}^p$ (the input space) to C, that associates each element z_i

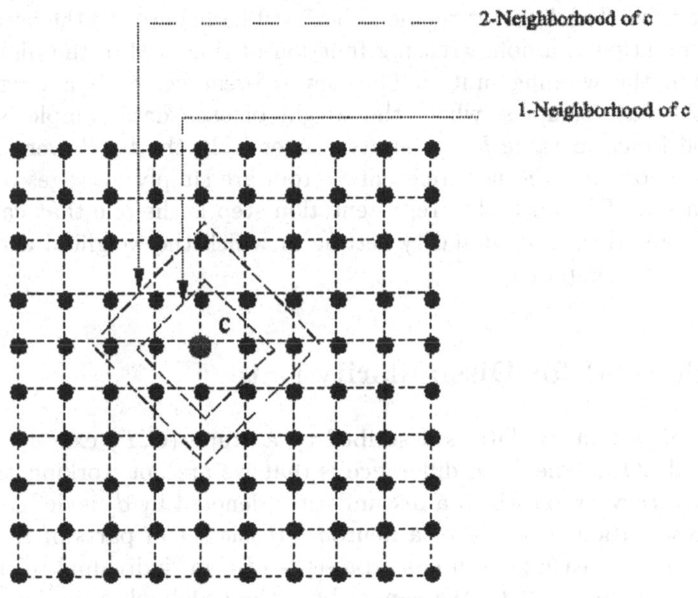

Fig. 1. Discrete topology of a two dimensional topological map (10×10 neurons), where each point represents a neuron. The diamonds show the 1-neighborhood and 2-neighborhood of neuron c.

of $\mathbb{R}^p$ to the neuron whose referent vector is "closest" to z_i (for the Euclidean distance). This function induces a partition $P = \{P_c; c = 1...m\}$ of the set of individuals where each part P_c is defined by: $P_c = \{z_i \in \Omega; f(z_i) = c\}$. This is the *affectation step*. It is quite clear that this step is rather easy to adapt to a dissimilarity setting.

After affectation, a *representation step* is performed. The algorithm updates the referent vectors by minimizing a cost function, denoted by $E(f, W)$. This function has to take into account the inertia of the partition P, while ensuring the topology preserving property. To achieve these two goals, it is necessary to generalize the inertia function of P by introducing the neighborhood notion attached to the map. In the case of individuals belonging to $\mathbb{R}^p$, this minimization can be done in a straightforward way. Indeed, new referent vectors are calculated as:

$$w_r^{t+1} = \frac{\sum_{i=1}^{n} h_{rc}(t) z_i}{\sum_{i=1}^{n} h_{rc}(t)}$$

where $c = \arg\min_r ||z_i - w_r||$ is the index of the best matching unit of the data sample z_i, $||\cdot||$ is the distance measure, typically the Euclidean distance, and t denotes the time. The $h_{rc}(t)$ is the neighborhood kernel around the winning unit c. This function is a nonincreasing function of time and of the distance of unit r from the winning unit c. The new referent vector is a weighted average of the data samples, where the weight of each data sample is the neighborhood function value $h_{rc}(t)$ at its winner c. In the batch version of the k-means algorithm, the new referent vectors are simply averages of the Voronoi data sets. Obviously, the representation step is the one that cannot be directly adapted to a dissimilarity setting in which the weighted average of data cannot be computed.

3 A Batch SOM for Dissimilarity Data

The Map for dissimilarity data is described by a graph (C, Γ) exactly as in the traditional SOM. The main difference is that we are not working on $\mathbb{R}^d$ but on an arbitrary set on which a dissimilarity (denoted by d) is defined.

The representation space L_c of a neuron c is the set of parts of Ω with a fixed cardinality q: each neuron c is represented by an "individual referent" $a_c = \{z_{j_1}, ..., z_{j_q}\}$, for $z_{j_i} \in \Omega$. We denote by a the codebook of individuals, i.e., the list $a = \{a_c; c = 1, ..., m\}$ of the individual referents of the map. In classical SOM each referent vector evolves in the entire input space $\mathbb{R}^p$. In our approach each neuron has a finite number of representations.

We define a new dissimilarity d^T from $\Omega \times P(\Omega)$ to $\mathbb{R}^+$ by

$$d^T(z_i, a_c) = \sum_{r \in C} K^T(\delta(c, r)) \sum_{z_j \in a_r} d^2(z_i, z_j).$$

This dissimilarity is based on a positive kernel function K. This function is such that $\lim_{|\delta| \to \infty} K(\delta) = 0$ and this allows one to transform the sharp graph distance between two neurons on the map ($\delta(c, r)$) into a smooth distance. The K is used to define a family of functions K^T parameterized by T, with $K^T(\delta) = K(\delta/T)$. As for the traditional SOM, T is used to control the size of the neighborhood (see Thiria and et al., 2002). When the parameter T is small, there are few neurons in the neighborhood. A simple example of K^T is defined by $K^T(\delta) = \exp(-\delta^2/T^2)$.

During the learning, we minimize the following cost function E by alternating the affectation step and the representation step:

$$E(f, a) = \sum_{z_i \in \Omega} d^T(z_i, a_{f(z_i)}) = \sum_{z_i \in \Omega} \sum_{r \in C} K^T(\delta(f(z_i), r)) \sum_{z_j \in a_r} d^2(z_i, z_j). \quad (1)$$

This function calculates the adequacy between the partition induced by the affectation function and the map referents a.

During the affectation step, the affectation function f assigns each individual z_i to the nearest neuron; in terms of the dissimilarity d^T,

$$f(z_i) = \text{argmin}_{c \in C} d^T(z_i, a_c). \tag{2}$$

This affectation step decreases the E criterion.

During the representation step, we have to find the new codebook for individuals a^* that represents the set of observations in the best way in terms of E. This optimization step can be realized independently for each neuron. Indeed, we minimize the m following functions:

$$E_r = \sum_{z_i \in \Omega} K^T(\delta(f(z_i), r)) \sum_{z_j \in a_r} d^2(z_i, z_j). \tag{3}$$

In the classical batch version, this minimization of the E function is immediate because the positions of the referent vectors are the averages of the data samples weighted by the kernel function.

3.1 The Algorithm

Initialization: At iteration $k = 0$, choose an initial individuals codebook a^0. Fix $T = T_{max}$ and the total number of iterations N_{iter}

Iteration: At iteration k, the set of individual referents of the previous iteration a^{k-1} is known. Calculate the new value of T:

$$T = T_{max} * (\frac{T_{min}}{T_{max}})^{k/N_{\text{iter}-1}}.$$

▶ **affectation step:** Update the affectation function f_{a^k} associated to the a^{k-1} codebook. Assign each individual z_i to the referent as defined in equation (2).

▶ **representation step:** Determine the new codebook a^{k*} that minimizes the $E(f_{a^k}, a)$ function (with respect to a), and a_c^{k*} is defined from equation (3).

Repeat **Iteration** until $T = T_{min}$.

4 Experiments

In all our experiments the representation space L_c of a neuron c is one individual, i.e., $q = 1$.

4.1 Simulated Data

The data are distributed in $\mathbb{R}^3$ and represent a geometric form of a cylinder. There are 1000 individuals. The input data is a Euclidean distance matrix and the map contains (20×3) neurons. In the following figures we present the training data and the evolution of the map during the training with the proposed algorithm. Figure 2 is the initial random map. In the final map, shown in figure 5, there is good quantification while preserving the topology.

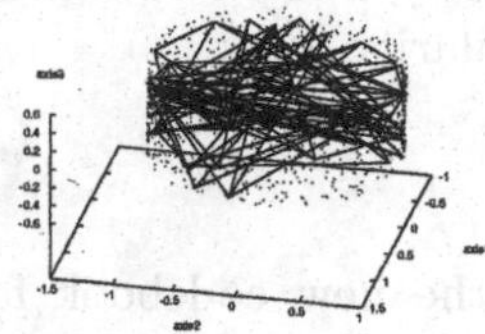

Fig. 2. The initial map neurons (random initialization) and the data.

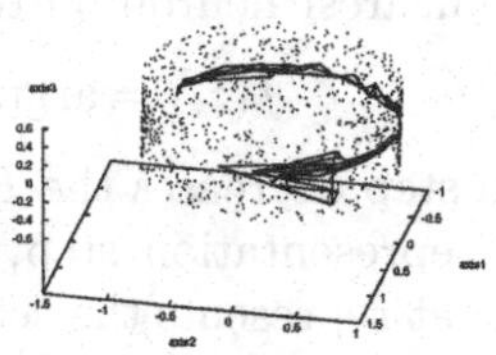

Fig. 3. The map after 50 iterations.

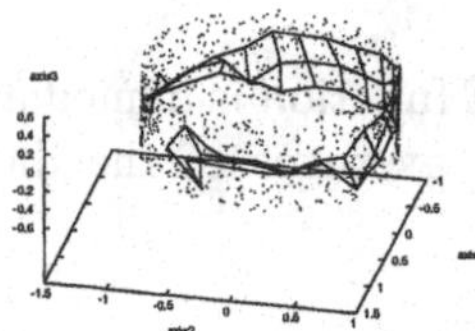

Fig. 4. The map after 100 iterations.

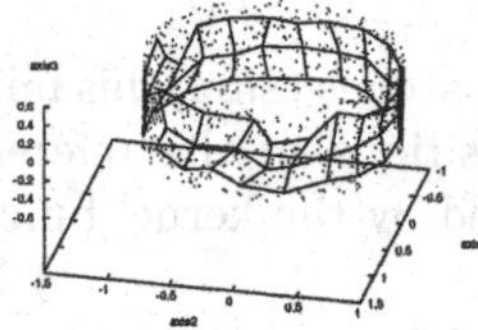

Fig. 5. The final map.

4.2 Real-World Data

The next example is a classification problem of spectrometric data from the food industry. Each observation is the near-infrared absorbance spectrum of a meat sample (finely choped), recorded on a Tecator Infratec Food and Feed Analyser. More precisely, an observation consists of a 100-channel spectrum of absorbances in the wavelength range 850-1050 nm (figure 6). There are 215 spectra in the database. In order to validate the behaviour of the proposed algorithm, we make use of another variable, which measures the fat content of each meat sample (the range of this variable is from 2% to 59%). This variable is deeply linked to the shape of the spectrum, and so the obtained classification should be consistent with the fat value. In the following experiments, all the maps contain 8×2 neurons.

In this experiment, we use the L^2-norm as a dissimilarity between spectra: $\| f \|^2 = \int (f(t))^2 \, dt$. The exact calculation of the integral is approximated by numerical integration (the trapezoidal rule). In Fig. 7, we show the result obtained by the proposed algorithm. Each square (which is associated to one class) is drawn with an intensity which is calculated with respect to the mean of the fat content of spectra belonging to the class (black for low fat value, white for high fat value).

Although the obtained classification seems to respect quite well the fat variable (low fat values on the left, and high fat values on the right), the result is not totally satisfactory; there is a class with high fat value located between two classes with lower fat value. As we can see in the next experiment, this is mainly due to a choice of an maladapted metric. Indeed, in the

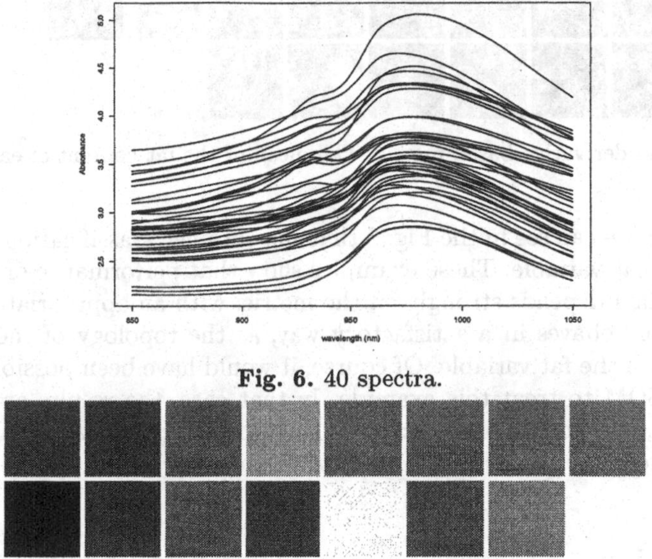

Fig. 6. 40 spectra.

Fig. 7. L^2-norm: the mean of the fat content of each class.

next experiment, we use as the dissimilarity a semi-metric based on the second derivative of the spectrum: $\| f \|_{d^2}^2 = \int (f^{(2)}(t))^2 \, dt$, where $f^{(2)}$ denotes the second derivative of f. Ferraty and Vieu (2002) point out that the second derivative of the spectrum is in general more informative than spectrum itself. In order to apply this functional approach, we differentiate each spectrum using a numerical formula (this estimation is consistent, as spectra are very smooth). Each derivative is therefore represented by a vector of 100 components as with the original data (Fig. 8). The integration is done according to the same procedure as the first experiment.

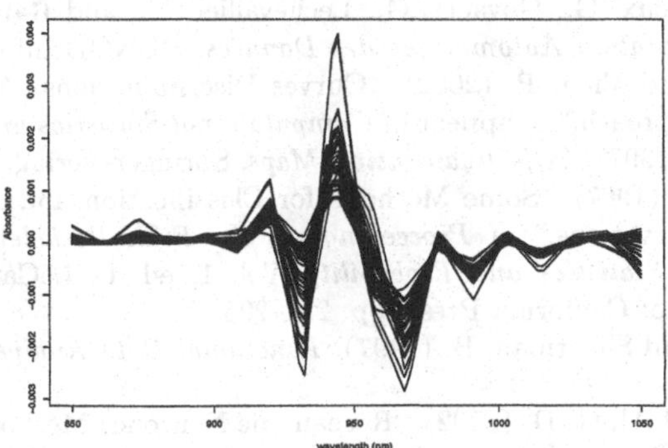

Fig. 8. Second derivatives of the 40 spectra.

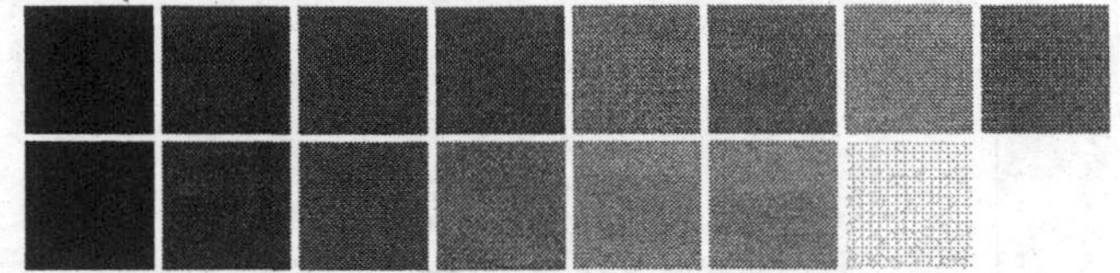

Fig. 9. Second derivative-based metric: The mean of the fat content of each class.

This time, we can see in the Fig. 9 that the obtained classification respects perfectly the fat variable. These examples show that performance of the proposed algorithm depends strongly on the metric: with an appropriate metric, the algorithm behaves in a satisfactory way, as the topology of the map is consistent with the fat variable. Of course, it would have been possible to use a standard SOM to treat this example. In that case, the results are in fact quite similar. Our goal in presenting this spectrometric application is to show both the validity of this approach, and its flexibility.

5 Conclusion

Compared to other clustering methods, self-organizing maps allow an easy visualisation of the obtained classification thanks to the preservation of the topology. The extension of SOMs to dissimilarity data is straightforward, and gives a very general tool which can be applied to various type of data without any adaptation. The results obtained on both simulated and real-world data are satisfactory.

References

1. de Reyniès, A. (2003). *Classification et Discrimination en Analyse de Données Symboliques*, Ph.D. thesis, Université Paris Dauphine.
2. Diday, E., Celeux, G., Govaert, G., Lechevallier, Y., and Ralambondrainy, H. (1989). *Classification Automatique des Données,* DUNOD Informatique, Paris.
3. Ferraty, F., and Vieu, P. (2002). "Curves Discriminations: A Nonparametric Functional Approach," to appear in *Computational Statistics and Data Analysis.*
4. Kohonen, T. (1997). *Self-Organisation Maps*, Springer-Verlag, New York.
5. MacQueen, J. (1967). "Some Methods for Classification and Analysis of Multivariate Observations," in *Proceedings of the Fifth Berkeley Symposium on Mathematical Statistics and Probability*, Vol. 1, ed. L. LeCam et al., Berkeley:University of California Press, pp. 281–296.
6. Ramsay, J., and Silverman, B. (1997). *Functional Data Analysis*, Springer Verlag, New York.
7. Thiria, S., and Al, G. D. (2002). "Réseaux de Neurones Méthodologie et Applications," Eyrolles, Paris.

Another Version of the Block EM Algorithm

Mohamed Nadif[1] and Gérard Govaert[2]

[1] Université de Metz, France
nadif@iut.univ-metz.fr
[2] Université de Technologie de Compiègne, France
gerard.govaert@utc.fr

Abstract: While most clustering procedures aim to construct an optimal partition of objects or, sometimes, of variables, there are other methods, called block clustering methods, which consider simultaneously the two sets and organize the data into homogeneous blocks. Recently, we have proposed a new mixture model called a *block mixture model* that addresses this situation. Our model allows one to embed simultaneous clustering of objects and variables through a mixture approach. We use maximum likelihood (ML) to implement the method, and have developed a new EM algorithm to estimate the parameters of this model. This requires an approximation of the likelihood and we propose an alternating-optimization algorithm, which is compared to another version of EM based on an interpretation given by Neal and Hinton. The comparison is performed through numerical experiments on simulated binary data.

1 Block Mixture Model and EM algorithm

Let $\mathbf{x}$ denote a $n \times r$ data matrix defined by $\mathbf{x} = \{(x_i^j); i \in I \text{ and } j \in J\}$, where I is a set of n objects (rows, observations, cases) and J is a set of r variables (columns, attributes). In contrast with standard clustering techniques such as hierarchical clustering, k-means, or self-organizing maps, block clustering (also called biclustering) provides a *simultaneous* clustering of the rows and columns of a data matrix. The basic idea of these methods consists in making permutations of objects and variables in order to draw a correspondence structure on $I \times J$.

Previous work by Hartigan (1975), Bock (1979) and Govaert (1983) has proposed algorithms dedicated to different kinds of matrices. But now, block clustering has emerged as an important challenge in data mining context. In the text mining field, Dhillon (2001) has proposed a spectral block clustering method that exploits the duality between rows (documents) and columns (words). In the analysis of microarray data where data are often presented as matrices of expression levels of genes under different conditions, block clustering of genes and conditions has permitted analysts to overcome the problem of the choice of similarity on both sets found in conventional clustering methods (Cheng and Church, 2000). Recently, we have proposed a *block mixture model* which takes into account the block clustering situation and allows one to embed it in a mixture approach (Govaert and Nadif, 2003a).

In the following, we represent a partition $\mathbf{z}$ of the sample I into g clusters either by the vector $(z_1, \ldots, z_n)$, where $z_i \in \{1, \ldots, g\}$ indicates the component of the observation i, or, when convenient, by the classification matrix $(z_{ik}, i = 1, \ldots, n, k = 1, \ldots, g)$ where $z_{ik} = 1$ if i belongs to cluster k and is 0 otherwise. We will use similar notation for a partition $\mathbf{w}$ of the set J into m clusters.

1.1 Definition of the Model

For the classical mixture model, we have shown (Govaert and Nadif, 2003a) that the probability density function of a mixture sample $\mathbf{x}$ defined by $f(\mathbf{x}; \boldsymbol{\theta}) = \prod_{i=1}^n \sum_{k=1}^g p_k \varphi(\mathbf{x}_i; \boldsymbol{\alpha}_k)$, where the p_k are the mixing proportions, the $\varphi(\mathbf{x}_i; \boldsymbol{\alpha}_k)$ are the densities of each component k, and $\boldsymbol{\theta}$ is defined by $(p_1, \ldots, p_g, \boldsymbol{\alpha}_1, \ldots, \boldsymbol{\alpha}_g)$, can be written as

$$f(\mathbf{x}; \boldsymbol{\theta}) = \sum_{\mathbf{z} \in \mathcal{Z}} p(\mathbf{z}; \boldsymbol{\theta}) f(\mathbf{x}|\mathbf{z}; \boldsymbol{\theta}), \tag{1}$$

where $\mathcal{Z}$ denotes the set of all possible partitions of I in g clusters, $p(\mathbf{z}; \boldsymbol{\theta}) = \prod_{i=1}^n p_{z_i}$ and $f(\mathbf{x}|\mathbf{z}; \boldsymbol{\theta}) = \prod_{i=1}^n \varphi(\mathbf{x}_i; \boldsymbol{\alpha}_{z_i})$. With this formulation, the data matrix $\mathbf{x}$ is assumed to be a sample of size one from a random $n \times r$ matrix.

To study the block clustering problem, we extend formulation (1) to a block mixture model defined by the probability density function $f(\mathbf{x}; \boldsymbol{\theta}) = \sum_{\mathbf{u} \in U} p(\mathbf{u}; \boldsymbol{\theta}) f(\mathbf{x}|\mathbf{u}; \boldsymbol{\theta})$ where U denotes the set of all possible partitions of $I \times J$ and $\boldsymbol{\theta}$ is the parameter of this mixture model. By restricting this model to a set of partitions of $I \times J$ defined by a product of partitions of I and J, which we assume are independent, we obtain the following decomposition:

$$f(\mathbf{x}; \boldsymbol{\theta}) = \sum_{(\mathbf{z}, \mathbf{w}) \in \mathcal{Z} \times \mathcal{W}} p(\mathbf{z}; \boldsymbol{\theta}) p(\mathbf{w}; \boldsymbol{\theta}) f(\mathbf{x}|\mathbf{z}, \mathbf{w}; \boldsymbol{\theta})$$

where $\mathcal{Z}$ and $\mathcal{W}$ denote the sets of all possible partitions $\mathbf{z}$ of I and $\mathbf{w}$ of J.

Now, extending the latent class principle of local independence to our block model, the x_i^j are assumed to be independent once $\mathbf{z}_i$ and $\mathbf{w}_j$ are fixed; then, we have $f(\mathbf{x}|\mathbf{z}, \mathbf{w}; \boldsymbol{\theta}) = \prod_{i=1}^n \prod_{j=1}^r \varphi(x_i^j; \boldsymbol{\alpha}_{z_i w_j})$ where $\varphi(x, \boldsymbol{\alpha}_{k\ell})$ is a probability density function defined on the set of real numbers $\mathbb{R}$. Denoting

$\boldsymbol{\theta} = (\mathbf{p}, \mathbf{q}, \boldsymbol{\alpha}_{11}, \ldots, \boldsymbol{\alpha}_{gm})$ where $\mathbf{p} = (p_1, \ldots, p_g)$ and $\mathbf{q} = (q_1, \ldots, q_m)$ are the vectors of probabilities p_k and q_ℓ that a row and a column belong to the kth component and to the ℓth component, respectively, we obtain a block mixture model with the following probability density function

$$f(\mathbf{x}; \boldsymbol{\theta}) = \sum_{(\mathbf{z},\mathbf{w}) \in \mathcal{Z} \times \mathcal{W}} \prod_{i=1}^{n} p_{z_i} \prod_{j=1}^{r} q_{w_j} \prod_{i=1}^{n} \prod_{j=1}^{r} \varphi(x_i^j; \boldsymbol{\alpha}_{z_i w_j}). \tag{2}$$

1.2 Block EM Algorithm

To estimate the parameters of the block mixture model, we propose to maximize the log-likelihood $L(\boldsymbol{\theta}; \mathbf{x}) = \log(f(\mathbf{x}; \boldsymbol{\theta}))$ by using the EM algorithm (Dempster, Laird and Rubin, 1977). To describe this algorithm, we define the complete log-likelihood, also called the classification log-likelihood, $L_C(\mathbf{z}, \mathbf{w}; \boldsymbol{\theta}) = L(\boldsymbol{\theta}; \mathbf{x}, \mathbf{z}, \mathbf{w}) = \log f(\mathbf{x}, \mathbf{z}, \mathbf{w}; \boldsymbol{\theta})$ which can be written

$$\begin{aligned} L_C(\mathbf{z}, \mathbf{w}; \boldsymbol{\theta}) = & \sum_{i=1}^{n} \sum_{k=1}^{g} z_{ik} \log p_k + \sum_{j=1}^{r} \sum_{\ell=1}^{m} w_{j\ell} \log q_\ell \\ & + \sum_{i=1}^{n} \sum_{j=1}^{r} \sum_{k=1}^{g} \sum_{\ell=1}^{m} z_{ik} w_{j\ell} \log \varphi(x_i^j; \boldsymbol{\alpha}_{k\ell}). \end{aligned}$$

The EM algorithm maximizes $L(\boldsymbol{\theta}; \mathbf{x})$ iteratively by maximizing the conditional expectation $Q(\boldsymbol{\theta}, \boldsymbol{\theta}^{(c)})$ of the complete log-likelihood given the previous estimate $\boldsymbol{\theta}^{(c)}$ and $\mathbf{x}$:

$$\begin{aligned} Q(\boldsymbol{\theta}, \boldsymbol{\theta}^{(c)}) = & \sum_{i=1}^{n} \sum_{k=1}^{g} P(z_{ik} = 1 | \mathbf{x}, \boldsymbol{\theta}^{(c)}) \log p_k + \sum_{j=1}^{r} \sum_{\ell=1}^{m} P(w_{j\ell} = 1 | \mathbf{x}, \boldsymbol{\theta}^{(c)}) \log q_\ell \\ & + \sum_{i=1}^{n} \sum_{j=1}^{r} \sum_{k=1}^{g} \sum_{\ell=1}^{m} P(z_{ik} w_{j\ell} = 1 | \mathbf{x}, \boldsymbol{\theta}^{(c)}) \log \varphi(x_i^j; \boldsymbol{\alpha}_{k\ell}). \end{aligned}$$

Unfortunately, difficulties arise due to the dependence structure in the model, specifically, in the determination of $P(z_{ik} w_{j\ell} = 1 | \mathbf{x}, \boldsymbol{\theta}^{(c)})$, and approximations are required to make the algorithm tractable.

A first approximation can be obtained by using the Classification ML approach with the block CEM algorithm (Govaert and Nadif, 2003a) which adds to the E-step a classification C-step. But this approach leads to biased parameter estimates.

An improved approximation can be obtained by using, as in the standard Markov field situation, a pseudo-likelihood. The term "pseudo-likelihood" was introduced (Besag, 1975) to refer to the product of conditional probabilities. Here, we approximate $P(z_{ik} w_{j\ell} = 1 | \mathbf{x}, \boldsymbol{\theta}^{(c)})$ by the product

$$P(z_{ik} = 1 | \mathbf{x}, \boldsymbol{\theta}^{(c)}) P(w_{j\ell} = 1 | \mathbf{x}, \boldsymbol{\theta}^{(c)})$$

and if we note

$$c_{ik}^{(c)} = P(z_{ik} = 1|\mathbf{x}, \boldsymbol{\theta}^{(c)}) \quad \text{and} \quad d_{j\ell}^{(c)} = P(w_{j\ell} = 1|\mathbf{x}, \boldsymbol{\theta}^{(c)}),$$

then the expectation $Q'(\boldsymbol{\theta}, \boldsymbol{\theta}^{(c)})$ takes the following form:

$$\sum_{i=1}^{n}\sum_{k=1}^{g} c_{ik}^{(c)} \log p_k + \sum_{j=1}^{r}\sum_{\ell=1}^{m} d_{j\ell}^{(c)} \log q_\ell + \sum_{i=1}^{n}\sum_{j=1}^{r}\sum_{k=1}^{g}\sum_{\ell=1}^{m} c_{ik}^{(c)} d_{j\ell}^{(c)} \log \varphi(x_i^j; \boldsymbol{\alpha}_{k\ell}).$$

The maximization of $Q'(\boldsymbol{\theta}, \boldsymbol{\theta}^{(c)})$ cannot be done explicitly. To solve this problem, we proposed (Govaert and Nadif, 2003b) to maximize alternately the conditional expectations of the complete-data log-likelihood $Q'(\boldsymbol{\theta}, \boldsymbol{\theta}^{(c)}|\mathbf{d})$ and $Q'(\boldsymbol{\theta}, \boldsymbol{\theta}^{(c)}|\mathbf{c})$ where $\mathbf{c}$ and $\mathbf{d}$ are the matrices defined by the c_{ik}'s and the $d_{j\ell}$'s. We have shown that these conditional expectations are associated, respectively, to the classical mixture models

$$\sum_{k=1}^{g} p_k \psi_k(\mathbf{u}_i; \boldsymbol{\theta}, \mathbf{d}) \quad \text{and} \quad \sum_{\ell=1}^{m} q_\ell \psi_\ell(\mathbf{v}^j; \boldsymbol{\theta}, \mathbf{c}) \tag{3}$$

where $\mathbf{u}_i = (u_i^1, \ldots, u_i^m)$ and $\mathbf{v}^j = (v_1^j, \ldots, v_g^j)$ are vectors of sufficient statistics and ψ_k and ψ_ℓ are the probability density functions of the sufficient statistics. Performing these separate maximizations using the EM algorithm gives a modified algorithm, called EM(1):

1. Start from $\mathbf{c}^{(0)}$, $\mathbf{d}^{(0)}$ and $\boldsymbol{\theta}^{(0)}$.
2. Compute $(\mathbf{c}^{(c+1)}, \mathbf{d}^{(c+1)}, \boldsymbol{\theta}^{(c+1)})$ starting from $(\mathbf{c}^{(c)}, \mathbf{d}^{(c)}, \boldsymbol{\theta}^{(c)})$:
   a) Compute $\mathbf{c}^{(c+1)}, \mathbf{p}^{(c+1)}, \alpha^{(c+\frac{1}{2})}$ by using the EM algorithm on the data $(\mathbf{u}_1, \ldots, \mathbf{u}_n)$, starting from $\mathbf{c}^{(c)}, \mathbf{p}^{(c)}, \alpha^{(c)}$.
   b) Compute $\mathbf{d}^{(c+1)}, \mathbf{q}^{(c+1)}, \alpha^{(c+1)}$ by using the EM algorithm on the data $(\mathbf{v}^1, \ldots, \mathbf{v}^r)$, starting from $\mathbf{d}^{(c)}, \mathbf{q}^{(c)}, \alpha^{(c+\frac{1}{2})}$.
3. Repeat Step 2 until convergence.

Note that the block CEM algorithm described in Govaert and Nadif (2003a) is a variant of EM(1). In each of steps 2(a) and 2(b), it is sufficient to add a C-step which converts the c_{ik}'s and $d_{j\ell}$'s to a discrete classification before performing the M-step by assigning each object and each variable to the cluster to which it has the highest posterior probability of belonging.

2 Another Version of the Block EM Algorithm

As pointed out by Hathaway (1986) in the classical mixture model context, the EM algorithm can be viewed as an alternating maximization of the following fuzzy clustering criterion:

$$F_C(\mathbf{c}; \boldsymbol{\theta}) = L_C(\mathbf{c}; \boldsymbol{\theta}) + H(\mathbf{c})$$

where $\mathbf{c}$ denotes a rectangular $n \times g$ data matrix which expresses a fuzzy partition, $L_C(\mathbf{c};\boldsymbol{\theta}) = \log f(\mathbf{x},\mathbf{c};\boldsymbol{\theta}) = \sum_{i=1}^{n}\sum_{k=1}^{g} c_{ik}\log(p_k\varphi(\mathbf{x}_i;\boldsymbol{\alpha}_k))$ is the fuzzy completed log-likelihood, and $H(\mathbf{c}) = -\sum_{i=1}^{n}\sum_{k=1}^{g} c_{ik}\log c_{ik}$ is the entropy function. Using the Neal and Hinton (1998) interpretation which extends the Hathaway approach to whatever model is used with the EM algorithm, one obtains that the maximization of the likelihood by EM is equivalent to an alternated maximization in $\mathbf{c},\mathbf{d}$ and $\boldsymbol{\theta}$ of the function

$$F_C(\mathbf{c},\mathbf{d};\boldsymbol{\theta}) = E(L_C(\mathbf{z},\mathbf{w};\boldsymbol{\theta})|\mathbf{c},\mathbf{d}) + H(\mathbf{c}) + H(\mathbf{d}).$$

Using the pseudo-likelihood approximation

$$P(z_{ik}w_{j\ell} = 1|\mathbf{c},\mathbf{d}) \approx P(z_{ik} = 1|\mathbf{c},\mathbf{d})P(w_{j\ell} = 1|\mathbf{c},\mathbf{d}) = c_{ik}d_{j\ell},$$

the expectation $E(L_C(\mathbf{z},\mathbf{w};\boldsymbol{\theta})|\mathbf{c},\mathbf{d})$ takes the form

$$\sum_{i=1}^{n}\sum_{k=1}^{g} c_{ik}\log p_k + \sum_{j=1}^{r}\sum_{\ell=1}^{m} d_{j\ell}\log q_\ell + \sum_{i=1}^{n}\sum_{j=1}^{r}\sum_{k=1}^{g}\sum_{\ell=1}^{m} c_{ik}d_{j\ell}\log\varphi(x_i^j;\boldsymbol{\alpha}_{k\ell})$$

which can be written

$$E(L_C(\mathbf{z},\mathbf{w};\boldsymbol{\theta})|\mathbf{c},\mathbf{d}) = L_C(\mathbf{c},\mathbf{d};\boldsymbol{\theta}).$$

Finally, to estimate the parameters of the model, we propose the fuzzy clustering criterion

$$F'_C(\mathbf{c},\mathbf{d};\boldsymbol{\theta}) = L_C(\mathbf{c},\mathbf{d};\boldsymbol{\theta}) + H(\mathbf{c}) + H(\mathbf{d}).$$

An iteration of the standard EM algorithm can therefore be expressed in terms of the function F'_C as follows:

- E-step: Set $\mathbf{c}^{(c+1)}$, $\mathbf{d}^{(c+1)}$ to the $\mathbf{c}$, $\mathbf{d}$ that maximize $F'_C(\mathbf{c},\mathbf{d};\boldsymbol{\theta}^{(c)})$.
- M-step: Set $\boldsymbol{\theta}^{(c+1)}$ to the $\boldsymbol{\theta}$ that maximizes $F'_C(\mathbf{c}^{(c+1)},\mathbf{d}^{(c+1)};\boldsymbol{\theta})$.

Note that the computation of $\mathbf{c}^{(c)}$ and $\mathbf{d}^{(c)}$ can be only done separately. Because of the following relations

$$\begin{cases} F'_C(\mathbf{c},\mathbf{d};\boldsymbol{\theta}) = F'_C(\mathbf{c};\boldsymbol{\theta}|\mathbf{d}) + g(\mathbf{d},\mathbf{q}) \\ F'_C(\mathbf{c},\mathbf{d};\boldsymbol{\theta}) = F'_C(\mathbf{d};\boldsymbol{\theta}|\mathbf{c}) + g(\mathbf{c},\mathbf{p}) \end{cases}$$

where $F'_C(\mathbf{c};\boldsymbol{\theta}|\mathbf{d}) = L_C(\mathbf{c};\boldsymbol{\theta}|\mathbf{d}) + H(\mathbf{c})$ and $F'_C(\mathbf{d};\boldsymbol{\theta}|\mathbf{c}) = L_C(\mathbf{d};\boldsymbol{\theta}|\mathbf{c}) + H(\mathbf{d})$ are two conditional fuzzy criteria associated, respectively, to the classical mixture models (3), we use the E-step on the intermediate mixture models. In contrast, in the M-step, the computation of $\boldsymbol{\theta}$ is direct and can be performed without any complication. This leads to a second algorithm, denoted EM(2), with the following steps:

1. Start from $\mathbf{c}^{(0)}$, $\mathbf{d}^{(0)}$ and $\boldsymbol{\theta}^{(0)}$, initial values of $\mathbf{c}$, $\mathbf{d}$ and $\boldsymbol{\theta}$.

2. Compute $(\mathbf{c}^{(c+1)}, \mathbf{d}^{(c+1)})$ starting from $\boldsymbol{\theta}^{(c)}$ by iterating steps (a) and (b) until convergence:
   a) Compute $\mathbf{c}^{(c+1)}$ by using the E-step on the data $(\mathbf{u}_1, \ldots, \mathbf{u}_n)$ starting from $\mathbf{d}^{(c)}, \mathbf{p}^{(c)}, \alpha^{(c)}$ to maximize $F'_C(\mathbf{c}; \boldsymbol{\theta}|\mathbf{d})$.
   b) Compute $\mathbf{d}^{(c+1)}$ by using the E-step on the data $(\mathbf{v}^1, \ldots, \mathbf{v}^r)$ starting from $\mathbf{c}^{(c)}, \mathbf{q}^{(c)}, \alpha^{(c)}$ to maximize $F'_C(\mathbf{d}; \boldsymbol{\theta}|\mathbf{c})$.
3. Compute $\boldsymbol{\theta}^{(c+1)} = (\mathbf{p}^{(c+1)}, \mathbf{q}^{(c+1)}, \alpha^{(c+1)})$.
4. Repeat the steps (2) and (3) until convergence.

In the ML approach of classical mixture models, after estimating the parameter $\boldsymbol{\theta}$ one can give a probabilistic clustering of the n objects in terms of their fitted posterior probabilities of component membership and thus obtain a partition by using a C-step that assigns each object to the mixture component for which it has the highest posterior of probability of belonging. Here, in the two versions of Block EM, this procedure is not direct: the calculus of posterior probabilities starting from the parameter is not tractable. A simple solution is to use the probabilities c_{ik} and $d_{j\ell}$ obtained at the end of the block EM algorithm.

3 Numerical Experiments

To illustrate the behavior of our algorithms and to compare them, we studied their performances for the Bernoulli block mixture model

$$f(\mathbf{x}; \boldsymbol{\theta}) = \sum_{(\mathbf{z},\mathbf{w}) \in \mathcal{Z} \times \mathcal{W}} \prod_{i=1}^{n} p_{\mathbf{z}_i} \prod_{j=1}^{r} q_{\mathbf{w}_j} \prod_{i=1}^{n} \prod_{j=1}^{r} \varphi(x_i^j; \alpha_{z_i w_j})$$

where $\alpha_{k\ell} \in (0,1)$ and $\varphi(x; \alpha_{k\ell}) = (\alpha_{k\ell})^x (1 - \alpha_{k\ell})^{1-x}$.

We selected nine kinds of data arising from 3×2-component mixture models corresponding to three degrees of overlap (well separated (+), moderately separated (++), or ill-separated (+++)) of the clusters and three sizes of the data matrix (small: 100×60, moderate: 200×120, and large: 300×150).

The degree of overlap can be measured by the true error rate corresponding to the block mixture model. Its computation being theoretically difficult, we used Monte Carlo simulations (500 samples) and evaluated the error rate by comparing the true partitions in the simulation to those estimated by applying a Classification step. But the Classification step is not as direct as in the classical mixture model and, in these simulations, we used a modified version of the block Classification EM algorithm in which the parameter $\boldsymbol{\theta}$ is fixed to the true value $\boldsymbol{\theta}^0$. The parameters were chosen to obtain error rates in $[0.01, 0.05]$ for the well-separated case, in $[0.12, 0.17]$ for the moderately-separated case, and in $[0.22, 0.27]$ for the ill-separated case. For each of these nine data structures, we generated 30 samples; for each sample, we ran the both EM(1) and EM(2) 20 times, starting from the same initial conditions, and found the estimates from each method. To summarize the behavior of these algorithms, we computed the likelihood, the error rates, and the total number of iterations for each simulation. Table 1 reports the mean and standard of these measures computed from the 30 samples.

Table 1. Comparison between EM(1) and EM(2): means and standard errors (in parentheses) of likelihood, error rates, and number of iterations for the two algorithms

size	degree of overlap	Likelihood		error rates		number of iterations	
		EM(1)	EM(2)	EM(1)	EM(2)	EM(1)	EM(2)
	+	-3838.7	-3838.8	0.05	0.05	108.93	164.93
		(29.45)	(29.45)	(0.03)	(0.03)	(47.34)	(96.97)
(100,60)	++	-3945.4	-3948.2	0.13	0.15	135.67	180.50
		(31.38)	(34.40)	(0.03)	(0.08)	(57.26)	(99.30)
	+++	-3999.8	-4001.2	0.32	0.34	490.87	557.40
		(24.93)	(25.05)	(0.13)	(0.12)	(244.86)	(846.18)
	+	-15556.3	-15556.3	0.01	0.02	36.53	60.10
		(64.40)	(64.39)	(0.01)	0.01	(5.94)	(18.42)
(200,120)	++	-16153.7	-16154.4	0.13	0.13	222.30	224.20
		(57.07)	(60.12)	(0.02)	(0.02)	(91.76)	(149.06)
	+++	-16202.0	-16205.0	0.30	0.33	648.70	439.37
		(40.42)	(40.45)	(0.08)	(0.11)	(305.54)	(456.60)
	+	-29676.3	-29679.3	0.04	0.04	49.00	90.90
		(111.17)	(111.73)	(0.01)	(0.01)	(6.08)	(30.22)
(300,150)	++	-30324.3	-30334.1	0.15	0.20	340.47	262.67
		(68.34)	(78.54)	(0.02)	(0.11)	(105.82)	(133.52)
	+++	-30502.5	-30508.9	0.26	0.31	1082.90	374.67
		(64.14)	(66.71)	(0.10)	(0.14)	(552.76)	(213.29)

The main points of comparison that arise from these simulation experiments are the following:

- When the clusters are not ill-separated, then both versions give the same results and in terms of maximization of the likelihood, EM(1) is better. Moreover, we notice that the average number of iterations for EM(1) is smaller than for EM(2).
- When the clusters are ill-separated, we recommend EM(1) because it outperforms EM(2) even though the average number of iterations is larger.

Thus on grounds of computation and accuracy, EM(1) is preferred.

4 Conclusion

Considering the problem of parameter estimation under the maximum likelihood approach, we have followed the Neal and Hinton strategy and have proposed new versions of the block EM algorithm to fit the block mixture model. Our methods are based on the EM algorithm, applied alternately to data matrices with reduced sizes. Even if both versions do not maximize the likelihood, as in the classical mixture model situation, but instead provide only an approximation of the likelihood for the block mixture model, these methods give encouraging results on simulated binary data. The first version, EM(1), appears to be clearly better than EM(2).

References

1. Besag, J. (1975). "Statistical Analysis of Lattice Systems," *The Statistician*, **24**, 179–195.
2. Bock, H.-H. (1979). "Simultaneous Clustering of Objects and Variables," in *Analyse des Données et Informatique*, ed. E. Diday, Rocquencourt:INRIA, pp. 187–203.
3. Cheng, Y. and Church, G. (2000). "Biclustering of Expression Data," *Proceedings of ISMB*, 93–103.
4. Dempster, A. P., Laird, N. M., and Rubin, D. B. (1977). "Maximum Likelihood from Incomplete Data Via the EM Algorithm (with discussion)," *Journal of the Royal Statistical Society, Series B*, **39**, 1–38.
5. Dhillon, I. S. (2001). "Co-Clustering Documents and Words Using Bipartite Spectral Graph Partitioning," *Proceedings of the Seventh ACM SIGKDD Conference*, 269–274.
6. Govaert, G. (1983). *Classification Croisée.* Thèse d'État, Université Paris 6, France.
7. Govaert, G. and Nadif, M. (2003a). "Clustering with Block Mixture Models," *Pattern Recognition*, **36**, 463–473.
8. Govaert, G. and Nadif, M. (2003b). "An EM Algorithm for the Block Mixture Model," submitted.
9. Hartigan, J. A. (1975). *Clustering Algorithms.* Wiley, New York.
10. Hathaway, R. (1986). "Another Interpretation of the EM Algorithm for Mixture Distributions," *Statistics & Probability Letters*, **4**, 53–56.
11. Neal, R. M. and Hinton, G. E. (1998). "A View of the EM Algorithm That Justifies Incremental, Sparse, and Other Variants," in *Learning in Graphical Models*, ed. M. I. Jordan, Dordrecht: Kluwer Academic Publishers, pp. 355–368.

Controlling the Level of Separation of Components in Monte Carlo Studies of Latent Class Models

José G. Dias

Instituto Superior de Ciências do Trabalho e da Empresa, Portugal
jose.dias@iscte.pt

Abstract: The paper proposes a new method to control the level of separation of components using a single parameter. An illustration for the latent class model (mixture of conditionally independent multinomial distributions) is provided. Further extensions to other finite mixture models are discussed.

1 Introduction

The level of separation of components of finite mixture models has been extensively studied, because it has strong implications on the model selection and estimation. For example, it influences the ability of information criteria to identify the correct model that has generated the data (see, e.g., Nadif and Govaert, 1998), the speed of convergence of the EM algorithm (Dempster et al., 1977; McLachlan and Krishnan, 1997), the precision of asymptotic standard errors of parameter estimates (Wedel, 2001), and the quality of the classification of observations into clusters.

Despite the importance of controlling the level of separation of components in Monte Carlo studies, the approach has been based on ad hoc procedures. For example, Wedel and DeSarbo (1995) generate randomly parameters of the first component, and obtained other components by adding successively 0.2 and 0.4 in low and high level of separation respectively. Nadif and Govaert (1998) proceeds in a similar way, defining three levels of separation (well-separated, moderately separated, and ill-separated mixture components), but parameters defining the first component are fixed as well. These procedures set parameters at specific points of the parameter space, keeping a fixed distance between them (constraint on the parameter space) and, consequently, do not truly represent the level of separation of components in Monte Carlo studies. Indeed, there are sets of parameters with different distances between parameters characterizing the components but still with the same level of separation. Another difficulty concerns the definition of the (fixed) distance to use. Moreover, for some distributions (e.g., Bernoulli and multinomial models) the parameter space is a subset of $\Re^d$, where simulated values can fall outside of the parameter space.

The paper proposes a new method that controls the level of separation of components using a single parameter. It is applied to the latent class model (mixture of conditionally independent multinomial/Bernoulli distributions). Results from a Monte Carlo study are discussed, and extensions to other finite mixture models proposed. The level of separation of components depends on other factors such as the sample size (n), the number of variables (J), and the number of categories (L_j) as well. Because those factors can be directly controlled in Monte Carlo studies, the method proposed here for the latent class model is based exclusively on the separation of the parameters which characterize each component, as it has been done by others.

The paper is organized as follows: Section 2 presents the latent class model using the finite mixture framework; Section 3 introduces the proposed method for controlling the level of separation of components in Monte Carlo studies of latent class models; Section 4 presents Monte Carlo simulations that show the performance of the method; and Section 5 discusses implications and further extensions.

2 The Latent Class Model

Let Y_1, Y_2,...,Y_J represent J observed variables; and y_{ij} indicates the observed value for variable j in observation i, with $i = 1, ..., n$, $j = 1, ..., J$. The finite mixture framework assumes the existence of a discrete latent variable with S categories that indicates the unobserved class or cluster that generated each observation. Let Z_i index the class or component that generated observation i, with $Z_i \in 1, ..., S$. Then the finite mixture model with S components for the observation $\mathbf{y}_i = (y_{i1}, ..., y_{iJ})$ is defined by $f(\mathbf{y}_i; \varphi) = \sum_{s=1}^{S} P(Z_i = s) f(\mathbf{y}_i | Z_i = s)$. Writing the *a priori* probability of belonging to component s as $\pi_s = P(Z_i = s)$, and $f_s(\mathbf{y}_i; \theta_s) = f(\mathbf{y}_i | Z_i = s)$, one gets

$$f(\mathbf{y}_i; \varphi) = \sum_{s=1}^{S} \pi_s f_s(\mathbf{y}_i; \theta_s),$$

where $\varphi = (\pi_1, ..., \pi_{S-1}, \theta_1, ..., \theta_S)$, with $\pi_s > 0$ and $\sum_{s=1}^{S} \pi_s = 1$.

The latent class model (LCM) assumes that manifest variables are discrete (Clogg, 1995). For nominal data, Y_j has L_j categories, and $y_{ij} \in \{1, ..., L_j\}$. From the local independence assumption—the J manifest variables are independent given the latent variable—one has $f_s(\mathbf{y}_i; \theta_s) = \prod_{j=1}^{J} f_s(y_{ij}; \theta_{sj})$. The category l can be associated with a binary variable defined by the indicator function $I(y_{ij} = l) = 1$, and 0 otherwise. Assuming the multinomial distribution for y_{ij}, it follows that

$$f_s(\mathbf{y}_i;\theta_s) = \prod_{j=1}^{J}\prod_{l=1}^{L_j} \theta_{sjl}^{I(y_{ij}=l)},$$

where $\theta_{sjl} = P(Y_{ij} = l \mid Z_i = s)$ is the probability that observation i belonging to component s has category l in variable j. Note that $\sum_{l=1}^{L_j} \theta_{sjl} = 1$. Thus, the LCM is a finite mixture of conditionally independent multinomial distributions, given by

$$f(\mathbf{y}_i;\varphi) = \sum_{s=1}^{S} \pi_s \prod_{j=1}^{J}\prod_{l=1}^{L_j} \theta_{sjl}^{I(y_{ij}=l)}.$$

The LCM presents problems of identifiability. A necessary condition for identifiability derives from the maximum number of estimable parameters, which is limited by the number of unique patterns minus 1, i.e., $\prod_{j=1}^{J} L_j > S\left[\sum_{j=1}^{J}(L_j - 1) + 1\right]$. For a discussion of the identifiability of the latent class model, see, e.g., Goodman (1974). Maximum likelihood estimates of the parameters of the LCM and its asymptotic standard errors are straightforward to obtain using the EM algorithm (c.f. Everitt and Hand, 1981; de Menezes, 1999).

3 The Proposed Method

Instead of defining a finite set of values for θ or generating randomly the first component and obtaining the others by adding a constant value, we generate θ using the following sampling procedure for the latent class model:

1. Draw θ_{1j} from the Dirichlet distribution with parameters $(\phi_1, ..., \phi_{L_j})$;
2. Draw θ_{sj} from the Dirichlet distribution with parameters $(\delta\theta_{1j1}, ..., \delta\theta_{1jL_j})$, $s = 2, ..., S$.

The Dirichlet distribution is confined to the interval $[0, 1]$. For the vector $\omega = (\omega_1, \omega_2, ..., \omega_k)$ with parameters $(\xi_1, ..., \xi_k)$, the Dirichlet distribution has density function

$$p(\omega_1, \omega_2, ..., \omega_k) = \frac{\Gamma(\xi_0)}{\prod_{j=1}^{k}\Gamma(\xi_j)} \prod_{j=1}^{k} \omega_j^{\xi_j - 1},$$

where $\Gamma(\cdot)$ is the gamma function and $\xi_0 = \sum_{j=1}^{k} \xi_j$. The expected value and variance of ω_j are $E(\omega_j) = \xi_j/\xi_0$ and $V(\omega_j) = [\xi_j(\xi_0 - \xi_j)]/[\xi_0^2(\xi_0 + 1)]$, respectively.

We set $(\phi_1, ..., \phi_{L_j}) = (1, ...1)$, which corresponds to the uniform distribution for θ_{1j} over [0, 1]. For $s = 2, ..., S$, we have

$$E(\theta_{sjl}) = \theta_{1jl}$$
$$V(\theta_{sjl}) = \frac{\theta_{1jl}\,(1-\theta_{1jl})}{\delta+1}.$$

On average all components are centered at the same parameter value generated from a uniform distribution (the first component). The parameter δ enables us to control the separation of the components. As δ increases, the variance decreases, and consequently the level of separation of components decreases too. As $\delta \to \infty$, all components tend to share the same parameters.

This procedure assumes that parameters θ of the LCM are sampled from a superpopulation defined by the hyperparameters δ and $(\phi_1, ..., \phi_{L_j}), j = 1, ..., J$, and thus defines a hierarchical (Bayesian) structure.

4 Monte Carlo Study

In this Monte Carlo study, the sample size ($n = 200, 2000$), number of components ($S = 2, 3$) and level of separation of components based on θ ($\delta = 0.01$, 0.1, 1, 10, 100, 1000) are controlled, which corresponds to a 6×2^2 factorial design. Fixed factors are set as: equal component sizes ($\pi_s = 1/S$), and 6 binary variables ($J = 6$; $L_j = 2$). We performed 1000 replications within each cell.

The level of separation of components is assessed using an entropy-based measure (see, e.g., Wedel and Kamakura, 2000) defined as

$$E_S = 1 + \frac{\sum_{i=1}^{n}\sum_{s=1}^{S} p_{is}\log p_{is}}{n\log S},$$

where the posterior probability that observation i was generated by component s is

$$p_{is} = \frac{\pi_s f_s(\mathbf{y}_i;\theta_s)}{\sum_{h=1}^{S}\pi_h f_h(\mathbf{y}_i;\theta_h)}.$$

Here E_S is a relative measure of entropy defined in $[0, 1]$. Values close to 1 (or 0) indicate that the estimated posterior probabilities are close to 0 (or 1, hence almost identical) for each component and consequently components are (or are not) well separated.

As a consequence of the randomness of the process (only the expected values and variances are ensured determined), it happens that a small number of outlier samples occurs, and thus those samples may not express the level of separation desired. An option is to apply a robust procedure that classifies a sample from δ as an outlier sample whenever its relative entropy is below $\max\left\{0, Q_2^\delta - 2.5 \times (Q_2^\delta - Q_1^\delta)\right\}$ or above $\min\left\{1, Q_2^\delta + 2.5 \times (Q_3^\delta - Q_2^\delta)\right\}$, where Q_i^δ is the ith quartile of E_S based on pre-samples (say of size 50) generated from δ. Note that the factor 2.5 defines very flexible whiskers for this

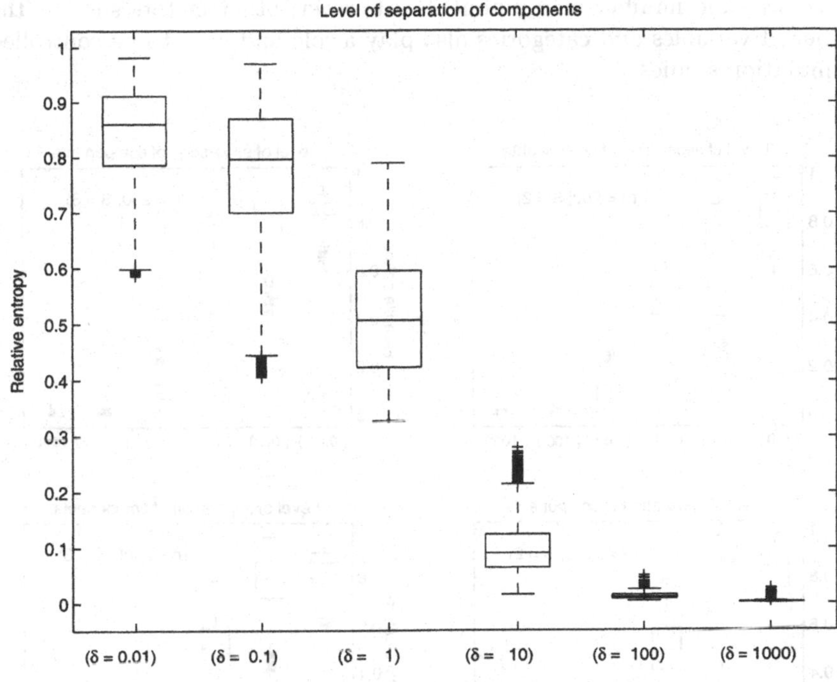

Fig. 1. Aggregate results

procedure. When this is used, extreme samples are excluded, and the sampling procedure is repeated.

Results from our simulation study are summarized in Table 1 and Figure 1. We observe that $\delta = 0.01$ presents results close to $\delta = 0.1$. For $\delta = 100$ and $\delta = 1000$, there is very small heterogeneity between components, and this is not too far from $\delta = 10$ (Figure 1). For this setting, three levels of δ (0.1, 1, 10) cover the different levels of separation of components. The overall percentage of outliers is 8.93%. The percentage is particularly high for $\delta = 1$, which may slow down the sampling procedure.

Table 1. Summary results (relative entropy).

	$\delta = 0.01$	$\delta = 0.1$	$\delta = 1$	$\delta = 10$	$\delta = 100$	$\delta = 1000$
1st quartile	0.787	0.700	0.423	0.064	0.008	0.001
Median	0.861	0.797	0.507	0.091	0.011	0.001
3rd quartile	0.913	0.870	0.595	0.125	0.015	0.002
Outliers (%)	12.08	6.85	20.47	3.07	7.22	3.90

Figure 2 shows results for the factorial design. We observe that δ controls the level of separation of components, and is generally robust to changes in sample size and number of components. However, other factors such as the number of variables and categories also play a role and have to be controlled in simulation studies.

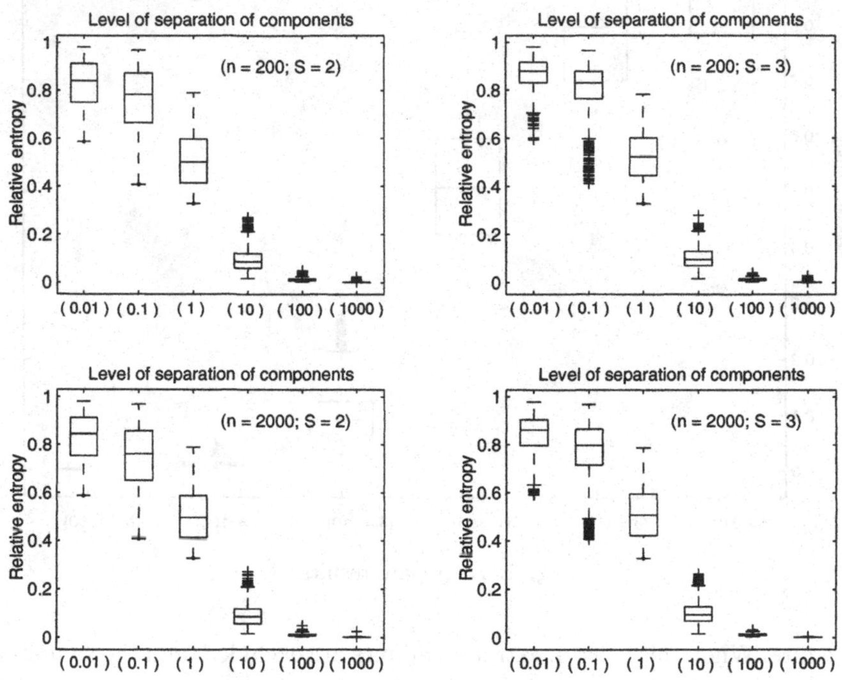

Fig. 2. Design-based results.

5 Discussion and Conclusions

This study shows how the level of separation of components can be successfully controlled for purposes of Monte Carlo studies using a simple method and avoiding ad hoc procedures such as fixing the value of parameters. We conclude that three levels of δ—low ($\delta = 0.1$), medium ($\delta = 1$), and high ($\delta = 10$)—give good coverage of the level of separation of components in the LCM setting. For simulation studies with two levels of separation of components, our results suggest that the use of $\delta = 0.1$ and $\delta = 10$ are appropriate for low and high levels of separation respectively. Further Monte Carlo simulations are needed to evaluate the performance of this method in the context of the LCM, controlling other factors such as size of components and the number of variables.

Extensions of this research concern the definition of level of separation of components for other finite mixture models such as Gaussian mixture models or mixture of linear models. The same idea—that the proposal distribution ensures that each component has the same expected value of parameters of the first component, but the variance is function of an additional parameter—can be applied, with a different distribution, to generate the parameters. For example, for the finite mixture of Poisson distributions defined by $f(y_i;\varphi) = \sum_{s=1}^{S}\pi_s\mathcal{P}(y_i;\lambda_s)$ the level of separation of the parameter components (based on $\lambda = (\lambda_1, ..., \lambda_S)$) is controlled by simulating the parameter λ_s, $s = 2, ..., S$ from $p(\lambda_s;\lambda_1,\delta) = \mathcal{G}(\delta, \delta/\lambda_1)$, $\delta > 0$, where $\mathcal{G}(\cdot,\cdot)$ is the gamma distribution. Then, the expected value and variance are $E(\lambda_s) = \lambda_1$ and $V(\lambda_s) = (\lambda_1)^2/\delta$, respectively, for $s = 2, ..., S$. As before, as δ increases, variance decreases, and consequently the separation of components decreases too. As $\delta \to \infty$, all components tend to share the same parameter (λ_1).

Whenever Monte Carlo studies concern parameter recovery, summary statistics of Monte Carlo studies have to take into account that the proposed method adds parameter variation to the sample variation The same applies for first component random parameters as in Wedel and DeSarbo (1995)). However, in applications such as comparing the performance of model selection criteria, the technique is straightforward and gives better coverage of the parameter space by sampling from different populations from the same superpopulation.

Acknowledgements

The author is also affiliated with the Faculty of Economics and the Population Research Centre, University of Groningen, The Netherlands. This research was supported by Fundação para a Ciência e Tecnologia Grant no. SFRH/BD/890/2000 (Portugal). The author is thankful to Jeroen Vermunt for his helpful comments on early drafts of the manuscript.

References

1. Clogg, C. C. (1995). "Latent Class Models," in *Handbook of Statistical Modeling for the Social and Behavioral Sciences*, eds. G. Arminger, C. C. Clogg, and M. E. Sobel, New York:Plenum Press, pp. 311–359.
2. de Menezes, L. M. (1999). "On Fitting Latent Class Models for Binary Data: The Estimation of Standard Errors," *British Journal of Mathematical and Statistical Psychology*, 49–168.
3. Dempster A. P., Laird, N. M., Rubin, D. B. (1977). "Maximum Likelihood From Incomplete Data Via the EM Algorithm (with Discussion)," *Journal of the Royal Statistical Society B*, **39**, 1–38.
4. Everitt, B. S. and Hand, D. J. (1981). *Finite Mixture Distributions*, Chapman & Hall, London.

5. Goodman, L. A. (1974). "Exploratory Latent Structure Analysis Using Both Identifiable and Unidentifiable Models," *Biometrika*, **61**, 215–231.
6. McLachlan, G. J. and Krishnan, T. (1997). *The EM Algorithm and Extensions*, John Wiley & Sons, New York.
7. Nadif, M. and Govaert, G. (1998). "Clustering for Binary Data and Mixture Models - Choice of the Model," *Applied Stochastic Models and Data Analysis*, **13**, 269–278.
8. Wedel, M. (2001). "Computing the Standards Errors of Mixture Model Parameters with EM when Classes are Well Separated," *Computational Statistics*, **16**, 539–558.
9. Wedel, M., and Kamakura, W. A. (2000). *Market Segmentation. Conceptual and Methodological Foundations*, 2nd ed., Kluwer Academic Publishers, Boston.
10. Wedel, M., and DeSarbo, W.S. (1995). "A Mixture Likelihood Approach for Generalized Linear Models," *Journal of Classification*, **12**, 21–55.

Fixing Parameters in the Constrained Hierarchical Classification Method: Application to Digital Image Segmentation

Kaddour Bachar[1] and Israël-César Lerman[2]

[1] Ecole Supérieure des Sciences Commerciales d'Angers, France
k.bachar@essca.asso.fr
[2] IRISA-Université de Rennes 1, France
lerman@irisa.fr

Abstract: We analyse the parameter influence of the likelihood of the maximal link criteria family (LLA hierarchical classification method) in the context of the CAHCVR algorithm (Classification Ascendante Hiérarchique sous Contrainte de contiguïté et par agrégation des Voisins Réciproques). The results are compared to those obtained with the inertia criterion (Ward) in the context of digital image segmentation. New strategies concerning multiple aggregation in the class formation and contiguity notion are positively evaluated in terms of algorithmic complexity.

1 Introduction

One of the most important objectives in data classification concerns the treatment of very large data sets. These can be provided by many fields. One of them is image processing. We are interested here in the problem of image segmentation. The proposed approach is derived from hierarchical classification methodology under a given contiguity constraint.

The data set is defined by all the pixels of a fixed image. The contiguity definition for a given pixel is obtained from a notion of spatial neighbouring in the image. This notion extends in a natural way to pixel classes. On the other hand, we accept as given, a description of the data units (the pixels here) by numerical variables. Thus the luminance variable is considered for grey level images. Indeed hierarchical classification enables you to obtain different "natural" segmentations by cutting the classification tree at suitable levels.

In order to solve the hierarchical classification problem an efficient and specific algorithm, called CAHCVR, has been set up. CAHCVR (Classification Ascendante Hiérarchique sous Contrainte de contiguïté et par aggrégation des Voisins Réciproques) is an ascendant hierarchical classification algorithm which works under a contiguity constraint by successive agglomeration the reciprocal neighbouring class couples relative to a dissimilarity measure between classes (Friedman, Baskett, and Shustek, 1975; Bachar, 1994; Bachar, 1998; Lerman, 2001; and Bachar, 2003). Two types of dissimilarity indices have been implemented and compared. The former is the classical Ward criterion (Ward, 1963) corresponding to the moment of inertia, which we denote by D. The second is defined by the family of criteria associated with the likelihood of the maximal probabilistic link included in the Likelihood Linkage Analysis (LLA) hierarchical classification method (Lerman (1991), Nicolaü (1996)). This family or an instance of it is denoted below by LL. Based upon experimental results from digital images, a new parameter has been introduced for this family. This concerns a threshold for the minimal value retained of the probabilistic index between data units. Precisely, one of the main purposes of this work consists of fixing a parameterization scale for the LLA method in order to obtain the "best" image segmentation according to expert "eyes."

Relative to the inversion phenomenon about the obtained indexed tree the respective behaviours of the two criteria (D and LL) are essentially different. Inversion can occur with the inertia criterion, but is impossible by nature with LL (see Section 5). We study and compare two alternatives for the CAHCVR algorithm; binary and multiple. The binary version consists of joining classes class couple by class couple. Whereas for the multiple version several classes can be related at the same time. In the latter case the minimal value of the class dissimilarities occurs more that once. These two algorithmic versions are presented in Section 2. In Section 3 we present an adequate adaptation of the likelihood of the maximal link criteria family in case of a planary contiguity constraint on the image pixels. The scale of relevant values for the LL parameters, as experimentally proved, are mentioned in Section 4. The inversion definition with respect to the criterion type is given in Section 5. Furthermore, two notions of planary contiguity constraint are defined in this section. Their respective effects are considered in Section 6 which is devoted to the comparison between different experimental results. Section 7 draws general conclusions.

2 Binary and Multiple Aggregation with CAHCVR

The first phase of the binary CAHCVR algorithm consists of determining all the adjacent couples of points, according to a given connected contiguity graph G_0, such that each element of a given couple is the closest to the other one in terms of a dissimilarity notion. Ward's inertia criterion has already been employed (Bachar, 1998). These couples are called adjacent reciprocal neighbours (RN).

The second phase aggregates all the RN adjacent couples one-by-one in order to form new classes. Both phases are performed alternately until all the elements have been grouped into a unique class. The update of the contiguity condition is performed only at the end of the two previous phases. The vertices of the new graph consist of new vertices associated with new classes and those associated with elements not incorporated into the new classes. The edges of the new graph are defined by extension: if x and y are two adjacent vertices in the preceding graph, the x-class is adjacent to the y-class. This update conserves the connectivity nature of the graph; the connectivity ensures, in particular, the convergence of the algorithm. In other words, it will always be possible to gather all the elements into one class.

2.1 The Multiple CAHCVR Clgorithm

The multiple CAHCVR algorithm is a faster variant of the previous algorithm. Indeed, our experimental results show that for every step of the binary CAHCVR algorithm several pairs of reciprocal neighbouring classes achieve the smallest dissimilarity "at the same time" (Lerman (1989)). The binary procedure chooses only one pair of classes. The non-uniqueness of the class formation for a given stage implies that the final classification tree is not unique: in the context of image segmentation we are frequently led to propose several different segmentations of a same image.

In the multiple CAHCVR algorithm one merges, in one step, all reciprocal neighbouring adjacent classes and obtains the same minimal dissimilarity. One takes advantage of the previous algorithmic organization by considering a binary construction of the classification tree. One obtains, as a consequence, a unique result (the result by binary aggregation is not always unique) and more especially one accelerates the speed of the process. In our different experiments we also systematically opted for the principle of multiple aggregation.

3 The Likelihood of the Maximal Link Criterion: Contiguity Graphs

The Likelihood of the Maximal Link criterion (LL criterion) of similarity between classes refers to a probability scale. This scale can be directly associated with a dissimilarity measure between classes in the form of a quantity of information. Following a very general construction, such a criterion can be applied to clustering both the set of variables and the set of described objects (Lerman, 1991). Relative to a variable j ($1 \leq j \leq p$) and to a pair of contiguous objects $\{i, i'\}$ (i.e., $(i, i') \in G_0$), and in agreement with the expert's perception, one defines the raw contribution $s^j(i, i')$ of the variable j to the comparison of the objects i and i'. For any given j, one calculates the average $moy(s^j)$ and the variance $v(s^j)$ of $s^j(i, i')$ on G_0. The normalized contribution of the variable j with the comparison of the two objects i and i' is defined by $S^j(i, i') = (s^j(i, i') - moy(s^j))/\sqrt{v(s^j)}$. The sum of the normalized contributions is then:

$$S(i,i') = \sum_{j=1}^{p} S^j(i,i'). \tag{1}$$

This measurement is again normalized on G_0, to obtain $Q_s(i,i')$. The probabilistic measurement is then $P(i,i') = \phi(Q_s(i,i'))$ where ϕ denotes the Gaussian cumulative distribution function. For the probabilistic measurements $\{P(i,i')|(i,i') \in G_0\}$ one can substitute measurements information dissimilarity:

$$\{\delta(i,i') = -log_2(P(i,i')|(i,i') \in G_0)\}. \tag{2}$$

If $\alpha(A,B)$ represents the number of edges joining the two classes A and B , the new dissimilarity measure between two classes A and B is given by:

$$\Delta_\epsilon(A,B) = \alpha^\epsilon(A,B) \times \min\{\delta(x,y)|(x,y) \in A \times B, (x,y) \in G_0\}. \tag{3}$$

As a special case, if G_0 is complete then $\alpha(A,B) = card(A) \times card(B)$; in this case, one recovers the more classical measurement of the likelihood of the maximal link criterion (Lerman, 1991).

4 The Parameters ϵ and π

The ϵ is a positive real parameter between 0 and 1. Two values of ϵ can be distinguished: $\epsilon = 1$ ("Pure" *LL*) and $\epsilon = 0.5$. In the case where G_0 is complete, the value $\epsilon = 0.5$ corresponds to the geometric average between $card(A)$ and $card(B)$. The most suitable values for our context (image segmentation) are located, according to the image, between 0.35 and 0.5.

Another parameter π also proved to be fundamental. This concerns the value of the probability index P from which one allows the possibility of merging two clusters. To obtain this, we choose to put, for all couples $(x,y) \in G_0$,

$$P(x,y) = \begin{cases} P(x,y) & \text{if } P(x,y) > \pi \\ \eta & \text{if } P(x,y) \leq \pi \end{cases}$$

where η is sufficiently small. In this way, and for classification purposes, we do not discriminate among the values of probabilistic indices less than π. In our experiments the value defined by $\pi = 0.45$ proved to be adequate.

5 Contiguity and Inversion

In a planary image, two pixels are adjacent in the sense of called "cont1" if and only if there is not an intermediate pixel. Therefore, in the sense of "cont1," a pixel (the summit of a related contiguity graph of which one edge translates the contiguity between 2 pixels) has a maximum of 8 pixels adjacent to it.

In a sense called "cont2," two pixels are adjacent if the Hamming distance (in the planary image) is equal to 1 as well. Thus, in the sense of "cont2," a pixel has a maximum of 4 pixels that are adjacent to it (if it is very close the boundary image it has 3 adjacent pixels; and if it is situated at the corner of the image it has 2 adjacent pixels). The transmissibility of "cont2" is ensured by transitivity—see Fig. 1.

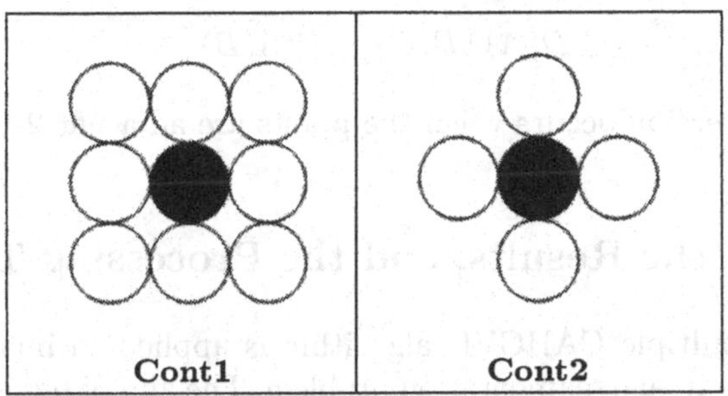

Fig. 1. The two notions of contiguity.

The LL measurement of dissimilarity Δ_ϵ between two classes A and B depends on the number of edges joining the two classes. It does not depend on the masses of these two classes, in contrast to the inertia criterion D. This shows that the LL measurement does not produce any inversion (see Fig. 2).

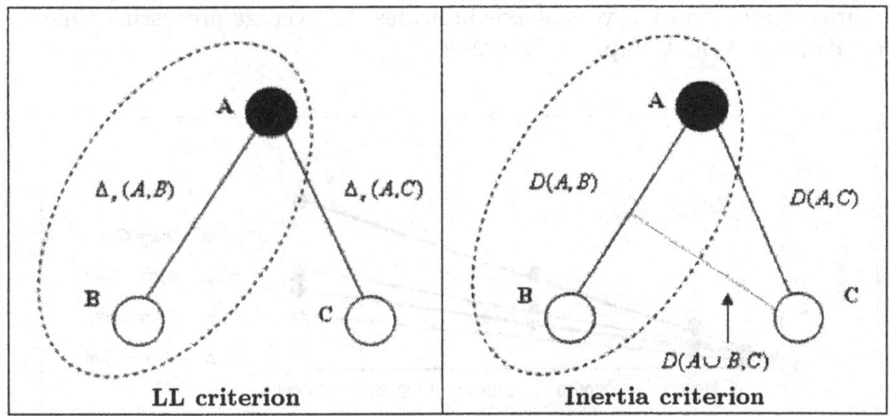

Fig. 2. An example of inversion.

Indeed, if we suppose that $\Delta_\epsilon(A,C) > \Delta_\epsilon(A,B)$ and B and C are not adjacent (in accordance with the classic configuration of a possible inversion of the type defined by Fig. 2), we always have:

$$\Delta_\epsilon(A \cup B, C) = \alpha^\epsilon(A \cup B, C) \times \min\{\delta(x,y) | (x,y) \in A \cup B \times C \cap G_0\}$$
$$\Delta_\epsilon(A \cup B, C) = \Delta_\epsilon(A, C) > \Delta_\epsilon(A, B).$$

But, using the classic inertia criterion (which considers the masses of A, B, and C), we can obtain:

$$D(A \cup B, C) < D(A, B).$$

Note that no inversion occurs when the points are adjacent 2-by-2.

6 The Data, the Results, and the Processing Time

The proposed multiple CAHCVR algorithm is applied to image analysis in order to solve the image segmentation problem. The aim of segmentation of an image is the identification of boundaries between the objects that constitute the image. The contiguity notion is then natural here: the pixels are on a plane. The segmentation of an image is a partition of the pixel set which can be obtained after classification under the contiguity constraint. The segmentation criteria employ, through the dissimilarity indices, the variables describing the image pixels.

Figure 3 shows the acceleration of the CAHCVR algorithm when we choose the contiguity constraint "cont2" and the strategy of multiple aggregation (the LL criterion). The horizontal axis indicates the number of pixels of the pictures treated and the verical axis indicates the average processing time in seconds (on a NEC Computer-1200Mhz).

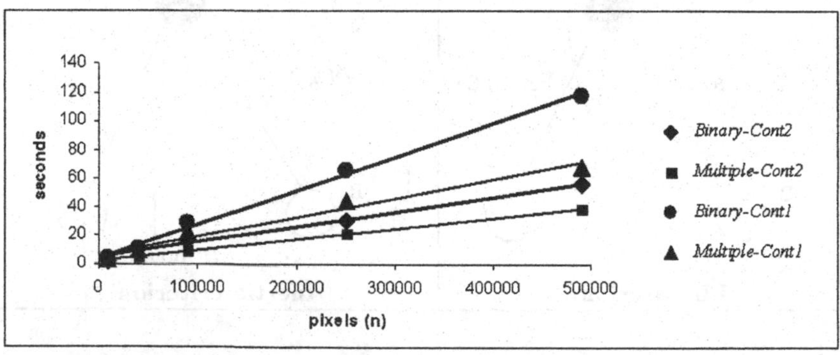

Fig. 3. Average processing time (seconds) as a function of image size.

Two satellite pictures (gratefully obtained from the IGN) have been treated. The first is called "sat3," has n=758×419 pixels, and is shown in Fig. 4. The second is called "sat2," has n=459×686 pixels, and is shown in Fig. 12.

The unique attribute kept for the segmentation is the luminance variable of the pixel (grey-level).

CAHCVR with Δ_ϵ or D can be used for any number of attributes on blocks of pixels. The results obtained with both criteria are comparable. The criterion type (I, inertia, or LL, Likelihood of the Link) and the class number are indicated in brackets for the different figures associated with the different segmentations. Different parameters for the LL criterion are considered in these figures. The best results are achieved with $\epsilon = 0.5$ and the contiguity constraint "cont2." Following these last parameters, several values of π are tried: $\pi = 0.4$ (Figs. 7, 10, 14), $\pi = 0.45$ (Fig. 6), and $\pi = 0.5$ (Fig. 8).

We note some visual differences. In the picture sat3 (Fig. 5) (according to the choice of a segmentation into 32 classes), zones 1 and 3 are better defined by Δ_ϵ (Fig. 8) than by D (Fig. 9); in contrast, zones 2 and 4 are more clearly identified by D. Larger numbers of classes (700 classes here) accentuate the spread more with D (Fig. 11) than with Δ_ϵ (Fig. 10).

In the image sat2 (Fig. 13), zones 3, 4 and 5 are well identified with D (Fig. 15); zones 3 and 4 are in the same class (Fig. 14). On the other hand one has a better definition of zone 1 with Δ_ϵ (Fig. 14).

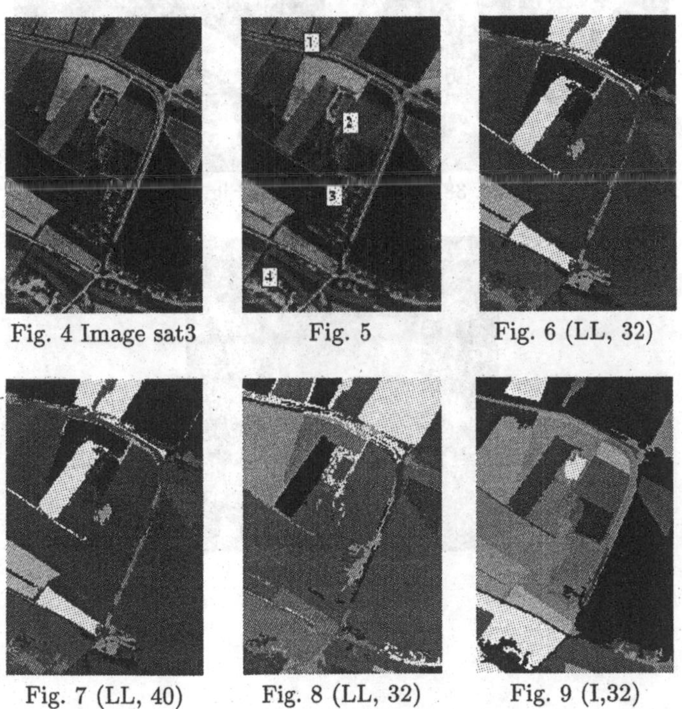

Fig. 4 Image sat3 Fig. 5 Fig. 6 (LL, 32)

Fig. 7 (LL, 40) Fig. 8 (LL, 32) Fig. 9 (I,32)

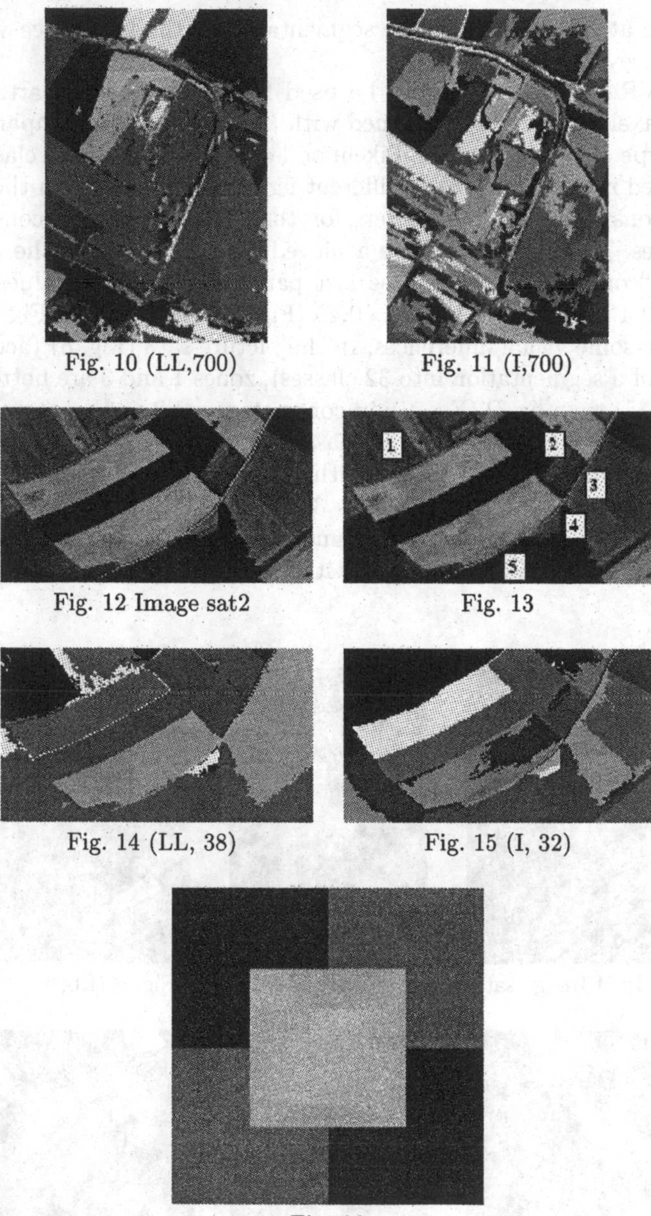

Fig. 10 (LL,700)

Fig. 11 (I,700)

Fig. 12 Image sat2

Fig. 13

Fig. 14 (LL, 38)

Fig. 15 (I, 32)

Fig. 16

7 Conclusion

Our methodology is very general and does not depend on the image segmentation field. It can be applied every time a contiguity constraint has to be satisfied in the merged clusters.

In this work experimental results have shown that the complexity processing time of binary version of CAHCVR is a linear function with respect to the image size. This confirms the theoretical aspects previously considered (Bachar, 1998). The multiple aggregation and the contiguity constraint "cont2" give the best processing times. Relative to binary aggregation, multiple aggregation gives approximately a 50% gain in processing time. On the other hand, the contiguity constraint "cont2" enables a 70% savings of computing time in relation to "cont1." A theoretical justification of these improvements can be established; "cont2" also notably improves the result quality. This quality is clearly influenced by a minute fitting of ϵ and π values. An accurate comparison of the results obtained by Δ_ϵ and D in terms of quality is not an easy task. This is because we do not have an a priori clear knowledge concerning the tested images (theses images are "natural"). Such a priori knowledge could be given by a systematic labelling of all pixels. This is what we have endeavoured to do by simulating simple and structured images in which this a priori knowledge is present (see Fig. 16 for an example). All the distinct segments defined in this artificial image have been perfectly identified with the D criterion as well as by Δ_ϵ.

References

1. Bachar, K. (1994). "Contribution en Analyse Factorielle et en CAH sous Contraintes de Contiguïté.," Ph.D Thesis, University of Rennes 1, France.
2. Bachar, K., and Lerman, I-C. (1998). "Statistical Conditions for a Linear Complexity for an Algorithm of Hierarchical Classification Under Constraint of Contiguity," in *Advances in Data Science and Classification*, eds. A. Rizzi, M. Vichi, and H.-H. Bock, Berlin:Springer, pp. 131–136.
3. Bachar, K., and Lerman, I-C. (2003). "Étude d'un Comportement Paramétré de CAHCVR sur des Données Réelles en Imagerie numérique," SFC'2003, Neuchâtel, Switzerland:Presses Académiques, pp. 63–66.
4. Friedman, J. H., Baskett, F., and Shustek, L. J. (1975). "An Algorithm for Finding Nearest Neighbours," *IEEE Transactions on Computers*, **C-24**, 1000–1006.
5. Lerman, I-C. (1989). "Formules de Réactualisation en Cas d'Agrégations Multiples," *Operations Research*, **23**, 151–163.
6. Lerman, I-C. (1991). "Foundations of the Likelihood Linkage Analysis (LLA) Classification Method," *Applied Stochastic Models and Data Analysis*, **7**, 63–76.
7. Lerman, I-C., Bachar, K. (2001). "Agrégations Multiples et Contraintes de Contiguïté dans la CAH Utilisant les Voisins Réciproques et le Critère VL," in *Actes du VIII-ème Congrès de la Société Francophone de Classification*, Guadeloupe:SFC'2001, pp. 232–237.

8. Costa Nicolaü, F., and Bacelar-Nicolaü, H. (1996). "Some Trends in the Classification of Variables," in *Data Science, Classification and Related Methods*, eds. C. Hayashi, N. Ohsumi, K. Yajima, Y. Tanaka, H.-H. Bock, Y. Baba, Berlin:Springer, pp. 89–98.
9. Ward, J. H. (1963). "Hierarchical Grouping to Optimise an Objective Function," *Journal of the American Statistical Association*, **58**, 238–244.

New Approaches for Sum-of-Diameters Clustering

Sarnath Ramnath, Mynul H. Khan, and Zubair Shams

St. Cloud State University, U.S.A.
sarnath,mkhan@eeyore.stcloudstate.edu, zubairshams@yahoo.com

Abstract: It was shown recently that by employing ideas from incremental graph connectivity the asymptotic complexity of sum-of-diameters bipartitioning could be reduced. This article further exploits this idea to develop simpler algorithms and reports on an experimental comparison of all algorithms for this problem.

1 Introduction

A general question facing researchers in many areas of inquiry is how to organize observed data into meaningful structures, that is, to develop taxonomies. Clustering of data helps to solve this problem by partitioning large sets of data into clusters of smaller sets of similar data. Most often the differences between pairs of entities are considered to partition the entire data set (Hansen and Jaumard, 1987). The maximum dissimilarity between any two entities within one cluster is called the *diameter* of the cluster.The idea of using *diameter* as a measure of the goodness of the partition was suggested by Delattre and Hansen (1980). In cases, where homogeneity of the clusters is desirable, partitioning the entities in clusters such that the sum of the diameters of the clusters are minimized is much more effective.

The minimum sum of diameters clustering problem is described as follows (Ramnath, 2002):

Input: *A set of n items,* $i_1, i_2, ... i_n$ *and an integer k; associated with each pair* (i_i, i_j) *is a length* l_{ij}*, which represents the distance between* i_i *and* i_j*.*

Output: *A partitioning of the set into k subsets, such that the sum of the diameters of the subsets is minimized.*

The input can be represented as a weighted graph where each item is represented by a vertex and the distance between any two items is identified by the weight of the edge that connects the corresponding vertices. The output is partitioning of the vertex set into k clusters $C_0, C_1, ..., C_{k-1}$ with diameters $D_0, D_1, ..., D_{k-1}$ respectively, that minimizes the sum of all diameters (Ramnath, 2002).

Brucker showed that the problem of partitioning a set of entities into more than two clusters, such that the sum of the diameters is minimized, is NP-complete (Brucker, 1978). Doddi et al. gave the first approximation algorithms for general k-clustering that minimizes the sum of diameters (Doddi et al., 2000). For the rest of the paper we will concentrate our discussion on the case k=2. To minimize the sum of diameters, Hansen and Jaumard developed an $O(n^6)$ algorithm which they later improved to $O(n^3 logn)$ (Hansen and Jaumard, 1987). Recently, Ramnath (2002) proposed a new set of algorithms that use an incremental approach in solving this problem. One of his algorithms run in $O(n^3)$ and the other one run in $O(mn)$ time. Although these algorithms are asymptotically faster, they involve maintenance of non-trivial data structures which sometimes involve large hidden constants. It is therefore useful to obtain a practical implementation and compare running times to get a better picture.

In this paper, we examine some of the implementation issues surrounding all these algorithms. This has resulted in some simplifications of the algorithms (Section 3). In addition we have applied the incremental approach to develop a new clustering algorithm that is very efficient in practice (Section 4) and a generalized algorithm that minimizes any function of diameters in $O(n^4)$ time (Section 6).

2 Preliminaries

A set of n entities and the dissimilarity between a pair of entities can be represented by a weighted graph $G = (V, E)$ with n vertices and m edges. The ith vertex is denoted v_i and edge between v_i and v_j is represented by e_{ij}. The dissimilarity between the vertices v_i and v_j is represented by the length l_{ij}. We want to partition the set of vertices into two clusters C_0 and C_1 where the diameter of cluster C_0 is equal to some value d_0 and the diameter of cluster C_1 is equal to d_1 such that the sum of diameters, $d_0 + d_1$, is minimized. By definition of diameter, there is no pair of vertices in C_0 such that the edge between them has length greater than d_0 and there is no pair of vertices in C_1 for which the connecting edge has length greater than d_1. Without loss of generality it can be assumed that $d_0 \geq d_1$.

The algorithms that find the minimum sum of diameters follow the structure of the generic algorithm discussed below:

Generic Algorithm

1. For a graph-function pair (G, w), let w: $E \to R$ be a mapping that assigns a real-valued weight to each edge.
2. Identify all edge lengths that are possible candidates for d_0 and d_1.

3. For each candidate of d_0, identify the smallest d_1 value such that there exists a partitioning of the graph into two clusters with diameters d_0 and d_1.
4. Find the pair (d_0, d_1) for which the sum, (d_0+d_1) is minimum.
5. **end.**

All the algorithms identify the set of possible candidates for d_0 by growing a maximum spanning tree (Hansen and Jaumard, 1987). However, they use different approaches when it comes to search for the smallest d_1 for each d_0 in Step 3. We denote as d_{min}, the length of the edge that completed the first odd cycle in the maximum spanning tree. d_{min} can be found in $O(n^2)$ time using Kruskal's algorithm (Hansen and Jaumard, 1987). Let $d_m, d_{m-1}, ..., d_{min}, ..., d_1$ be the edges of G sorted in non-increasing order of edge lengths. The sequence $d_m ... d_{min}$ is denoted S_0 and the sequence $d_{min} ... d_1$ is denoted S_1.

For any (d_0, d_1) pair, the partition needs to satisfy the following three invariants, which can be captured as a 2CNF expression (Hansen and Jaumard, 1987).

1. If for some edge e_{ij}, $l_{ij} > d_0$, corresponding vertices v_i and v_j cannot be in the same cluster. Therefore, v_i and v_j are assigned the following boolean values: x_i=0, x_j=1 or x_i=1, x_j=0. This gives us 2 boolean constraints, viz., $(x_i \vee x_j)$ and $(x_i \vee x_j)$. Refer to $(x_i \vee x_j)$ as a *Type0* constraint and $(\neg x_i \vee \neg x_j)$ as a *Type1* constraint.
2. If for some edge e_{ij}, $d_0 \geq l_{ij} > d_1$, both v_i and v_j cannot be in cluster C_1. This implies either x_i=0 or x_j =0 i.e., we have only constraint $(\neg x_i \vee \neg x_j)$.
3. If for some edge e_{ij}, $d_1 \geq l_{ij}$, there is no constraint because there is no restriction on which cluster v_i or v_j would belong to.

The 2CNF expression can be represented by a directed graph that has vertices x_i and $\neg x_i$ corresponding to the assignment x_i=1 and x_i=0, respectively (Aspvall et al., 1979). Satisfiability of this is checked by looking for directed cycles containing x_i and $\neg x_i$ which can be done in $O(n)$ time if we have the transitive closure. The following lemma establishes how this can be done in $O(1)$ time if we use the incremental approach.

Lemma 1. *Consider a situation we have a satisfiable expression to which we add a constraint. Let it be that the addition of the constraint adds directed edges from x_i to $\neg x_j$ and x_j to $\neg x_i$. Then for any k, there exists a cycle containing x_k and $\neg x_k$ only if there exists a cycle containing x_i and $\neg x_i$ and there exists a cycle containing x_j and $\neg x_j$.*

Computing Step 3 of the Generic Algorithm: Hansen's algorithm runs in $O(mnlogn)$ time by n performing binary searches on S_1 (Hansen and Jaumard, 1987). Both of Ramnath's algorithms compute step 3 as follows: *To decide a 2-SAT instance, we construct a directed graph. In this digraph we have to look at $O(n)$ pairs of entries to check if any of these pairs falls in the same*

SCC (Strongly Connected Component). By maintaining a transitive closure or decompositions of the digraph into SCCs, this check can be performed with $O(n)$ queries, each requiring $O(1)$ time.

There are at most p instances of d_0, viz., $l_1, l_2, ..., l_p$ where $l_1 > l_2 > ... > l_p$. In the process of finding d_1 for each d_0, we can either start with $d_0 = l_1$ and then decrease d_0 all the way down to l_p, or we can start with $d_0 = l_p$ and increase to l_1. If we choose the former, we perform $O(n)$ inserts and $O(m)$ deletes; this is the approach that Ramnath uses for $O(n^3)$ algorithm. If we choose the latter, we maintain the decomposition of the constraint graph into SCCs in such a way that each deletable edge requires $O(m)$ operations and each non-deletable edge requires $O(n)$ operations.

The new algorithm also works incrementally but does not maintain either the transitive closure or the decompositions of the digraph into *SCCs*. Details of this are in Section 4.

3 Implementation Issues

Hansen and Jaumard's $O(n^3 logn)$ Algorithm: For each d_0 candidate in S_0, the algorithm carries out a binary search on the ordered set S_1 to find a d_1 value. For each (d_0, d_1) pair that is considered, we construct a 2-CNF expression consisting of *Type0* constraints of length greater than d_0 and *Type1* constraints for all edges of length greater than d_1. The check for satisfiability of the 2-CNF expression is done using the algorithm described in Aspvall et al. (1979).

Ramnath's $O(n^3)$ Algorithm: The algorithm (Ramnath, 2002) works by dynamically maintaining a transitive closure of the constraint graph. The existence of both x_i and $\neg x_i$ in the same *SCC* can be found in $O(1)$ time.

The algorithm works as follows:

1. Add edges for all *Type1* constraints into the graph.
2. While there are more edges in S_0.
   a) Add edges for the *Type0* constraints from S_0 into the graph in decreasing order of edge length until we get an unsatisfiable expression.
   b) Remove edges from S_1 in increasing order of edge length until the satisfiability is restored.
   c) Record (d_0, d_1) pair.

Since the order in which edges in S_1 are to be deleted is known, algorithm has a perfect lookahead for deletions. Ramnath's approach exploits this lookahead to obtain the dynamic connectivity of the data structure.

Some of the concepts are given below from Ramnath (2002) to assist our further discussion:

1. Deletion Time Stamp *(DTS)*: Associated with each edge is a *DTS* that gives the order in which the edge will be deleted, the edge with largest

DTS being the next to be deleted. Edges that will never be deleted have a $DTS = 0$.
2. Current Time Stamp *(CTS)*: When we delete an edge, the *CTS* is decremented. A *CTS* of i indicates that the graph has i deletable edges. When we add a deletable edge, *CTS* is incremented.
3. Connectivity Number *(CN)*: For each pair of vertices (u, v) we have a *CN* that gives us the measure of the number of deletes needed to eliminate all paths from u to v.

The following observations lead to simplifications of the implementation of this algorithm.

Step 1 can be simplified due to the structure of the constraint graph. The constraint graph initially remains empty. *Type1* constraints are added in step 1 to all the edges that are greater than d_{min}, in non-increasing order. Since all the edges that are added are non-deletable, their *DTS* must be zero. It follows that *CN* and *CTS* values must also be zero. Therefore, the following computations can be avoided:*For all pairs of vertices* (p, q) *such that* $CTS < CN(p) < \infty$, *set* $CN(p, 1) = \infty$ *(Ramnath, 2002)*. And, *For each pair of vertices* (x, y), $CN\ (x, y) = min(\ CN(x, y),\ max(CN(x, u),\ CN(v, y),\ t))$ *(Ramnath, 2002)*. Now, the edges that are created by adding *Type1* constraints to the edge lengths greater than d_{min}, are given *CN* values equal to their *DTS* values because at this point all the paths consist of only two vertices. Thus it avoids the operations associated with updating the *CN* values every time we add a new path. Also, since *DTS* and *CN* values are given incrementally, it avoids computing the following statement: *if* $CTS \geq t$ *(t* is the *DTS* of the most recent edge), *increment the DTS for each that has a current DTS value* $\geq t$. *For each pair of vertices* (p, q) *with* $CN \geq t$, *increment* $CN(p, q)$. As a result of these, we simplified the computation in step 1. Although for more general case Ramnath suggested in Ramnath (2002) that any insertion could be done in $O(n^2)$ time, in this case we see that *Type1* insertions in step 1 are done in $O(1)$ time.

In Hansen and Jaumard approach every $(x_i, \neg x_i)$ pair must be checked to ensure the satisfiability of the constraint graph. However, checking satisfiability can be simplified in the incremental/decremental approach by applying *lemma* as follows: If the recently added constraint corresponds to the edge e_{ij}, then check if there is a path from x_i to $\neg x_i$; if it exists, then check for a path from $\neg x_i$ to x_i.

Ramnath's $O(mn)$ Algorithm: Unlike the previous algorithm, this algorithm maintains a collection of all *SCC*s in the constraint graph. The algorithm shows better performance for sparse cluster graphs. The approach used to maintain the decomposition of the graph into *SCC*s adapts a basic technique from Cicerone et al. (1998).

Let $G(V, E)$ be a graph for which we are maintaining decomposition into *SCC*s. The following concepts from Ramnath (2002) are needed to simplify the presentation.

1. Priority of a vertex: A vertex $v_i \in V$ is assigned a priority i.
2. Whenever a deletable edge (v_i, v_j) is inserted into a graph, a dummy vertex a_{ij} (called an enode) is introduced. a_{ij} has the priority $DTS(e_{ij})+ \mid V \mid$.
3. With each *SCC*, we associate a positive integer, which is the highest priority of all the vertices in the *SCC*.

The algorithm thenworks as follows:

1. Insert the *Type1* and *Type0* constraints for all edges of length greater than d_{min} value. The *Type0* constraints must be inserted as deletable edges.
2. While there are more edges in S_1,
   a) Add edges for the *Type1* constraints for edges in S_1 in decreasing order of edge length until we get an unsatisfiable expression
   b) Remove *Type0* constraints from S_0 in increasing order of edge length until the satisfiability is restored.
   c) Record the (d_0, d_1) pair.

The operation for inserting a deletable edge and verifying the satisfiability of the constraint graph given in Ramnath (2002) can therefore be simplified to the following:

1. *DTS* is assigned to the deletable edges incrementally, that is, the last deletable edge will have the largest *DTS*. Therefore, the most recently created *enode* will have the largest priority among the enodes that are in the graph. Thus, the following steps suffice to deal with the insertion of a deletable edge, from node u to node v, with *DTS* t:
   a) Create an enode a, and add directed edges from u to a and from a to v.
   b) Do a forward *BFS* (Breadth First Search) and a backward *BFS* from a, and enumerate the items in a_{scs} by taking the intersection of the sets of nodes visited by the two traversals.
2. Checking the satisfiability of the constraint graph can be simplified using lemma as we did in the $O(n^3)$ algorithm.

4 A New Algorithm

First, add *Type1* constraints to all the edges. Then add *Type0* constraints for edges that have length greater than d_{min}, in non-increasing order. Once the graph reaches the unsatisfiable state, keep deleting *Type1* edges until it becomes satisfiable.

1. Following *lemma*, checking satisfiability is done by carrying out Depth-First traversals from end-vertices of *Type0* edges inserted into the constraint graph. If the last constraint inserted was $(x_i \vee x_j)$, then perform *DFS* searches from x_i and $\neg x_i$ to check for paths from x_i to $\neg x_i$ and $\neg x_i$ to x_i respectively.

2. If both the above paths exist, delete a sufficient number of *Type1* edges so that either (i). all paths from x_i to $\neg x_i$ are disconnected or (ii). all paths from $\neg x_i$ to x_i are disconnected.

The algorithm works as follows:

1. Add edges for all *Type1* constraints into the graph.
2. While there are more edges in S_0
   a) Add edges for the *Type0* constraints from S_0 into the graph in non-increasing order of edge length until the expression becomes unsatisfiable.
   b) Record (d_0, d_1) pair.
   c) While (expression is unsatisfiable) loop.
   Let $(x_i \vee x_j)$ be the last *Type0* constraint added. Perform a depth first traversal from x_i with the following variation with each edge, e, inserted in the stack, store the minimum length of all edges present in the stack at that point (including e).When $\neg x_i$ is reached, the weight l_1, item on top of the stack gives the lightest edge that must be deleted in order to disconnect the path. If $\neg x_i$ is reached, perform a similar *DFS* from $\neg x_i$, if x_i is reached, we get l_2, the lightest edge on the path from $\neg x_i$ to x_i. Let $l = \min(l_1, l_2)$. Delete *Type1* constraints for all edges of weight less than or equal to l.
   End while;

In a situation where edge lengths are randomly assigned, this algorithm is very efficient. The reason for this appear to be similar to why quicksort performs well on random permutations.

5 Performance

Big-oh worst case analysis for the earlier algorithms have been given in Ramnath (2002). For a complete graph, Hansen's algorithm runs in $O(n^3 logn)$ time, whereas Ramnath's algorithms run in $O(n^3)$ time. The new algorithm has a worst case time of $O(n^4)$.

These algorithms were implemented in C++. The programs were compiled using GNU g++ compiler on a Digital AlphaServer 1000A 4/266 running Digital UNIX v4.0D with 256 MB of RAM. In comparing the performance of four algorithms, processor time used by each algorithm is counted. The performance is compared by using randomly generated input graphs of different numbers of vertices. Although the new algorithm is tightly close to $O(mn)$ algorithm in performance, it shows consistent better performance over $O(n^3 logn)$ and $O(n^3)$ algorithms. For any large number of vertices it appears to be the most feasible algorithm because of its simplicity, less overhead and minimal time of execution.

Table 1. Processor time used by the algorithms (in secs).

No. of Nodes	$O(n^3)$	$O(mn)$	$O(n^3 logn)$	New Algorithm
10	0.13	0.02	1.76	0.02
20	2.25	0.16	16.94	0.11
30	13.03	0.71	59.99	0.38
40	30.78	1.81	124.57	1.15
50	86.27	-	-	2.80
60	161.29	-	-	5.73
70	294.55	-	-	7.63
80	402.83	-	-	13.55

6 Generalization and Conclusion

The paper compares the running times of four different algorithms for sum-of-diameters bipartitioning. One aspect we have not considered here is parallelizability. Hansen's algorithm has a straightforward parallelization: Find the d_1 for each d_0 in parallel. Ramnath's $O(mn)$ algorithm and the new algorithm both have highly sequential structure. The $O(n^3)$ algorithm, on the other hand, uses matrix operations, the parallelization of which is very well understood. Further study would be needed to answer these questions.

Using the incremental approach we have also designed an algorithm than minimizes any function of the diameters. Due to space constraints, we present the following theorem without proof.

Theorem 1. *Given a cluster graph, a bipartition that minimizes any non-monotone function of the diameters can be computed in* $O(n^4)$ *time.*

References

1. Aspvall, B., Plass, M. F., and Tarjan, R. E. (1979). "A Linear-Time Algorithm for Testing the Truth of Certain Quantified Boolean Formulas," *Information Processing Letters*, **8**, 121–123.
2. Brucker, P. (1978). "On the Complexity of Clustering Problems," *Optimization and Operations Research*, Lecture Notes in Economics and Mathematical Systems, pp. 45–54.
3. Cicerone, S., Frigioni, D., Nanni, U., and Pugliese, F. (1998). "A Uniform Approach to Semi-Dynamic Problems on Diagraphs," *Theoretical Computer Science*, **203**, 69–90.
4. Delattre, M. and Hansen, P. (1980). "Bicriterion Cluster Analysis," *IEEE Transactions on Pattern Analysis and Machine Intelligence*, **4**, 277–291.
5. Doddi, S. R., Marathe, M. V., Ravi, S. S., Taylor, D. S., and WidMayer, P. (2000). "Approximation Algorithms for Clustering to Minimize the Sum of Diameters," in *Proceedings of the 7th Scandinavian Workshop on Algorithm Theory*, Lecture Notes in Computer Science, Berlin:Springer, pp. 237-250.

6. Hansen, P., and Jaumard, B. (1987). "Minimum Sum of Diameters Clustering," *Journal of Classification*, **2**, 277–291.
7. Ramnath, S. (2002). "Dynamic Digraph Connectivity Hastens Minimum Sum-of-Diameters Clustering," in *Proceedings of the 9th Scandinavian Workshop on Algorithm Theory*, Lecture Notes in Computer Science, Berlin:Springer, pp. 220–229.

Spatial Pyramidal Clustering Based on a Tessellation

Edwin Diday

Université Paris IX Dauphine, France
diday@ceremade.dauphine.fr

Abstract: Indexed hierarchies and indexed clustering pyramids are based on an underlying order for which each cluster is connected. In this paper our aim is to extend standard pyramids and their underlying one-to-one correspondence with Robinsonian dissimilarities to spatial pyramids where each cluster is "compatible" with a spatial network given by a kind of tessellation called "m/k-network". We focus on convex spatial pyramids and we show that they are in one-to-one correspondence with a new kind of dissimilarities. We give a building algorithm for convex spatial pyramids illustrated by an example. We show that spatial pyramids can converge towards geometrical pyramids. We indicate finally that spatial pyramids can give better results than Kohonen mappings and can produce a geometrical representation of conceptual lattices.

1 Introduction

Indexed hierarchies and ultrametrics yield to a one-to-one correspondence shown by (Johnson, 1967) and (Benzecri, 1973). Diday (1984, 1986) has introduced indexed clustering pyramids (which contain, as a special case, indexed hierarchies). In the same paper he has shown a one-to-one correspondence between indexed clustering pyramids and Robinsonian dissimilarities which generalize the one-to-one correspondence between indexed hierarchies and ultrametrics. These new concepts have been studied by several authors, for example Bertrand (1986), Durand and Fichet (1988), and Bertrand and Janowitz (2002). In order to build a clustering pyramid, several algorithms have been proposed by Diday (1984, 1986), Bertrand (1986, 1995), Aude (1999) for the standard case of classical variables and by Brito and Diday (1989), Brito (1991), and Rodriguez (2000) for the symbolic data case. Indexed clustering pyramids defined on a finite set Ω are based on an order O defined by a sequence $w_1,\ldots,w_n$ of elements of Ω. This order defines a chain of a graph G(O), whose nodes are all the elements w_i of Ω and the edges are defined by the pairs of consecutive elements w_i, w_{i+1} of the sequence. A clustering pyramid is then defined by a family of sets called "clusters"' stable for intersection which contains Ω and the singleton and for which each cluster is "connected" for a given order O. We say that a subset of Ω is connected in the graph G(O) iff any pair of elements can be connected by a chain of ordered elements of this subset. The length of a chain correspond to the number of its edges. The dissimilarity between two elements of G(O) is the number of edges of the smallest chain relating these elements. A subset A of Ω is "convex" if any smallest chain of G(O) connecting a pair of elements of A is inside A. subset A of Ω is "maximal" when an element is in A iff its dissimilarity to all of its elements is lower than its diameter. In this case we say that the clusters are "compatible" with an order. It appears that connectivity, convexity and maximally are identical in the case of a graph reduced to a chain like G(O), but they are different in the case of a graph G(M) defined by the nodes and edges of a tessellation M. In this paper we introduce a kind of tessellation called "m/k-network" which is a case of tessellation. It is a grid when m = k = 4. Spatial pyramids are based on a graph defined by an m/k -network for which each cluster of the pyramid is "convex". The "compatibility" between an order O and a dissimilarity which is expressed by a Robinsonian matrix ordered by O, is generalized to the compatibility between a dissimilarity and a grid M expressed by a "Yadidean matrix" ordered by M. A Yadidean matrix is a Robinsonian matrix in the very special case where G(M) is reduced to a chain. We generalize Robinsonian dissimilarities by "Yadidean dissimilarities." We show that such dissimilarities d are diameter conservative, which means that a diameter for a convex of the grid corresponds to a diameter for d. We show that there is a one-to-one correspondence between "indexed pyramids" and Yadidean dissimilarities and between "strictly indexed pyramids" and "strictly Yadidean dissimilarities." We give a building algorithm for convex spatial pyramids illustrated by an example. We show that spatial pyramids can converge towards geometrical pyramids. Finally, we conclude by giving some links with other fields by saying how spatial pyramids can improve Kohonen mappings and conceptual lattice representation.

2 A Kind of Tessellation: m/k-Networks

An m/k-network is defined by a network where i) m arcs defining m equal angles meet at each node and ii) smallest cycles contain k arcs of equal length. It is a kind of tessellation since it is a tiling pattern that covers space without leaving any gaps. Notice that any tessellation is not necessarily an m/k-network as shown in Fig. 1a which is a tessellation but not an m/k-network (as the three angles at each node are not equal) and Fig. 1.b where three m/k-networks are shown.

Instead of representing the clustered units on a line as in standard hierarchical or pyramidal clustering (Diday, 1984)), it is then possible to represent

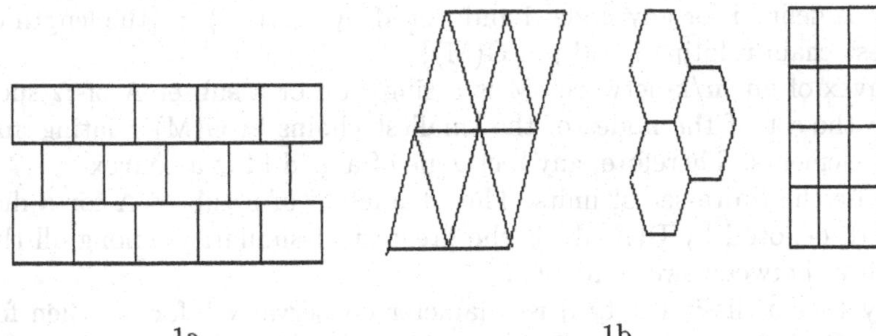

Fig. 1. (1a) Part of a tessellation and (1b) Part of a 6/3-network, 3/6-network and 4/4-network.

them on a surface or on a volume . It can be shown that on a surface there are only three possibilities for such a network: (m, k) = (6, 3), (m, k) = (4, 4), (m, k) = 3/6 which are shown in figure 2. If (m, k) = (4, 4), we get a usual grid of two dimensions where each smallest cycle is a square. If (m, k) = (12, 12) we get a grid of three dimensions where the smallest cycle are cubes. In order to simplify the presentation, most of the following results are expressed in the case (m, k) = (4, 4) (i.e. a grid).

3 Dissimilarity Induced by a Network and Convex, Maximal and Connected Subsets

We imbed Ω in an m/k-network M by associating to each element of Ω a node of M. In practice, this can be done in a "compact" way (i.e. without holes) which means that there are no nodes of M not associated with an element Ω surrounded by nodes associated with elements of Ω . In order to simplify, we denote by the same way the node of M associated with an element of Ω and this element. Hence, in the following, Ω is considered to be a set of nodes of an m/k -network M. More precisely in order to simplify, we consider that $|\Omega|$= np. This is always possible by taking the greatest n and p such that np$\leq |\Omega|$ and then, adding at the end, the remaining $|\Omega|$- np elements to their closest leave elements in the spatial pyramid obtained from the np chosen for building it for instance, by the algorithm given in Section 8.

A dissimilarity d defined on is a mapping: $\Omega \times \Omega \rightarrow [0, \infty)$ such that d(a, b) = d(b, a) $\geq$d(a, a) = 0 for all a, b$\in \Omega$. When d(a, b) = 0 implies a = b, d is called proper.

The length of a chain in an m/k-network will be considered to be the sum of the length of the edges which link two nodes of the chain. In the following, in order to simplify, all edges are considered to have the same length equal to 1. G(M) is the graph which has the same nodes and edges than M.

If we denote by M an m/k-network, the dissimilarity induced by M, denoted d_M, is defined for any nodes i and j of M by: d_M(i, j) = {the length of the smallest chain relating i and j in G(M)}.

A "convex of an m/k-network" M is a singleton or a subset A of Ω such that A be the set of the nodes of the smallest chains in G(M) relating any pair of its elements. Therefore, any rectangle of a grid M is a convex.

Let Ω be the finite set of units. The "diameter" of a subset A for a dissimilarity d, denoted by D(A, d), is the greatest dissimilarity among all the dissimilarities between two units of A.

We say that a dissimilarity d is "diameter conservative" for M when for any convex C of M we have: $D(C, d_M) = d_M(i, k) ==> D(C, d) = d(i, k)$. In that case we say that d is compatible with M.

4 Dissimilarity Matrix Induced by a Grid and Yadidean Matrices

A dissimilarity matrix induced by a grid (i.e. a 4/4-network) M for a dissimilarity d called a "d-grid matrix" is defined in the following way. Let M be a grid of n rows and p columns, $X_i = (x_{i1}, ..., x_{in})^T$ and $X_j = (x_{j1}, ..., x_{jn})^T$ be two row matrices associated with two parallel columns of M (see Fig. 2). We denote by $X_i X_j^T(d)$ the n×n matrix which contains in its generic term (i.e. in the entry of its kth row and mth column) the value $d(x_{ik}, x_{jm})$. The block matrix induced by M for a dissimilarity d (called also a "d-grid blocks matrix") is defined by a matrix $Z(d) = \{Z_{ij}(d)\}_{i,j\in\{1,...,p\}}$ where each term $Z_{ij}(d)$ is a block defined by the matrix $Z_{ij}(d) = X_i X_j^T(d)$. In other words, $Z(d) = \{X_i X_j^T(d)\}_{i,j\in\{1,...,p\}}$. Then, a "d-grid matrix" is a matrix $W(d)$ whose terms are the dissimilarities of the blocks $X_i X_j^T(d)$. More precisely, a d-grid matrix $W(d)$ is defined by:

$$W(d) = \{d(x_{ik}, x_{jm})\}_{i,j\in\{1,..,p\},k,m\in\{1,..,n\}}.$$

We recall that a Robinsonian matrix is symmetrical, its terms increase in row and column from the main diagonal and the terms of this diagonal are equal to 0.

A "Robinsonian by blocks matrix" is a d-grid block matrix $Z(d)$ such that:

1. It is symmetrical.
2. The matrices of its main diagonal $Z_{ii}(d) = X_i X_i^T(d)$ are Robinsonian.
3. The matrices $Z_{ij}(d) = X_i X_j^T(d)$ are symmetrical and increase in row and column from the main diagonal.

More precisely, these entries increase in j and decrease in i when $i < j$ (i.e., $X_{i+1}\, X_j^T(d) \leq X_i X_j^T(d), X_i X_j^T(d) \leq X_i X_{j+1}^T(d)$, in the upper part of $Z(d)$). It can be considered as a Robinsonian matrix "by blocks" as the

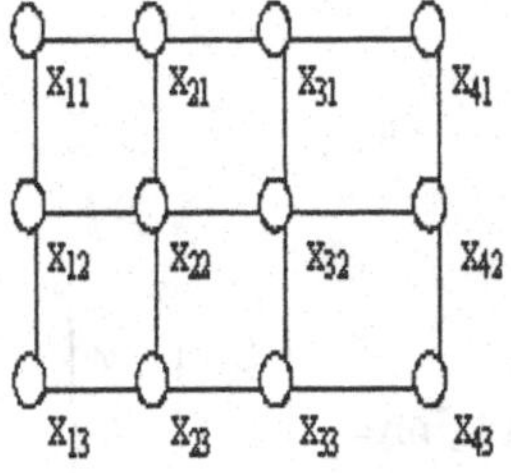

$X_1X_1^T(d)$	$X_1X_2^T(d)$	$X_1X_3^T(d)$	$X_1X_4^T(d)$
$X_2X_1^T(d)$	$X_2X_2^T(d)$	$X_2X_3^T(d)$	$X_2X_4^T(d)$
$X_3X_1^T(d)$	$X_3X_2^T(d)$	$X_3X_3^T(d)$	$X_3X_4^T(d)$
$X_4X_1^T(d)$	$X_4X_2^T(d)$	$X_4X_3^T(d)$	$X_4X_4^T(d)$

Fig. 2. The 9 nodes of a 3x4 grid and its "d-grid blocks matrix" Z(d) which is a "Robinson by blocks matrix" when the terms d(xik, xjm) i, j 1,..,p, k, m 1,..,n in the blocks Xi Xj T(d) i, j 1,..,p, constitute a Yadidean matrix

blocks $Z_{ij}(d) = X_iX_j^T(d)$ increase from the main diagonal of $Z(d)$defined by $\{Z_{ii}(d)\}_{i=1,n}$ as for a standard Robinsonian matrix.

We say that a d-grid matrix $Y(d) = \{d(x_{ik}, x_{jm})\}_{i,j\in\{1,\ldots,p\},k,m\in\{1,\ldots,n\}}$ induced by a grid M is Yadidean when the d-grid blocks matrix $Z(d) = \{X_iX_j^T(d)\}_{i,j\in\{1,\ldots,p\}}$ induced by M is Robinsonian by blocks. In Fig. 3, we show an example of such a matrix.

We say that a Yadidean matrix $Y(d)$ is strictly indexed when:

1. Two consecutive terms in a row or in a column of any matrix $X_iX_j^T(d)$ are never equal. In other words, for i and j fixed such that $i \le j$ we have not: $d(x_{ik}, x_{jm}) = d(x_{ik'}, x_{jm'})$ with $k = k' + 1$(or $k = k' - 1$) when $m = m'$ or $m = m' + 1$ (or $m = m' - 1$) when $k = k'$.
2. Two terms at the same position $d(x_{ik}, x_{jm})$, $d(x_{ik'}, x_{jm'})$ in two matrices $X_iX_j^T(d)$ and $X_{i'}X_{j'}^T(d)$ are never equal if the two matrices are consecutive in row or in column in the associated blocks matrix $Z(d)$. In other words, for m and k fixed, for i and j such that $i \le j$, we have not $d(x_{ik}, x_{jm}) = d(x_{ik'}, x_{jm'})$ with $i = i' + 1$ (or $i = i' - 1$) when $j = j'$ or $j = j' + 1$ (or $j = j' - 1$) when $i = i'$.
3. If the condition (1) or the condition (2) is not satisfied, this means that there is a convex C' strictly included in another convex C with same diameter. In that case we have the following third condition: C' is not the intersection of two (M, d)-maximals. In other words, if the diagonal of C' is (x_{ik}, x_{jm}) then in the Yadidean matrix the term $d(x_{ik}, x_{jm})$ it is not on the same row and column of two maximal (M, d)-convex (i.e. when i an j are fixed and k, m vary or when i and j vary and k, m are fixed).

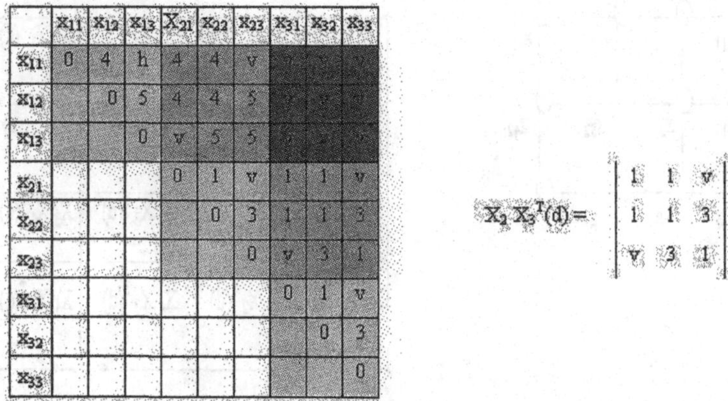

Fig. 3. The upper part of a Yadidean matrix Y(d) of a 3x3 grid when v 5 and the block matrix X2 X3T(d) of its associated Robinsonian by blocks matrix.

5 Some Properties of a Yadidean Matrix

A Yadidean matrix is not Robinsonian since its terms $\{d(x_{ik}, x_{jm})\}_{i,j}$ (for $j \in \{1, \ldots, p\}$, $k, m \in \{1, \ldots, n\}$ do not increase in the rows and columns from the main diagonal. Also, the maximal number of different terms in such a matrix is lower then in a Robinsonian matrix of the same size. For example, in a grid of n rows and p columns where there are np elements of Ω, there are $np(np-1)/2$ dissimilarities which can be different due to the symmetry of a dissimilarity or a Robinsonian matrix of $(np)^2$ elements. In a Yadidean matrix the $p(p-1)/2$ matrices $X_i X_j^T(d)$ are symmetrical which implies the equality of $(p(p-1)/2)(n(n-1)/2)$ dissimilarities. Hence, the number of possible different terms in such a Yadidean matrix is only $K(n,p) = np(np-1)/2 - (p(p-1)/2)(n(n-1)/2) = (np/4)(n+1)(p+1) - np$. A Yadidean matrix is a Robinsonian matrix in the case where $p = 1$, in this case $K(n, 1) = n(n-1)/2$ as expected. If $n = p$ the greatest number of different terms is $K(n,n) = n^2(n^2-1)/2 - [n(n-1)/2]^2 = n^2(n+3)(n-1)/4$.

Therefore, the maximal percentage of different values in a Yadidean matrix among all possible dissimilarities is $x = K(n,p)200/np(np-1) = 50 + 100(n+p-2)/2(np-1)$ in the general case and $x = 100K(n,n)(2/n^2(n^2-1)) = 50 + 100/(n+1)$ when $p = n$. Therefore, when n and p increases towards infinity, the number of different dissimilarities in a Yadidean matrix tends to be two times less then in a dissimilarity or a Robinson matrix, where all values are different in the upper part of these symmetrical matrices.

A "Yadidean dissimilarity" is a dissimilarity for which there exists a grid M such that its induced d-grid matrix $Y(d) = \{d(x_{ik}, x_{jm})\}_{i,j \in \{1,..,p\}, k,m \in \{1,..,n\}}$. is Yadidean. A "Strictly Yadidean dissimilarity" is a dissimilarity for which exists a grid such that its induced d-grid matrix is strictly Yadidean.

Proposition 1: A dissimilarity is compatible with a grid if and only if it is Yadidean.

Proof: First, let us show that if a dissimilarity is compatible with a grid, then it is Yadidean. Let d be a compatible dissimilarity with a grid M of n rows and p columns. We have to show, by definition of a Yadidean matrix $Y(d)$, that the d-grid blocks matrix $Z(d)$ induced by M satisfies the three conditions of a Robinson by blocks matrix. Figs. 2 and 4 can be used in order to follow more easily the proof.

i.) In order to show that $Y(d)$ is symmetrical, we have to prove (Fig. 4b), that for any $i, j \in \{1,,p\}$, we have $d(x_{ik}, x_{jm}) = d(x_{jk}, x_{im})$. This is the case as (x_{ik}, x_{jm}) and (x_{jk}, x_{im}) are the diagonals of the same convex C of the grid, defined by the nodes $(x_{ik}, x_{jm}, x_{im}, x_{jk})$. Therefore:

$D(C, d_M) = d_M(x_{ik}, x_{jm}) = d_M(x_{jk}, x_{im})$ which implies

$D(C, d) = d(x_{ik}, x_{jm}) = d(x_{jk}, x_{im})$ as d is compatible with the grid and so preserves the diameters.

ii.) The matrices $X_iX_i(d)$ are Robinsonian as they are symmetrical as d is symmetrical by definition, the terms of its main diagonal are equal to 0 as $d(x_{ik}, x_{ik}) = 0$. The other terms increase in row and column from the main diagonal as on a column X_i of the grid if $k < l < m$ and C is the connected set containing all the nodes x_{il} of this column of the grid which are between x_{ik} and x_{im}, we have $D(C, d_M) = d_M(x_{ik}, x_{im})$. So we have $D(C, d) = d(x_{ik}, x_{im})$ as d preserves the diameters. Therefore, $d(x_{ik}, x_{im}) \geq Max(d(x_{ik}, x_{il}), d(x_{il}, x_{im}))$, so $X_iX_i(d)$ increases in row (resp. in column) from the main diagonal as $d(x_{ik}, x_{im}) \geq d(x_{ik}, x_{il})$ (resp. $d(x_{ik}, x_{im}) \geq d(x_{il}, x_{lm})$) for any $i \in \{1,p\}$, $k, l, m \in \{1, n\}$ with $k < l < m$.

iii.) In order to prove that the matrices $X_iX_j^T(d)$ are symmetrical we have to prove that $X_iX_j^T(d) = X_jX_i^T(d)$. As the generic term of $X_iX_j^T(d)$ is $d(x_{ik}, x_{jm})$ for $k = 1, ..., n$; $m = 1, ..., n$ we have to prove that $d(x_{ik}, x_{jm})$ $= d(x_{im}, x_{jk})$. This has been already proved in i).

When i is smaller then j, we have now to show that the matrix $X_iX_j^T(d)$ increases in j. As its generic term is $d(x_{ik}, x_{jm})$, we have to show that:

$$d(x_{ik}, x_{j'm}) \leq d(x_{ik}, x_{jm}) \text{ if } j' < j.$$

This comes from the fact that the convex C of the grid defined by its diagonal x_{ik}, x_{jm} contains the convex C' of the grid defined by the diagonal $x_{ik}, x_{j'm}$, so

$$D(C', d_M) = d_M(x_{ik}, x_{j'm}) \leq D(C, d_M) = d_M(x_{ik}, x_{jm})$$

from which it follows that $D(C', d) = d(x_{ik}, x_{j'm}) \leq D(C, d_M) = d(x_{ik}, x_{jm})$ as d is diameter conservative. In the same way we can show that $X_iX_j^T(d)$ decreases in i.

Now we have to show that if a dissimilarity is Yadidean, then it is compatible with a grid. Let d be Yadidean for a grid G. If d was not compatible with G, a convex C would exist in the grid with diagonal x_{ik}, x_{jm} and another

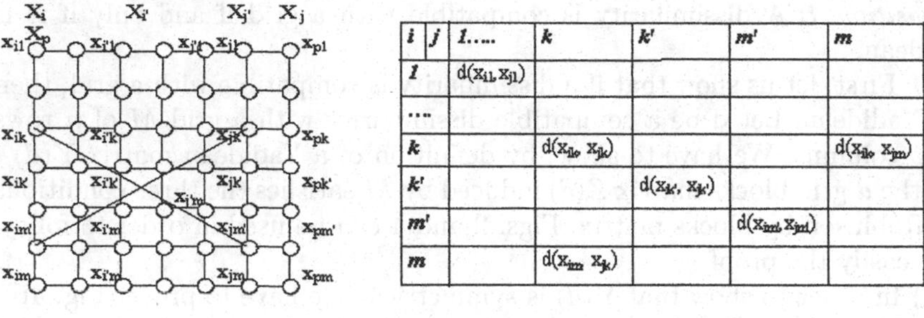

Fig. 4. Each xij is a node of the grid where the two diagonals of the convex xik, xim, xjm, xjk of the grid are represented. (b) This array represents some terms of the matrix XiXjT.

convex $C' \subset C$ with a diagonal $(x_{i'k'}, x_{j'm'})$ (see Fig. 4), such that the diameter would not be preserved, which means that: $D(C', d_M) \leq D(C, d_M)$ but $D(C, d) < D(C', d)$ which implies that we have $d(x_{ik}, x_{jm}) < d(x_{i'k'}, x_{j'm'})$. But as the grid matrix d-grid matrix induced from G is Yadidean, when $i < j$ (i.e. in the upper part of the matrix Y) we have $X_i X_j^T(d)$ decreasing in i and increasing in j. Moreover, inside $X_i X_j^T(d)$, $d(x_{ik}, x_{jm})$ is decreasing in k and increasing in m when $k < m$ (i.e. in the upper part of this matrix). Therefore, it results that $d(x_{i'k'}, x_{j'm'}) \leq d(x_{ik'}, x_{j'm'})$ as $X_{i'} X_{j'}^T(d) \leq X_i X_{j'}^T(d)$ when $i < i'$ in the upper part of a Yadidean matrix. For the same reason, we have also, $d(x_{ik'}, x_{j'm'}) \leq d(x_{ik'}, x_{jm'})$ as $X_i X_{j'}^T(d) \leq X_i X_j^T(d)$ when $j' < j$. We have also, $d(x_{ik'}, x_{jm'}) \leq d(x_{ik}, x_{jm'})$ as $k < k'$ in the matrix $X_i X_j^T(d)$ where $k < m$ (i.e. in the upper part of the matrix $X_i X_j^T(d)$) and finally $d(x_{ik}, x_{jm'}) \leq d(x_{ik}, x_{jm})$ as $m' < m$ in the same matrix $X_i X_j^T(d)$. Therefore, $d(x_{i'k'}, x_{j'm'}) \geq d(x_{ik}, x_{jm})$ which is in contradiction with the inequality (1) and shows that d must be Yadidean if it is compatible with the grid. □

6 Spatial Pyramids

A spatial pyramid on a finite set Ω is a set of subsets (called "level") of Ω satisfying the following conditions:

1. $\Omega \in P$
2. $\forall\, w \in \Omega, \{w\} \in P$.
3. $\forall\, (h, h') \in P\mathrm{x}P$, we have $h \cap h' \in P \cup \emptyset$
4. An m/k -network M of Ω exists for which any element of P belongs to a given set of subsets Q_M of M.

If Q_M is the set of convex of M, such an m/k-network M is called "convex compatible" with P and P is called a "convex pyramid". If we wish to give a height to each level of a pyramid, we need to introduce a mapping f from Q a set of subsets of Ω to $[0, \infty)$. We say that (Q, f) is a largely indexed set if $f : Q \longrightarrow [0, \infty)$ is such that: i) $\forall\ A, B \in Q, A \subset B$ (strict inclusion) $==>$ $f(A) \leq f(B)$ and ii) $f(A) = 0 \Leftrightarrow |A| = 1$. We say that Q is strictly indexed if i) is replaced by: i) $\forall\ A, B \in Q, A \subset B$ (strict inclusion) $==> f(A) < f(B)$

We say that Q is indexed if to i) and ii) a third condition is added: iii) $A \in Q, A \subset B \in Q$ and $f(A) = f(B)$ implies the existence of A_1 and A_2 in Q with $A \neq A_1$ and $A \neq A_2$ such that $A \equiv A_1 \cap A_2$.

Notice that strictly indexed (Q, f) are a case of indexed (Q, f) which are a case of largely indexed (Q, f).

If Q is a convex pyramid compatible with M and f is an index defined on the set of convex of M, the pair (Q, f) is an "indexed convex pyramid". If the index is large (strict) then the pyramid is largely (strictly) indexed.

Notice that there exists an equivalence relation R between indexed pyramids. We say that C is a maximal level of a convex pyramid or a f-maximal if it is a convex of the pyramid for which there does not exist a level C' such that C would be strictly included in C' and $f(C) = f(C')$. The binary relation R defined by $(P', f)R(P'', f)$ iff (P', f) and (P'', f) has the same set of f-maximal, is an equivalence relation. Therefore, each equivalence class of R contains a unique indexed pyramid defined by the set of f-maximal and their intersections. In other words, each equivalent class is composed by a set of largely indexed pyramids and one indexed pyramid. So, in the following, we consider the set of indexed pyramids, keeping in mind that it is equivalent to the elements of the set of equivalent classes of R.

In order to prove the following important result concerning the one to one correspondence between the indexed spatial pyramids and the Yadidean dissimilarities, we need to introduce some new notions.

A convex C of M is called a "maximal (M, d)-convex" if another convex C' of M such that $C' \subset C$ (strictly) and $D(C', d) = D(C, d)$ doesn't exist. In a Yadidean matrix $Y = \{d(x_{ik}, x_{jm})\}_{i,j\in\{1,p\},k,m\in\{1,n\}}$, such a convex C is easy to find as it is characterized by the fact that if its diameter is $D(C, d) = d(x_{ik}, x_{jm})$. If $i < j$ and $k < m$, then, the same value does not exist in any row or column smaller than k and higher than m if i and j are fixed (i.e. among the terms $d(x_{ik'}, x_{jm'})$ where $k' \leq k$ and $m' \leq m$ in the matrix $X_i X_j^T(d)$) and in any row or column lower than i and higher than j if k and m are fixed (i.e. among the matrices $X_{i'} X_{j'}^T(d)$ with $i' \leq i$ and $j' \geq j$). For example, in the Yadidean matrix shown in Fig. 2 the convex C_i of diameter $D(C_1, d) = d(x_{11}, x_{33}) = v$, $D(C_2, d) = d(x_{12}, x_{23}) = 5$, $D(C_2, d) = d(x_{21}, x_{32}) = 1$ defined by their diagonal (x_{11}, x_{33}), (x_{12}, x_{23}), (x_{21}, x_{32}), (in the grid whose columns are the elements of X_1, X_2, X_3) are maximal (M, d)-convex.

7 One-To-One Correspondence Between Indexed Convex Pyramids and Yadidean Dissimilarities

Let ICP be the set of indexed convex pyramids, convex compatible with M, D the set of proper dissimilarities on $\Omega x \Omega$. Let φ be a mapping: $ICP \longrightarrow D$ defined by $\varphi(\{P, f\}) = d$ such that $d(i, j) = \min\{f(A) : A \in P, i \in A, j \in A\}$. We show hereunder that with such a definition, d is a proper dissimilarity. Let be YD the set of proper Yadidean dissimilarities compatible with a grid M and IC the set of indexed convex of M. The mapping Ψ: $YD \longrightarrow IC$ is defined by $\Psi(d) = (Q, f)$, where Q is the set of maximal (M, d)-convex and their intersection and f is the index defined on the set of convex C_M of M by their diameters for d. In other words f is the mapping $C_M \longrightarrow [0, \infty)$ such that $f(A) = D(A, d)$. In the following, in order to simplify notations we denote $\varphi(\{P, f\})$ by $\Psi(P, f)$.

We have the following result. In order to simplify the proof we give it when M is a grid, but it can be generalized to the other m/k-networks:

Lemma 1: If $\varphi(P, f) = d$ then, for any convex A in M, we have $f(A) = D(A, d)$. Moreover, d is diameter preservative.

Proof: Let $\varphi(P, f) = d$. We denote $h(i, k)$ a convex of the pyramid containing i and k and such that $f(h(i, k)) = Min\{f(B)/B \in P, i \in B, k \in B\} = d(i, k)$. Let A be a convex of M with $i, k \in A$ such that $D(A, d_M) = d_M(i, k)$. As the convex $h(i, k)$ contains the diagonal of the convex A in the grid we have necessarily $A \subseteq h(i, k)$ and so $f(A) \leq f(h(i, k)) = d(i, k)$ (1) and $f(A) \leq D(A, d)$ (2) as $d(i, k) \leq D(A, d)$. We have also for any $i', k' \in A$, $d(i', k') = f(h(i', k')) \leq f(A)$ as $h(i', k') \subseteq A$, from which it results as $i, k \in A$ that $d(i, k) \leq f(A)$ (3) and $D(A, d) \leq f(A)$ (4). Hence, from (1) and (3) we get $d(i, k) = f(A)$ and from (2) and (4) we get $D(A, d) = f(A)$. Hence, $d(i, k) = D(A, d)$ and we have proved that $D(A, d_M) = d_M(i, k)$ implies $D(A, d) = d(i, k)$. Therefore d is diameter conservative. □

Lemma 2: We have $\varphi(P, f) = d \in YD$ and $\Psi(d) \in ICP$.

Proof: First $\varphi(P, f) = d \in YD$. This can be proved in the following way. It is easy to see that d is a proper dissimilarity as the symmetry comes directly from its definition and we have $d(x, x) = 0$ as $f(\{x\}) = 0$. Moreover, d is proper as from the definition of an index, we get: $d(i, j) = f(A) = 0 \Longleftrightarrow |A'| = 1 \Longleftrightarrow i \equiv j$. From the Lemma 1 we know that d is diameter conservative so d is compatible with the grid and therefore, from the proposition 1, it is Yadidean.

Second, $\Psi(d) = (P, f) \in ICP$. It is easy to see that and the singleton are in P as they are convex (M, d)-maximal because they cannot be strictly included in a convex of a same diameter. The third condition of the definition of a convex pyramid is satisfied as any intersection of the two elements of

P is in P because it is the intersection of a finite number of convex (M,d)-maximal. Therefore, by the definition of Ψ it is in P. Moreover the fourth condition is satisfied as the elements of P are convex of M, as they are convex (M,d)-maximal or intersection of such convex (the intersection of convex of a grid is empty or convex). Now, remains to prove that P is indexed by f. As $f(A)$ is by definition the diameter of A for d, we have necessarily $A \subset B ==> f(A) \leq f(B)$ *and* $f(A) = 0 \Longleftrightarrow A$ is a singleton as d is proper. Finally, by the definition of Ψ there cannot exist an element of P which is not the intersection of two different elements of P. So P is indexed by f. □

Theorem: The set of indexed convex pyramids is in a one-to-one correspondence with the set of Yadidean dissimilarities. This one-to-one correspondence is defined by φ or Ψ and moreover $\varphi = \Psi^{-1}$, $\Psi = \varphi^{-1}$.

Proof: We need to show that $\Psi \circ \varphi(P, f) = (P, f)$ and $\varphi \circ \Psi(d) = d$ from which it follows that φ and Ψ are a one to one correspondence between YD and IC and, moreover, $\Psi = \varphi^{-1}$, $\varphi = \Psi^{-1}$.

First $\Psi \circ \varphi(P, f) = (P, f)$. If we set $\varphi(P, f) = d$ and $\Psi(d) = (P', f')$ then, we have to prove that $(P, f) = (P', f')$. It results from the Lemma 1 the following equivalence: $\{A$ is (M,d)-maximal $\} \Longleftrightarrow$ {there does not exist B such that $A \subset B$ (strictly) and $D(A,d) = D(B,d)\} \Longleftrightarrow$ { there does not exist B such that $A \subset B$ (strictly) and $f(A) = f(B)\} \Longleftrightarrow \{A$ is f-maximal}. Therefore, the set of all (M,d)-maximal and their intersections which by definition of Ψ is P' is identical to the set of all f-maximal and their intersections which is P as by definition P is indexed by f. So $P \equiv P'$. We have also $f \equiv f'$ as from the Lemma 1, we know that $f(A) = D(a,d)$ and for any convex A of M we have by the definition of f', $f'(A) = D(a,d)$.

Second $\varphi \circ \Psi(d) = d$. If we set $\Psi(d) = (P, f)$ and $\varphi(P, f) = d'$ then we have to prove that $d = d'$. For any $i,j \in \Omega$, there exists a convex C of M such that $d_M(i,j) = D(C, d_M)$. As Ψ is defined on the set of Yadidean dissimlarities, it results from Proposition 1 that d is compatible with a grid M and so it is diameter conservative. Hence, as $d_M(i,j) = D(C, d_M)$ we have $d(i,j) = D(C,d)$. By definition of f when $\Psi(d) = (P, f)$, we get $f(C) = D(C,d)$ if C is a convex (M,d)-maximal. If C is not a convex (M,d)-maximal then, by definition, there exists a convex (M,d)-maximal C' such that $C \subset C'$ and $f(C') = f(C) = d(i,j)$. Therefore in any case, $f(C) = d(i,j)$ (1). Now, from $\varphi(P, f) = d'$ and the Lemma 1 we know that d' is diameter conservative. Therefore $d'(i,j) = D(C,d')$ as $d_M(i,j) = d(C,d_M)$. We know also from Lemma 1 that $f(C) = D(C,d')$. Hence, $f(C) = d'(i,j)$ and from (1) it results finally that $d(i,j) = d'(i,j)$. □

Corollary: The set of strictly indexed convex pyramids is in a one-to-one correspondence with the set of strictly Yadidean dissimilarities.

Proof: It follows directly from the preceding theorem and from the definition of strictly Yadidean dissimilarities, which implies that there does not exist two convexes with a same diameter such that one would strictly be included in the other, like in the strictly indexed convex pyramids $(P, f) = \Psi(d)$. □

8 A Spatial Convex Pyramidal Clustering Algorithm

Let $P(\Omega)$ be set of subsets of Ω. An aggregation index is a mapping $\delta : P(\Omega)xP(\Omega) \longrightarrow [0, \infty)$ which is symmetric and satisfies $\delta(\{x\}, \{x'\}) = d(x, x')$ where d is a given dissimilarity. There are many possible choices for δ, for instance, $\delta_{Max}(A, B) = Max\{d(a, b)/a \in A, b \in B\}$, for the "complete linkage." Two subsets A and B are called "mutual neighbors" in a set C of subsets of Ω, iff

$$\delta(A, B) = Min\{\delta(A, B')/B' \in C\} = \min\{\delta(A', B)/A' \in C\}.$$

Given an aggregation index δ and a dissimilarity d, the index f is defined by $f(h_i \cup h_j) = \delta(h_i, h_j)$.

A bottom-up convex spatial pyramidal clustering algorithm called SCAP, generalizing the CAP algorithm given in Diday (1984, 1986) is defined by the following steps. At thc bcginning the convex spatial pyramid P is empty.

1. Each element of Ω is considered as a class and added to P.
2. Each mutual neighbor class which can be merged in a new convex, among the set of classes already obtained and which have not been merged four times, is merged in a new class and added to P.
3. The process continue until all the elements of Ω are merged.
4. During the process:
5. Each time a new convex is created an order is fixed for its rows and columns.
6. Two convex cannot be merged if they are not connected.
7. A convex C' which is contained by another convex C and which does not contain a row or a column of the limit of C, cannot be aggregated with any convex external to C.

This algorithm can be applied to any kind of dissimilarity and aggregation index. By deleting all the classes which are not the intersection of two different classes of P the algorithm SCAP produces an indexed pyramid (P, f). In order to simplify, we apply SCAP in the following example in the case of a Yadidean dissimilarity.

Example: We take the Yadidean dissimilarity d shown in Fig. 2 and the aggregation index δ_{Max}, we obtain the following clusters at each step of the algorithm (see Fig. 5).

Step 1: All the $\{x_{ij}\}$for$i,j \in \{1,2,3\}$ constitute the first classes of the spatial pyramid.

Step 2: The obtained mutual neighbor convex are:

$$h_1 = \{x_{11}, x_{12}\},\ h_2 = \{x_{12}, x_{13}\},\ \ h_3 = \{x_{21}, x_{22}\},\ \ h_4 = \{x_{22}, x_{23}\},$$
$$h_5 = \{x_{31}, x_{32}\},\ h_6 = \{x_{32}, x_{33}\},\ \ h_7 = \{x_{11}, x_{21}\},\ \ h_8 = \{x_{21}, x_{31}\},$$
$$h_9 = \{x_{12}, x_{22}\},\ h_{10} = \{x_{22}, x_{32}\},\ h_{11} = \{x_{13}, x_{23}\},\ h_{12} = \{x_{23}, x_{33}\}$$

with $f(h_1) = 4$, $f(h_2) = 5$, $f(h_3) = 1$, $f(h_4) = 3$, $f(h_5) = 1$, $f(h_6) = 3$, $f(h_7) = 4$, $f(h_8) = 1$, $f(h_9) = 4$, $f(h_{10}) = 1$, $f(h_{11}) = 5$, $f(h_{12}) = 3$.

Step 3: The new mutual neighbor convex is:

$$h_{13} = \{h_1, h_3\} = \{\{x_{11}, x_{12}\}, \{x_{21}, x_{22}\}\},$$
$$h_{14} = \{h_3, h_5\} = \{\{x_{21}, x_{22}\}, \{x_{32}, x_{31}\}\},$$
$$h_{15} = \{h_2, h_4\} = \{\{x_{12}, x_{13}\}, \{x_{23}, x_{22}\}\},$$
$$h_{16} = \{h_4, h_6\} = \{\{x_{22}, x_{23}\}, \{x_{33}, x_{32}\}\}$$

with $f(h_{13}) = 4$,$f(h_{14}) = 1$,$f(h_{15}) = 5$, $f(h_{16}) = 3$.

Step 4: We obtain $h_{17} = \{h_{13}, h_{14}\}$, $h_{18} = \{h_{15}, h_{16}\}$ with $f(h_{17}) = v$ and $f(h_{18}) = v$.

Step 5: We obtain $f(h_{19}) = v$.

With this information we can build the indexed spatial pyramid shown in Fig. 5. This spatial convex pyramid is defined by

$$P = \{\{x_{ij}\}_{i,j \in \{1,..,p\}}, h_3, h_4, h_9, h_{10}, h_{13}, h_{14}, h_{15}, h_{16}, h_{19}\}$$

obtained by deleting all the convex strictly included in an obtained convex of same diameter and not intersection of (M,d)-maximal where d is the initial dissimilarity and M is the 3x3 grid. If $v = 5$, P is indexed. If $v > 5$, P is strictly indexed by definition. Notice that in the Yadidean matrix $Y(d)$ (see figure 3) when $v > 5$, the condition i) and ii) in order that it be strict are not satisfied but the condition iii) is satisfied and so it is a strict Yadidean matrix. If we add to P the convex h_1 for instance, we obtain a new spatial pyramid $P' = P \cup h_1$ which is equivalent to P in the equivalent relation R defined in section 6 as both pyramids has the same f-maximal. Notice also that $\varphi(P)$ and $\Psi(P')$ induce the same Yadidean matrix and so the same Yadidean dissimilarity. This would be the case for any equivalent spatial pyramid P' to P.

As the initial dissimilarity matrix is Yadidean, it would also be possible to apply a top-down algorithm in order to build P, by taking at each step the highest convex class (which is (M,d)-maximal or intersection of (M,d)-maximal) and its associating nodes in the 3×3 grid.

This algorithm can be extended to the case of a symbolical indexed pyramid for the Symbolic Data Analysis framework, (see Bock, Diday (2000), Billard, Diday (2003)) where the index is a mapping $f : Q_M \longrightarrow S$ where S is a set of symbolic objects partially ordered. In this case the same algorithm can

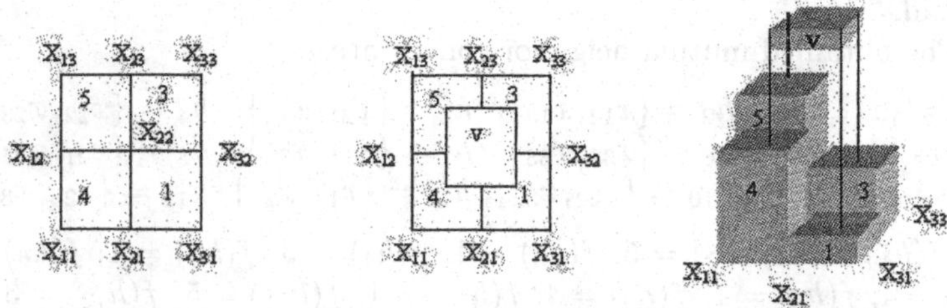

Fig. 5. Spatial Convex Pyramid obtained from the dissimilarity defined in figure 3

be applied with the restriction that at each level only the "complete symbolic objects" (Diday (1987, 1991), Diday, Brito (1989), Brito (1991), Rodriguez (2000)) are retained which means that the symbolic object associated to each class of the spatial convex pyramid must have an extent whose intent is itself.

9 Spatial Pyramid and Geometrical Pyramids

The aim of this section is to justify the name "Pyramid" in "Spatial Convex Pyramids." First we consider the spatial convex pyramid built on a grid of $3 \times 3 = 9$ nodes shown in Fig. 6a where each cell is a cube of size c. A vertical cut at its middle gives the standard clustering pyramid of Fig. 6b a horizontal view is shown in Fig. 6c. The spatial convex pyramid of Fig. 6a can be imbedded in the geometrical pyramid of height $H = 4c$ and of surface of the base $S = 4c \times 4c$ shown in Fig. 6d. The standard clustering pyramid of the Fig. 6b can be imbedded in the triangle of Fig. 6e obtained from a vertical cut of the geometrical pyramid and containing its top. The volume of a geometrical pyramid is: $VG = H\text{x}S/3$. So, in this case its volume is $VG = 4c \text{ x } 16c^2/3 = 64c^3/3$. The volume of the spatial convex pyramid is $VS = 9c^3 + 4c^3 + c^3 = 14c^3$ (1).

More generally if $h = nc$ is the height of the geometrical pyramid, its surface is $S = (nc)^2$ and so its volume is $VG = n^3c^3/3$. From (1), the volume of the imbedded spatial convex pyramid is $VS = c^3n(n-1)(2n-1)/6$. So we get $VG - VS = c^3n(n-1/3)/2$. Let $c = b/n$, we get: $VG - VS = (b^3/n^3)(n(n-1/3)/2 = b^3(1/2n - 1/6n^2)$. Therefore, when $n \longrightarrow \infty$, the volume of the spatial pyramid tends toward the volume of the geometrical pyramid. As the spatial convex pyramid is (by construction) included in the geometrical pyramid we can say finally that the spatial convex pyramid converges when $n \longrightarrow \infty$ towards the geometrical pyramid.

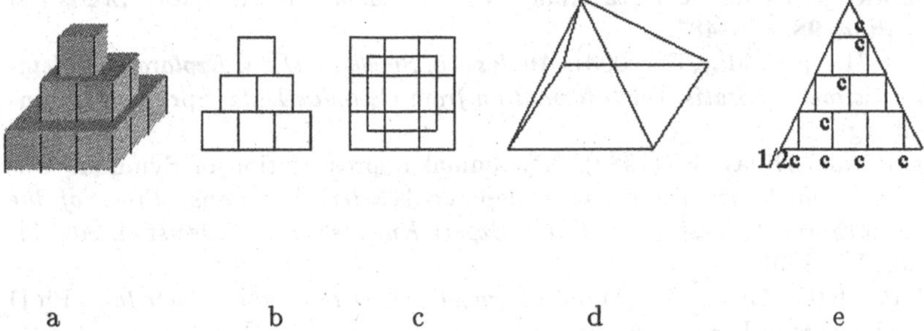

Fig. 6. The spatial convex pyramid shown in 6a converge towards the geometrical pyramid shown in 6d

10 Conclusion

We have shown that spatial pyramids compatible with a grid are in one-to-one correspondence with a kind of dissimilarity called Yadidean which can be rewritten in terms of a "Robinsonian matrix by blocks." This result can be extended under some assumptions (Diday 2003) to other kinds of k/m-networks and other families of spatial pyramids (for instance, instead of the convex, we can use the maximal clique or the connected subsets of the network). Many applications are possible, for instance, to give a geometrical representation of a conceptual lattice by a decomposition into spatial pyramids. In the case of huge data sets, it is possible to use as units the means obtained after a k-means clustering without the constraints imposed by a Kohonen mapping, and then to use the grid obtained from the Spatial Convex Pyramid as is done with the Kohonen mappings. On this grid it is also possible to project interactively the different levels of the pyramid. Many questions remain open such as how to get the closest Yadidean dissimilarity of a given dissimilarity.

References

1. Aude, J. C. (1999). *Analyse de Génomes Microbiens, Apports de la Classification Pyramidal,* Ph.D Thesis, Université Paris Dauphine, Paris.
2. Benzecri, J. P. (1973). *l'Analyse des Données: la Taxonomie*, Vol. 1, Dunod, Paris.
3. Bertrand, P., and Janowitz, M. F. (2002). "Pyramids and Weak Hierarchies in the Ordinal Model for Clustering," *Discrete Applied Mathematics*, **122**, 55–81.
4. Bertrand, P. (1986). *Etude de la Représentation Pyramidale,* Ph.D Thesis, Université Paris Dauphine, Paris.
5. Bertrand, P. (1995). "Structural Properties of Pyramidal Clustering," *DIMACS Series on Theoretical Computer Science*, **19**, pp. 35-53.

6. Billard L., and Diday, E. (2003). "From the Statistics of Data to the Statistics of Knowledge: Symbolic Data Analysis," *Journal of the American Statistical Association*, **98**, 470–487.
7. Bock, H.-H., and Diday, E. (2000). *Analysis of Symbolic Data: Exploratory Methods for Extracting Statistical Information from Complex Data*, Springer, Berlin-Heidelberg.
8. Brito, P., and Diday, E. (1989). "Pyramidal Representation of Symbolic Objects," in *Knowledge, Data and Computer-Assisted Decisions: Proc. of the NATO advanced Workshop on Data, Expert Knowledge and Decision*, eds. M. Schader, W. Gaul.
9. Brito, P. (1991). *Analyse de Données Symboliques et Pyramides d'héritage*, Ph.D Thesis, Université Paris Dauphine, Paris.
10. Diday, E. (1984). "Une Représentation Visuelle des Classes Empiétantes: Les Pyramides," *Rapport de Recherche INRIA, Rocquencourt, France*, **291**.
11. Diday, E. (1986). "Orders and Overlapping Clusters in Pyramids," in *Multidimensional Data Analysis*, eds. J. De Leeuw et al., Leiden:DSWO Press, pp. 201-234.
12. Diday, E. (1987). "Introduction á l'Approche Symbolique en Analyse des Données," in *Actes des Journées Symboliques-Numériques pour l'Apprentissage de Connaissances à Partir d'Observations*, eds. E. Diday and Y. Kodratoff, Université Paris-IX Dauphine, France.
13. Durand, C., and Fichet, B. (1988). "One-to-One Correspondance in Pyramidal Representation," in *Classification and Related Methods of Data Analysis*, ed. H.-H. Bock, Elsevier Science Publishers.
14. Janowitz, M. F. (1978). "An Order Theoretic Model for Cluster Analysis," *SIAM Journal of Applied Mathematics*, **34**, 55–72.
15. Johnson, S. C. (1967). "Hierarchical Clustering Schemes," *Psychometrika*, **32**, 241–254.
16. Rodriguez, R. O. (2000). *Classification et Modéles Linéaires en Analyse des Données Symboliques*, Ph.D Thesis, Université Paris Dauphine, Paris.

Part II

Modern Nonparametrics

Relative Projection Pursuit and its Application

Masahiro Mizuta and Shintaro Hiro

Hokkaido University, Japan
mizuta,hiro@cims.hokudai.ac.jp

Abstract: In this paper, we propose a new method of projection pursuit, relative projection pursuit (RPP), which finds 'interesting' low dimensional spaces different from reference data sets predefined by the user. In addition, as an application of the method, we develop a new dimension reduction method: sliced inverse regression with relative projection pursuit.

Recently, high dimensional datasets such as microarray gene data and point-of-sale data have become important. It is generally difficult to see the structure of data when the dimension of data is high. Therefore, many studies have invented methods that reduce high dimensional data to lower dimensional data. Among these methods, projection pursuit was developed by Friedman and Tukey (1974) in order to search for an 'interesting' linear projection of multidimensional data. They defined the degree of 'interestingness' as the difference between the distribution of the projected data and the normal distribution. We call this measure a *projection index*.

However, projection indices that measure the difference from the normal distribution do not always reveal interesting structure because interesting structure depends on the purpose of the analysis. According to the scientific situation that motivates the data analysis, 'uninteresting' structure is not always the normal distribution.

Relative projection pursuit allows the user to predefine a reference data set that represents 'uninteresting' structure. The projection index for relative projection pursuit measures the distance between the distribution of the projected target data set and that of the projected reference data set. We show the effectiveness of RPP with numerical examples and actual data.

1 Introduction

Projection pursuit was developed by Friedman and Tukey (1974) in order to search for the most 'interesting' linear projection of a dataset. Methods for dimension reduction with linear projection are fundamental in multidimensional data analysis. For example, principal components analysis (PCA) can detect linear structures in data. However, it is difficult to detect non-linear structures, such as toroidal data clusters, with PCA. Projection pursuit is widely viewed as an effective method which can find interesting structure, both linear and non-linear, in complex data.

In conventional projection pursuit, it is assumed that interesting structure is maximally different from the normal distribution. The reason that the normal distribution is uninteresting is because that for most high-dimensional data clouds, nearly all low-dimensional projections are approximately normal (Diaconis and Freedman, 1984). But this assumption is not always valid because uninteresting structure depends upon such factors as the purpose of analysis.

Sometimes we would like to find interesting features in a data set (say, the *target data set*) as compared to another data set (say, the *reference data set*). And it may be that the reference data set does not follow a normal distribution. In this case, the uninteresting structure is that of the reference data, not the normal distribution.

We therefore propose *relative projection pursuit* (RPP), which finds the most different structure from the distribution of the reference data set predefined by user. In this paper we develop RPP as an extension of conventional projection pursuit and definc a projection index, the *relative projection index*, which measures interestingness in terms of a reference dataset. In addition, with artificial data and real data, we show that RPP achieves good performance. Finally, we propose a method for sliced inverse regression (SIR) with RPP for the dimension reduction method. We also show the effectiveness of SIR with RPP through numerical examples.

2 Outline of Projection Pursuit

In general, it is difficult to define 'interestingness' as a unique concept. Hence we first define uninteresting structure and formulate interesting structure as any structure that is different. Conventional projection indices take uninteresting structure to follow a normal distribution. So projection pursuit searches for projection vectors that maximize projection indices which highlight deviations from the normal distribution.

2.1 Algorithm for Projection Pursuit

Projection pursuit is executed by the following steps:

(1) Standardize each sample vector $\mathbf{x}_i,\ i = 1, \ldots, n$ by an affine transformation to get $\tilde{\mathbf{x}}_i = \hat{\Sigma}_{xx}^{-1/2}(\mathbf{x}_i - \bar{\mathbf{x}})$, where $\hat{\Sigma}_{xx}$ and $\bar{\mathbf{x}}$ are the sample covariance matrix and the sample mean of the data, respectively.

(2) Choose an initial value of $\boldsymbol{\alpha}$, the projection direction vector.
(3) Search for a new $\boldsymbol{\alpha}$ to maximize a projection index through some method of nonlinear constrained optimization.
(4) Change the initial value of $\boldsymbol{\alpha}$, and repeat (3) a preset number of times.

2.2 Projection Index

We explain the Friedman projection index, the Hall projection index, and the Moment projection index as projection indices for conventional projection pursuit. In particular, we describe the Hall projection index in detail because our new projection index for relative projection pursuit is based on the concept behind the Hall index.

Friedman Projection Index

The one-dimensional Friedman projection index (Friedman, 1987) reduces the dimension of the target dataset to a unidimensional space. It is defined as

$$I(\boldsymbol{\alpha}) = \frac{1}{2}\sum_{j=0}^{J}(2j+1)\left[\frac{1}{n}\sum_{i=1}^{n}P_j(2\Phi(\boldsymbol{\alpha}^{\mathrm{T}}\mathbf{x}_i)-1)\right]^2,$$

where $P_j(\cdot)$ is a j-dimensional Legendre polynomial and $\Phi(\cdot)$ is the cumulative distribution function of the standard normal distribution.

The two-dimensional Friedman index is defined as

$$I(\boldsymbol{\alpha}_1,\boldsymbol{\alpha}_2) = \frac{1}{4}\sum_{j=0}^{J}\sum_{k=0}^{J-j}(2j+1)(2k+1)E^2\left[P_j(R_1)P_k(R_2)\right]-\frac{1}{4},$$

where

$$\begin{aligned} R_1 &= 2\Phi(Z_1)-1 \; R_2 = 2\Phi(Z_2)-1,\\ Z_1 &= \boldsymbol{\alpha}_1^{\mathrm{T}}X, \qquad Z_2 = \boldsymbol{\alpha}_2^{\mathrm{T}}X. \end{aligned}$$

Here $E[\cdot]$ denotes expectation and X denotes the target dataset arranged as a matrix with each column being an observation.

The Friedman projection index measures the difference between the estimated density function $f_{\boldsymbol{\alpha}}(Z)$, where $Z=\boldsymbol{\alpha}^{\mathrm{T}}X$ is a projection of the target data X, and the density function of standardized normal distribution $\phi(Z)$. Now, the target data X is standardized by the affine transformation and $\boldsymbol{\alpha}$ is projection direction vector. The difference is measured by

$$\int_{-1}^{1}(p_R(R)-p_U(R))^2\,dR = \int_{-1}^{1}p_R^2(R)dR-\frac{1}{2},$$

where $p_R(R)$ is the density function of R, $p_U(R)$ is the density function of the uniform distribution $U(-1,1)$, and $R=2\Phi(Z)-1$. With the transformation $R=2\Phi(Z)-1$, the standard normal distribution $N(0,1)$ is transformed into the uniform distribution $U(-1,1)$.

Hall Projection Index

We consider the Hall projection index (Hall, 1989) when the target dataset is projected into a one-dimensional space. The projection of the target data X by the projection direction vector $\boldsymbol{\alpha}$ under the condition that $\boldsymbol{\alpha}^{\mathrm{T}}\boldsymbol{\alpha} = 1$ is denoted by

$$Z = \boldsymbol{\alpha}^{\mathrm{T}} X.$$

Denote the density function of the projection by $f_{\boldsymbol{\alpha}}$. The Hall index is the integral of the square of the distance between the density function $f_{\boldsymbol{\alpha}}$ and the density function of the normal distribution. The one-dimensional Hall projection index is defined, in terms of densities, as

$$J^* \equiv \int_{-\infty}^{\infty} \{f_{\boldsymbol{\alpha}}(u) - \phi(u)\}^2 du.$$

In this definition, the density function is approximated by an orthogonal function expansion with Hermite functions. Then we can calculate the sample estimate of the one-dimensional Hall projection index as

$$I(\boldsymbol{\alpha}) = [\theta_0(\boldsymbol{\alpha}) - 2^{-1/2}\pi^{-1/4}]^2 + \sum_{j=1}^{J} \theta_j{}^2(\boldsymbol{\alpha}),$$

where

$$\theta_j(\boldsymbol{\alpha}) = n^{-1}\sum_{i=1}^{n} P_j(\boldsymbol{\alpha}^{\mathrm{T}} z_i)\phi(\boldsymbol{\alpha}^{\mathrm{T}} z_i),\ P_j(z) = \left(\frac{2}{j!}\right)^{1/2} \pi^{1/4} H_j(2^{1/2} z).$$

Here, $\phi(\cdot)$ is the standard normal density function and $H_j(\cdot)$ is the jth Hermite polynomial, given by

$$H_j(x) = (-1)^j \{\phi^2(x)\}^{-1} \frac{d^j}{dx^j} \phi^2(x).$$

The two-dimensional Hall projection index, in terms of densities, is defined as

$$J^* \equiv \int_{-\infty}^{\infty}\int_{-\infty}^{\infty} \{f_{\alpha_1,\alpha_2}(x_1,x_2) - \phi(x_1,x_2)\}^2 dx_1 dx_2,$$

where $f_{\alpha_1,\alpha_2}(x_1,x_2)$ is the density function of the bivariate projection when the target data are projected with two vectors $\boldsymbol{\alpha}_1, \boldsymbol{\alpha}_2$ and $\phi(x_1,x_2)$ is the density function of the two-dimensional normal distribution with mean zero and the identity covariance matrix. Then the sample form of the two-dimensional Hall projection index is

$$I(\boldsymbol{\alpha}_1,\boldsymbol{\alpha}_2) = \sum_{i=0}^{q}\sum_{j=0}^{q-i}\left\{\frac{1}{n}\sum_{m=1}^{n} h_i(\boldsymbol{\alpha}_1{}^{\mathrm{T}} x_m) h_j(\boldsymbol{\alpha}_2{}^{\mathrm{T}} x_m)\right\}^2$$
$$- \pi^{-1/2}\frac{1}{n}\sum_{m=1}^{n} h_0(\boldsymbol{\alpha}_1{}^{\mathrm{T}} x_m) h_0(\boldsymbol{\alpha}_2{}^{\mathrm{T}} x_m) + (4\pi)^{-1},$$

where

$$h_i(u) = (i!)^{-1/2}\pi^{1/4}2^{-(i-1)/2}H_i(u)\phi(u) \quad -\infty < u < \infty.$$

Moment Projection Index

The Moment projection index (Jones and Sibson, 1987) is developed from the property of the normal distribution that the third and higher cumulants are equal to zero. The third and the fourth cumulants are denoted by $k_3 = \mu_3$ and $k_4 = \mu_4 - 3$, respectively, where μ_3 and μ_4 are the third and the fourth moments of the distribution projected with vector $\boldsymbol{\alpha}$. Thus, the one-dimensional Moment index is

$$M = {k_3}^2 + \frac{1}{4}{k_4}^2.$$

Similarly, the two-dimensional Moment index is

$$M = ({k_{30}}^2 + 3{k_{21}}^2 + 3{k_{12}}^2 + {k_{03}}^2) + \frac{1}{4}({k_{40}}^2 + 4{k_{31}}^2 + 6{k_{22}}^2 + 4{k_{13}}^2 + {k_{04}}^2)$$

where k_{rs} is the (r, s)th cumulant of the variables. This index is sensitive to heavy-tailed distributions.

3 Relative Projection Pursuit

In this section, we describe relative projection pursuit (RPP). This method finds interesting structure with a new projection index that measures the distance between the distribution of a projection of the *target data set* and that of a projection of a *reference data set*; the latter is not restricted to be the normal distribution.

A data set which includes ‘uninteresting’ structure is defined as the reference data set by user. Relative projection pursuit is only different from the conventional projection pursuit in its definition of ‘interestingness’. Here, we develop the relative projection index in correspondence with classical techniques.

3.1 Relative Projection Index

We extend the concept of the Hall projection index to develop the *Hall-type relative projection index*. The Hall projection index is defined by a squared distance between the projected distribution and the normal distribution. We define the Hall-type relative projection index by a squared distance between the distribution of the target data set and the distribution of the reference data set. We denote the reference data set by Y_j, $j = 1, \dots, m$, and the density function of the one-dimensional projection of Y with vector $\boldsymbol{\alpha}$ by $g_{\boldsymbol{\alpha}}(x)$. Then the one-dimensional Hall-type relative projection index is defined as

$$I(\boldsymbol{\alpha}) = \int_{-\infty}^{\infty} \{f_{\boldsymbol{\alpha}}(x) - g_{\boldsymbol{\alpha}}(x)\}^2 dx$$
$$= \int_{-\infty}^{\infty} f_{\boldsymbol{\alpha}}^2(x)dx + \int_{-\infty}^{\infty} g_{\boldsymbol{\alpha}}^2(x)dx - 2\int_{-\infty}^{\infty} f_{\boldsymbol{\alpha}}(x)g_{\boldsymbol{\alpha}}(x)dx.$$

Here, we must use estimated density functions $f_{\boldsymbol{\alpha}}, g_{\boldsymbol{\alpha}}$ obtained from kernel density estimators. In kernel density estimation, we use the bandwidth $h = (4/3)^{1/5}\sigma n^{-1/5}$ (n is sample size) as obtained by Scott (1992, pp. 125–193) and the kernel function is the density of the standard normal distribution. The estimated density functions $f_{\boldsymbol{\alpha}}, g_{\boldsymbol{\alpha}}$ are:

$$f_{\boldsymbol{\alpha}}(x) = \frac{1}{n}\sum_{i=1}^{n} \frac{1}{\sqrt{2\pi}h_f} \exp\left\{-\frac{(x - X_i)^2}{2{h_f}^2}\right\},$$
$$g_{\boldsymbol{\alpha}}(x) = \frac{1}{m}\sum_{j=1}^{m} \frac{1}{\sqrt{2\pi}h_g} \exp\left\{-\frac{(x - Y_j)^2}{2{h_g}^2}\right\}.$$

Therefore,

$$\int_{-\infty}^{\infty} f_{\boldsymbol{\alpha}}^2(x)dx = \frac{1}{2\sqrt{\pi}n^2 h_f}\sum_{i=1}^{n}\sum_{j=1}^{n} \exp\left\{-\frac{(X_i - X_j)^2}{4{h_f}^2}\right\}$$
$$\int_{-\infty}^{\infty} g_{\boldsymbol{\alpha}}^2(x)dx = \frac{1}{2\sqrt{\pi}m^2 h_g}\sum_{i=1}^{m}\sum_{j=1}^{m} \exp\left\{-\frac{(Y_i - Y_j)^2}{4{h_g}^2}\right\}$$
$$\int_{-\infty}^{\infty} f_{\boldsymbol{\alpha}}(x)g_{\boldsymbol{\alpha}}(x)dx = \frac{1}{\sqrt{2\pi}nm\sqrt{{h_f}^2 + {h_g}^2}}\sum_{i=1}^{n}\sum_{j=1}^{m} \exp\left\{-\frac{(X_i - Y_j)^2}{2({h_f}^2 + {h_g}^2)}\right\}.$$

Thus the one-dimensional Hall-type relative projection index can be represented in the form

$$I(\boldsymbol{\alpha}) = \int_{-\infty}^{\infty} f_{\boldsymbol{\alpha}}^2(x)dx + \int_{-\infty}^{\infty} g_{\boldsymbol{\alpha}}^2(x)dx - 2\int_{-\infty}^{\infty} f_{\boldsymbol{\alpha}}(x)g_{\boldsymbol{\alpha}}(x)dx$$
$$= \frac{1}{2\sqrt{\pi}n^2 h_f}\sum_{i=1}^{n}\sum_{j=1}^{n} \exp\left\{-\frac{(X_i - X_j)^2}{4{h_f}^2}\right\} +$$
$$\frac{1}{2\sqrt{\pi}m^2 h_g}\sum_{i=1}^{m}\sum_{j=1}^{m} \exp\left\{-\frac{(Y_i - Y_j)^2}{4{h_g}^2}\right\} -$$
$$\frac{\sqrt{2}}{\sqrt{\pi}nm\sqrt{{h_f}^2 + {h_g}^2}}\sum_{i=1}^{n}\sum_{j=1}^{m} \exp\left\{-\frac{(X_i - Y_j)^2}{2({h_f}^2 + {h_g}^2)}\right\}.$$

Now consider the Hall-type relative projection index when the target dataset is projected into a two-dimensional space. We denote the density function of the projection of reference data set $Y_j, j = 1, \dots, m$ with projection vectors $\boldsymbol{\alpha}_1$, $\boldsymbol{\alpha}_2$ by $g_{\alpha_1,\alpha_2}(x_1, x_2)$. Then the two-dimensional Hall-type relative projection index is

$$
\begin{aligned}
I(\boldsymbol{\alpha}_1, \boldsymbol{\alpha}_2) &= \int_{-\infty}^{\infty}\int_{-\infty}^{\infty} \{f_{\alpha_1,\alpha_2}(x_1, x_2) - g_{\alpha_1,\alpha_2}(x_1, x_2)\}^2 dx_1 dx_2 \\
&= \int_{-\infty}^{\infty}\int_{-\infty}^{\infty} f^2_{\alpha_1,\alpha_2}(x_1, x_2) dx_1 dx_2 \; + \\
&\quad \int_{-\infty}^{\infty}\int_{-\infty}^{\infty} g^2_{\alpha_1,\alpha_2}(x_1, x_2) dx_1 dx_2 \; - \\
&\quad 2\int_{-\infty}^{\infty}\int_{-\infty}^{\infty} f_{\alpha_1,\alpha_2}(x_1, x_2) g_{\alpha_1,\alpha_2}(x_1, x_2) dx_1 dx_2.
\end{aligned}
$$

We obtain estimated density functions f_{α_1,α_2}, g_{α_1,α_2} by kernel density estimators as before. For these kernel density estimates, the kernel function is the density function of the standard normal distribution. The bandwidths are $h_i = \sigma_i n^{-1/6}$ $(i = 1, 2)$, $b_i = \sigma_i m^{-1/6}$ $(i = 1, 2)$, as shown in Scott (1992, pp. 125–193) to be optimal. Here n is the sample size of the target dataset and m is the size of the reference dataset. The estimated density functions are then

$$
\begin{aligned}
f_{\alpha_1,\alpha_2}(x_1, x_2) &= \frac{1}{n}\sum_{i=1}^{n} \frac{1}{2\pi h_1 h_2} \exp\left\{-\frac{(x_1 - \boldsymbol{\alpha}_1{}^{\mathrm{T}} X_i)^2}{2{h_1}^2} - \frac{(x_2 - \boldsymbol{\alpha}_2{}^{\mathrm{T}} X_i)^2}{2{h_2}^2}\right\}, \\
g_{\alpha_1,\alpha_2}(x_1, x_2) &= \frac{1}{m}\sum_{j=1}^{m} \frac{1}{2\pi b_1 b_2} \exp\left\{-\frac{(x_1 - \boldsymbol{\alpha}_1{}^{\mathrm{T}} Y_j)^2}{2{b_1}^2} - \frac{(x_2 - \boldsymbol{\alpha}_2{}^{\mathrm{T}} Y_j)^2}{2{b_2}^2}\right\}.
\end{aligned}
$$

Thus the two-dimensional Hall-type relative projection index $I(\boldsymbol{\alpha}_1, \boldsymbol{\alpha}_2)$ can be calculated as

$$
\begin{aligned}
&\frac{1}{4\pi n^2 h_1 h_2}\sum_{i=1}^{n}\sum_{k=1}^{n} \exp\left\{-\frac{(\boldsymbol{\alpha}_1{}^{\mathrm{T}} X_i - \boldsymbol{\alpha}_1{}^{\mathrm{T}} X_k)^2}{4{h_1}^2} - \frac{(\boldsymbol{\alpha}_2{}^{\mathrm{T}} X_i - \boldsymbol{\alpha}_2{}^{\mathrm{T}} X_k)^2}{4{h_2}^2}\right\} + \\
&\frac{1}{4\pi m^2 b_1 b_2}\sum_{j=1}^{m}\sum_{k=1}^{m} \exp\left\{-\frac{(\boldsymbol{\alpha}_1{}^{\mathrm{T}} Y_j - \boldsymbol{\alpha}_1{}^{\mathrm{T}} Y_k)^2}{4{b_1}^2} - \frac{(\boldsymbol{\alpha}_2{}^{\mathrm{T}} Y_j - \boldsymbol{\alpha}_2{}^{\mathrm{T}} Y_k)^2}{4{b_2}^2}\right\} - \\
&\frac{1}{\pi n m\sqrt{({h_1}^2 + {b_1}^2)({h_2}^2 + {b_2}^2)}}\sum_{i=1}^{n}\sum_{j=1}^{m} \exp\left\{\frac{(\boldsymbol{\alpha}_1{}^{\mathrm{T}} X_i - \boldsymbol{\alpha}_1{}^{\mathrm{T}} Y_j)^2}{2({h_1}^2 + {b_1}^2)} - \right. \\
&\qquad\qquad \left. \frac{(\boldsymbol{\alpha}_2{}^{\mathrm{T}} X_i - \boldsymbol{\alpha}_2{}^{\mathrm{T}} Y_j)^2}{2({h_2}^2 + {b_2}^2)}\right\}.
\end{aligned}
$$

3.2 Numerical Examples

We apply conventional projection pursuit and relative projection pursuit to an artificial dataset in order to investigate efficacy of the proposed method. Then we apply our method to actual data.

We use the squared multiple correlation coefficient to evaluate the distance between projection vectors obtained by relative projection pursuit and the true projection direction space in artificial data, following the example of Li (1991). The squared multiple correlation coefficient is defined as

$$R^2(\hat{\boldsymbol{\alpha}}_i) = \max_{\boldsymbol{\alpha} \in A} \frac{(\hat{\boldsymbol{\alpha}}_i{}^{\mathrm{T}} \Sigma_{xx} \boldsymbol{\alpha})^2}{\hat{\boldsymbol{\alpha}}_i{}^{\mathrm{T}} \Sigma_{xx} \hat{\boldsymbol{\alpha}}_i \cdot \boldsymbol{\alpha}^{\mathrm{T}} \Sigma_{xx} \boldsymbol{\alpha}},$$

where A is true projection direction space, $\boldsymbol{\alpha}$ is true projection direction vector in artificial data, $\hat{\boldsymbol{\alpha}}_i$ are estimated projection vectors, and Σ_{xx} is variance covariance matrix of the data.

Artificial Data

We generate a reference dataset with 1000 observations in $\mathbb{R}^{10}$. Each component of each vector is independent with a mixture-normal distribution; with probability .5 the value it is $N(-1.5, 0.25)$ and with probability .5 it is $N(1.5, 0.25)$. We next calculate the values of $\sin(x_1) + \cos(x_2) + \varepsilon$; $\varepsilon \sim N(0, 0.2^2)$ for the data and extract the subset of the data which satisfies the condition $-\frac{2}{3} < \sin(x_1) + \cos(x_2) + \varepsilon < \frac{2}{3}$. This subset is the target dataset and has 334 observations. Figures 1 and 2 show scatterplots of the target and reference datasets, respectively.

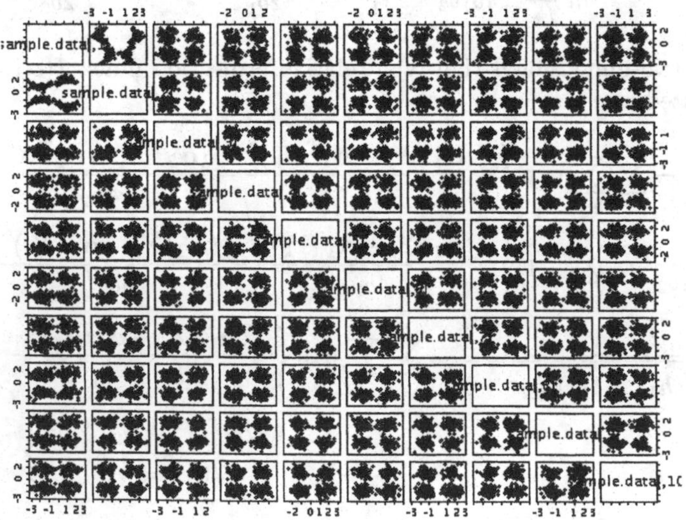

Fig. 1. Scatterplot of the target data.

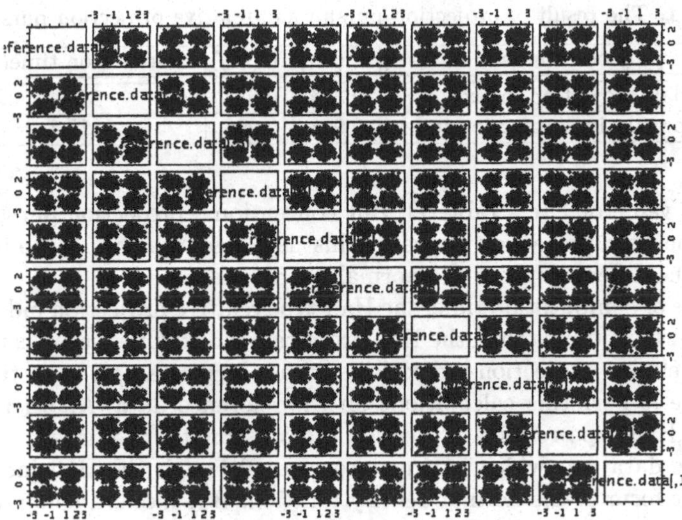

Fig. 2. Scatterplot of the reference data.

We apply RPP to this problem and estimate the 'interesting' projection vectors the squared multiple correlation coefficients of those vectors. The steps are:

(1) Standardize the artificial data.
(2) Assign initial values to the projection vectors as uniform random numbers.
(3) Calculate the $\boldsymbol{\alpha}_1$, $\boldsymbol{\alpha}_2$ which maximize the projection index. We use a quasi-Newton method in nonlinear optimization to maximize the index.
(4) Calculate the squared multiple correlation coefficients of the estimates of $\boldsymbol{\alpha}_1, \boldsymbol{\alpha}_2$.
(5) Change the initial value of estimates of the projection vectors, and repeat steps (3) and (4) 100 times. Then find the projection vectors that maximize the projection index among the 100 optimized projection vectors.

Result

We now compare the result of conventional projection pursuit with the Hall index to relative projection pursuit with the Hall-type relative projection index. By construction, the target data differ from the reference data in the space generated by the first two components.

Table 1 shows the squared multiple correlation coefficient of estimated projection vectors and the computation time for one initial value to converge to the local optimum. In this example, the true projection direction is the space generated by $\boldsymbol{\beta}_1 = (1, 0, 0, 0, 0, 0, 0, 0, 0, 0)$, $\boldsymbol{\beta}_2 = (0, 1, 0, 0, 0, 0, 0, 0, 0, 0)$. This is used when we calculate the squared multiple correlation coefficient.

Relative projection pursuit detects the true projection direction space because the values of the squared multiple correlation coefficients almost equal

Table 1. The result of projection pursuit and relative projection pursuit.

projection index	$R^2(\boldsymbol{\alpha}_1)$	$R^2(\boldsymbol{\alpha}_2)$	computation time(sec)
Hall projection index	0.304	0.687	54.3
Hall-type relative projection index	0.998	0.998	1112.1

the correct value of 1 (cf. Table 1). But conventional projection pursuit does not find the true projection space in this data because the method always measures the difference from the normal distribution.

In terms of computation time, the Hall-type relative projection index takes much longer to optimize than the Hall projection index. One reason is that the Hall-type relative projection index deals with a larger sample than the Hall-index, since it performs calculations on the reference data. Another reason is that the Hall-type relative projection index estimates the density function of reference data set, which is time-intensive, although the Hall index uses the analytic form of the normal density function. But modern computers are sufficiently fast that this difference is not very important—the difference in runtime is about 1 minute for Hall's method versus 20 minutes for RPP.

Actual Data

To apply the method to real data, we use the Faculty Salary Data collected by the American Association of University Professors (AAUP, 1994). The data are from an annual faculty salary survey of American colleges and universities. The number of variables reported is 13 and the data size is 1161. Table2 describes the variables used in the analysis.

We now apply relative projection pursuit to the data of Type I (Doctoral-Level Institutions). In this example, we search for 'interesting' two-dimensional projection direction spaces of the data of Type I. We use the 10 variables $x_1, \ldots, x_{10}$ shown in the Table 2 as the explanatory variables and we define the data set of all types of universities and colleges as the reference data set. Observations which include missing data are deleted and so we have 1074 observations from the original survey of 1161 institutions.

Result

Now consider what 'interesting' structure is detected. We display four scatterplots that show the distributions in the estimated projection direction space using RPP (Fig. 3).

A coordinate of each of the scatterplots in Fig. 3 is $(x, y) = (\boldsymbol{\alpha}_1{}^{\mathrm{T}} X, \boldsymbol{\alpha}_2{}^{\mathrm{T}} X)$ where X is the sample. First, we try to interpret what projection vectors $\boldsymbol{\alpha}_1, \boldsymbol{\alpha}_2$ represent. From Table 3, the estimate of $\boldsymbol{\alpha}_1$, has components $a_4 = 0.358$ and $a_7 = 0.833$ that are larger than the other components. Since these elements are the weights on Average Compensation of Full Professors and Number of Full Professors, respectively, we guess the vector $\boldsymbol{\alpha}_1$

Table 2. Variables in AAUP Faculty Salary Data. The variable Type in the fourth line has three values: Type I is a Doctoral-Level Institution, Type IIA is a Comprehensive Institution, and TypeIIB is a General Baccalaureate Institution.

name of variable	meaning of variable
FICE	FICE (Federal ID number)
College.name	College name
State	State (postal code)
Type	Type (I, IIA, or IIB)
x_1	Average salary - full professors
x_2	Average salary - associate professors
x_3	Average salary - assistant professors
x_4	Average compensation - full professors
x_5	Average compensation - associate professors
x_6	Average compensation - assistant professors
x_7	Number of full professors
x_8	Number of associate professors
x_9	Number of assistant professors
x_{10}	Number of instructors

represents the treatment of full professors. And for $\boldsymbol{\alpha}_2$, the components $a_4 = 0.642, a_5 = 0.328, a_7 = -0.414$ and $a_9 = -0.400$ are larger than the other elements. These put weight on Average Compensation of Full Professors, Average Compensation of Associate Professors, the Number of Full Professors, and the Number of Assistant Professors, respectively. We guess that $\boldsymbol{\alpha}_2$ provides a general sense of the salary at the universities and colleges.

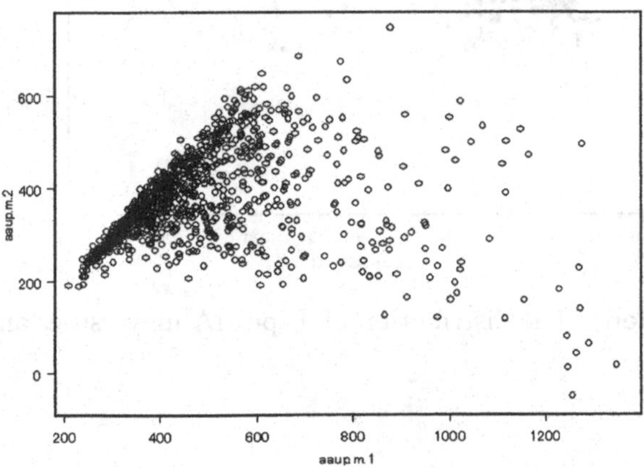

Fig. 3. The scatterplots of the projections obtained in the estimated projection direction space. The distribution of reference data set (all type universities and colleges).

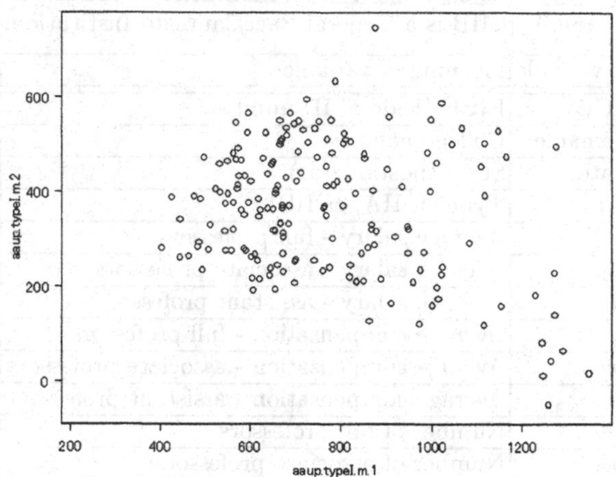

Fig. 3 (continued). The distribution of target data set (Type I universities and colleges).

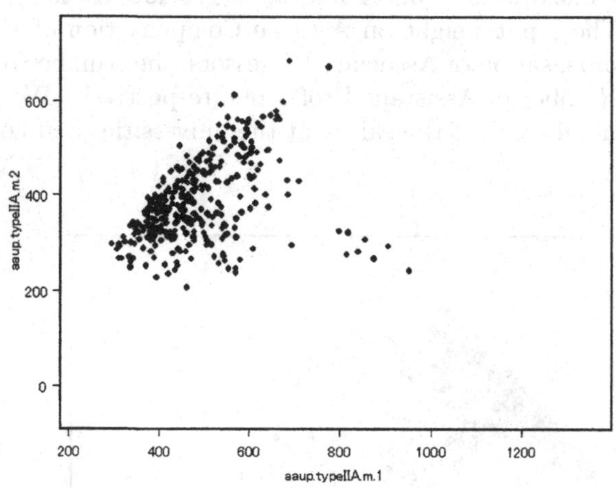

Fig. 3 (continued). The distribution of Type IIA universities and colleges.

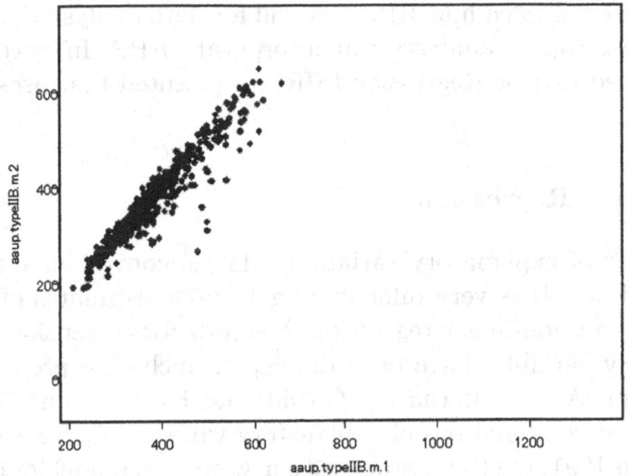

Fig. 3 (continued). The distribution of Type IIB universities and colleges.

Table 3 shows the projection vectors which are estimated with the 2-dimensional Hall-type relative projection index. The space generated the estimated values of α_1 and α_2 is the one that finds the most difference between the distributions of Type I universities (Doctoral-Level Institutions) and the distribution of all types of universities and colleges (Types I, IIA, and IIB).

Table 3. The result of relative projection pursuit with the 2-dimensional Hall-type relative projection index.

vector	elements of projection vector $(a_1, a_2, a_3, a_4, a_5, a_6, a_7, a_8, a_9, a_{10})$
α_1	$(0.216, -0.003, -0.027, 0.358, 0.135, -0.022, 0.883, -0.029, -0.098, -0.121)$
α_2	$(0.164, -0.207, -0.181, 0.642, 0.328, -0.197, -0.414, 0.049, -0.400, -0.072)$

If we take account of the interpretation of α_1 and α_2, we see from the scatterplots in Fig. 3 that universities and colleges of Type I (Doctoral-Level Institutions) do not have a strong relation between α_1 and α_2 as compared with the distribution of all type universities and colleges. In the scatterplot of Type IIB universities and colleges, we see positive correlation between α_1 and α_2, which indicates that the treatment of full professors and general faculty is associated. In the Type I universities, many universities pay full professors well and also employ many full professors, even if the scale of the university is small. In fact, doctoral-level universities and colleges hire notable professors at a large salary irrespective of the scale.

We can find the above 'interesting' structure from the distribution of samples in estimated projection direction space. Conventional projection pursuit cannot find this structure.

4 Application of Relative Projection Pursuit

The previous section showed how RPP is useful for data analysis. This section shows that more complex analyses can incorporate RPP. In particular, an algorithm for Sliced Inverse Regression (SIR) is presented that uses RPP; we call it SIRrpp.

4.1 Sliced Inverse Regression

When the number of explanatory variables is large, conventional regression analysis breaks down. It is very difficult to get stable estimates of the coefficients, especially in non-linear regression. Methods for dimension reduction of the explanatory variables have been developed, including projection pursuit regression and ACE (Alternating Conditional Expectation). These two methods find linear combinations of explanatory variables under a special regression model. In 1991, Li (1991) proposed a new general model for dimension reduction called the SIR model (Sliced Inverse Regression); it assumes:

$$y = f(\boldsymbol{\beta}_1^T \mathbf{x}, \boldsymbol{\beta}_2^T \mathbf{x}, \ldots, \boldsymbol{\beta}_K^T \mathbf{x}, \varepsilon),$$

where $\mathbf{x}$ is the vector of p explanatory variables, $\boldsymbol{\beta}_k$, $k = 1, ldots, K$ are unknown vectors, ε is independent of $\mathbf{x}$, and f is an arbitrary unknown function on $\mathbf{R}^{K+1}$. The purpose of SIR is to estimate the vectors $\boldsymbol{\beta}_k$ when this model holds. If we can estimate the $\boldsymbol{\beta}_k$ vectors, then we can reduce the dimension of $\mathbf{x}$ to K. Hereafter, we shall refer to any linear combination of the $\boldsymbol{\beta}_k$ vectors as effective dimension reduction (e.d.r.) direction.

Li developed an algorithm called SIR1 to derive the e.d.r. directions. When the distribution of $\mathbf{X}$ is elliptically symmetric, the centered inverse regression $E[\mathbf{X}|y] - E[\mathbf{X}]$ is contained in the linear subspace spanned by $\boldsymbol{\beta}_k^T \Sigma_{XX}$, $k = 1, \ldots, K$, where Σ_{XX} denotes the covariance matrix of $\mathbf{X}$. The SIR1 algorithm for the data $(y_i, \mathbf{x}_i)$, $i = 1, \ldots, n$, is:.

SIR1 algorithm

1. Sphere $\mathbf{X}$: $\tilde{\mathbf{x}}_i = \hat{\Sigma}_{\mathbf{xx}}^{-1/2}(\mathbf{x}_i - \bar{\mathbf{x}})$ for $i = 1, \ldots, n$, where $\hat{\Sigma}_{\mathbf{xx}}$ is the sample covariance matrix and $\bar{\mathbf{x}}$ is the sample mean.
2. Divide range of y into H slices, $I_1, \ldots, I_H$; let the proportion of the y_i that falls in slice h be $\hat{p}_h$.
3. Within each slice, compute the sample mean of the $\tilde{\mathbf{x}}_i$ observations, and denote these by $\hat{\mathbf{m}}_h$, so $\hat{\mathbf{m}}_h = n\hat{p}_h{}^{-1} \sum_{y_i \in I_h} \tilde{\mathbf{x}}_i$.
4. Conduct a (weighted) principal component analysis for the data $\hat{\mathbf{m}}_h$ in the following way: form the weighted covariance matrix $\hat{V} = \sum_{h=1}^{H} \hat{p}_h \hat{\mathbf{m}}_h \hat{\mathbf{m}}_h^T$, then find the eigenvalues and the eigenvectors for $\hat{V}$.
5. Let the K largest eigenvectors of $\hat{V}$ be $\hat{\boldsymbol{\eta}}_k$, $k = 1, \ldots, K$. Output $\hat{\boldsymbol{\beta}}_k = \hat{\Sigma}_{\mathbf{xx}}^{-1/2} \hat{\boldsymbol{\eta}}_k$ $(k = 1, 2, \cdots, K)$ for the estimated of e.d.r. directions.

The main idea of SIR1 is to use $E[\mathbf{X}|y]$. The $E[\mathbf{X}|y]$ is contained in the space spanned by the e.d.r. directions, but there is no guarantee that the $E[\mathbf{X}|y]$ span the space. To address this, Li also proposed another algorithm, called SIR2, that uses $\mathrm{Cov}[\mathbf{X}|y]$.

4.2 Sliced Inverse Regression with Projection Pursuit

Mizuta (1999) proposed an algorithm for the SIR model using projection pursuit (SIRpp). SIRpp uses the conditional distribution $X|y$, as follows:

SIRpp Algorithm

1. Same as Step 1 of SIR1 algorithm.
2. Same as Step 2 of SIR1 algorithm.
3. Conduct projection pursuit in the K dimensional space for each slice. We get H projections: $(\boldsymbol{\alpha}_1^{(h)}, \ldots, \boldsymbol{\alpha}_K^{(h)})$, $h = 1, \ldots, H$.
4. Let the K largest eigenvectors of $\hat{V}$ be $\hat{\boldsymbol{\eta}}_k$, $k = 1, \ldots, K$. Output

$$\hat{\boldsymbol{\beta}}_k = \hat{\Sigma}_{\mathbf{xx}}^{-1/2} \hat{\boldsymbol{\eta}}_k \quad k = 1, 2, \ldots, K$$

for estimates of the e.d.r. directions, where

$$\hat{V} = \sum_{h=1}^{H} w(h) \sum_{k=1}^{K} \boldsymbol{\alpha}_k^{(h)} \boldsymbol{\alpha}_k^{(h)T}$$

and $w(h)$ is a weight determined by the size of the slice and the projection pursuit index.

Steps 1 and 2 are the same as those of SIR1. The H projections in Step 3 are regarded as e.d.r. directions on the coordinates of $\tilde{\mathbf{X}}$. We get H projections and combine them into $\hat{V}$ in Step 4; this is similar to a singular value decomposition.

4.3 Sliced Inverse Regression with Relative Projection Pursuit

We can construct a new SIR algorithm with relative projection pursuit; we call this SIRrpp. The algorithm for SIRrpp is almost the same as for SIRpp except in Step 3.

SIRrpp Algorithm

1. Same as Step 1 of SIRpp algorithm.
2. Same as Step 2 of SIRpp algorithm.
3. Assign the whole dataset to the reference dataset and assign each slice in turn, which is a subset of whole dataset, to the target dataset. Conduct a relative projection pursuit in K dimensional space for each slice. We get H projections $(\boldsymbol{\alpha}_1^{(h)}, \cdots, \boldsymbol{\alpha}_K^{(h)})$.

4. Same as Step 4 of SIRpp algorithm.

Note that we do not make assumptions about the distribution of the explanatory variables.

We evaluate the SIRrpp algorithm on $n = 1000$ independent simulated observations $\mathbf{x} \in \mathbb{R}^{10}$. The functional relationship is

$$y = \sin(x_1) + \cos(x_2) + \varepsilon$$

so eight components of the observations are irrelevant. In the simulation, each component of $\mathbf{x}$ is independent and drawn from a mixture normal, $(.5)N(-1.5,(0.5)^2)+(.5)N(1.5,(0.5)^2)$. And ε is $N(0,0.2^2)$ and independent of the $\mathbf{x}$. In this framework, the ideal e.d.r. directions are contained in the space spanned by two vectors: $(1,0,0,0,0,0,0,0,0,0)$ and $(0,1,0,0,0,0,0,0,0,0)$.

Table 4 shows the results of relative projection pursuit on each slice of the data. All projections are practically e.d.r. directions: $(\alpha,\beta,0,0,0,0,0,0,0,0)$, and $\alpha^2+\beta^2=1$. In Step 4 of the SIRrpp algorithm, we get these eigenvalues of $\hat{V}$: 1.04, 0.63 0.50, 0.34, 0.18, 0.15, 0.09,0.017, 0.003, 0. The first and second eigenvalues are large and the rest are almost zero. The first and second eigenvectors of $\hat{V}$ are almost perfect:

(-0.9678,-0.1512,0.0170,0.0138,0.0094,0.1596, -0.1140,0.0073,0.0253,0.0251)
(0.1515,-0.9115,-0.1860,-0.0933,-0.2699,0.1293,0.0654,0.0170,0.0083,0.0931).

Table 4. Result of SIRrpp.

slices	projections
slice 1	(0.83,-0.36,-0.13,-0.06,0.07,0.23,-0.08,-0.21,0.07,0.22)
	(0.55,0.51,0.16,0.19,-0.01,-0.29,0.04,0.35,-0.15,-0.38)
slice 2	(0.99,0.02,0.05,-0.03,0.01,0.02,-0.002,-0.06,0.02,0.08)
	(-0.09,0.39,0.09,-0.36,-0.17,0.02,0.28,-0.44,0.48,0.41)
slice 3	(0.54,0.69,-0.02,0.03,0.48,0.03,-0.03,0.04,-0.02,-0.003)
	(-0.29,-0.37,0.08,-0.05,0.87,-0.04,-0.002,0.05,0.05,-0.03)
slice 4	(0.71,-0.07,-0.05,-0.13,-0.02,0.08,0.67,-0.06,-0.03,-0.10)
	(0.01,0.67,0.04,0.61,0.34,0.04,0.19,0.05,-0.15,0.02)
slice 5	(0.65,-0.25,-0.14,0.11,-0.08,-0.68,0.07,0.13,-0.03,0.02)
	(0.21,0.63,0.24,-0.39,0.27,-0.27,-0.18,-0.40,0.13,0.01)

5 Concluding Remarks

In this paper, we propose relative projection pursuit and SIRrpp. This extends previous work by allowing the researcher to propose models for uninteresting projection directions that are different from those whose projected distributions are approximately normal. This is useful when the search for a direction in which the projected distribution of a subset of the variables is different from the distribution of the entire data. This is the basic idea of relative projection pursuit, and we have developed SIRrpp as an application of this idea. There are many ways to adapt relative projection pursuit to other kinds of data analysis.

Mizuta and Minami (2000) have derived the conditional distribution $\mathbf{X}|y$ under the SIR model and have shown that SIRpp is able to derive e.d.r. directions when the distribution of $\mathbf{X}$ is normal. It may be that a similar result holds for SIRrpp when the conditional distribution of $\mathbf{X}$ is not normal.

References

1. AAUP (1994). Faculty Salary Data. `http://lib.stat.cmu.edu/index.php`.
2. Diaconis, P., Freedman, D. (1984). "Asymptotics of Graphical Projection Pursuit," *Annals of Statistics*, **12**, 793–815.
3. Friedman, J.H. (1987). Exploratory projection pursuit. *Journal of the American Statistical Association*, No.82, 249–266.
4. Friedman, J.H., Tukey, J.W. (1974). "A Projection Pursuit Algorithm for Exploratory Data Analysis," *IEEE Transactions on Computation*, C-23, **9**, 881–890.
5. Hall, P. (1989). "On Polynomial-Based Projection Indices for Exploratory Projection Pursuit," *Annals of Statistics*, **17**, 589–605.
6. Jones, M.C., Sibson, R. (1987). "What is projection pursuit?" (with discussion), *Journal of the Royal Statistical Society, Series A*, **150**, 1–36.
7. Li, K.-C.. (1991). "Sliced Inverse Regression for Dimension Reduction," *Journal of the American Statistical Association*, **86**, 316–327 .
8. Mizuta, M. (1999). "Sliced Inverse Regression with Projection Pursuit," in *Applied Stochastic Models and Data Analysis*, eds. H. Bacelar-Nicolau, F. C. Nicolau, and J. Janssen, J., Berlin:Springer, pp. 51–56.
9. Mizuta, M. (2002). "Relative Projection Pursuit," in *Data Analysis, Classification, and Related Methods*, eds. K. Jajuga, A. Sokolowski, and H.-H. Bock, Berlin:Springer, pp. 122-130.
10. Mizuta, M., Minami, H. (2000). "An Algorithm with Projection Pursuit for Sliced Inverse Regression Model," in *Data Analysis, Classification, and Related Methods*, eds. H. A. L. Kiers, J.-P. Rasson, P. Groenen, M. Schader, Berlin:Springer, pp. 255–260.
11. Scott, D.W. (1992). *Multivariate Density Estimation*, Wiley, New York.

Priors for Neural Networks

Herbert K. H. Lee

University of California at Santa Cruz, USA
herbie@ams.ucsc.edu

Abstract: Neural networks are commonly used for classification and regression. The Bayesian approach may be employed, but choosing a prior for the parameters presents challenges. This paper reviews several priors in the literature and introduces Jeffreys priors for neural network models. The effect on the posterior is demonstrated through an example.

1 Introduction

Neural networks are a popular tool for nonparametric classification and regression. They offer a computationally tractable model that is fully flexible, in the sense of being able to approximate a wide range of functions (such as all continuous functions). Many references on neural networks are available (Bishop, 1995, Fine, 1999, and Ripley, 1996). The Bayesian approach is appealing as it allows full accounting for uncertainty in the model and the choice of model (Lee, 2001 and Neal, 1996). An important decision in any Bayesian analysis is the choice of prior. The idea is that your prior should reflect your current beliefs (either from previous data or from purely subjective sources) about the parameters before you have observed the data. This task turns out to be rather difficult for a neural network, because in most cases the parameters have no interpretable meaning, merely being coefficients in a basis expansion (a neural network can be viewed as using an infinite set of location-scale logistic functions to span the space of continuous functions). The model for neural network regression is:

$$y_i = \beta_0 + \sum_{j=1}^{k} \beta_j \frac{1}{1+\exp\left(-\gamma_{j0} - \sum_{h=1}^{r} \gamma_{jh} x_{ih}\right)} + \varepsilon_i \,,$$

where k is the number of logistic basis functions (hidden nodes), r is the number of explanatory variables (inputs), and ε_i are i.i.d. Gaussian error. The parameters of this model are k (the number of hidden nodes), β_j

for $j \in \{0, \ldots, k\}$ (linear coefficients for the basis functions), and γ_{jh} for $j \in \{1, \ldots, k\}$, $h \in \{0, \ldots, r\}$ (location-scale parameters to create the basis functions). For a classification problem, the fitted values from the neural network are transformed into a multinomial likelihood via the softmax function, i.e., $p_{ig} = \exp(\hat{y}_{ig}) / \sum_{h=1}^{q} \exp(\hat{y}_{ih})$, where g indexes the q possible categories, $g \in \{1, \ldots, q\}$.

In general, the parameters of a neural network have no intuitive interpretations, as they are merely coefficients of a basis expansion. Lee (2003) provides a discussion of the few specific cases when the parameters have physical meaning, as well as graphic example of how the parameters become uninterpretable in even the simplest situations. Another example of interpretation difficulties can be found in Robinson (2001). He provides an example (pp. 19–20) of two fitted three-node neural networks which give very similar fitted curves, yet have completely different parameter values. We again see that there is no clear link between parameter values and their interpretations.

This paper will review a variety of proposals for neural network priors, introduce Jeffreys priors, and provide an example comparing these priors.

2 Proper Priors

A common class of priors in the literature for neural networks are hierarchical proper priors. A *proper* prior is one that is a valid probability distribution, putting probability one on the whole domain of the distribution. The alternative is an *improper* prior as discussed in the next section. Hierarchical priors are useful for neural networks because of the lack of interpretability of the parameters. Adding levels to the hierarchy reduces the influence of the choice made at the top level, so the resulting prior at the bottom level (the original parameters) will be more diffuse, more closely matching the lack of available information about the parameters themselves. This approach can let the data have more influence on the posterior.

Müller and Rios Insua (1998) proposed a three-stage hierarchical model with a relatively simple structure. Prior distributions are chosen to be conditionally conjugate. A tool for visualizing a hierarchical prior is a directed acyclic graph (DAG), where the arrows show the flow of dependency. For this model, the DAG is shown in Figure 1. The priors are Gaussian for β_j and μ_β, multivariate Gaussian for $\boldsymbol{\gamma}_j$ and $\boldsymbol{\mu}_\gamma$, inverse-gamma for σ^2 and σ_β^2, and inverse-Wishart for $\mathbf{S}_\gamma$.

Neal (1996) suggests a more complex model. The DAG diagram of his prior is shown in Figure 2. Each of the network parameters (β_j and γ_{jh}) is treated as a Gaussian with mean zero and its own standard deviation which is the product of two hyperparameters, one for the originating node of the link in the graph, and one for the destination node. For example, the weight for the first input to the first hidden node, γ_{11}, has distribution $N(0, \sigma_{in,1} * \sigma_{a,1})$, where $\sigma_{in,h}$ is the term for the links from the hth input and $\sigma_{a,j}$ is the term for the

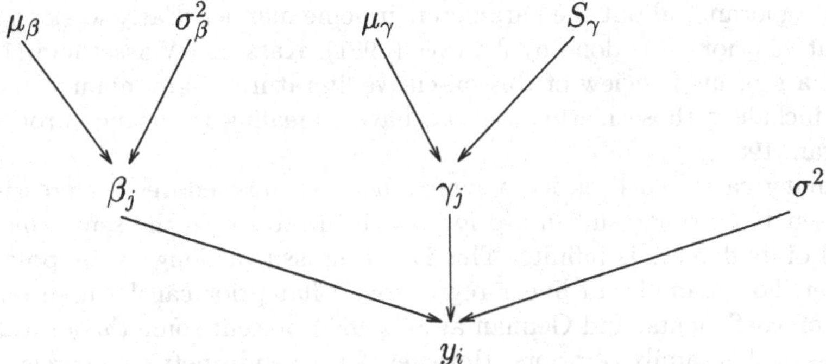

Fig. 1. DAG for the Müller and Rios Insua prior

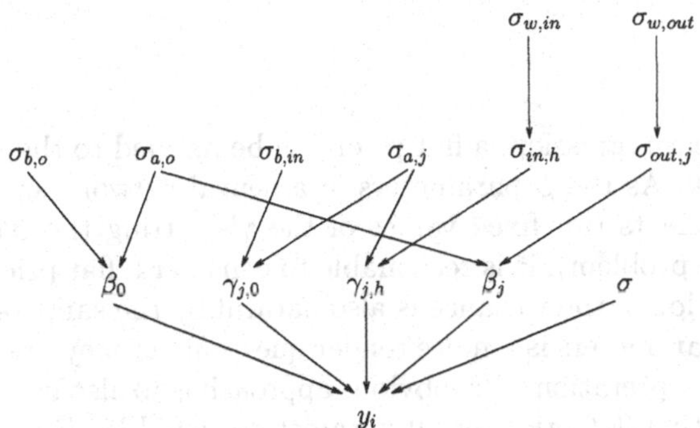

Fig. 2. DAG for the Neal prior

links into the jth hidden node; the weight from the first hidden node to the output (i.e. the regression coefficient), β_1, has distribution $N(0, \sigma_{out,1} * \sigma_o)$, where $\sigma_{out,j}$ is the term for the links from the jth hidden node, and σ_o is the term for links to the output node. For all of the new σ parameters and for the original σ of the error term, there is an inverse-gamma distribution. There is another set of hyperparameters that must be specified for the inverse-gamma priors on these σ parameters.

3 Noninformative Priors

As was demonstrated in Lee (2003), the parameters of a neural network are typically not interpretable. This makes choosing an informative prior difficult. The previous section introduced various hierarchical priors defined to be proper, yet an attempt was made to let them be diffuse enough that they do not contain too much information, since one would not want to use a highly informative prior that may not come close to one's actual beliefs, or lack thereof. An alternative approach is to use a noninformative prior, one that attempts to quantify ignorance about the parameters in some manner. Early work on noninformative priors was done by Jeffreys (1961). Kass and Wasserman (1996) provide a thorough review of this extensive literature. Many noninformative priors, including those in this section, have appealing invariance properties (Hartigan, 1964).

In many cases, such as for a neural network, procedures for creating a noninformative prior result in a prior that is improper, in the sense that the integral of its density is infinite. This is not an issue as long as the posterior is proper. For example, in linear regression, a flat prior can be used on the regression coefficients, and Gelman at al. (1995) present some theoretical advantages of this family of priors. However, for a neural network, careless use of improper priors will result in an improper posterior, so measures will need to be taken to prevent this problem.

3.1 Flat Priors

Just as with linear regression, a flat prior can be applied to the parameters of a neural network. As the β parameters of a neural network are analogous to regression coefficients (for fixed values of the γ's, fitting the β's is exactly a linear regression problem), it is reasonable to consider a flat prior for them. A flat prior on the log of the variance is also natural by the same reasoning. The prior for the γ parameters is a more tender question, as they are the ones that are lacking in interpretation. One obvious approach is to also use a flat prior for them. The resulting flat prior for all parameters would be $P(\boldsymbol{\gamma}, \boldsymbol{\beta}, \sigma^2) \propto \sigma^{-2}$. Since the prior is improper, the normalizing constant is arbitrary. A major problem with this prior is that it leads to an improper posterior. There are two ways in which things can go wrong: linear independence and tail behavior (Lee, 2003). Some additional notation is necessary. Denote the basis functions evaluated at the data points (i.e., the outputs of the hidden layer) as

$$\Gamma_{ij} = \left[1 + \exp\left(-\gamma_{j0} - \sum_{h=1}^{r} \gamma_{jh} x_{ih}\right)\right]^{-1} \tag{1}$$

with $\Gamma_{i0} = 1$ and let $\boldsymbol{\Gamma}$ be the matrix with elements (z_{ij}). Thus the fitting of the vector $\boldsymbol{\beta}$ is a least-squares regression on the design matrix $\boldsymbol{\Gamma}$, $\hat{\mathbf{y}} = \boldsymbol{\Gamma}^t \boldsymbol{\beta}$.

To understand the linear independence problem, consider the linear regression parallel. When using the standard noninformative prior for linear regression, the posterior will be proper as long as the design matrix is full rank (its columns are linearly independent). For a neural network, we need the k logistic basis functions to be linearly independent, i.e., we need $\boldsymbol{\Gamma}$ to be full rank. A straightforward way to ensure linear independence is to require that the determinant of $\boldsymbol{\Gamma}^t \boldsymbol{\Gamma}$ is positive.

The second possible problem is that unlike in most problems, the likelihood does not necessarily go to zero in the tails, converging to non-zero constants in some infinite regions. If the tails of the prior also do not go to zero, the posterior will not have a finite integral. An obvious way to avoid this problem is to bound the parameter space for γ. It is worth noting that truncating the parameter space tends to not have much impact on the posterior, as the fitted functions being eliminated are numerically indistinguishable (in double precision) from those in the valid range of the parameter space.

Thus instead of using the flat prior introduced above, a restricted flat prior should be used:

$$P(\gamma, \boldsymbol{\beta}, \sigma^2) \propto \frac{1}{\sigma^2} \mathrm{I}_{\{(\gamma, \boldsymbol{\beta}, \sigma^2) \in \boldsymbol{\Omega}\}}$$

where $\mathrm{I}_{\{\}}$ is an indicator function, and $\boldsymbol{\Omega}$ is the parameter space restricted such that $\left|\boldsymbol{\Gamma}^T \boldsymbol{\Gamma}\right| > C$ and $|\gamma_{jh}| < D$ for all j, h, where $C > 0$ and $D > 0$ are constants with C small and D large. Lee (2003) shows that this restricted flat prior guarantees a proper posterior, as well as showing that the "interesting" parts of the parameter space are the same under the restricted and unrestricted priors, and thus the posteriors are essentially the same, in the sense that they are both asymptotically globally and locally equivalent.

3.2 Jeffreys Priors

Flat priors are not without drawbacks. In particular, if the problem is re-parameterized using a non-linear transformation of the parameters, then the same transformation applied to the prior will result in something other than a flat prior. Jeffreys (1961) introduced a rule for generating a prior that is invariant to differentiable one-to-one transformations of the parameters. The Jeffreys prior is the square root of the determinant of the Fisher information matrix:

$$P_J(\boldsymbol{\theta}) = \sqrt{|I(\boldsymbol{\theta})|} \tag{2}$$

where the Fisher information matrix, $I(\boldsymbol{\theta})$, has elements

$$I_{ij}(\boldsymbol{\theta}) = \mathrm{Cov}_{\boldsymbol{\theta}} \left[\left(\frac{\partial}{\partial \theta_i} \log f(\mathbf{y}|\boldsymbol{\theta}) \right) \left(\frac{\partial}{\partial \theta_j} \log f(\mathbf{y}|\boldsymbol{\theta}) \right) \right] \tag{3}$$

where $f(\mathbf{Y}|\boldsymbol{\theta})$ is the likelihood and the expectation is over $\mathbf{Y}$ for fixed $\boldsymbol{\theta}$. Often the Jeffreys prior is intuitively reasonable and leads to a proper posterior. Occasionally the prior may fail to produce a reasonable or even proper posterior (e.g., Berger et al., 2001 and Jeffreys, 1961), which also turns out to be the case for a neural network.

Jeffreys (1961) argued that it is often better to treat classes of parameters as independent, and compute the priors independently (treating parameters from other classes as fixed). To distinguish this approach from the previous one which treated all parameters collectively, the collective prior (Equation 2) is referred to as the *Jeffreys-rule prior*. In contrast, the *independence Jeffreys prior* (denoted P_{IJ}) is the product of the Jeffreys-rule priors for each class of parameters independently, while treating the other parameters as fixed. In the case of a neural network, separate Jeffreys-rule priors would be computed for each of γ, β, and σ^2, and the independence Jeffreys prior is the product of these separate priors.

The next step is to compute the Fisher information matrix. We shall consider only univariate regression predictions here, but these results are readily extended to a multivariate regression or classification scenario. For notational and conceptual simplicity, it is easier to work with the precision, $\tau = \frac{1}{\sigma^2}$, the reciprocal of the variance. Thus our parameter vector is $\boldsymbol{\theta} = (\boldsymbol{\gamma}, \boldsymbol{\beta}, \tau)$ and the full likelihood is

$$f(\mathbf{y}|\boldsymbol{\theta}) = f(\mathbf{y}|\mathbf{x}, \boldsymbol{\gamma}, \boldsymbol{\beta}, \tau) = (2\pi)^{-n/2}\tau^{n/2} \exp\left\{-\frac{\tau}{2}(\mathbf{y} - \boldsymbol{\Gamma}^t\boldsymbol{\beta})^t(\mathbf{y} - \boldsymbol{\Gamma}^t\boldsymbol{\beta})\right\},$$

where $\boldsymbol{\Gamma}$ is as defined in Equation (1). The loglikelihood, without the normalizing constant, is

$$\log f = \frac{n}{2}\log\tau - \frac{\tau}{2}(\mathbf{y} - \boldsymbol{\Gamma}^t\boldsymbol{\beta})^t(\mathbf{y} - \boldsymbol{\Gamma}^t\boldsymbol{\beta}).$$

The individual elements of the information matrix are given by Equation (3), and it is straightforward to show that:

$$Cov_{\boldsymbol{\theta}}\left(\frac{\partial}{\partial\beta_j}\log f(\mathbf{y}|\boldsymbol{\theta}), \frac{\partial}{\partial\beta_g}\log f(\mathbf{y}|\boldsymbol{\theta})\right) = \tau\sum_{i=1}^{n}\Gamma_{ij}\Gamma_{ig}$$

$$Cov_{\boldsymbol{\theta}}\left(\frac{\partial}{\partial\beta_j}\log f(\mathbf{y}|\boldsymbol{\theta}), \frac{\partial}{\partial\gamma_{gh}}\log f(\mathbf{y}|\boldsymbol{\theta})\right) = \tau\beta_g\sum_{i=1}^{n}x_{ih}\Gamma_{ij}\Gamma_{ig}(1-\Gamma_{ig})$$

$$Cov_{\boldsymbol{\theta}}\left(\frac{\partial}{\partial\gamma_{jh}}\log f(\mathbf{y}|\boldsymbol{\theta}), \frac{\partial}{\partial\gamma_{gl}}\log f(\mathbf{y}|\boldsymbol{\theta})\right) =$$

$$\tau\beta_j\beta_g\sum_{i=1}^{n}x_{ih}x_{il}\Gamma_{ij}(1-\Gamma_{ij})\Gamma_{ig}(1-\Gamma_{ig})$$

$$Cov_{\boldsymbol{\theta}}\left(\frac{\partial}{\partial\beta_j}\log f(\mathbf{y}|\boldsymbol{\theta}), \frac{\partial}{\partial\tau}\log f(\mathbf{y}|\boldsymbol{\theta})\right) = 0$$

$$Cov_{\boldsymbol{\theta}}\left(\frac{\partial}{\partial\gamma_{jh}}\log f(\mathbf{y}|\boldsymbol{\theta}), \frac{\partial}{\partial\tau}\log f(\mathbf{y}|\boldsymbol{\theta})\right) = 0$$

$$Var_{\boldsymbol{\theta}}\left(\frac{\partial}{\partial\tau}\log f(\mathbf{y}|\boldsymbol{\theta})\right) = \frac{n}{2\tau^2}.$$

To combine these into the matrix $I(\boldsymbol{\theta})$, the exact ordering of parameters within $\boldsymbol{\theta} = (\boldsymbol{\gamma}, \boldsymbol{\beta}, \tau)$ must be specified. The $\boldsymbol{\beta}$ section of $k+1$ elements are $(\beta_0, \dots, \beta_k)$ and the final element is τ, but $\boldsymbol{\gamma}$ is a matrix. In the presentation here, it appears as row-order, so that

$$\boldsymbol{\gamma} = (\gamma_{10}, \gamma_{11}, \gamma_{12}, \dots, \gamma_{1r}, \gamma_{20}, \gamma_{21}, \dots, \gamma_{2r}, \gamma_{30}, \gamma_{31}, \dots).$$

Now define the n x $(r+1)\,k$ matrix $\mathbf{G}$ to have elements $G_{ij} = \beta_g x_{ih}\Gamma_{ig}(1-\Gamma_{ig})$ where g is the integer part of $\frac{j}{r+1}$ and h is the remainder, i.e., $h = j-(r+1)*g$. With this notation, the full Fisher information matrix is

$$I(\boldsymbol{\theta}) = \begin{bmatrix} \tau \mathbf{G}^t\mathbf{G} & \tau \mathbf{G}^t\boldsymbol{\Gamma} & 0 \\ \tau \boldsymbol{\Gamma}^t\mathbf{G} & \tau \boldsymbol{\Gamma}^t\boldsymbol{\Gamma} & 0 \\ 0 & 0 & \frac{n}{2\tau^2} \end{bmatrix}.$$

Thus the Jeffreys-rule prior is

$$P_J(\boldsymbol{\theta}) \propto \tau^{((r+2)k-1)/2} \begin{vmatrix} \mathbf{G}^t\mathbf{G} & \mathbf{G}^t\boldsymbol{\Gamma} \\ \boldsymbol{\Gamma}^t\mathbf{G} & \boldsymbol{\Gamma}^t\boldsymbol{\Gamma} \end{vmatrix}^{1/2}.$$

The prior is stated as a proportionality because any constants are irrelevant since the prior is improper. The large power on τ seems rather odd, and so Jeffreys would probably recommend the independence prior instead, as this situation is similar to the linear regression setting where analogous problems occur with the prior for the precision. The independence Jeffreys prior is simpler in form, as the Jeffreys-rule prior for $\boldsymbol{\beta}$ with other parameters fixed is a flat prior.

$$P_{IJ}(\boldsymbol{\theta}) \propto \frac{1}{\tau} \left|\mathbf{F}^t\mathbf{F}\right|^{1/2},$$

where $\mathbf{F}$ is just $\mathbf{G}$ without any of the β_g terms, i.e., $F_{ij} = x_{ih}\Gamma_{ig}(1 - \Gamma_{ig})$ where g is the integer part of $\frac{j}{r+1}$ and h is the remainder. It is unfortunate that both of these priors are improper, and both lead to improper posteriors. For any particular dataset, it is possible to construct an infinite region of the γ space such that all of the entries of $\boldsymbol{\Gamma}$ are nonnegative and its columns are linearly independent. Thus $\left|\boldsymbol{\Gamma}^t\boldsymbol{\Gamma}\right| > 0$ over this infinite region, so the integral of $\left|\boldsymbol{\Gamma}^t\boldsymbol{\Gamma}\right|$ over the whole parameter space will be infinite. This same region of the parameter space also leads to strictly positive $|\mathbf{F}^t\mathbf{F}|$ and $\begin{vmatrix} \mathbf{G}^t\mathbf{G} & \mathbf{G}^t\boldsymbol{\Gamma} \\ \boldsymbol{\Gamma}^t\mathbf{G} & \boldsymbol{\Gamma}^t\boldsymbol{\Gamma} \end{vmatrix}$. One can also find ranges of $\boldsymbol{\beta}$ so that the likelihood is larger than some positive constant over this same region of the $\boldsymbol{\gamma}$ parameter space. Thus the posterior will also be improper, for both the Jeffreys-rule prior and the independence Jeffreys prior. As with the flat prior, this can be worked around by suitably truncating the parameter space.

4 Hybrid Priors

Some of the priors proposed in the literature combine elements of proper priors and noninformative priors. A basic prior for a neural network would be to combine the noninformative priors for $\boldsymbol{\beta}$ and σ^2 with independent normal priors for each γ_{jh}, i.e., $P(\boldsymbol{\beta}) \propto 1$, $P(\sigma^2) \propto \frac{1}{\sigma^2}$, $P(\gamma_{jh}) \sim N(0, \nu)$. This prior gives a proper posterior, and it is notable because it is equivalent to using *weight decay*, a popular (non-Bayesian) method in machine learning for reducing overfitting. The usual specification of weight decay is as penalized maximum likelihood, where there is a penalty of $||\gamma_j||/\nu$ for each of the hidden nodes. Thus instead of maximizing only the likelihood $f(\mathbf{y}|\boldsymbol{\theta})$, one might maximize $f(\mathbf{y}|\boldsymbol{\theta}) - \sum_j \sum_h \gamma_{jh}^2/\nu$, which results in shrinkage of the parameters toward zero. The β_j parameters could also be shrunk if desired. Of course, the choice of ν is important, and various rules of thumb have been developed. Just as with ridge regression, this penalized maximum likelihood approach is equivalent to using a simple prior in a Bayesian context.

Robinson (2001, 2001b) proposes priors for parsimony on an effective domain of interest. He starts with the basic weight decay prior above, adds one level of hierarchy, putting an inverse-gamma prior with parameters a and b on ν, and then notes that ν can be integrated out leaving the marginal prior distribution for γ_j as a multivariate t, i.e., $P(\gamma_j) \propto \left(1 + b^{-1}||\gamma_j||^2\right)^{-(a+r)/2}$. Parsimony is then imposed either through orthogonality or additivity by adding appropriate penalty terms to the prior.

MacKay (1992) takes an empirical Bayes approach. Starting with a simple two-stage hierarchical model, he attempts to use flat and improper priors at the top level. Since this would lead to an improper posterior, he uses the data to fix the values for these hyperparameters (α_m and ν) at their posterior modes. This approach is essentially using a data-dependent prior for a one-stage model, and represents a slightly different approach to get around putting too much information in the prior for parameters that do not have straightforward interpretations.

5 Example Comparing Priors

To demonstrate some of the differences between the priors discussed in this paper, Figure 3 shows the posterior means for several choices of prior. The data are from Breiman and Friedman (1985) and the goal is to model groundlevel ozone concentration (a pollutant) as a function of several meteorological variables. Only day of the year is used here so that the results can be plotted and visually interpreted. A regression example was chosen because it can be easily visualized, but the consequences translate to classification problems as well. Included are the proper priors of Müller and Rios Insua and of Neal, two noninformative priors (flat and independence Jeffreys), and the hybrid weight decay prior. The Neal and weight decay priors have user-specified hyperparameters that greatly affect the behavior of the resulting posteriors, and values were picked here just as examples. The suggested default levels of Müller and Rios Insua were used, and the noninformative priors do not need user specification.

Figure 3 shows that the posterior mean fit can have a wide variety of behaviors depending on the choice of prior. This weight decay prior produces the most shrinkage, resulting in a very smooth posterior mean. The Müller and Rios Insua is also highly informative and results in a smooth fit. In contrast, the other priors result in posterior means with more features that try to capture more of the variability in the data.

It is important to note that the weight decay and Neal priors can be adjusted by using different choices of hyperparameters. The examples provided

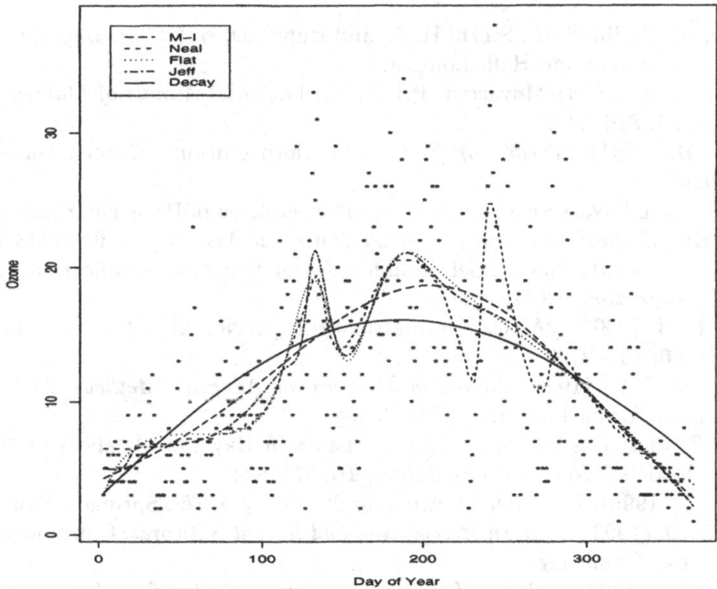

Fig. 3. Comparison of priors.

here are meant to show a large part of the range of their flexibility. The weight decay prior has limiting cases with full shrinkage (the posterior mean is just a constant at the mean of the data) and no shrinkage (equivalent to the flat prior). The pictured plot shows a large amount of shrinkage (a more informative prior). The Neal prior similarly has a wide range, with the pictured plot representing very little shrinkage, but it could also be tuned to produce a large amount of shrinkage.

Acknowledgments

This work was supported by National Science Foundation grant DMS 0233710.

References

1. Berger, J. O., De Oliveira, V., and Sans 6, B.. (2001). "Objective Bayesian Analysis of Apatially Correlated Data," *Journal of the American Statistical Association*, **96**, 1361–1374.
2. Bishop, C. M. (1995). *Neural Networks for Pattern Recognition.* Clarendon, Oxford.
3. Breiman, L. and Friedman, J. H. (1985). "Estimating Optimal Transformations for Multiple Regression and Correlation," *Journal of the American Statistical Association*, **80**, 580–619.

4. Fine, T. L. (1999). *Feedforward Neural Network Methodology.* Springer, New York.
5. Gelman, A., Carlin, J. B., Stern, H. S., and Rubin, D. B. (1995). *Bayesian Data Analysis.* Chapman and Hall, London.
6. Hartigan, J. A. (1964). "Invariant Prior Distributions," *Annals of Mathematical Statistics*, **35**, 836–845.
7. Jeffreys, H. (1961). *Theory of Probability* (third edition). Oxford University Press, New York.
8. Kass, R. E., and Wasserman, L. (1996). "The Selection of Prior Distributions by Formal Rules," *Journal of the American Statistical Association*, **91**, 1343–1370.
9. Lee, H. K. H. (2001). "Model Selection for Neural Network Classification," *Journal of Classification*, **18**, 227–243.
10. Lee, H. K. H. (2003). "A Noninformative Prior for Neural Networks," *Machine Learning*, **50**, 197–2152.
11. MacKay, D. J. C. (1992). *Bayesian Methods for Adaptive Methods.* Ph.D. dissertation, California Institute of Technology.
12. Müller, P., and Rios Insua, D. (1998). "Issues in Bayesian Analysis of Neural Network Models," *Neural Computation*, **10**, 571–592.
13. Neal, R. M. (1996). *Bayesian Learning for Neural Networks.* Springer, New York.
14. Ripley, B. D. (1993). *Pattern Recognition and Neural Networks.* Cambridge University Press, Cambridge.
15. Robinson, M. (2001). *Priors for Bayesian Neural Networks.* Master's thesis, Department of Statistics, University of British Columbia.
16. Robinson, M. (2001b). "Priors for Bayesian Neural Networks," in *Computing Science and Statistics*, eds. E. Wegman, A. Braverman, A. Goodman, and P. Smythe, **33**, 122–127.

Combining Models in Discrete Discriminant Analysis Through a Committee of Methods

Ana Sousa Ferreira

Universidade de Lisboa, Portugal
asferreira@fpce.ul.pt

Abstract: In this paper we are concerned with combining models in discrete discriminant analysis in the small sample setting. Our approach consists of an adaptation to discriminant analysis of a method for combining models introduced in the neural computing literature (Bishop, 1995). For combining models we consider a single coefficient obtained in a fuzzy classification rule context and we evaluate its performance through numerical experiments (Sousa Ferreira, 2000).

1 Introduction

In discrete discriminant analysis each object is described by p discrete variables and is assumed to belong to one of K exclusive groups $G_1, G_2, ..., G_K$ with prior probabilities $\pi_1, \pi_2, ..., \pi_K$ $(\sum_{i=1}^{K} \pi_i = 1)$.

The purpose of discriminant analysis methods is to derive a classification rule to assign, in the future, objects, described with the p discrete variables, but with unknown group membership, to one of the K groups. To obtain this classification rule a n-dimensional training sample $X = (x_1, ..., x_n)$ is used for which the group membership of each object is known.

Then, the Bayes classification rule assigns an individua observed vector $\mathbf{x}$ to G_{K^*} if

$$\pi_{K^*} P(\mathbf{x}|G_K) \geq \pi_l P(\mathbf{x}|G_l), \text{ for } l = 1, ..., K$$

where $\mathbf{x}$ is a p-dimensional observation and $P(\mathbf{x}|G_K)$denotes the conditional probability function for the l-th group. Usually, the conditional probability functions are unknown and are estimated on the basis of the training sample.

In this paper, we are concerned with discrete discriminant analysis in the small sample setting, with K=2 groups. In this context, most of the discrete discrimination methods are expected to perform poorly due to the high-dimensional problem.

This is the reason why we propose a classification rule designed by combining discriminant analysis models in a way introduced in the neural computing literature (Bishop, 1995). This combining model has been introduced in a fuzzy classification rule context and has an intermediate position between the full multinomial model and the first order independence model hereunder described. We call this model the committee of methods (CMET).

The main aim of this approach is to obtain a better prediction performance and more stable results.

For the sake of simplicity, we focus on binary data in our presentation.

2 Discrete Discriminant Analysis

For discrete data, the most natural model is to assume that the conditional probability function $P(\mathrm{x}|G_K)$, where $\mathbf{x} \in \{0,1\}^p$ and $k = 1, ..., K$, are multinomial probabilities. In this case, the conditional probabilities are estimated by the observed frequencies. Godstein and Dillon(1978) call this model the full multinomial model (FMM). This model involves 2^{p-1} parameters in each group. Hence, even for moderate p, not all of the parameters are identifiable.

One way to deal with the curse of dimensionality consists of reducing the number of parameters to be estimated. The first-order independence model (FOIM) assumes that the binary variables are independent in each group G_k, $k = 1, ..., K$. Then, the number of parameters to be estimated for each group is reduced from 2^{p-1} to p. This method is simple but may be unrealistic in some situations.

Since we are mainly concerned with small or very small sample sizes, we encounter a problem of sparseness in which some of the multinomial cells may have no data in the training sets. Hand (1982) has noticed that the choice of the smoothing method is not very important so that computationally less demanding methods may be used. Then, we suggest smoothing the observed frequencies with a parameter λ, as follows:

$$\widehat{P}(x|\lambda, B) = \frac{1}{n}\sum_{i=1}^{n} \lambda^{p-||x-x_i||}(1-\lambda)^{||x-x_i||}$$

where $\lambda = 1.00$ implies no smoothing
and $\lambda = .99, .95$ or $.90$ according to the training sample size.

3 Combining Models in Discrete Discriminant Analysis

Nowadays combining models has became a common approach in several fields, such as regression, neural networks, discriminant analysis, and so forth (cf. Celeux and Mkhadri, 1992; Breiman, 1995; Bishop, 1995; Leblanc and Tibshirani, 1996; Raftery, 1996; Sousa Ferreira et al., 1999, 2000)

In discrete discriminant analysis, we have to deal with a problem of dimensionality in many circumstances. This problem is due to sparseness and to the large number of parameters to be estimated even in the simplest models. Thus, most of the discrete discrimination methods could be expected to perform poorly.

Combining models is a natural approach to reduce this problem. The advantage of this strategy is that it can lead to significant improvements in the results, while demanding a little additional computational effort.

In this paper we investigate the performance of an approach adapted from the committees of networks presented by Bishop (1995). We consider a simple linear combination

$$\sum_{m=1}^{2} P_k^m(\mathrm{x})\beta_m$$

where $P_k^m(\mathrm{x})$ is the conditional probability function for the k-group and the model m. An intuitive combination method is to propose a single coefficient β producing an intermediate model between the full multinomial model and the first order independence model:

$$\widehat{P}_k(\mathrm{x}|\beta) = (1-\beta)\widehat{P}_M(\mathrm{x}|G_k) + \beta\widehat{P}_I(\mathrm{x}|G_k)$$

where $\widehat{P}_M(\mathrm{x}|G_k)$ is the conditional probability function for the k-group and the full multinomial model, estimated by cross-validation and $\widehat{P}_I(\mathrm{x}|G_k)$ is the conditional probability function for the k-group and the first order independence model, estimated by cross-validation.

Thus, the problem is to estimate the coefficient of the combination. Different strategies to obtain β estimate can be proposed. In this work, we use the committee of methods model (CMET) hereunder described.

4 The Committee of Methods (CMET)

Let consider a two class discriminant analysis problem and two different classifications rules obtained from a n-dimensional training sample, $X = (\mathrm{x}, \mathrm{y})$, where each x_i is a p-dimensional vector and y_i is a binary indicator scalar of the class membership. That is to say, y_i is one if the observation i becomes from G_1 and zero otherwise.

We denote $r_m(\mathrm{x}) = (r_m(x_1), ..., r_m(x_n))$ the output of the mth model under consideration, $m \in \{1, 2\}$, and we can consider two situations:

- each $r_m(x_i)$ is a binary scalar indicating the class to which the observation i is assigned;
- each $r_m(x_i)$ is the first group conditional probability for the observation i, knowing x_i, of belonging to the first group, approximated by the model m: $\mathbf{0} \leq r_m(x_i) \leq \mathbf{1}$ and $\sum_{k=1}^{2} r_m(x_i) = \mathbf{1}$.

The first situation is called the "hard classification rule situation" and the second the "fuzzy classification rule situation."

Then, the committee of models proposed by Bishop (Bishop, 1995) takes the form

$$r_{COM} = \sum_{m=1}^{2} \beta_m r_m(\mathrm{x}), \text{ with } \sum_{m=1}^{2} \beta_m = 1.$$

In the "hard classification rule situation" the function h(x) to be approximated is the true classification vector t but for the "fuzzy classification rule situation" the function h(x) to be approximated is the conditional expectation of y knowing x.

Since, in the present study, we are interested on combining two models (the first-order independence model, FOIM, and the full multinomial model, FMM) in the two class case, the hard classification rule is useless, because the committee model reduces to the average of the two models. Thus, in this framework, we focus attention on the fuzzy classification rule.

In this context, following Bishop (Bishop, 1995), the committee of the fuzzy classification rule leads to the error

$$E = \sum_{j=1}^{2} \sum_{l=1}^{2} \beta_j \beta_l C_{jl}, \text{ with } l, j \in \{1, 2\},$$

where the general term of matrix C is estimated by

$$C_{jl} = \tfrac{1}{n} \sum_{i=1}^{n} \left(r_j(x_i) - y_i\right)^T \left(r_l(x_i) - y_i\right) \text{ with } l, j \in \{1, 2\}.$$

Thus, the coefficient of the combination takes de form

$$\beta_m = \frac{\sum_{l=1}^{2} \left(C^{-1}\right)_{ml}}{\sum_{j=1}^{2} \sum_{l=1}^{2} \left(C^{-1}\right)_{jl}}.$$

5 Numerical Experiments

The efficiency of the model CMET has been investigated on both real and simulated binary data. These studies showed that good performances can be expected from CMET in a setting for which sample sizes are small or very small and population structures are identical in the two classes.

However, for the sake of simplicity, we only present, in this article, the application to real data, which is concerned with our professional applied field: Psychology and Education Sciences.

We investigate the performance of the present approach CMET, compared with others models: FOIM, FMM and KER (Kernel Discriminant Analysis), where the smoothing parameter λ has been set to 0.95.

5.1 The Psychological Data

The question of how well-being comes about has been studied with a focus on people's actual life experiences. The goal of the present study is to explore the impact of playing with pets on psychological well-being among older people (Dourado et al., 2003).

Our data set consists of 80 older adults (mean age=72 yrs., s.d.= 6 yrs.) from both sexes, evaluated by a Psychological Well-Being Scale (Ryff, 1989) adapted for the Portuguese population. This sample is divided into two groups: 40 elderly persons who have pets (G_1) and 40 elderly persons who don't have pets (G_2).

The Psychological Well-Being Scale is organized in six key dimensions: Autonomy, Environmental Mastery, Personal Growth, Positive Relations with Others, Purpose in Life, and Self-Acceptance. In this work the scores obtained for each older adult in the six dimensions were taken as binary data.

Since the sample is small, we estimate the misclassification risk by half-sampling. In Table 1 we summarize the results of the four methods for this data set.

For each method, we give the misclassification risk estimated by half-sampling and the prior probabilities were taken to be equal, $\pi_k = .5$ (k=1,2).

Table 1. Estimated set misclassification risk and parameter values for the psychological data.

	FOIM	FMM	KER	CMET	CMET
Half-sampling	30%	41%	32%	25%	25%
λ			.95	1.00	.95
β				.5553	.4930

Note that this data set is not very sparse (2^6=64 states and 80 observations) but, even so, the CMET model provides the lowest test estimates of the misclassification risk. On the basis of this study we can conclude that the involvement of playing with pets among older people can contribute for psychological well-being and thus, perhaps, for more successful aging.

6 Conclusions

We have presented a method for the two-class case in discrete discriminant analysis. As we know, sparseness is the main problem of discrete discriminant analysis, particularly when sample sizes are small or very small. The numerical experiments showed that the estimates obtained for β, through CMET, are very stable, producing almost always a really intermediate model between the full multinomial model and the first-order independence model. Also, those studies allow us to remark that this approach is not sensitive to the problem of sparseness and thus there is no need for smoothing the observed frequencies.

Thus, we can conclude that CMET could be quite effective for discrete discriminant analysis in a small samples setting.

Acknowledgements

This work has been partially supported by the Franco-Portuguese Scientific Programme "Analyse des Données pour le Data Mining" MSPLLDM-542-B2 (Embassy of France and Portuguese Ministry of Science and Superior Education - GRICES), co-directed by H. Bacelar-Nicolau and G. Saporta and the Multivariate Data Analysis research team of CEAUL/FCUL directed by H. Bacelar-Nicolau.

References

1. Breiman, L. (1995). "Stacked Regression," *Machine Learning*, **24**, 49–64.
2. Bishop, C. M. (1995). *Neural Networks For Pattern Recognition*, Oxford University Press.
3. Celeux, G., and Mkhadri, A. (1992). "Discrete Regularized Discriminant Analysis," *Statistics and Computing*, **2**, 143–151.
4. Dourado, S., Mohan, R., Vieira, A., Sousa Ferreira, A., and Duarte Silva, M. E. (2003). "Pets and Well-being Among Older People (in Portuguese)," in *Book of Abstracts of V National Symposium of Psychological Research*, Lisbon.
5. Goldstein, M., and Dillon, W. R. (1978). *Discrete Discriminant Analysis*, John Wiley and Sons, New York.
6. Hand, D. J. (1982). *Kernel Discriminant Analysis*, Research Studies Press, Wiley, Chichester.
7. Leblanc, M., and Tibshirani, R. (1996). "Combining Estimates in Regression and Classification," *Journal of the American Statistical Association*, **91**, 1641–1650.
8. Raftery, A. E. (1996). "Approximate Bayes Factors and Accounting for Model Uncertainty in Generalised Linear Models," *Biometrika*, **83**, 251–266.
9. Ryff, C. D. (1989). "Happiness Is Everything, Or Is It? Explorations on the Meaning of Psychological Well-Being," *Journal of Personality and Social Psychology*, **57**, 1069–1081.
10. Sousa Ferreira, A., Celeux, G., and Bacelar-Nicolau, H. (1999). "Combining Models in Discrete Discriminant Analysis by a Hierarchical Coupling Approach," in *Proceedings of the IX International Symposium of ASMDA (ASMDA 99)*, eds. H. Bacelar-Nicolau, F. Costa Nicolau, and J. Janssen), Lisbon:INE, pp. 159–164.
11. Sousa Ferreira, A., Celeux, G., and Bacelar-Nicolau, H. (2000). "Discrete Discriminant Analysis: The Performance of Combining Models by a Hierarchical Coupling Approach," in *Proceedings of the 7th Conference of the International Federation of Classification Societies (IFCS 2000)*, eds. H. Kiers, J.-P. Rasson, P. Groenen, M. Schader, Berlin:Springer, pp. 181–186.
12. Sousa Ferreira, A. (2000). *Combining Models in Discrete Discriminant Analysis*, Ph.D. Thesis (in Portuguese), New Univ. Lisbon, Lisbon.

Phoneme Discrimination with Functional Multi-Layer Perceptrons

Brieuc Conan-Guez[1,2] and Fabrice Rossi[1,2]

[1] INRIA-Rocquencourt, France
brieuc.conan-guez@inria.fr
[2] Université Paris Dauphine, France
rossi@ufrmd.dauphine.fr

Abstract: In many situations, high dimensional data can be considered as sampled functions. We recall in this paper how to implement a Multi-Layer Perceptron (MLP) on such data by approximating a theoretical MLP on functions thanks to basis expansion. We illustrate the proposed method on a phoneme discrimination problem.

1 Introduction

Functional Data Analysis (cf. Ramsay and Silverman, 1997) is a framework which aims at improving traditional data analysis techniques when individuals are described by functions. This approach, contrary to its multivariate counterpart, takes advantage of internal data structure to produce results that are often more pertinent. The most obvious structure, in the functional context, is of course the regularity of the observed individuals: for example, in some spectrometric applications from food industry, each individual is described by a spectrum (say 100 channels). The shape of these spectra are very smooth, and is handled in a natural way by the functional techniques. Another example of structure which can not be treated without a functional prior-knowledge is the periodicity; for example, in Ramsay and Silverman(1997), the authors study the evolution of the Canadian temperature over one year. These data present strong sinusoidal patterns, which are taken into account by the functional framework.

In this paper, we recall the properties of the Functional Multi-Layer Perceptron (FMLP) based on a projection step. This model is in fact a natural extension of standard MLPs to the functional context, and its properties were studied from a theoretical point of view in some earlier works (see for example Rossi and Conan-Guez (2002) and Rossi and Conan-Guez(2003)). In this paper, we focus on comparing our model to standard MLPs in a real application.

Our problem is a discrimination task on phoneme data which is very similar to the one studied in Hastie, Buja, and Tibshirani (1995).

2 Functional Multi-Layer Perceptrons

An n input MLP neuron is characterized by a fixed activation function, T, a function from $\mathbb{R}$ to $\mathbb{R}$, by a vector from $\mathbb{R}^n$ (the weight vector, w), and by a real-valued threshold, b. Given a vector input $x \in \mathbb{R}^n$, the output of the neuron is $N(x) = T(w'x + b)$.

In the proposed approach, we restrict ourselves to the case where inputs belong to the Hilbert space $L^2(\mu)$ (with μ a finite positive Borel measure). In this framework, the extension of numerical neurons to functional inputs is straightforward. Indeed, we consider two functions f and g, elements of $L^2(\mu)$. The f is the input function, and g is called the *weight function* (g has the same meaning as w for the numerical neuron). The output of the functional neuron is $N(f) = T(\int fg\, d\mu + b)$ (where T is a function from $\mathbb{R}$ to $\mathbb{R}$ and b is real).

The MLP architecture can be decomposed into neuron layers: the output of each layer (i.e., the vector formed by the output of neurons belonging to this layer) is the input to the next layer. As a functional neuron gives a numerical output, we can define a functional MLP by combining numerical neurons with functional neurons. The first hidden layer of the network consists exclusively in functional neurons (defined thanks to weight functions g_i), whereas subsequent layers are constructed exclusively with numerical neurons. For instance, an one hidden layer functional MLP with real output computes the following function:

$$H(f) = \sum_{i=1}^{k} a_i T\left(\int g_i f\, d\mu + b_i\right) \tag{1}$$

where a_i, b_i are real values, and f, g_i are elements of $L^2(\mu)$.

3 Projection-Based Approach

This section reviews the key ideas behind the FMLP methodology, discussing the mathematical formulation, useful approximations, and links to related techniques.

3.1 Parametric Approach

As stated above, the FMLP evaluation relies on the computation of all the integrals $\int g_i f\, d\mu$ of the first hidden layer. Unfortunately, in practice these integrals cannot be calculated exactly, as g_i and f are arbitrary functions of $L^2(\mu)$. One way to deal with this problem is to use a regularized representation of f and g_i in place of the true functions.

Let $(\phi_p)_{p\in\mathbb{N}^*}$ be a topological basis of $L^2(\mu)$, and let Π_P be the projection operator on the subspace spanned by the P first elements of the basis (denoted $\text{span}(\phi_1, ..., \phi_P)$); i.e., $\Pi_P(f) = \sum_{p=1}^{P}(\int f\phi_p\, d\mu)\phi_p$. Thanks to this projection step, simplification occurs in the FMLP evaluation—it is no longer necessary to deal with the real input function f as well as to compute $H(f)$. We can just consider the projection $\Pi_P(f)$ as the FMLP input, and our only concern is the evaluation of $H(\Pi_P(f))$. A second simplification can be applied to our model; we restrict the choice of weight functions to $\text{span}(\phi_1, ..., \phi_P)$. Therefore, for the weight function $g = \sum_{q=1}^{P} \alpha_q\phi_q$, the integral can be rewritten in the following form:

$$\int g\Pi_P(f)\, d\mu = \sum_{q=1}^{P}\sum_{p=1}^{P}(\int \phi_p f\, d\mu)\alpha_q \int \phi_p\phi_q\, d\mu = \alpha^T \Lambda\beta \tag{2}$$

where $\Lambda = (\int \phi_p\phi_q d\mu)_{p,q}$, and $\beta = (\int \phi_p f\, d\mu)_p$.

In this expression, each $\int \phi_p f\, d\mu$ is computed during the projection step (more precisely, an approximate value as explained in 3.2). The $\int \phi_p\phi_q\, d\mu$ are independant of the α_q as well as the input functions, and therefore their evaluation can be done once and for all. Depending on the basis used to represent weight functions and input functions, this evaluation can bc performed either exactly, or approximately.

Using linear models to represent weight functions allows the FMLP to be parameterized by a finite number of numerical parameters. Hence the FMLP training can be performed with traditional optimization algorithms.

3.2 Approximation of the Projection

As explained in 3.1, the proposed method aims at computing $H(\Pi_P(f))$. Unfortunaltely, due to our limited knowledge of f (f is known only by a finite number of input/output pairs), the computation of $\Pi_P(f)$ is not possible in practice. To overcome this problem, we substitute, for the FMLP evaluation of the real projection $\Pi_P(f)$, an empirical one defined as follows.

Each observed f is described by a list of values $(x_j, f(x_j) + \varepsilon_j)_{0\leq j\leq m}$, where ε_j is the evaluation error on f at the observation point x_j (see Rossi and Conan-Guez (2002) for a detailed probabilistic description). It should be noted that the number of evaluation points m is free to vary from one function to another.

Let $\Pi_P(f)_m$, an element of $L^2(\mu)$, be the unique minimizer $\sum_{p=1}^{P} \beta_p\phi_p$ of $\sum_{j=1}^{m}(f(x_j) + \varepsilon_j - \sum_{p=1}^{P} \beta_p\phi_p(x_j))^2$; this is defined by the Moore-Penrose inverse. Thanks to this empirical projection, a second simplification occurs in the FMLP evaluation: after the substitution of the input function f by its projection $\Pi(f)$ in section 3.1, we can now focus on computing $H(\Pi_P(f)_m)$ rather than $H(\Pi_P(f))$.

3.3 Link with Classical MLPs

In section 3.1 we showed that the evaluation of the integral of a functional neuron reduces to an algebraic computation: $\int g\Pi_P(f)_m \, d\mu = \alpha^T \Lambda \beta_m$ where β_m is the coordinates of $\Pi_P(f)_m$. In fact, as we shall see now, the calculation of a functional neuron is equivalent to the one for its numerical counterpart. Indeed, as $\{\phi_p\}$, $0 \leq p \leq P$, is a free system, then Λ is a full rank matrix. Therefore if we choose an arbitrary vector of coefficients c, we can define a function t by:

$$t = \sum_{q=1}^{P} d_q \phi_q$$

with $d = \Lambda^{-1} c$ such that

$$\int t \, \Pi_m(f) \, d\mu = \sum_{q=1}^{P} c_q \beta_{m,q}.$$

Therefore a linear combination of the (approximate) coordinates of f on $\text{span}(\phi_1, \ldots, \phi_P)$ is always equal to the scalar product of $\Pi_m(f)$ with a well chosen weight function t. From a practical point of view, we can submit the coordinates of $\Pi_m(f)$ to a standard MLP, and the prediction made by this model will be totally equivalent to the one made from an FMLP. Consequently we see that our functional approach doesn't require specific software developement—an existing neural network library can be easily used to implement FMPs.

3.4 Theoretical Properties

We studied from a theoretical point of view the proposed model in earlier works (Rossi and Conan-Guez, 2002; Rossi and Conan-Guez, 2003). We showed that FMLPs possess two important properties:

- the FMLP based on a projection step is a universal approximator, in the sense that for any real-valued continuous function F defined on a compact K of $L^2(\mu)$, there exists P, the size of the truncated basis (the basis is fixed), and H a FMLP, such that F is approximated by $H o \Pi_P$ to a given precision (the set of functions $H o \Pi_P$ is dense in $C(K, \mathbb{R})$ for the uniform norm);
- the FMLP based on a projection step is consistent, in the sense that if we estimate the model parameters on a finite number of input functions, each one known from to a finite list of observations, these estimators converge to the theoretical parameters as the number of functions as well as the number of observation points tend to infinity (more precisely, the number of observations needed to achieve a given precision depends on the number of functions).

4 Experiment

The problem we adress in this paper is a discrimination task for phoneme data. This dataset can be found in the TIMIT database and was studied by Hastie, Buja, and Tibshirani (1995) and Ferraty and Vieu (2002). The data are log-periodograms corresponding to recording phonemes of 32 ms duration. The goal of this experiment is to discriminate five different patterns corresponding to five different phonemes ("sh" as in "she," "dcl" as in "dark," "iy" as in "she," "aa" as in "dark," and "ao" as in "water"). These phonemes are part of the first sentence of the speech corpus. Each speaker (325 in the training set and 112 in the test set) is recorded at a 16-kHz sampling rate; we use only the first 256 frequencies. Finally, the training set contains 3340 spectra, whereas the test set contains 1169 spectra.

classes	aa	ao	dcl	iy	sh
training	519	759	562	852	648
test	176	263	195	311	224

Table 1. Number of phonemes in the training/test set.

Table 1 describes the distribution of each phoneme in the training set as well as in the test set. In Fig. 1, we draw five spectra of the phoneme "sh." We see that the spectra are very noisy.

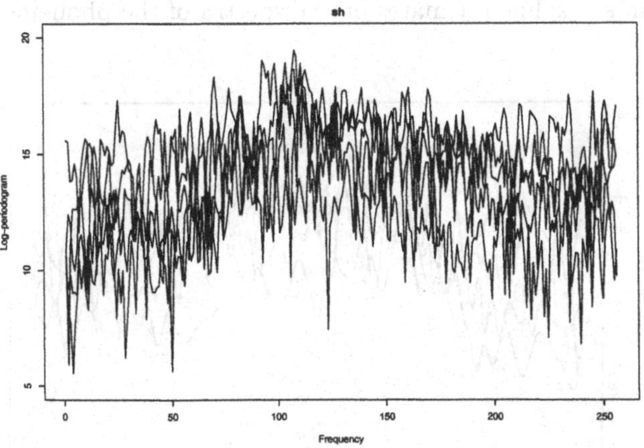

Fig. 1. 5 Log-Periodograms for the "sh" phoneme.

4.1 Multivariate and Functional Approach

We compare the projection-based FMP to standard MLPs. As it can be seen in the following part, both models are in many ways very similar. The main difference lies in the data pre-processing—the FMLP uses a functional pre-treatement, whereas the standard MLP relies on raw pre-processing. It should be noted that apart from this practical difference, the functional model has a theoretical framework which does not exist for the multivariate model (e.g., consistency in Section 3.4).

Each spectrum is a vector of 256 components. In the case of the standard MLP, we compute the principal component analysis on these spectra and we retain a fixed number of eigenvectors according to the explained variance criterion. More precisely, each eigenvector that explains more than 0.5% of the total variance is retained. The criterion finds 11 eigenvectors. The projection components are then centered and scaled to have unit variance. We finally submit these vectors to a standard MLP.

In the case of the FMLP, functions are first smoothed by a standard roughness penalty technique; the estimation of each curve is done by a spline with a penalty on the second derivative of the estimate (function `smooth.spline` in R). After this fitting step, each estimate is then sampled on 256 equally-spaced points. The vector is then submitted to a principal component analysis, and the number of retained eigenfunctions is done according to the same explained variance criterion as above—we found 10 eigenfunctions. This technique of smoothing the data before the PCA is well described in Ramsay and Silverman(1997). This functional approach allows the data to speak while adding a functional constraint which gets rid of the noise in the observed functions. In Fig. 2, we can see spline estimates of five spectra of the phoneme "sh."

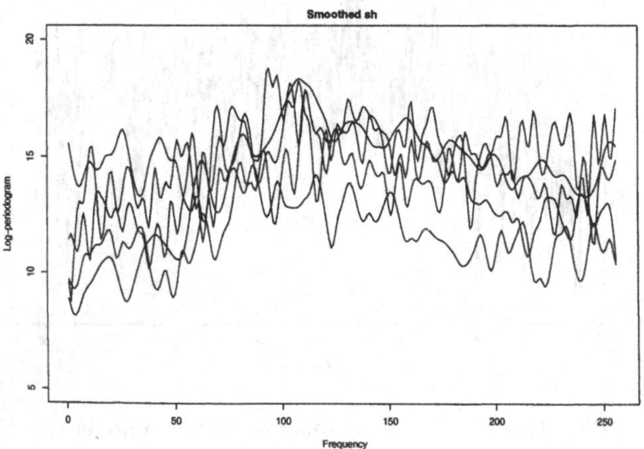

Fig. 2. 5 Log-Periodograms for the smoothed "sh" phoneme.

After a centering and scaling stage, we submit the sample from each spline to a standard MLP (which is equivalent to the functional approach explained in Section 3.3). In Figs. 3 and 4, we show the PCA for both approaches.

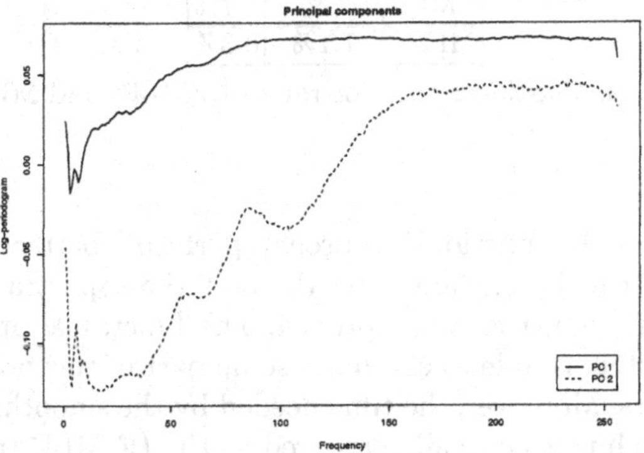

Fig. 3. The first two eigenvectors for the multivariate approach.

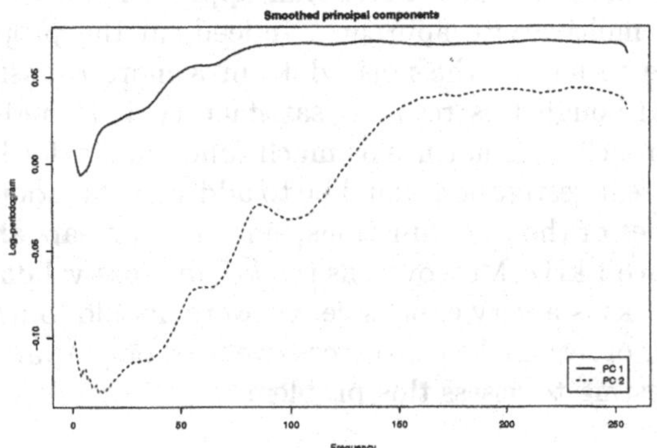

Fig. 4. The first two eigenfunctions for the functional approach.

The MLP training is done thanks to a weight decay technique—we add to the error function a penalty term which constrains model parameters to be small (the penalty is the L^2-norm of parameter vector). In order to find the best model, we therefore have to choose the best architecture (the number of hidden neurons in the MLP) as well as the smoothing parameter (which controls the weight decay). This can be done by a k-fold cross-validation technique. In our case, we choose k equal to 4, mainly for computational reasons. For the multivariate approach, 4 neurons are chosen, whereas for the functional one, 5 neurons are chosen (the range of hidden neurons for the k-

fold cross-validation runs from 3 to 7). The results obtained are summarized in Table 2.

set	training	test
FMLP	7 %	7.7%
MLP	7.1%	8.3%

Table 2. Classification error rates of FMLPs and MLPs.

As can be seen, the functional approach performs better than the multivariate one. This can be explained by the fact that spectra are very noisy, which penalizes the multivariate approach. The functional approach, thanks to its smoothing step, is able to eliminate some part of this noise, which leads to improved results. Moreover, the time needed by the smoothing phase of the functional approach is very small compared to the (F)MLP training time.

5 Conclusion

In this paper, we showed that a functional approach can be valuable when compared to the multivariate approach. Indeed, in the proposed example, the FMLP is able to handle the noisy data in a more robust way than the standard MLP. Although this result is satisfactory, it should be noted that the proposed approach does not use as much functional prior knowledge as it could. So one future investigation would be to add some functional penalties on the high frequencies of the eigenfunctions, since human ears are less sensitive to frequencies above 1 kHz. Moreover, as the k-fold cross-validation associated with neural networks is a very expensive, we were unable to use it in order to choose the number of retained eigenvectors (we used only a variance criterion). It would be interesting to assess this problem.

References

1. Ferraty, F., and Vieu, P. (2002). "Curves Discrimination: A Nonparametric Functional Approach," to appear in *Computational Statistics and Data Analysis.*
2. Hastie, T., Buja, A., and Tibshirani, R. (1995). "Penalized Discriminant Analysis," *Annals of Statistics* **23**, 73–102.
3. Ramsay, J., and Silverman, B. (1997). *Functional Data Analysis,* Springer Series in Statistics, Springer, New York.
4. Rossi, F., and Conan-Guez, B. (2002). "Multi-Layer Perceptrons for Functional Data Analysis: A Projection-Based Approach," in *Artificial Neural Networks—ICANN 2002*, ed. J. Dorronsoro, International Conference, Lecture Notes in Computer Science, Berlin:Springer, pp. 661-666.

5. Rossi, F., and Conan-Guez, B. (2003). "Functional Multi-Layer Perceptron: A Nonlinear Tool for Functional Data Analysis," Technical Report 0331, September, LISE/CEREMADE, http://www.ceremade.dauphine.fr/.

PLS Approach for Clusterwise Linear Regression on Functional Data

Cristian Preda[1] and Gilbert Saporta[2]

[1] Université de Lille 2, France
cpreda@univ-lille2.fr
[2] Conservatoire National des Arts et Métiers, France
saporta@cnam.fr

Abstract: The Partial Least Squares (PLS) approach is used for the clusterwise linear regression algorithm when the set of predictor variables forms an L_2-continuous stochastic process. The number of clusters is treated as unknown and the convergence of the clusterwise algorithm is discussed. The approach is compared with other methods via an application to stock-exchange data.

1 Introduction

Let us consider the following regression problem: The response variable Y is numerical and the predictor set is a stochastic process $\mathbf{X} = (X_t)_{t\in[0,T]}$, $T > 0$. For example, $(X_t)_{t\in[0,T]}$ can represent temperature curves observed during a period of time $[0, T]$ and Y the amount of crops. Here there are an infinite number of predictors for Y. The Partial Least Squares (PLS) approach (Wold et al., 1984) gives better results than other tools for linear regression on a stochastic process (Preda and Saporta, 2002). In this paper we propose an improvement and extension of this technique by combining PLS regression on a stochastic process and clusterwise regression.

Clusterwise linear regression supposes that the points of each cluster are generated according to some linear regression relation; given a dataset $\{(x_j, y_j)\}_{j=1}^{n}$ the aim is to find simultaneously an optimal partition $\mathcal{G}$ of data into K clusters, $1 \leq K < n$, and regression coefficients $(\alpha, \beta) = \{(\alpha^i, \beta^i)\}_{i=1}^{K}$ within each cluster which maximize the overall fit. We write that $j \in \{1, \ldots, n\}$ is an element of the cluster $i \in \{1, \ldots, K\}$ by $\mathcal{G}(j) = i$. For each element j of the cluster i we consider the linear model $y_j = \alpha^i + \langle \beta^i, x_j \rangle + \epsilon_{ij}$. Then, the optimization problem associated with the clusterwise linear regression is:

$$(\mathcal{G}, (\alpha, \beta)) = \text{argmin} \sum_{i=1}^{K} \sum_{j:\mathcal{G}(j)=i} \epsilon_{ij}^2.$$

In such a model, the parameters that have to be estimated are the number of clusters (K), the regression coefficients for each cluster $\{(\alpha^i, \beta^i)\}_{i=1}^K$, and the variance of residuals ϵ_{ij} within each cluster. Charles (1977) and Spaeth (1979) propose methods for estimating these parameters considering a kind of piecewise linear regression based on the least squares algorithm of Bock (1969). The algorithm is a special case of k-means clustering with a criterion based on the minimization of the squared residuals instead of the classical within-cluster dispersion. The estimation of local models $\{(\alpha^i, \beta^i\}_{i=1}^K$ could be a difficult task (the number of observations is less than the number of explanatory variables, causing multicollinearity). Solutions such as clusterwise principal component regression (PCR) or ridge regression are considered in Charles (1977). Other approaches based on mixtures of distributions are developed in DeSarbo and Cron (1988) and Hennig (1999).

We propose to use PLS estimators (Wold et al., 1984) for regression coefficients of each cluster in the particular case where the set of explanatory variables forms a stochastic process $\mathbf{X} = (X_t)_{t\in[0,T]}$, $T > 0$. The paper is divided into three parts. Clusterwise linear regression algorithm is presented in the first part. In the second part we recall some tools for linear regression on a stochastic process (PCR, PLS) and justify the choice for the PLS approach. The clusterwise linear regression algorithm adapted to PLS regression as well as aspects related to the prediction problem are given here and represent the main results of this work. In the last part we present an application of the clusterwise PLS regression to stock-exchange data and compare the results with those obtained by other methods such as Aguilera et al. (1998) and Preda and Saporta (2002).

2 Clusterwise Linear Regression

Let $\mathbf{X} = (X_j)_{j=1}^p$, for $p \geq 1$, be a real random vector and let Y be a real random variable defined on the same probability space $(\Omega, \mathcal{A}, P)$. We assume that $\mathbf{X}$ and Y are of second order.

The clusterwise linear regression of Y on $\mathbf{X}$ states that there exists a random variable $\mathcal{G}$, $\mathcal{G} : \Omega \to \{1, 2, \ldots, K\}$, $K \in \mathbf{N} - \{0\}$ such that :

$$\begin{aligned} E(Y|\mathbf{X} = x, \mathcal{G} = i) &= \alpha^i + \beta^i x, \\ V(Y|\mathbf{X} = x, \mathcal{G} = i) &= \sigma_i^2 > 0, \forall x \in \mathbf{R}^p, \forall i = 1, \ldots K, \end{aligned} \tag{1}$$

where E and V stand for expectation and variance, respectively, and (α^i, β^i) are the regression coefficients associated to the cluster i, $i = 1, \ldots, K$.

Let us denote by $\hat{Y}$ the approximation of Y given by the global linear regression of Y on $\mathbf{X}$, and let $\hat{Y}^i = \alpha^i + \beta^i \mathbf{X}$ be the approximation of Y given by the linear regression of Y on $\mathbf{X}$ within the cluster i, $i = 1, \ldots, K$, and set

$$\hat{Y}^L = \sum_{i=1}^{K} \hat{Y}^i \mathbf{1}_{\mathcal{G}=i},$$

where $\mathbf{1}_{\mathcal{G}=i}(j) = 1$ if j belongs to the cluster i and is 0 else (L stands for "Local"). Then the following decomposition formula holds (Charles, 1977):

$$\begin{aligned} \mathrm{V}(Y-\hat{Y}) &= \mathrm{V}(Y-\hat{Y}^L)+\mathrm{V}(\hat{Y}^L-\hat{Y}) \\ &= \sum_{i=1}^{s} \mathbf{P}(\{\mathcal{G}=i\})\mathrm{V}(Y-\hat{Y}^i|\mathcal{G}=i)+\mathrm{V}(\hat{Y}^L-\hat{Y}). \end{aligned} \tag{2}$$

Thus, the residual variance of the global regression is decomposed into a part of residual variance due to linear regression within each cluster and another part representing the distance between predictions given by global and local models. This formula defines the criterion for estimating the local models used in the algorithms of Charles (1977) and Bock (1969).

2.1 Estimation

Let us consider K fixed and suppose that the homoscedasticity hypothesis holds; i.e., $\sigma_i^2 = \sigma^2$, $\forall i = 1, \dots K$. Charles (1977) and Bock (1969) use the following criterion for estimating $\mathcal{L}(\mathcal{G})$ and $\{\alpha^i, \beta^i\}_{i=1}^K$:

$$\min_{\{\alpha^i,\beta^i\}_{i=1}^K,\mathcal{L}(\mathcal{G})} \left\{\mathrm{V}(Y-\hat{Y}^L)\right\}. \tag{3}$$

If n data points $\{x_i, y_i\}_{i=1}^n$ have been collected, the cluster linear regression algorithm finds simultaneously an optimal partition of the n points, $\hat{\mathcal{G}}$ (an estimate of $\mathcal{L}(\mathcal{G})$), and the regression models for each cluster (element of the partition) $(\hat{\alpha}, \hat{\beta} = \{\hat{\alpha}^i, \hat{\beta}^i\}_{i=1}^K$, which minimize the criterion:

$$\mathcal{V}(K,\hat{\mathcal{G}},\hat{\alpha},\hat{\beta}) = \sum_{i=1}^{K} \sum_{\hat{\mathcal{G}}(j)=i} \left(y_j - (\hat{\alpha}^i + \hat{\beta}^i x_j)\right)^2. \tag{4}$$

Notice that under classical hypotheses on the model (i.e., residuals within each cluster are considered independent and normaly distributed) this criterion is equivalent to maximization of the likelihood function (Hennig 2000).

In order to minimize (4), the clusterwise linear regression algorithms iterates the following two steps :

i) For given $\hat{\mathcal{G}}$, $\mathcal{V}(K,\hat{\mathcal{G}},\hat{\alpha},\hat{\beta})$ is minimized by the LS-estimator $(\hat{\alpha}^i, \hat{\beta}^i)$ from the points (x_j, y_j) with $\hat{\mathcal{G}}(j) = i$.

ii) For given $\{\hat{\alpha}^i, \hat{\beta}^i\}_{i=1}^K$, $\mathcal{V}(K,\hat{\mathcal{G}},\hat{\alpha},\hat{\beta})$ is minimized according to

$$\hat{\mathcal{G}}(j) = \operatorname{argmin}_{i\in\{1,\dots,K\}} \left(y_j - (\hat{\alpha}^i + \hat{\beta}^i x_j)\right)^2. \tag{5}$$

That is, $\mathcal{V}(K,\hat{\mathcal{G}},\hat{\alpha},\hat{\beta})$ is monotonely decreasing if the steps *i)* and *ii)* are carried out alternately:

$$\underbrace{\hat{\mathcal{G}}_0 \Rightarrow (\hat{\alpha}_0, \hat{\beta}_0)}_{\mathcal{V}_0} \Rightarrow_{\geq} \underbrace{\hat{\mathcal{G}}_1 \Rightarrow (\hat{\alpha}_1, \hat{\beta}_1)}_{\mathcal{V}_1} \Rightarrow_{\geq} \ldots \Rightarrow_{\geq} \underbrace{\hat{\mathcal{G}}_l \Rightarrow (\hat{\alpha}_l, \hat{\beta}_l)}_{\mathcal{V}_l} \Rightarrow_{\geq} \ldots \quad (6)$$

where the index of each quantity denotes the iteration number, $\hat{\mathcal{G}}_0$ being an initial partition of the n data points.

In the following section we are interested in estimating the regression coefficients of each cluster in the particular case where the set of explanatory variables forms a stochastic process $\mathbf{X} = (X_t)_{t\in[0,T]}$, $T > 0$.

3 Functional Data: The PLS Approach

Let $\mathbf{X} = (X_t)_{t\in[0,T]}$ be a random process and $\mathbf{Y} = (Y_1, \ldots, Y_p)$, $p \geq 1$, be a random vector defined on the same probability space $(\Omega, \mathcal{A}, P)$. We assume that $(X_t)_{t\in[0,T]}$ and $\mathbf{Y}$ are of second order, $(X_t)_{t\in[0,T]}$ is L_2-continuous, and for any $\omega \in \Omega$, $t \mapsto X_t(\omega)$ is an element of $L_2([0,T])$. Without loss of generality we also assume $E(X_t) = 0$, $\forall t \in [0,T]$ and $E(Y_i) = 0\ \forall i = 1, \ldots, p$.

3.1 Some Tools for Linear Regression on Functional Data

It is well known that the approximation of $\mathbf{Y}$ obtained by the classical linear regression on $(X_t)_{t\in[0,T]}$, $\hat{\mathbf{Y}} = \int_0^T \beta(t) X_t dt$ is such that β is in general a distribution rather than a function of $L_2([0,T])$ (Saporta, 1981). This difficulty appears also in practice when one tries to estimate the regression coefficients, $\beta(t)$, using a sample of size N. Indeed, if $\{(\mathbf{Y}_1, \mathbf{X}_1), (\mathbf{Y}_2, \mathbf{X}_2), \ldots (\mathbf{Y}_N, \mathbf{X}_N)\}$ is a finite sample of $(\mathbf{Y}, \mathbf{X})$, the system

$$\mathbf{Y}_i = \int_0^T X_i(t)\beta(t)dt, \quad \forall i = 1, ..., N$$

has an infinite number of solutions (Ramsay and Silverman, 1997). Regression on principal components (PCR) of $(X_t)_{t\in[0,T]}$ (Deville, 1978) and the PLS approach (Preda and Saporta, 2002) give satisfactory solutions to this problem.

Linear Regression on Principal Components (PCR)

Also known as the Karhunen-Loève expansion, the principal component analysis (PCA) of the stochastic process $(X_t)_{t\in[0,T]}$ consists in representing X_t as:

$$X_t = \sum_{i\geq 1} f_i(t)\xi_i, \quad \forall t \in [0,T], \quad (7)$$

where the set $\{f_i\}_{i\geq 1}$ (the principal factors) forms an orthonormal system of deterministic functions of $L_2([0,T])$ and $\{\xi_i\}_{i\geq 1}$ (the principal components) are uncorrelated zero-mean random variables (Deville, 1974). The principal factors $\{f_i\}_{i\geq 1}$ are solutions of the eigenvalue equation:

$$\int_0^T C(t,s)f_i(s)\,ds = \lambda_i f_i(t), \tag{8}$$

where $C(t,s) = \mathrm{cov}(X_t, X_s)$, $\forall t, s \in [0,T]$. Therefore, the principal components $\{\xi_i\}_{i\geq 1}$ defined as $\xi_i = \int_0^T f_i(t)X_t\,dt$ are the eigenvectors of the Escoufier operator, $\mathbf{W}^X$, defined by

$$\mathbf{W}^X Z = \int_0^T E(X_t Z)X_t\,dt, \quad Z \in L_2(\Omega). \tag{9}$$

The process $(X_t)_{t\in[0,T]}$ and the set of its principal components, $\{\xi_k\}_{k\geq 1}$, span the same linear space. Thus, the regression of $\mathbf{Y}$ on $(X_t)_{t\in[0,T]}$ is equivalent to the regression on $\{\xi_k\}_{k\geq 1}$ and we have $\hat{\mathbf{Y}} = \sum_{k\geq 1} \lambda_k^{-1} E(\mathbf{Y}\xi_k)\xi_k$.

In practice we need to choose an approximation of order q, $q \geq 1$:

$$\hat{\mathbf{Y}}_{PCR(q)} = \sum_{k=1}^{q} \frac{E(\mathbf{Y}\xi_k)}{\lambda_k}\xi_k = \int_0^T \hat{\beta}_{PCR(q)}(t)X_t\,dt. \tag{10}$$

But the use of principal components for prediction is heuristic because they are computed independently of the response. The difficulty in choosing the principal components used for regression is discussed in detail in Saporta (1981).

PLS Regression on a Stochastic Process

The PLS approach offers a good alternative to the PCR method by replacing the least squares criterion with that of maximal covariance between $(X_t)_{t\in[0,T]}$ and $\mathbf{Y}$ (Preda and Saporta, 2002).

PLS regression is an iterative method. Let $X_{0,t} = X_t$, $\forall t \in [0,T]$ and $\mathbf{Y}_0 = \mathbf{Y}$. At step q, $q \geq 1$, of the PLS regression of $\mathbf{Y}$ on $(X_t)_{t\in[0,T]}$, we define the qth PLS component, t_q, by the eigenvector associated to the largest eigenvalue of the operator $\mathbf{W}_{q-1}^X \mathbf{W}_{q-1}^Y$, where $\mathbf{W}_{q-1}^X$ and $\mathbf{W}_{q-1}^Y$ are the Escoufier's operators associated to $(X_{q-1,t})_{t\in[0,T]}$ and $\mathbf{Y}_{q-1}$, respectively. The PLS step is completed by the ordinary linear regression of $X_{q-1,t}$ and $\mathbf{Y}_{q-1}$ on t_q. Let $X_{q,t}$, $t \in [0,T]$ and $\mathbf{Y}_q$ be the random variables which represent the error of these regressions: $X_{q,t} = X_{q-1,t} - p_q(t)t_q$ and $\mathbf{Y}_q = \mathbf{Y}_{q-1} - \mathbf{c}_q t_q$.

Then, for each $q \geq 1$, $\{t_q\}_{q\geq 1}$ forms an orthogonal system in $L_2(X)$ and the following decomposition formulas hold:

$$\mathbf{Y} = \mathbf{c}_1 t_1 + \mathbf{c}_2 t_2 + \ldots + \mathbf{c}_q t_q + \mathbf{Y}_q,$$
$$X_t = p_1(t)t_1 + p_2(t)t_2 + \ldots + p_q(t)t_q + X_{q,t}, \quad t \in [0,T].$$

The PLS approximation of $\mathbf{Y}$ by $(X_t)_{t\in[0,T]}$ at step q, $q \geq 1$, is given by:

$$\hat{\mathbf{Y}}_{PLS(q)} = \mathbf{c}_1 t_1 + \ldots + \mathbf{c}_q t_q = \int_0^T \hat{\beta}_{PLS(q)}(t) X_t \, dt, \tag{11}$$

and de Jong (1993) shows that for a fixed q, the PLS regression fits better than PCR, that is,

$$R^2(\mathbf{Y}, \hat{\mathbf{Y}}_{PCR(q)}) \leq R^2(\mathbf{Y}, \hat{\mathbf{Y}}_{PLS(q)}). \tag{12}$$

In Preda and Saporta (2002) we show the convergence of the PLS approximation to the approximation given by the classical linear regression:

$$\lim_{q\to\infty} E(\|\hat{\mathbf{Y}}_{PLS(q)} - \hat{\mathbf{Y}}\|^2) = 0. \tag{13}$$

In practice, the number of PLS components used for regression is determined by cross-validation (Tenenhaus, 1998).

We note that because $(X_t)_{t\in[0,T]}$ is a continous-time stochastic process, in practice we need a discretization of the time interval in order to obtain a numerical solution. Preda (1999) gives such an approximation. Thus, if $\Delta = \{0 = t_0 < t_1 < \ldots < t_p = T\}$, $p \geq 1$, is a discretization of $[0, T]$, consider the process $(X_t^{\Delta})_{t\in[0,T]}$ defined as:

$$X_t^{\Delta} = \frac{1}{t_{i+1} - t_i} \int_{t_i}^{t_{i+1}} X_t \, dt, \quad \forall t \in [t_i, t_{i+1}), \quad \forall i = 0, ..., p-1. \tag{14}$$

Denote by m_i the random variable $(t_{i+1} - t_i)^{-1} \int_{t_i}^{t_{i+1}} X_t \, dt$, $i = 0, \ldots, p-1$ which represents the time-average of X_t on the interval $[t_i, t_{i+1})$. Then, the approximation of the PLS regression on $(X_t)_{t\in[0,T]}$ by that on $(X_t^{\Delta})_{t\in[0,T]}$ is equivalent to the PLS regression on the finite set $\{m_i\sqrt{t_{i+1} - t_i}\}_{i=0}^{p-1}$.

For some fixed p, we give in Preda (1999) a criterion for the choice of the optimal discretization Δ according to the approximation given in (14).

3.2 The Clusterwise PLS Approach

When the predictor variables form a stochastic process $\mathbf{X} = (X_t)_{t\in[0,T]}$, i.e., the x_i are curves, then classical linear regression is not adequate to give estimators for the linear models within clusters, $\{\alpha^i, \beta^i\}_{i=1}^K$ (Preda and Saporta, 2001). We propose to adapt the PLS regression for the clusterwise algorithm in order to overcome this problem. Thus, the local models are estimated using the PLS approach given in the previous section. Notice that PCR and Ridge Regression approaches are discussed for the discrete case (finite number of predictor variables) in Charles (1977).

Let us denote by $\hat{\mathcal{G}}_{PLS,s}$ and $\{\hat{\alpha}^i_{PLS,s}, \hat{\beta}^i_{PLS,s}\}_{i=1}^K$ the estimators at step s of the clusterwise algorithm using the PLS regression. However, a natural question arises: Is the clusterwise algorithm still convergent in this case?

Indeed, the LS criterion is essential in the proof of the convergence of the algorithm (Charles, 1977). The following proposition justifies the use of the PLS approach in this context:

Proposition 1. *For each step s of the clusterwise PLS regression algorithm there exists a pozitive integer $q(s)$ such that $\hat{\mathcal{G}}_{PLS,s}$ and $\{\hat{\alpha}^i_{PLS,s}, \hat{\beta}^i_{PLS,s}\}_{i=1}^K$ given by the PLS regressions using $q(s)$ PLS components preserve the decreasing monotonicity of the sequence $\{\mathcal{V}(\hat{\mathcal{G}}_{PLS,s}, \{\hat{\alpha}^i_{PLS,s}, \hat{\beta}^i_{PLS,s}\}_{i=1}^K)\}_{s\geq 1}$.*

Proof. Let $s \geq 1$ and $\left(\hat{\mathcal{G}}_{PLS,s}, \{\hat{\alpha}^i_{PLS,s}, \hat{\beta}^i_{PLS,s}\}_{i=1}^K\right)$ be the estimators given by the clusterwise PLS algorithm at the step s. From (5) we have

$$\mathcal{V}(\hat{\mathcal{G}}_{PLS,s}, \{\alpha^i_{PLS,s}, \beta^i_{PLS,s}\}_{i=1}^K) \geq \mathcal{V}(\hat{\mathcal{G}}_{PLS,s+1}, \{\hat{\alpha}^i_{PLS,s}, \hat{\beta}^i_{PLS,s}\}_{i=1}^K).$$

On the other hand, from (13), there exists $q(s+1)$ such that:

$$\mathcal{V}(\hat{\mathcal{G}}_{PLS,s+1}, \{\alpha^i_{PLS,s}, \beta^i_{PLS,s}\}_{i=1}^K) \geq \mathcal{V}(\hat{\mathcal{G}}_{PLS,s+1}, \{\hat{\alpha}^i_{PLS,s+1}, \hat{\beta}^i_{PLS,s+1}\}_{i=1}^K),$$

where $\{\hat{\alpha}^i_{PLS,s+1}, \hat{\beta}^i_{PLS,s+1}\}_{i=1}^K$ are the estimators of the regression coeficients within each cluster using $q(s+1)$ PLS components. Thus the proof is complete.

In our experience, the number of PLS components given by cross-validation with thereshold higher thant 0.9 (Tenenhaus, 1998) provides a good approximation for $q(s)$ from Proposition 1.

We now denote by $\hat{\mathcal{G}}_{PLS}$, $\{\hat{\alpha}^i_{PLS}, \hat{\beta}^i_{PLS}\}_{i=1}^K$ the estimators given by the clusterwise algorithm using the PLS regression.

Prediction

Given a new data point (x_{i^*}, y_{i^*}) for which we have only the observation of x_{i^*}, the prediction problem of y_{i^*} is reduced to the problem of pattern recognition: To which cluster does the point (x_{i^*}, y_{i^*}) belong? A rule that uses the k-nearest neighbours approach is proposed by Charles (1977) as follows.

Let m, M be two positive integers such that $m \leq M$. For each $k \in [m, M]$ let

- N_k be the set of the k nearest neighbours of x_{i^*},
- $n_j(k) = |G^{-1}(j) \cap N_k|$, $\forall j \in 1, \ldots, K$,
- $J(k) = \{j \in \{1, \ldots, K\} : n_j(k) = \max_{l=1,\ldots,K} n_l(k)\}$,
- $\eta_j = \sum_{k=m}^M \mathbf{1}_{J(k)}(j)$.

Then,

$$\mathcal{G}(i^*) = \text{argmax}_j \eta_j. \tag{15}$$

Therefore,

$$\hat{y}_{i^*} = \hat{\alpha}^{\hat{\mathcal{G}}(i^*)}_{PLS} + \int_0^T \hat{\beta}^{\hat{\mathcal{G}}(i^*)}_{PLS}(t) x_{i^*}(t)\, dt. \tag{16}$$

It is important to notice that the properties of the clusterwise PLS regression do not change if $\mathbf{Y}$ is a random vector of finite or infinite dimension. When $\mathbf{Y} = \{X_t\}_{t\in[T,T+a]}$, the clusterwise PLS regression is used to predict the future of the process from its past. We will consider this situation in the following application to stock exchange data. The number of clusters is considered unknown. Charles (1977) proposes to choose K observing the behavior of the decreasing function $c(K) = V(Y - \hat{Y}^L)/V(Y)$. Other criteria based on the decomposition formula (2) are proposed in Plaia (2001). Hennig (1999) gives some approximations of K based on the likelihood function.

4 Application to Stock Exchange Data

The clusterwise PLS regression on a stochastic process presented in the previous sections is used to predict the behavior of shares at a certain lapse of time. We have developed a C++ application which implements the clusterwise PLS approach, by varying the number of clusters and using cross-validation.

We have 84 shares quoted at the Paris stock exchange, for which we know the whole behavior of the growth index during one hour (between 10:00 and 11:00). Notice that a share is likely to change every second. We also know the evolution of the growth index of a new share (denoted by 85) between 10:00 and 10:55. The aim is to predict the way that the share will behave between 10:55 and 11:00 using the clusterwise PLS approach built with the other 84 shares.

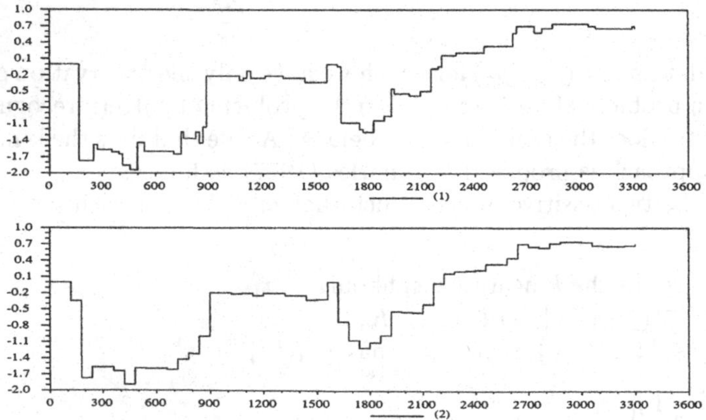

Fig. 1. Evolution of the share 85. The top graph is before approximation, and the bottom is after approximation.

We use the approximation given in (14) by taking an equidistant discretization of the interval $[0, 3600]$ (time expressed in seconds) in 60 subintervals. Figure 1 gives the evolution of the share 85 in $[0, 3300]$ before and after this approximation. The forecasts obtained will then match the average level of the growth index of share 85 considered on each interval $[60 \cdot (i-1), 60 \cdot i)$, $i = 56, \ldots, 60$.

The same data are used in Preda and Saporta (2002) where the global PCR and PLS regressions are fitted. We denote by CW-PLS(k) the clusterwise PLS regression with k clusters, and by PCR(k) and PLS(k) the global regression on the first k principal components and on the first k PLS components, respectively.

Considering the cross-validation approach (thereshold = 0.95) we obtain the following results :

	$\hat{m}_{56}(85)$	$\hat{m}_{57}(85)$	$\hat{m}_{58}(85)$	$\hat{m}_{59}(85)$	$\hat{m}_{60}(85)$	SSE
Observed	**0.700**	**0.678**	**0.659**	**0.516**	**-0.233**	-
PLS(2)	0.312	0.355	0.377	0.456	0.534	0.911
PLS(3)	0.620	0.637	0.677	0.781	0.880	1.295
PCR(3)	0.613	0.638	0.669	0.825	0.963	1.511
CW-PLS(3)	0.643	0.667	0.675	0.482	0.235	0.215
CW-PLS(4)	0.653	0.723	0.554	0.652	-0.324	0.044
CW-PLS(5)	0.723	0.685	0.687	0.431	-0.438	0.055

Using the sum of squared errors (SSE) as measure of fit, let us observe that the clusterwise models give better results than the global analysis. The models with 4 and 5 clusters predict the crash of share 85 for the last 5 minutes, whereas the global models do not. For the model with 4 clusters, the estimation of the distribution of $\mathcal{G}$ is $(17/84, 32/84, 10/84, 25/84)$, with the point 85 belonging to the first cluster.

5 Conclusions

The clusterwise PLS regression on a stochastic process offers an interesting alternative to classical methods of clusterwise analysis. It is particularly adapted to solve multicollinearity problems for regression and also when the number of observations is smaller than the number of predictor variables, which is often the case in the context of the clusterwise linear regression.

References

1. Aguilera, A. M., Ocaña, F., and Valderrama, M. J. (1998). "An Approximated Principal Component Prediction Model for Continuous-Time Stochastic Process," *Applied Stochastic Models and Data Analysis*, **11**, 61–72.

2. Bock, H.-H. (1969). "The Equivalence of Two Extremal Problems and Its Application to the Iterative Classification of Multivariate Data," in *Lecture notes, Mathematisches Forschungsinstitut Oberwolfach.*
3. Charles, C. (1977). *Régression Typologique et Reconnaissance des Formes*, Ph.D. disseration, Université Paris IX, Paris, France.
4. DeSarbo, W. S. and Cron, W. L. (1988). "A Maximum Likelihood Methodology for Clusterwise Linear Regression," *Journal of Classification*, **5**, 249–282.
5. Deville, J. C. (1974). "Méthodes Statistiques et Numériques de l'Analyse Harmonique," *Annales de l'INSEE (France)*, **5**, 3–101.
6. Deville, J. C. (1978). "Analyse et Prévision des Séries Chronologiques Multiples Non Stationnaires," *Statistique et Analyse des Données (France)*, **3**, 19–29.
7. Hennig, C. (1999). "Models and Methods for Clusterwise Linear Regression," *Classification in the Information Age*, Berlin:Springer, pp. 179–187.
8. Hennig, C. (2000). "Identifiability of Models for Clusterwise Linear Regression," *Journal of Classification*, **17**, 273–296.
9. Plaia, A. (2001). "On the Number of Clusters in Clusterwise Linear Regression," in *Proceedings of the Xth International Symposium on Applied Stochastic Models and Data Analysis*, pp. 847–852.
10. Preda, C. (1999). "Analyse Factorielle d'un Processus: Problèmes d'Approximation et de Régression," doctoral thesis, Université de Lille 1, Lille, France.
11. Preda, C., and Saporta, G. (2002). "Régression PLS sur un Processus Stochastique," *Revue de Statistique Appliquée*, **50**, 27–45.
12. Ramsay, J. O., and Silverman, B. W. (1997). *Functional Data Analysis*, Springer-Verlag, New York.
13. Saporta, G. (1981). "Méthodes Exploratoires d'Analyse de Données Temporelles," Cahiers du B.U.R.O, Technical Report 37, Université Pierre et Marie Curie, Paris, France.
14. Spaeth, H. (1979). "Clusterwise Linear Regression," *Computing*, **22**, 367–373.
15. Tenenhaus, M. (1998). *La Régression PLS: Théorie et Pratique.* Editions Technip, Paris.
16. Wold, S., Ruhe, A. and Dunn III, W. J. (1984). "The Collinearity Problem in Linear Regression: The Partial Least Squares (PLS) Approach to Generalized Inverses," *SIAM Journal on Scientific and Statistical Computing*, **5**, 765–743.

On Classification and Regression Trees for Multiple Responses

Seong Keon Lee

Chuo University, Japan
sklee@grad.math.chuo-u.ac.jp

Abstract: The tree method can be extended to multivariate responses, such as repeated measures and longitudinal data, by modifying the split function so as to accommodate multiple responses. Recently, some decision trees for multiple responses have been constructed by other researchers. However, their methods have limitations on the type of response, that is, they allow only continuous or only binary responses. Also, there is no tree method to analyze polytomous and ordinal responses.

In this paper, we will modify the tree for the univariate response procedure and suggest a new tree-based method that can analyze any type of multiple response by using Generalized Estimating Equations (GEE) techniques.

1 Introduction

In many clinical trials and marketing research problems, multiple responses are often observed on individual subjects. Unfortunately, most tree-based algorithms handle only one target variable at a time. So, if more than one correlated responses are observed, they cannot give a reasonable result to analysts.

Some decision trees for multiple responses have been constructed by Segal (1992) and Zhang (1998). Segal (1992) suggested a tree that can analyze continuous longitudinal response using Mahalanobis distance for within-node homogeneity measures. Zhang (1998) suggested a tree that can analyze multiple binary responses using a generalized entropy criterion that is proportional to the maximum likelihood of the joint distribution of multiple binary responses (Cox, 1972; Zhao and Prentice, 1990).

Also, in classical statistics, when researchers want to analyze data that arise from a longitudinal or clustered design, models for discrete-type outcomes generally require a different approach. However, there are a variety of standard likelihood-based approaches to analysis when the outcome variables are approximately multivariate normal, so Liang and Zeger (1986) formalized an approach to this problem using generalized estimating equations (GEE) to extend the generalized linear model (GLM) to a regression setting with correlated observations within subjects.

In this paper, we will show that the decision tree method can be extended to multiple responses, such as repeated measures and longitudinal data, by modifying the split function so as to accommodate multiple responses and applying GEE techniques to finding splits. This method has no limitations for the data type of the responses, while previous methods have limitations on theirs. Therefore, this method would be called the "generalized multivariate decision tree." In Section 2, we shall consider the difficulties in analyzing multiple polytomous and ordinal responses. We shall propose a multivariate decision tree that can analyze any type of responses using GEE techniques in Section 3. Finally, using simulation data and well-known data sets, we shall investigate the performance of the split criterion.

2 Trees for Multivariate Polytomous and Ordinal Data

One of the famous multivariate decision trees was suggested by Segal (1992) and Zhang (1998). Their methods are good approaches for multiple responses. But they could not provide the methodology for correlated discrete responses, such as multinomial or count responses.

Of course, the homogeneity measure $h(\tau_L)$ suggested by Zhang (1998) can be further extended to analyze longitudinal binary responses and polytomous responses. For longitudinal data, the time trend can be incorporated into the parameters of the equation of homogeneity suggested by Zhang. But it is indicated that there are computational issues associated with rapidly increasing numbers of parameters to be estimated when dealing with polytomous or ordinal responses. For polytomous responses, additional parameters corresponding to various levels of the outcomes can be included. For instance, the component $\Psi' y$ can be replaced with

$$\sum_{k=1}^{q} \sum_{l=1}^{c_k - 1} \Psi_{kl} I(y_k = l),$$

where c_k is the number of levels for y_k, $k = 1, ..., q$, and $I(\cdot)$ is the indicator function. As we can see, for polytomous responses the parameters that should be estimated increase substantially. So the implementation requires signficant computational effort.

To avoid computational effort, we will consider another statistical methodology that can easily analyze any type of correlated responses.

3 Multivariate Decision Trees Using GEE Techniques

I shall extend the idea of Chaudhuri (1995) to a multivariate decision tree. He suggested the general recursive partitioning methodology for *univariate responses.* His paper consists of following recursive steps: (i) the univariate model and parameters are estimated from the data in each node by a low order polynomial using maximum likelihood, and (ii) each node is split into two sub-nodes using a criterion based on the distributions of the covariate vectors according to the signs of the residuals.

Similarly, in this section a decision tree that can analyze *multiple responses* using GEE techniques will be proposed. The basic step of this method is to first fit the statistical model using GEE in each node, and find the best split using the residuals. The recursive process is given as follows:

(1) Fit the marginal regression model, using GEE techniques at each parent node.

(2) Let μ_{ij} be the estimated value of y_{ij}. The Pearson residual e_{ij} is calculated for each y_{ij} in the node according to

$$e_{ij} = \frac{(y_{ij} - \mu_{ij})}{(v(\mu_{ij}))^{1/2}}.$$

(3) Calculate r_i, i.e., the average of e_{ij} on each observation, or

$$r_i = \frac{1}{k} \sum_j e_{ij}.$$

(4) Observations with nonnegative r_i are classified as belonging to one group and the remainder to a second group.

(5) The two-sample t-statistics and chi-squared statistics to test for differences between the two groups along each covariate axis are computed.

(6) The covariate selected to split the node is the one with the largest absolute t-statistic. The cut-point for the selected covariate is the weighted (by the inverse of the standard deviation) average of the two group means along the covariate. Observations with covariate values less than or equal to the cut-point are channeled to the left sub-node and the remainder to the right sub-node.

(7) After a large tree is constructed, a nested sequence of sub-trees is obtained by progressively deleting branches according to the pruning method of Breiman, Friedman, Olshen, and Stone (1984), with residual deviance replacing apparent error in the cost-complexity function.

(8) The sub-tree with the smallest cross-validation estimate of deviance is selected.

The characteristics of the proposed method are, first, this split selection strategy performs model fitting only once at each node. The task of finding the best split is reduced to a classification problem by grouping the covariate vectors into two classes according to the signs of the residuals. Second, the highest ranking covariate is interpreted as the direction in which lack of model fit is greatest and is selected to split the node.

Through the above methodology, we can generalize previous methods; that is, Segal's and Zhang's methods can be obtained by setting the "identity link" and "logit link" in the GEE setting, respectively. Also, this methodology extends the general regression tree proposed by Chaudhuri (1995) to multivariate problems by using GEE techniques. Moreover, our proposed method can handle both correlated numeric and categorical multiple responses including ordinal and polytomous data, so that it could be called the *generalized multivariate decision tree.*

4 Application for Multiple Count Responses

Count data appear in many applications; e.g, as the number of certain events within a fixed period of time (insurance claims, accident, deaths, births, and so forth). Epileptic seizure data from Thall and Vail (1990) is concerned with the treatment of people suffering from epileptic seizure episodes. These data are also analyzed in Diggle, Liang, and Zeger (1994). The data consist of the number of epileptic seizures in an eight-week baseline period, before any treatment, and in each of four two-week treatment periods, in which patients received either a placebo or the drug Progabide in addition to other therapy.

The data on epileptic seizures shows correlation within the four time periods considered in the study, as shown in Table 1.

Table 1. Correlation matrix of number of epileptic seizures.

Period 1	1.000	0.688	0.544	0.717
Period 2	0.688	1.000	0.670	0.762
Period 3	0.544	0.670	1.000	0.713
Period 4	0.717	0.762	0.713	1.000

Since the response variables are count data, i.e., number of epileptic seizures, the Poisson distribution should be the first choice for the distribution of response. Hence, the data should be analyzed by using the GEE method with log link. The working correlation should be set as unstructured in each split.

To explain this tree methodology simply, the process of finding the best split in root node will be briefly shown. After the fitting of a marginal regression model at root node, the sign of the average of residuals should be examined for every study subject. Then, the subjects should be classified according to whether they are negative or not. In this example the "minus" group had 38 subjects and "plus" group has 20 subjects. And then, as shown in Tables 2 and 3, the t-values and corresponding significance probabilities should be obtained for a test for differences in mean between the two groups in each covariate. Through these results, it is found that the baseline count, i.e., the number of epileptic seizures in an eight-week baseline period, is the most significant covariate (P-value < 0.0001) and it should be used for the first splitting variable. Then, to find the split point, the mean of the baseline in the two groups and the weighted average of the two group means should be calculated. Consequently the split point is

$$25.21 \times \frac{15.78}{23.39 + 15.78} + 36.65 \times \frac{23.39}{15.78 + 24.39} = 32.04.$$

Therefore, the first split of this analysis is whether baseline is greater than 32.04 or not, and the resulting numbers of subjects in the child nodes are 38 and 20, respectively. Similar steps are then carried out on each node.

Table 2. Mean of the baseline counts in the two groups at root node.

Group	Obs.	Mean	Std.	Min	Max
- sign	38	25.21	23.39	6.00	111.00
+ sign	20	36.65	15.78	9.00	66.00

Table 3. The t-test of differences in mean: root node.

t-test				Equality of Variances		
Variable	Variance	t-value	Pr > $\lvert t\rvert$	Variable	F-value	Pr>F
Treatment	Equal	0.38	0.7045	Treatment	1.01	0.9482
	Unequal	0.38	0.7050			
Baseline	Equal	-3.93	0.0001	Baseline	2.20	< 0.0001
	Unequal	-4.41	< 0.0001			
Age	Equal	1.41	0.1592	Age	1.15	0.4739
	Unequal	1.38	0.1688			

The tree that results from this analysis is shown in Fig. 1. Figure 1 suggests that "number of epileptic seizures in an eight-week baseline period" is the first splitting variable for the number of epileptic seizures in each of the four two-week treatment periods with the P-value of the t-test less than 0.0001.

To examine the average node profiles in Figure 2, patients in terminal nodes 1 and 2 have lower number of epileptic seizures in each of the four two-week treatment. The number of epileptic seizure in node 5 is increasing, although node 4 is decreasing. Terminal node 4 contains the patients who have values for "number of eplieptic seizures in baseline period" between 16.01 and 32.04 and for whom "treatment" is Progabide, although the "treatment" value in node 5 is a placebo. So, we can find the treatment effect of the drug Progabide here.

An advantage of the GEE tree that can be found here is that one can consider not only average profile but also the time trend in interpreting results, as shown in Fig. 3.

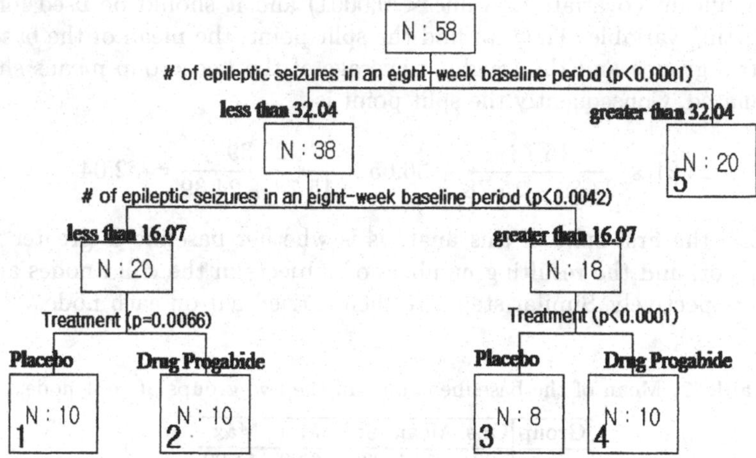

Fig. 1. Tree structure using GEE: Log Link.

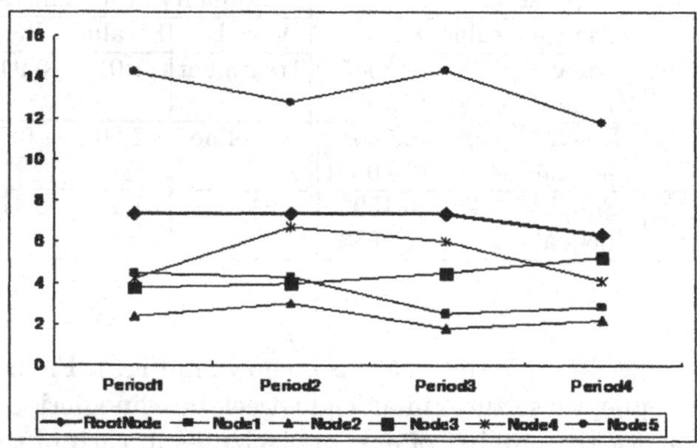

Fig. 2. Average profiles of the number of epileptic seizures within each node of the tree presented in Figure 1.

5 Conclusion and Discussion

We have introduced and described a tree-based technique for the analysis of multiple responses using GEE. By applying GEE techniques for finding

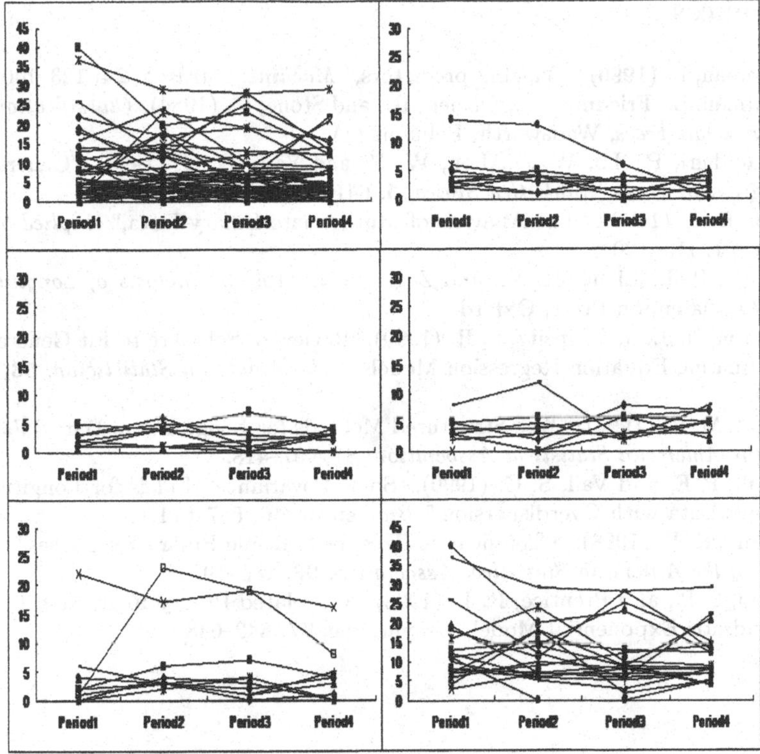

Fig. 3. Patterns of the number of epiletic siezures for all individuals in the root and terminal nodes of the tree presented in Figure 1.

splits, we have shown that the decision tree method can be extended to repeated measures and longitudinal data by modifying the split function so as to accommodate multiple responses. Compared to previous multivariate decision tree methods that have limitations on the type of response, the proposed method can analyze any type of multiple responses by using GEE techniques. Hence, we shall call it the *generalized multivariate decision tree*.

To produce good results by using our tree method, we need to consider carefully the choice of model for the correlation structure of the responses. Horton and Lipsitz (1999) indicated that if the number of observations per cluster is small in a balanced and complete design, then an *unstructured* matrix is recommended. For datasets with mistimed measurements, it may be reasonable to consider a model where the correlation is a function of the time between observations (i.e., *M-dependent* or *autoregressive*). For datasets with clustered observations (i.e., rat litters), there may be no logical ordering for observations within a cluster and an *exchangeable* structure may be most appropriate.

References

1. Breiman, L. (1996). "Bagging predictors," *Machine Learning*, **24**, 123–140.
2. Breiman, L., Friedman, J., Olshen, R., and Stone, C. (1984). *Classification and Regression Trees*, Wadsworth, Belmont CA.
3. Chaudhuri, P., Lo, W. D., Loh, W. Y. and Yang C. C. (1995). "Generalized Regression Trees," *Statistica Sinica*, **5**, 641–666.
4. Cox, D. R. (1972). "The Analysis of Multivariate Binary Data," *Applied Statistics*, **21**, 113–120.
5. Diggle, P. J., Liang, K. Y., and Zeger, S. L. (1994). *Analysis of Longitudinal Data*, Clarendon Press, Oxford.
6. Horton, N. J., and Lipsitz, S. R. (1999). "Review of Software to Fit Generalized Estimating Equation Regression Models," *The American Statistician*, **53**, 160–169.
7. Segal, M. R. (1992). "Tree-Structured Methods for Longitudinal Data," *Journal of the American Statistical Association*, **87**, 407–418.
8. Thall, P. F. and Vail, S. C. (1990). "Some Covariance Models for Longitudinal Count Data with Overdispersion," *Biometrics*, **46**, 657–671.
9. Zhang, H. P. (1998). "Classification Tree for Multiple Binary Responses," *Journal of the American Statistical Association*, **93**, 180–193.
10. Zhao, L. P., and Prentice, R. L. (1990). "Correlated Binary Regression Using a Quadratic Exponential Model," *Biometrika*, **77**, 642–648.

Subsetting Kernel Regression Models Using Genetic Algorithm and the Information Measure of Complexity

Xinli Bao and Hamparsum Bozdogan

The University of Tennessee at Knoxville, U.S.A.
{xbao, bozdogan}@utk.edu

1 Introduction

Recently in statistical data mining and knowledge discovery, kernel-based methods have attracted attention by many researchers. As a result, many kernel-based methods have been developed, particularly, a family of regularized least squares regression models in a *Reproducing Kernel Hilbert Space (RKHS)* have been developed (Aronszajn, 1950). The *RKHS* family includes *kernel principal component regression K-PCR* (Rosipal et al. 2000, 2001), *kernel ridge regression K-RR* (Saunders et al., 1998, Cristianini and Shawe-Taylor, 2000) and most recently *kernel partial least squares K-PLSR* (Rosipal and Trejo 2001, Bennett and Emrechts 2003). Rosipal et al. (2001) compared the *K-PLSR*, *K-PCR* and *K-RR* techniques using conventional statistical procedures and demonstrated that "*K-PLSR achieves the same results as K-PCR, but uses significantly fewer and qualitatively different components*" through computational experiments.

In this paper, we focus our attention on the *K-PLSR*. We develop a novel computationally feasible subset selection method for *K-PLSR* and show how to select an appropriate kernel function when the original data are nonlinearly mapped into a feature space $\mathcal{F}$. To our knowledge up to now in the literature of kernel based-methods, there is no practical method for choosing the best kernel function for a given data set. Further, as stated by Bennett and Emrechts (2003), "*K-PLSR exhibits the elegance that only linear algebra is required, once the kernel matrix has been determined.*" So, the choice of the kernel function is very important and crucial which determines the kernel matrix and hence any result obtained depend on such a choice.

In this paper, for the first time we address this challenging unsolved problem. In doing so, we develop and introduce a genetic algorithm (GA) and hybridize the GA with the information complexity criterion in choosing the appropriate kernel function for a given particular data set, and then in finding the best subset *K-PLSR* and *K-PCR* models. We compare the performances of these two approaches using both training and testing data sets.

We demonstrate our new approach using a real benchmark data set and on a simulated example to illustrate the versatility and the utility of the new approach.

2 Kernel PLSR and Kernel PCR in RKHS

A *RKHS* is defined by a positive definite kernel function

$$K : R^m \times R^m \to R \tag{1}$$

on pairs of points in data space.

If these kernel functions satisfy the Mercer's condition (Mercer, 1909), and (Cristianini and Shawe-Taylor, 2000), they correspond to non-linearly mapping the data in a higher dimensional *feature* space $\mathcal{F}$ by a map

$$\Phi : R^m \to \mathcal{F} \text{ (feature space)}, \tag{2}$$

where $\Phi(\mathbf{x}) = [\phi_1(\mathbf{x}), \ldots, \phi_M(\mathbf{x})]'$ (M could be infinite), and taking the dot product in this space (Vapnik, 1995):

$$K(x, y) = <\Phi(\mathbf{x}), \Phi(\mathbf{y})> . \tag{3}$$

This means that any linear algorithm in which the data only appears in the form of dot products $< \mathbf{x}_i, \mathbf{x}_j >$ can be made nonlinear by replacing the dot product by the kernel function $K(\mathbf{x}_i, \mathbf{x}_j)$ and doing all the other calculations as before. In other words, each data point is mapped nonlinearly to a higher dimensional feature space. A linear regression function is used in the mapped space corresponding to a nonlinear function in the original input space. In the dual space, the mapped data only appears as dot products and these dot products can be replaced by kernel functions.

The main idea is that this new approach enables us to work in the feature space without having to map the data into it. Some examples of valid, that is, satisfying Mercer's (1909) condition kernel functions are:

1. The *simple polynomial kernel:*

$$K(\mathbf{x}_i, \mathbf{x}_j) = (< x_i, x_j > +1)^d \tag{4}$$

2. The *Gaussian kernel:*

$$K(\mathbf{x}_i, \mathbf{x}_j) = exp[-\frac{||\mathbf{x}_i - \mathbf{x}_j||^2}{(2\sigma^2)}] \tag{5}$$

3. The *PE kernel* (a generalization of Gaussian kernel, Liu and Bozdogan 2004):

$$K(\mathbf{x}_i, \mathbf{x}_j) = exp[-(\frac{||\mathbf{x}_i - \mathbf{x}_j||^2}{r^2})^{\beta}] \tag{6}$$

4. *Hyperbolic tangent* or *sigmoid kernel:*

$$K(\mathbf{x}_i, \mathbf{x}_j) = tanh[a < \mathbf{x}_i, \mathbf{x}_j >] \tag{7}$$

which all correspond to a dot product in a high dimensional feature space.

The *partial least squares regression* (*PLSR*) model in matrix form can be defined as

$$Y = XB + E, \tag{8}$$

where Y is a $(n \times p)$ matrix of responses, X is an $(n \times k)$ matrix of predictor or input variables, B is a $(k \times p)$ matrix of the regression coefficients, and E is an $(n \times p)$ matrix of random errors similar to the multivariate regression model.

Kernel Partial Least Squares Regression (K-PLSR) Model: Let Φ be a matrix of input variables whose i-th row is the vector $\Phi(\mathbf{x}_i)$. To develop the *kernel partial least squares K-PLSR*, we define the kernel function as $K(\mathbf{x}_i, \mathbf{x}_j) = \Phi(\mathbf{x}_i)'\Phi(\mathbf{x}_j)$ with the most commonly used kernels listed above. It is easy to see that $\Phi'\Phi$ represents the $(n \times n)$ *kernel* or *Gram matrix* K of the cross dot products between all the mapped input data points $\{\Phi(\mathbf{x}_i)\}_{i=1}^n$. Thus, instead of an explicit nonlinear mapping, we use the kernel function K.

Let T and U be component matrices extracted from KYY' and YY', where Y is the response of training data set. In the *K-PLSR* mode, we can write the matrix of regression coefficients as

$$\widehat{B} = \Phi' U(T'KU)^{-1}T'Y. \tag{9}$$

To make prediction on the training data, we can write the predicted Y as

$$\widehat{Y} = \Phi\widehat{B} = KU(T'KU)^{-1}T'Y = TT'Y. \tag{10}$$

In the case when we have $p = 1$ response variable, the above *K-PLSR* results reduce to

$$\widehat{\beta} = \Phi' U(T'KU)^{-1}T'y \tag{11}$$

and

$$\widehat{y} = \Phi\widehat{\beta} = KU(T'KU)^{-1}T'y = TT'y. \tag{12}$$

The estimated covariance matrix of the coefficients is given by

$$\widehat{Cov}(\widehat{\beta}) = \widehat{\sigma}^2(T'KU)^{-1}, \text{ where } \widehat{\sigma}^2 = \frac{1}{n}(\widehat{\varepsilon}'\widehat{\varepsilon}) \tag{13}$$

is the estimated error variance of the *K-PLSR*.

Kernel Principal Component Regression (K-PCR) Model: In *K-PCR*, let P denote the matrix of principal components extracted from the covarinace matrix $\Sigma = (1/n)\Phi'\Phi$. Then the principal component regression can be written as:

$$Y = Bv + E, \tag{14}$$

E is the matrix of random errors, $B = \Phi P$ and the *least squares estimate* of the coefficients v is

$$\widehat{v} = (B'B)^{-1}B'Y. \tag{15}$$

In the case when we have $p = 1$ response variable, the above *K-PCR* result reduces to

$$\widehat{v} = (B'B)^{-1}B'y, \tag{16}$$

and its corresponding estimated covariance matrix of the coefficients is

$$\widehat{Cov}(\widehat{v}) = \widehat{\sigma}^2(P'P)^{-1}, \text{ where } \widehat{\sigma}^2 = \frac{1}{n}(\widehat{\varepsilon}'\widehat{\varepsilon}) \tag{17}$$

is the estimated error variance of the *K-PCR*.

3 Akaike's Information Criterion (AIC) and Bozdogan's Information Complexity (ICOMP) Criterion

Cross-validation techniques can be used to determine the adequacy of the individual components to enter the final model (Wold, 1978). Rosipal and Trejo (2001) used R^2 and the *prediction error sum of squares* (*PRESS*) statistic for model selection. These do not take model complexities into account. In this paper, we use an informational approach in evaluating the models. An information criterion is used to compare various competing models. Information criteria provide a tradeoff between the model complexity in terms of number of parameters needed to estimate and the ability of the model to explain the data. In particular we introduce Akaike's information criterion and Bozdogan's information complexity criterion for the *K-PLSR* and *K-PCR* models.

Akaike's (1973) *information criterion* (*AIC*) is based on estimating the expected *Kullback-Leibler* (1951) information for regression models and can be written as

$$AIC = n\ln(2\pi) + n\ln\left(\hat{\sigma}^2\right) + n + 2\,(k+1)\,, \tag{18}$$

where n is the number of observations, k is the number of predictors and plus one is for the constant term in the model, and $\hat{\sigma}^2$ is the estimated error variance. A model is chosen if the *AIC* value is the smallest among all the competing models.

Bozdogan (1988, 1990, 1994, 2000, and 2004) has developed a new entropic statistical complexity criterion called *ICOMP* for model selection in general linear and nonlinear regression models. The *ICOMP* criterion resembles *AIC*, but incorporates a different measure of the complexity of the model into the penalty term.

Since for the *K-PLSR* and *K-PCR* models we are dealing with orthogonal design or model matrices, in this paper we introduce another version of

ICOMP(IFIM) which is useful in orthogonal least squares. This new version of *ICOMP(IFIM)* is obtained by approximating the entropic complexity

$$C_1(\widehat{\mathcal{F}}^{-1}) = \frac{s}{2}\log[\frac{trace(\widehat{\mathcal{F}}^{-1})}{s}] - \frac{1}{2}\log\left|\widehat{\mathcal{F}}^{-1}\right| \tag{19}$$

where $s = \dim(\widehat{\mathcal{F}}^{-1}) = rank(\widehat{\mathcal{F}}^{-1})$, using the Frobenius norm characterization of complexity $C_F(\widehat{\mathcal{F}}^{-1})$ of *IFIM* given by

$$C_F(\widehat{\mathcal{F}}^{-1}) = \frac{1}{s}\left\|\widehat{\mathcal{F}}^{-1}\right\|^2 - \left(\frac{tr\,\widehat{\mathcal{F}}^{-1}}{s}\right)^2 \tag{20}$$

$$= \frac{1}{s}tr(\widehat{\mathcal{F}}^{-1\prime}\widehat{\mathcal{F}}^{-1}) - \left(\frac{tr\,\widehat{\mathcal{F}}^{-1}}{s}\right)^2 \tag{21}$$

$$= \frac{1}{s}\sum_{j=1}^{s}(\lambda_j - \overline{\lambda}_a)^2,$$

where λ_j, $j = 1, 2, \ldots, s$, are the eigenvalues, and $\overline{\lambda}_a$ denotes the arithmetic mean of these eigenvalues of $\widehat{\mathcal{F}}^{-1}$ (see, van Emden 1971, and Bozdogan, 1990). In terms of the eigenvalues, we now define this approximation as

$$C_{1F}(\widehat{\mathcal{F}}^{-1}) = \frac{s}{4}\frac{C_F(\widehat{\mathcal{F}}^{-1})}{(\frac{tr(\widehat{\mathcal{F}}^{-1})}{s})^2} = \frac{1}{4\overline{\lambda}_a^2}\sum_{j=1}^{s}(\lambda_j - \overline{\lambda}_a)^2. \tag{22}$$

We note that $C_{1F}(\cdot)$ is a second order equivalent measure of complexity to the original $C_1(\cdot)$ measure. Also, we note that $C_{1F}(\cdot)$ is scale-invariant and $C_{1F}(\cdot) \geq 0$ with $C_{1F}(\cdot) = 0$ only when all $\lambda_j = \overline{\lambda}$.Also, $C_{1F}(\cdot)$ measures the relative variation in the eigenvalues.

Based on the above, we now define *ICOMP(IFIM)* for the *K-PLSR* and *K-PCR* models as

$$ICOMP(IFIM)_{1F} = n\ln(2\pi) + n\ln(\widehat{\sigma}^2) + n + 2C_{1F}\left(\widehat{\mathcal{F}}^{-1}\right), \tag{23}$$

where

$$\widehat{\mathcal{F}}^{-1}_{K-PLSR} = \begin{bmatrix} \widehat{\sigma}^2(T'KU)^{-1} & 0 \\ 0' & \frac{2\widehat{\sigma}^4}{n} \end{bmatrix}, \text{ and } \widehat{\mathcal{F}}^{-1}_{K-PCR} = \begin{bmatrix} \widehat{\sigma}^2(P'P)^{-1} & 0 \\ 0' & \frac{2\widehat{\sigma}^4}{n} \end{bmatrix}. \tag{24}$$

With *ICOMP(IFIM)*, complexity is viewed as the degree of interdependence instead of the number of parameters in the model. By defining the complexity this way, $ICOMP(IFIM)$ provides a more judicious penalty term than AIC. For more details on $ICOMP(IFIM)$, we refer the readers to Bozdogan (2000). We can also use Schwarz's (1978) Bayesian information criterion SBC.

4 Genetic Algorithm For Model Selection

A genetic algorithm has been widely used in problems where large numbers of solutions exist. It is an intelligent random search algorithm based on evolutionary ideas of natural selection and genetics. It follows the principles first laid down by Charles Darwin of survival of the fittest. The algorithm searches within a defined search space to solve a problem. It has outstanding performance in finding the optimal solution for problems in many different fields.

The GA presented here is based on the work of Luh, Minesky and Bozdogan (1997), which in turn basically follows Goldberg (1989). The algorithm is implemented using the following steps:

1. *Implementing a genetic coding scheme*

The first step of the GA is to represent each subset model as a binary string. A binary code of 1 indicating presence and a 0 indicating absence. Every string is of the same length, but contain different combinations of predictor variables, for example, a binary string of 10010 represents a model including variable x_1 and x_4, but excluding x_2, x_3 and x_5.

2. *Generating an initial population of the models*

The initial population consists of randomly selected models from all possible models. We have to choose an initial population of size N. Our algorithm allows one to choose any population size. The best population size to choose depends on many different factors and requires further investigation.

3. *Using a fitness function to evaluate the performance of the models in the population*

A fitness function provides a way of evaluating the performance of the models. We use the $ICOMP$ information criteria defined in the previous section as the fitness function. We also compare the results with AIC as fitness function. In general, the analyst has the freedom of using any appropriate model selection criterion as the fitness functions.

4. *Selecting the parents models from the current population*

This step is to choose models to be used in the next step to generate new population. The selection of parents' models is based on the natural selection. That is, the model with better fitness value has greater chance to be selected as parents. We calculate the difference:

$$\Delta ICOMP_{(i)}(IFIM) = ICOMP(IFIM)_{Max} - ICOMP(IFIM)_{(i)} \quad (25)$$

for $i = 1, ..., N$, where N is the population size. Next, we average these differences; that is, we compute

$$\overline{\Delta ICOMP(IFIM)} = \frac{1}{N}\sum_{i=1}^{N} \Delta ICOMP_{(i)}(IFIM). \quad (26)$$

Then the ratio of each model's difference value to the mean difference value is calculated; that is, we compute

$$\Delta ICOMP_{(i)}(IFIM)/\overline{\Delta ICOMP(IFIM)}. \quad (27)$$

This ratio is used to determine which models will be included in the mating pool. The chance of a model being mated is proportional to this ratio. In other words, a model with a ratio of two is twice as likely to mate as a model with a ratio of one. The process of selecting mates to produce offspring models continues until the number of offsprings equals the initial population size. This is called the proportional selection or fitting. For this see Bozdogan (2004).

5. *Produce offspring models by crossover and mutation process*

The selected parents are then used to generate offsprings by performing crossover and/or mutation process on them. Both the crossover and mutation probability is determined by the analyst. A higher crossover probability will on one hand introduce more new models into the population in each generation, while on the other hand remove more of the good models from the previous generation. A mutation probability is a random search operator. It helps to jump to another search area within the solutions' scope. Lin and Lee (1996) states that mutation should be used sparingly because the algorithm will become little more than a random search with a high mutation probability.

There are different ways of performing the crossover, for example, uniform crossover, single point crossover and two-point crossover. Interested readers are referred to Goldberg (1989) for more details. The method of crossover is also determined by the analyst.

5 Computational Results

In this section, we report our computational results on a real benchmark polymer dataset using our three-way hybrid approach between *K-PLSR-K-PCR, GA* and *ICOMP(IFIM)*. The source of this data comes from Ungar (1995) which has been used in his several other publications. This dataset is called *"polymer plant data"* which is taken from a polymer test plant. It

Table 1. Choice of the best kernel function with model selection criteria.

	K-PLSR			*K-PCR*		
Kernels	*AIC*	*SBC*	*ICOMP*	*AIC*	*SBC*	*ICOMP*
$(< x_i, x_j >)$	−976.39	−957.37	−772.26	−705.8	−699.98	−627.52
$(< x_i, x_j > +1)^2$	−1105.9	−1084.8	−926.38	**−754.02**	**−741.93**	**−659.34**
Gaussian	**−1146.6**	**−1127.7**	**−983.30**	−700.82	−695.69	−618.86

has been disguised by linearly transforming the data. This dataset has also been used in Rosipal and Trejo (2001). We chose this data set because *"it is claimed that this dataset is particularly good for testing the robustness of nonlinear modeling methods to irregularly spaced data."* This data set has 10 input variables (or predictors) and 4 output (or response) variables, and $n = 61$ observations.

In our analysis, we use polynomial kernel with degree $d = 1$, and 2, and the Gaussian kernel. In the case of degree $d = 1$ for the polynomial kernel, the model reduces to the *usual linear multiple regression model*. First we optimize the GA over the choice of kernel functions to determine the best choice using all the 4 response variables and 10 predictors. Our results are given in Table 1 below.

Looking at Table 1 we note that for *K-PLSR* all the criteria are minimized under the Gaussian kernel, whereas for *K-PCR* all the criteria are minimized under the polynomial kernel of degree $d = 2$. Next, we compare the *K-PLSR* results with those of *K-PCR* at the micro-level on the *mean squared error* (*MSE*) yardstick to see the performance of these two approaches in the accuracy of the parameter estimates. In carrying out such optimization, the computational cost and complexity is almost null for this data size.

In *K-PLSR*, we pick the best combination of the input variables and extract the same number of components as the number of input variables. While in *K-PCR*, we pick the best subset of components. We could pick the best number of components in *K-PLSR* to further improve its performance.

Of the original $n = 61$ observations, 41 observations are used as training set and the remaining 20 observations are used as testing data set. We ran univariate *K-PLSR* and *K-PCR* using polynomial kernel of degree 2 and the Gaussian kernel. For this data set the usual linear regression model data does not perform well in terms of MSE. In fact MSE's are the largest under linear regression model as compaired to the kernel methods. In fact the linear regression model performance the worst for this data set. Therefore, we only report our results for the polynomial kernel degree 2 and for the Gaussian kernel.

For the GA runs, we chose the following GA parameters:

Table 2. The results from one run of the GA for *K-PLSR using information criteria.*

Kernel Method			*K-PLSR*			
Kernel Function	Criteria		y_1	y_2	y_3	y_4
Polynomial Kernel degree=2	*MSE*	Training	0.00315	0.0020	0.0018	*0.001581*
		Testing	0.001509	0.0018	0.0032	*0.0020601*
	AIC	Training	-102.56	-121.21	-123.82	**-130.69**
		Testing	-47.67	-49.398	-57.689	**-63.464**
	SBC	Training	-90.567	-108.98	-113.11	**-116.4**
		Testing	-40.7	-34.62	-42.515	**-56.607**
	ICOMP	Training	-104.28	-123.45	-126.24	**-133.51**
		Testing	-22.798	-52.122	-41.174	**-58.283**
Gaussian	*MSE*	Training	0.0020839	0.0018	0.0017	*0.0012*
		Testing	0.0073735	0.001604	0.0014046	*0.0009*
	AIC	Training	-124.98	-122.41	-132.94	**-140.68**
		Testing	-51.857	-51.948	-56.217	**-63.968**
	SBC	Training	-107.84	-109.17	-113.94	**-123.55**
		Testing	-41.9	-22.307	-45.588	**-54.011**
	ICOMP	Training	-123.85	-125.81	-130.68	**-138.49**
		Testing	-50.733	-49.414	-70.348	**-78.053**

Number of generations	= 15
Population size	= 20
Probability of crossover p_c	= 0.75
Probability of mutation p_m	= 0.01

Consequently, the GA needs to compute only models among all possible subset models. The choices of these parameters here are merely for demonstration purposes. One can set other parameter values also. For one run of the GA, our results are given in Tables 2 and 3 below.

Looking at Tables 2 and 3, we see that comparing *K-PLSR* and *K-PCR*, *K-PLSR* gives more consistent and better results than *K-PCR* both on the training dataset and the testing dataset. Gaussian kernel gives better result than the other kernels. *K-PLSR* provides the best prediction for the response y_4. The best predictors for y_4 are x_2, x_3, x_4, x_5, x_6, x_7, x_8, x_9 and x_{10}. The *mean squared error* (*MSE*) in this case for both the training and testing datasets are much smaller than other choices. We rank order the choices of responses, it is in the order $y_4 \succ y_3 \succ y_2 \succ y_1$.

6 Conclusions and Discussion

In this paper, we have outlined a novel approach of subset selection in kernel based methods. We demonstrated that the GA is a powerful optimization tool for *K-PLSR* and *K-PCR* in *RHKS*. The best model is located by the GA

Table 3. The results from one run of the GA for *K-PCR using information criteria.*

Kernel Method			*K-PCR*			
Kernel Function	Criteria		y_1	y_2	y_3	y_4
Polynomial Kernel degree=2	*MSE*	Training	0.0039384	0.0025633	*0.002395*	*0.0024704*
		Testing	0.0022728	0.0069298	*0.0017671*	*0.0025379*
	AIC	Training	-90.663	-108.27	-111.06	**-116.43**
		Testing	-44.977	-22.681	-50.011	**-52.543**
	SBC	Training	-73.527	-91.137	-93.921	**-99.292**
		Testing	-35.02	-12.724	-40.054	**-42.586**
	ICOMP	Training	-100.24	-117.85	-120.64	**-126.01**
		Testing	-10.682	11.614	-15.716	**-18.249**
Gaussian	*MSE*	Training	0.016148	0.011496	0.0048291	*0.0038671*
		Testing	0.0120	0.003487	0.0053295	*0.0070*
	AIC	Training	-41.095	-56.11	-87.181	-96.346
		Testing	-20.13	-45.282	-29.465	-26.598
	SBC	Training	-33.966	-52.683	-78.613	-85.435
		Testing	-20.292	-43.291	-24.486	-19.202
	ICOMP	Training	-48.759	-63.835	-98.251	-108.16
		Testing	10.8	-38.117	-5.4016	-2.0674

by examining only a very small portion of all possible models in the model landscape.

In the context of our small example using the polymer data set, we showed that the *K-PLSR* model chosen by the GA with *AIC*, *SBC*, and *ICOMP*(*IFIM*) as the fitness function performs better than the *K-PCR* model. With our approach we can now provide a practical method for choosing the best kernel function for a given data set which was not possible before in the literature of kernel based-methods.

In real world applications, we frequently encounter data sets with hundreds and thousands of variables. We believe our approach is a viable means of data mining and knowledge discovery via the kernel based regression methods.

Due to restricted page limitations of this paper, technical details of our derivations have been omitted. Also in a short paper such as this, we intentionally avoided the performance of the GA with that of Simulated Annealing (SA) or some other optimization method. The results of such studies including simulation examples, will be reported and published elsewhere.

References

1. Akaike, H. (1973). "Information theory and an extension of the maximum likelihood principle," in *Second international symposium on information theory*, eds. B. N. Petrov and F. Csáki, Académiai Kiadó, Budapest, pp. 267–281.
2. Aronszajn, N. (1950). "Theory of reproducing kernels," *Transactions of the American Mathematical Society*, ***68***, 337–404.

3. Bennett, K. P. and Emrechts, M. J. (2003). "An optimization perspective on kernel partial least squares regression," in *Advances in Learning Theory: Methods, Models and Applications,* eds. J. Suykens, G. Horvath, S. Basu, C. Micchelli, J. Vandewalle, NATO Science Series III: Computer & Systems Sciences, Volume 190, IOS Press, Amsterdam, pp. 227–250.
4. Bozdogan, H. (1988). "ICOMP: A new model-selection criterion," in *Classification and Related Methods of Data Analysis,* ed. H. Bock, Amsterdam, Elsevier Science Publishers B. V. (North Holland), pp. 599–608.
5. Bozdogan, H. (1990). "On the information-based measure of covariance complexity and its application to the evaluation of multivariate linear models," *Communications in Statistics Theory and Methods,* **19**, 221–278.
6. Bozdogan, H. (1994). "Mixture-model cluster analysis using a new informational complexity and model selection criteria," in *Multivariate Statistical Modeling,* ed. H. Bozdogan, Vol. 2, Proceedings of the First US/Japan Conference on the Frontiers of Statistical Modeling: An Informational Approach, Kluwer Academic Publishers, the Netherlands, Dordrecht, pp. 69–113.
7. Bozdogan, H. (2000). "Akaike's information criterion and recent developments in information complexity," *Journal of Mathematical Psychology,* **44**, 62–91.
8. Bozdogan, H. (2004). "Intelligent statistical data mining with information complexity and genetic algorithm," in *Statistical Data Mining and Knowledge Discovery,* ed. H. Bozdogan, Chapman and Hall/CRC, pp. 15–56.
9. Cristianini, N. and Shawe-Taylor, J. (2000). *An introduction to Support Vector Machines,* Cambridge University Press.
10. Goldberg, D. E. (1989). *Genetic Algorithm in Search, Optimization, and Machine Learning,* Addison-Wesley, New York.
11. Kullback, S. and Leibler, R. (1951). "On information and sufficiency." *Ann. Math. Statist.*, **22**, 79–86.
12. Lin, C-T. and Lee, C.S.G. (1996). *Neural Fuzzy Systems,* Upper Saddle River, Prentice Hall.
13. Liu, Z. and Bozdogan, H. (2004). "Kernel PCA for Feature extraction with information complexity," in *Statistical Data Mining and Knowledge Discovery,* ed. H. Bozdogan, Chapman and Hall/CRC.
14. Mercer, J. (1909). "Functions of positive and negative type and their connection with the theory of integral equations," *Philosophical Transactions Royal Society London,* **A209**, 415–446.
15. Rosipal, R. and Trejo, L. (2001). "Kernel partial least squares regression in reproducing kernel Hilbert space." *Journal of Machine Learning Research,* **2**, 97–123.
16. Rosipal R., M. Girolami, and L.J. Trejo (2000). "Kernel PCA for feature extraction of event-related potentials for human signal detection performance," in *Proceedings of ANNIMAB-1 Conference*, Gotegorg, Sweden, pp. 321–326.
17. Rosipal, R., M. Girolami, L.J. Trejo and A. Cichocki. (2001). "Kernel PCA for feature extraction and de-noising in non-linear regression," *Neural Computing and Applications,* **10**.
18. Saunders C., A. Gammerman, and V. Vovk. (1998). "Ridge regression learning algorithm in dual variables," in *Proceedings of the 15th International Conference on Machine Learning*, Madison, Wisconsin, pp. 515–521.
19. Ungar, L. H. (1995). UPenn ChemData Repository. Philadelphia, PA. Available electronically via ftp://ftp.cis.upenn.edu/pub/ungar/chemdata.

20. Van Emden, M. H. (1971). *An Analysis of Complexity.* Mathematical Centre Tracts, Amsterdam, 35.
21. Vapnik, V. (1995). *The Nature of Statistical Learning Theory*, Springer-Verlag, New York.
22. Wold, S. (1978). "Cross-validatory estimation of the number of components in factor and principal components models," *Technometrics*, **20**, 397–405.

Cherry-Picking as a Robustness Tool

Leanna L. House and David Banks

Duke University, U.S.A.
{house,banks}@stat.duke.edu

Abstract. When there are problems with data quality, it often happens that a reasonably large fraction is good data, and expresses a clear statistical signal, while a smaller fraction is bad data that shows little signal. If it were possible to identify the subset of the data that collectively expresses a strong signal, then one would have a robust tool for uncovering structure in problematic datasets. This paper describes a search strategy for finding large subsets of data with strong signals. The methodology is illustrated for problems in regression. This work is part of a year-long program in statistical data mining that has been organized by SAMSI, the new National Science Foundation center for research at the interface of statistics and applied mathematics.

1 Introduction

The world is full of bad data. Most important datasets contain outliers and errors. For survey data, it is generally appropriate to assume that a significant proportion of the responses are so flawed as to be irrelevant or even damaging to the analysis. Industrial and scientific data are usually a little better, but often a misleading portion of the data come from some aberrant measuring instrument or non-representative situation.

To address this problem, statisticians invented robust methodologies. Most of these (e.g., the L, M, R, and S families) were designed to handle rather simple parameter estimation problems, and the strategies often do not generalize to complex applications such as the use of regression trees, or factor analysis, or multidimensional scaling.

We examine a different type of approach, in which one searches among all subsets of the sample in order to find the subsample that has a strong statistical signal. This signal can be characterized in terms of lack-of-fit (for regression) or minimum stress (for multidimensional scaling); other applications have analogous measures. A desirable subsample is one that contains a large fraction of the data and which has the lowest lack-of-fit measure among all subsets of comparable size.

Obviously, this strategy encounters significant obstacles in practice. First, it is a hard combinatorial problem to efficiently search the list of all possible subsets, even if the search is restricted to subsets of a given size. Second, when fitting models that require significant computation, it can quickly become too expensive to evaluate many different subsets. Third, it is unclear how to make inference on the appropriate level of lack-of-fit (or the analogous measure in more general applications) given that one is trying to cherry-pick the best possible subset of the data.

The first two problems are addressed through smart stochastic search strategies. This raises a number of operational issues which are discussed in detail later in the next section. These issues become especially troublesome in the context of very large datasets, such as federal survey data, microarray data, and transaction data; unfortunately, such datasets are particularly prone to suffer from data quality problems.

The third problem is less susceptible to principled solution. We consider two options: prespecification of the fraction of the sample that will be used, and inspection of a plot of lack-of-fit against subsample size. The second option looks for a knee in the curve that corresponds to the subset size at which one is forced to begin including bad data.

In the context of previous statistical work, our approach is most akin to the S-estimators introduced by Rousseeuw and Yohai (1987), which built upon Tukey's proposal of the shorth as an estimate of central tendency (cf. Andrews et al., 1972, and Rousseeuw and Leroy, 1987). Our key innovations are that instead of focusing upon parameter estimates we look at complex model fitting, and also we focus directly upon subsample selection. See Davies (1987, 1990) for more details on the asymptotics of S-estimators and the difficulties that arise from imperfect identification of bad data.

In the context of previous computer science work, our procedure is related to one proposed by Li (2002). That paper also addresses the problem of finding good subsets of the data, but it uses a chi-squared criterion to measure lack-of-fit and applies only to discrete data applications. Besides offering significant generalization, we believe that the two-step selection technique described here enables substantially better scalability in realistically hard computational inference.

2 Regression Analysis Example

Consider first the standard multiple regression problem. One has n observations $(Y_i, \boldsymbol{X}_i)$ and wants to fit a linear model

$$Y_i = \beta_0 + \beta_1 X_{i1} + \ldots + \beta_p X_{ip} + \epsilon_i$$

where the errors ϵ_i are independent $N(0, \sigma^2)$ random variables. The only unique feature of our problem is that we believe a (potentially large) fraction of the data is spurious, and those data have either no linear relationship or show a different relationship than the rest of the data.

One strategy is to prespecify a proportion of the sample that we want to describe by a linear model. For example, in many applications it seems quite reasonable to find the best linear model that explains 80% of the data. In that case, our job is to search among the $\binom{n}{[.8n]}$ subsets that contain 80% of the sample in order to find the subset that has the largest R^2 value (here $[\cdot]$ denotes the integer part of the argument).

The maximum R^2 criterion uses sum-of-squares as the measure of fit, and is the example used throughout this section. But other possibilities include minimizing the sum of the absolute deviations, or incorporating a complexity penalty on the fit such as Mallow's C_p statistic (1973) or Akaike's Information Criterion (1973). Our methodology extends immediately to such alternatives. The only caveat is that the measure of lack-of-fit should not depend strongly upon the sample size, for reasons discussed in subsection 2.2.

To find the best 80% of the data, we start with a set small subsamples of size $p+2$. This is the minimum size that allows us to fit a model for $\boldsymbol{X} \in \mathbb{R}^p$ and still obtain a lack-of-fit measure. For each subsample we sequentially add sample points, according to a protocol described below. Done properly, there is a strong probability that one of the subsamples will eventually grow to contain nearly all of the good data.

We emphasize that the procedure used entails a stochastic choice of starting sets, followed by application of a selection algorithm to extend those sets. The stochastic starting sets allow us to make a probabilistic guarantee about the chance of having at least one good starting subsample. But the results of the selection algorithm depend slightly upon the order in which the cases are considered, and thus the final result does not quite enjoy the same probabilistic guarantee.

Since we do not enumerate and test all possible subsamples of size $[.8n]$, we cannot ensure that the globally optimal solution is found. But simulation results, some of which are summarized below, indicate that this strategy usually leads to acceptable conclusions. The method applies to a wider range of situations than do competing techniques, such as S-estimators. And the method avoids some of the awkward geometric approximations, such as minimum-volume ellipsoids (cf. Hawkins, 1993), that are used to make S-estimates computable for high-dimensional datasets.

2.1 Choosing the Initial Subsamples

To begin we select the minimum number of samples d needed to guarantee, with probability c, that at least one of the subsamples contains only "good" data. In the regression setting, when a sample contains only good data, all of the data follow the linear relationship that is hypothesized to hold for the majority of the sample.

We begin by drawing the starting subsamples S_i, $i = 1, \ldots, d$ at random with replacement from the set of all n observations. If we let Q be the proportion of data that are thought to be good, then for our application, the number of starting subsamples (each of size $p + 2$) must satisfy:

$$\begin{aligned} c &= \mathbb{P}[\text{ at least one of } S_1, \ldots, S_d \text{ is all good }] \\ &= 1 - \mathbb{P}[\text{ all of } S_1, \ldots, S_d \text{ are bad}] \\ &= 1 - \prod_{i=1}^{d} \mathbb{P}[\ S_i \text{ is bad }] \\ &= 1 - (1 - Q^{p+2})^d. \end{aligned}$$

Thus if one wants to be 95% certain that at least one initial sample is good when 20% of the data are spurious, then we have $p = 1$, $Q = .8$ and $c = .95$. Solving for d means solving

$$.95 = 1 - [1 - (.8)^3]^d$$

which, in integers, means that one must have at least $d = 5$ starting subsamples.

This calculation should be slightly modified when n is small relative to p since we do not want to permit the same observation to appear twice in the same subsample. In that case drawing with replacement gives an inaccurate approximation to d. Instead, one can use finite population methods. The calculation of d becomes slightly more complicated; when p is very large, one needs to use numerical techniques to find d.

2.2 Extending the Initial Subsamples

Using two steps, we extend each of the initial subsamples S_i. If k equals the desired proportion of data we wish to summarize, then the extension process continues until, during or before step 2, the size of n_i of S_i is greater than or equal to $[kn]$.

For each S_i in turn, the first step runs through all the sample values not already in that subsample. If including the observation in S_i reduces the lack-of-fit measure, or increases it by only some prespecified small amount η, then the sample value is added to the subsample and the size of S_i increases by one. At the end of the first step, each observation has been considered and either added to the subsample or not. If at any stage the size n_i of S_i equals $[kn]$, the algorithm stops.

The second step only adds one observation to the subsample in each pass. It searches over the entire set of observations not already in S_i and finds the value that increases the lack-of-fit by the smallest amount. It adds that observation to S_i, and then goes back through the remaining sample to find the next best value to add. Step 2 repeats until n_i equals $[kn]$.

The following pseudo-code describes this algorithm. We use LOF$(\cdot)$ to denote a generic lack-of-fit measure.

Pseudocode for a Two-Step Selection

```
Step 1: Fast Search
Initialize: Draw d random samples S_i of size p + 2 (with replacement).

Search over all observations:
    Do for all samples S_i:
        Do for observations Z_j = (Y_j, X_j):
            If Z_j ∈ S_i goto next j
            If LOF(Z_j ∪ S_i) < η add Z_j to S_i.
            If n_i = [kn] stop.
        Next j
    Next i.

Step 2: Slow Search
Search over all observations:
    Do for all samples S_i:
        Do for observations Z_j = (Y_j, X_j):
            If Z_j ∈ S_i goto next j
            If LOF(Z_j ∪ S_i) < min_j LOF(Z_j ∪ S_i) add Z_j to S_i.
            If n_i = [kn] stop.
        Next j
    Next i.
```

This algorithm starts with a fast search that adds data points quickly, then reverts to a slower search in step 2 that adds data points more carefully. The intent is to balance the need for computational speed against the risk of adding bad data. The main concern is the possibility of a "slippery slope" that allows bad data to enter into a subsample S_i. One does not want a selection that only slightly increases the lack-of-fit to lower the standard so that one gets a subsequent selection that also slightly increases the lack-of-fit, with the end result that a chain of marginally satisfactory selections eventually produces a subsample that contains bad data.

Two vital inputs for the algorithm are the lack-of-fit measure and the choice of η, the tolerated increase in lack-of-fit during step 1. The lack-of-fit measure should not depend strongly upon the sample size; the lack-of-fit values should be comparable as n_i increases. Our choice of R^2 for the measure ensures this, and most alternative measures are either approximately comparable or can be scaled to achieve this.

The choice of η offers one way to enforce comparability, by making η depend upon n_i. But this is awkward in practice and it is easier to find a comparable lack-of-fit measure and use a constant value of η. To avoid subjectivity in the algorithm, η=0 is a legitimate selection. For $\eta = 0$, one only accepts points in step 1 that strictly improve the fitness measure. On the other hand, the value of η can be determined empirically by inspection of a histogram of 100 lack-of-fit values obtained by adding 100 random data points to an initial subsample of size $p + 2$.

The spirit of this two-step algorithm can be implemented in other ways. Our choices reflect an emphasis on speed, and so we accept the risk of suboptimal selections. If one had no time constraints, then one might imagine running step 2 only, so that at each stage one only chooses the very best observation from the pool to be added to S_i. But that clearly requires $d(n-p-2)$ separate reviews of the entire pool, which is hard when n is large or the calculation of the lack-of-fit measure is complex.

Another modification of the algorithm mimics the stepwise rule for variable selection in regression. One might first search for an observation that increases lack-of-fit by the smallest amount, and then re-examine all the elements of S_i to determine whether, after the new observation has been added, any of the previous observations contributes disproportionately to lack-of-fit and thus might be removed. Again, this modification can dramatically increase runtime.

2.3 Choosing the Best Extended Sample

After extending all the initial subsamples to final subsamples of size $[kn]$, we now choose the one that has the lowest lack-of-fit. It is often useful to make a box-plot of the lack-of-fit values, just to determine how much difference the cherry-picking approach has made in fitting the final model. In an exploratory mode, this can help one estimate Q, the fraction of good data in the sample, and that leads to the determination of k, the fraction of the data that one chooses to use in fitting the model.

Similarly, it is often helpful to look at a plot of lack-of-fit against the order of entry of the observations for each of the initial subsamples. If the initial subsample has only good data, then one typically sees a long plateau with a sudden knee when the lack-of-fit measure increases swiftly as more and more bad data are included. An example of this is shown in Fig. 2 of section 2.4, in the context of regression.

2.4 Simulation Results

To examine the performance of the two-step algorithm in the context of regression we generated nine datasets (three groups three) of 100 observations. In each dataset, the good data satisfied $Y = 3X+2+\epsilon$. The X values were simulated independently from uniform distribution on $[0, 10]$. The ϵ values were mutually independent normal random variables with mean 0 and variance 9.

In a real-world setting, the true proportion of good data (Q) is unknown. Thus, it is hard to guess what fraction k of the data one should try to model.

One approach is to guess a good value of k based upon knowledge of the scientific context; another approach is to continue to add observations until there is a bend in the curve shown in Fig. 2, indicating that adding additional observations degrades the fit. In hopes of assessing both approaches, the simulation study explores a range of values for Q when k is held at .8. In all cases the number of initial subsamples was calculated under the assumption that $Q = .9$, even when the true value is lower. Table 1 shows the results from this experiment; the column labeled "n^a" gives the result from the direct application of the algorithm until the prespecified fraction k has been obtained, whereas the column labeled "n^*" gives the number of observations in the final dataset after inspecting a plot of lack-of-fit against subsample size. If an obvious increase in lack-of-fit occurs at a given sample size, the final sample is reduced from n^a to n^* accordingly.

Table 1 shows the results of taking values for the estimated Q and k that either equal or exceed the true proportion of good data in the sample; the latter cases are the most problematic, since then the algorithm is forced to select bad data. The columns labeled "% Good Obs.^{a}" and "% Good Obs.*" respectively indicate the percent of good data within the final sample before and after the inspection of the lack-of-fit plot.

The leftmost graph of Figure 2 plots the lack-of-fit against subsample size when $Q = .9$, $k = .8$, and Std. Dev. = 4. Given 100% of the sample generated from the algorithm are good, the plot depicts a relatively flat plateau. However, when $Q = .7$, $k = .8$, and Std. Dev. = 4, the plotted curve slopes downward indicating bad data exist within the final sample. But an obvious change point or knee does not exist, so we opt not to remove any observations from the sample.

To observe a plot when a knee would certainly occur, we ran one more simulation. Given $Q = .7$, $k = .8$, and Std. Dev. = 10, the rightmost graph of Figure 2 plots the lack-of-fit versus subsample size. Notice the vivid change point when the sample size is 70. As documented in Table 1, the subsample is reduced accordingly.

3 Discussion

Modern computer-intensive statistics fits complex models. But complex models are so flexible that they can be strongly influenced by outliers and (even worse) clusters of bad data.

To address this problem, we propose a procedure that searches among the sample to find a large subset for which a statistical model can be fit without much lack-of-fit. Thus we "cherry pick" the best data for the model of interest, minimizing the chance that bad data will distort the inference.

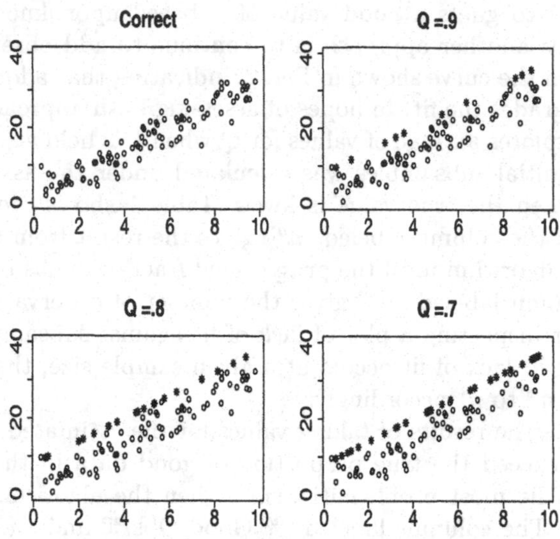

Fig. 1. Scatterplots of clean (upper left) and error induced data. Q percent of the observations are skewed by the addition of 2 times the standard deviation. The symbol "*" represents unclean observations.

Table 1. Compare 10 data quality scenarios for regression

True Q	Est. Q	Std. Dev.	k	n^a	% Good Obs.^{a}	n^*	% Good Obs.*	final R^2
	0.9	2	0.8	80	0.9625	80	0.9625	0.938
.9	0.9	3	0.8	80	0.9875	80	0.9875	0.929
	0.9	4	0.8	80	1.0000	80	1.0000	0.941
	0.9	2	0.8	80	0.9375	80	0.9375	0.918
.8	0.9	3	0.8	80	0.9750	80	0.9750	0.903
	0.9	4	0.8	80	0.9875	80	0.9875	0.884
	0.9	2	0.8	80	0.7625	80	0.7625	0.912
.7	0.9	3	0.8	80	0.8375	80	0.8375	0.865
	0.9	4	0.8	80	0.8500	80	0.8500	0.840
0.7	0.9	10	0.8	80	0.8750	70	1.0000	0.911

We illustrate the procedure in the context of multiple regression, where lack-of-fit is measured by $1 - R^2$. The procedure successfully distinguished good data from bad data in simulated situations, and did so without excessive computational burden in the combinatorial search of the sample.

The procedure we describe extends easily to almost any statistical application, requiring only some measure of fit. There is a natural graphical tool for determining when one has found essentially all of the good data, and that tool performed well in the studies reported here. Subsequent work will extend

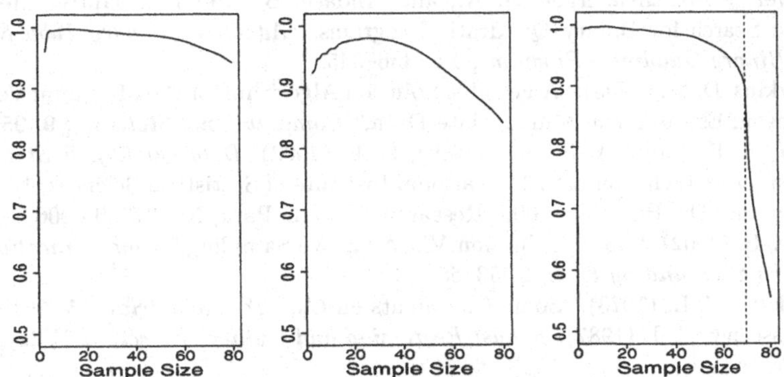

Fig. 2. In regression setting, plotting R^2 versus sample size: (left)true $Q = .9$ and Std. Dev.=4, (middle) true $Q = .7$ and Std. Dev.=4, (right) true $Q = .7$ and Std. Dev.=10. Notice point at which erroneous information appears in right plot; $n^* = 70$

this technique to other situations and provide a more thorough study of the search strategy.

Finally, we note that the proposed approach seems ideal for complex data mining situations in which the sample contains many different kinds of structure (e.g., multiple regression lines, clusters of different shapes and locations, mixture models). One can apply the method described in this paper iteratively, so that the first iteration fits a model to the largest portion of the data consistent with the model, then one removes the fitted data and uses the technique again to fit a new model to the second largest portion of the data. Proceeding in this way, one can extract different kinds of structure in an automatic way.

References

1. Akaike, H. (1973). "Information Theory and an Extension of the Maximum Likelihood Priciple," *Second International Symposium on Information Theory*, 267–281.
2. Andrews, D. F., Bickel, P. J., Hampel, F. R., Huber, P. J., Rogers, W. H., and Tukey, J. W. (1972). *Robust Estimates of Location: Survey and Advances.* Princeton University Press.
3. Davies, P. L. (1987). "Asymptotic Behaviour of S-Estimates of Multivariate Location Parameters and Dispersion Matrices," *Annals of Statistics*, **15**, 1269–1292.
4. Davies, P. L. (1990). "The Asymptotics of S-Estimators in the Linear Regression Model," *Annals of Statistics*, **18**, 1651–1675.
5. Franke, J., H ardle, W., and Martin, R. D. (1984). "Robust and Nonlinear Time Series Analysis", in *Lecture Notes in Statistics 26.* Springer-Verlag, New York.

6. Glover, F., Kochenberger, G. A., and Alidaee, B. (1998). "Adaptive Memory Tabu Search for Binary Quadratic Programs," *Adaptive Memory Tabu Search for Binary Quadratic Programs*, **11**, 336–345.
7. Hawkins, D. M. (1993). "A Feasible Solution Algorithm for the Minimum Volume Ellipsoid Estimator in Multivariate Data," *Computational Statistics*, **9**, 95–107.
8. Karr, A. F., Sanil, A. P., and Banks, D. L. (2002). *Data Quality: A Statistical Perspective* Tech. Report 129, National Institute of Statistical Sciences, 19 T.W. Alexander Dr. PO Box 14006, Research Triangle Park, NC 27709-4006.
9. Li, X-B. (2002). "Data Reduction Via Adaptive Sampling," *Communications in Information and Systems*, **2**, 53–68.
10. Mallows, C. L. (1973). "Some Comments on C_p," *Technometrics*, **15**, 661–675.
11. Rousseeuw, P. J. (1987). *Robust Regression and Outliers Detection.* Wiley, New York.

Part III

Classification and Dimension Reduction

Academic Obsessions and Classification Realities: Ignoring Practicalities in Supervised Classification

David J. Hand

Imperial College, England
texttttd.j.hand@imperial.ac.uk

Abstract: Supervised classification methods have been the focus of a vast amount of research in recent decades, within a variety of intellectual disciplines, including statistics, machine learning, pattern recognition, and data mining. Highly sophisticated methods have been developed, using the full power of recent advances in computation. Many of these methods would have been simply inconceivable to earlier generations. However, most of these advances have largely taken place within the context of the classical supervised classification paradigm of data analysis. That is, a classification rule is constructed based on a given 'design sample' of data, with known and well-defined classes, and this rule is then used to classify future objects. This paper argues that this paradigm is often, perhaps typically, an over-idealisation of the practical realities of supervised classification problems. Furthermore, it is also argued that the sequential nature of the statistical modelling process means that the large gains in predictive accuracy are achieved early in the modelling process. Putting these two facts together leads to the suspicion that the apparent superiority of the highly sophisticated methods is often illusory: simple methods are often equally effective or even superior in classifying new data points.

1 Introduction

In supervised classification one seeks to construct a rule which will allow one to assign objects to one of a prespecified set of classes based solely on a vector of measurements taken on those objects. Construction of the rule is based on a 'design set' or 'training set' of objects with known measurement vectors and for which the true class is also known: one essentially tries to extract from the design set the information which is relevant in defining the classes in terms of the given measurements. It is because the classes are known for the members of this initial data set that the term 'supervised' is used: it is as if a 'supervisor' has provided these class labels.

Such problems are ubiquitous and, as a consequence, have been tackled in several different research areas including statistics, machine learning, pattern recognition, and data mining. The challenges encountered in constructing such rules (data summarisation, inference, generalisability, overfitting, etc.) are the same as those encountered in other areas of data analysis, so that the domain of supervised classification has served as a proving ground for progress in wider theoretical and practical arenas. For these multiple reasons, a tremendous variety of algorithms and models has been developed for the construction of such rules. A partial list includes linear discriminant analysis, quadratic discriminant analysis, regularised discriminant analysis, the naive Bayes method, logistic discriminant analysis, perceptrons, neural networks, radial basis function methods, vector quantization methods, nearest neighbour and kernel nonparametric methods, tree classifiers such as CART and C4.5, support vector machines, rule-based methods, and many others. New methods, new variants on existing methods, and new algorithms for existing methods, including developments such as genetic algorithms, are being developed all the time. In addition, supplementary tools such as techniques for variable selection, multiply the number of possibilities. Furthermore, general theoretical advances have been made which have resulted in improved performance at predicting the class of new objects. These include such methods as bagging, boosting, and other techniques for combining disparate classifiers. Also, apart from the straightforward development of new rules, theory and practice has been developed for performance assessment: a variety of different criteria have been proposed, and estimators developed and their properties explored. These include criteria such as misclassification rate and the area under the Receiver Operating Characteristic curve, and estimation issues such as how best to avoid the bias which results if the criteria are estimated directly from the data used to construct the rule.

Despite the substantial and dramatic progress in this area over the last few decades, work is still continuing rapidly. In part this is because of new computational developments permitting the exploration of new ideas, and in part it is because of new application domains arising. Examples of the latter are problems in genomics and proteomics, where often there are relatively few (e.g. perhaps a few tens) of cases, but many thousands of variables. In such situations the risk of overfitting is substantial and new classes of tools are required. General references to work on supervised classification include Hand (1981, 1997), Ripley (1996), Webb (2002), Hand (2003c).

The situation to date thus appears to be one of very substantial theoretical progress, leading to deep theoretical developments, which have led to increased predictive power in practical applications. However, it is the contention of this paper that much of this progress, especially the more recent apparent progress, is misleading and illusory. In particular, I will argue that the above 'progress' has taken place in the context of a narrowly defined classical paradigm of supervised classification, and that this often fails to take account of aspects of the classification problems which are sufficiently important that they may render meaningless the apparent improvements made in recent years. This paper builds on earlier work described in Hand (1996, 1998, 1999, 2003).

The paper is in two parts. The first explores the relationship between increased complexity of a classification rule and improved predictive power in practical applications. I contend that the marginal improvement of predictive power decreases dramatically once some fairly crude approximations to the underlying distributions have been made. In particular, this means that the slight improvements in classification accuracy claimed for recent developments are indeed only very slight. The second part of the paper then argues that real classification problems involve issues not captured by the conventional paradigm of static distributions with well-defined classes and objectives. For example, I assert that the relevant distributions are often not static, but evolve over time, that the classes often have a subjective and indeed arbitrary component in their definition, and that the criteria used to fit the models are often irrelevant to the real objectives.

Putting these arguments together, I conclude that the failure to capture real aspects of the problems means that often the claimed slight marginal improvements in classification accuracy are swamped by more substantial changes, leading overall to degradation in classifier performance. Put another way, the modern tools are squeezing information from the design data about the distributions from which these data arose, and are solving problems which miss important aspects of the real problem, to the extent that future classification accuracy is often reduced rather than improved. One consequence of all of this is that the apparent superiority of the highly sophisticated methods is often illusory: simple methods are often equally effective or even superior in classifying new data points.

The phenomenon is related to the phenomenon of overfitting. The aim of supervised classification is to construct a rule to predict the classes of new objects. To do this, one estimates the relevant distributions from the design sample, (typically) assuming that this is a random sample from these distributions. Such estimation treads a fine line between providing a biased estimate of the distributions (through using an oversimple model which fails to reflect the intricacies of the functions) and overfitting the design data, reflecting the idiosyncrasies of these data, rather than the shapes of the underlying distributions. Overfitting is thus purely an inferential statistical phenomenon, with its resolution hinging on choosing the right class of models for the estimation—neither too complex nor too simple. In contrast, this paper is concerned with the fact that the distributions from which the design data are chosen fail to represent properly the future distributions to which the classification rule will be applied. This may be because of changes ('drift') in these distributions, or for other reasons.

2 Marginal Improvements

2.1 A Simple Regression Example

Science and scientific folklore have many variants of a law which says that the marginal returns decrease dramatically with increased effort. One example of such a law is the *80:20 law* or *Pareto's Principle*, which, in its original form, says that about 80% of the wealth of a country is controlled by 20% of the people. The basic principle, which the Italian economist Pareto called a 'predictable imbalance' has been applied in numerous other economic and business situations. Another example, also arising in economics, is the *law of diminishing returns*, which asserts 'that under certain circumstances the returns to a given additional quantity of labour must necessarily diminish' (Cannan, 1892).

Statistical modelling is typically a sequential process: one constructs a model, explores its inadequacies, and refines it. The refinement may take the form of adding extra terms to the existing model, leaving the parameters of the existing model as they are, or it may take the form of re-estimating the parameters of the expanded model. In either case, we can compare the predictive accuracy of the earlier model with that of the expanded model, and see how much improvement has resulted from the increase in model complexity. Generally, though there will be exceptions, the marginal improvement will decrease as the model complexity increases: the initial crude versions of the model will explain the largest portions of the uncertainty in the prediction. This is not surprising: one tries to gain as much as one can with the early models.

Although this paper is chiefly concerned with supervised classification problems, it is illuminating to examine a simple regression case. Suppose that we have a single response variable y, which is to be predicted from p variables $(x_1, ..., x_p)^T = \mathbf{x}$. To illustrate the ideas, suppose also that the correlation matrix of $(\mathbf{x}^T, y)^T$ has the particular form

$$\boldsymbol{\Sigma} = \begin{bmatrix} \Sigma_{11} & \Sigma_{12} \\ \Sigma_{21} & \Sigma_{22} \end{bmatrix} = \begin{bmatrix} (1-\rho)\mathbf{I} + \rho\mathbf{1}\mathbf{1}^T & \boldsymbol{\tau} \\ \boldsymbol{\tau}^T & 1 \end{bmatrix}, \tag{1}$$

with $\Sigma_{11} = (1-\rho)\mathbf{I} + \rho\mathbf{1}\mathbf{1}^T$, $\Sigma_{12} = \Sigma_{21}^T = \boldsymbol{\tau}$, and $\Sigma_{22} = 1$, where $\mathbf{I}$ is the $p \times p$ identity matrix, $\mathbf{1} = (1, ..., 1)^T$ of length p, and $\boldsymbol{\tau} = (\tau, ..., \tau)^T$ of length p. That is, the correlation between each pair of predictor variables is ρ, and the correlation between each predictor variable and the response variable is τ. Suppose also that ρ, $\tau \geq 0$. This condition is not necessary for the argument which follows—it merely allows us to avoid some detail.

By symmetry, the linear combination of the x_i which has the maximum correlation with y is obtained with equal weights on the x_i. A little algebra shows this correlation to be

$$R = \frac{p\tau}{(p + p\rho(p-1))^{1/2}}. \tag{2}$$

Since $R^2 \leq 1$ we obtain a constraint on the relationship between τ and ρ:

$$\tau^2 \leq \rho + \frac{1}{p}(1-\rho), \tag{3}$$

from which it follows that $(1-p)^{-1} \leq \rho$, a condition which is automatically satisfied when $p > 1$ since, for simplicity, we are assuming $\rho \geq 0$.

Let $V(p)$ be the conditional variance of y if there are p predictor variables, as above. Now, the conditional distribution of y given $\mathbf{x}$ has variance

$$\Sigma_{22} - \Sigma_{21}\Sigma_{11}^{-1}\Sigma_{12} \tag{4}$$

and

$$\Sigma_{11}^{-1} = [(1-\rho)\mathbf{I} + \rho\mathbf{1}\mathbf{1}^T]^{-1} = \frac{1}{1-\rho}\left\{\mathbf{I} - \frac{\rho\mathbf{1}\mathbf{1}^T}{1+(p-1)\rho}\right\} \tag{5}$$

when $(1-\rho)^{-1} < \rho < 1$. Hence

$$\begin{aligned} V(p) &= 1 - \boldsymbol{\tau}^T \frac{1}{1-\rho}\left\{\mathbf{I} - \frac{\rho\mathbf{1}\mathbf{1}^T}{1+(p-1)\rho}\right\}\boldsymbol{\tau} \\ &= 1 - \frac{p\tau^2}{1-\rho} + \frac{\rho p^2\tau^2}{(1+(p-1)\rho)(1-\rho)}. \end{aligned} \tag{6}$$

From this it follows that the reduction in conditional variance of y due to adding an extra predictor variable, x_{p+1}, also correlated ρ with the other predictors and τ with the response variable, is

$$X(p+1) = V(p) - V(p+1) = \frac{\tau^2}{1-\rho} + \frac{\rho\tau^2}{1-\rho}\left[\frac{p^2}{1+(p-1)\rho} - \frac{(p+1)^2}{1+p\rho}\right]. \tag{7}$$

Note that ρ must satisfy the condition $(1-(p+1))^{-1} \leq \rho$, having increased p by 1, but, again, our assumption that $\rho \geq 0$ means that this is automatically satisfied.

We now want to consider two cases:

Case 1: when the predictor variables are uncorrelated: $\rho = 0$. From (7), we obtain $X(p+1) = \tau^2$. That is, if the predictor variables are mutually uncorrelated, and each is correlated τ with the response variable, then each additional predictor reduces the variance of the conditional variance of y given the predictors by τ^2. (Of course, from (3) this is only possible up to a maximum of p predictors.)

Case 2: $\rho > 0$. Plots of $V(p)$ for $\tau = 0.5$ and for a range of ρ values are shown in Figure 1. When there is reasonably strong mutual correlation between the predictor variables, the earliest ones contribute substantially more to the reduction in variance remaining unexplained than do the later ones. The case $\rho = 0$ consists of a diagonal straight line. In the case $\rho = 0.9$ almost all of the variance in the response variable is explained by the first chosen predictor.

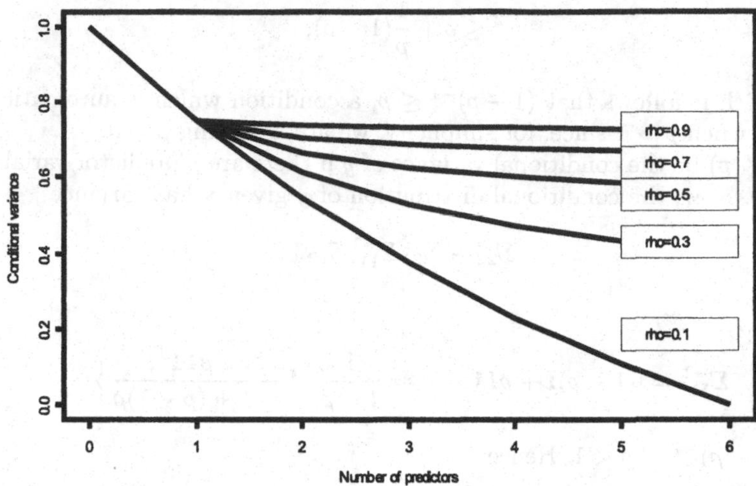

Fig. 1. Conditional variance of response variable as additional predictors are added. $\tau = 0.5$ and a range of values of ρ are shown.

This example shows that the reduction in conditional variance of the response variable decreases with each additional predictor we add, even though each predictor has an identical correlation with the response variable (provided this correlation is greater than zero). The reason for the reduction is, of course, the mutual correlation between the predictors: much of the predictive power of a new predictor has already been accounted for by the existing predictors.

In real applications, the situation is generally even more pronounced than in this illustration. Usually, in real applications, the predictor variables are not identically correlated with the response, and the predictors are selected sequentially, beginning with those which maximally reduce the conditional variance. In a sense, then, the example above provides a lower bound on the phenomenon: in real applications the initial gains are even greater.

2.2 Effectiveness of Simple Classifiers

Now let us return to our main concern of classification. For illustrative purposes, let us use misclassification rate as the performance criterion (similar arguments apply with other criteria). Ignoring issues of overfitting, additional variables cannot lead to an increase in misclassification rate. The simplest model is that which uses no predictors, leading, in the two-class case, to a misclassification rate of $m_0 = \pi_0$, where π_0 is the prior probability of the smallest class. Suppose that a predictor variable is now introduced which has the effect of reducing the misclassification rate to $m_1 < m_0$. Then the scope for further improvement is only m_1. If $m_1 < (m_0 - m_1)$, then future additions necessarily improve things by less than the first predictor variable. More generally, if a model with p parameters reduces the misclassification rate by $(m_0 - m_1)$, then no matter how many more parameters one adds, one cannot further reduce the misclassification rate by more than m_1 . In fact, things are even more extreme than this: one cannot further reduce the misclassification rate by more than $(m_1 - m_b)$, where m_b is the Bayes error rate. At each step, the maximum possible increase in predictive power is decreased, so it is not surprising that, in general at each step the additional contribution to predictive power decreases.

Although the literature contains examples of artificial data which simple models cannot separate (e.g. intertwined spirals or chequerboard patterns), such data sets are exceedingly rare in practice. Conversely, in the two class case, although few real data sets have exactly linear decision surfaces, it is common to find that the centroids of the predictor variable distributions of the classes are different, so that a simple linear surface can do surprisingly well as an estimate of the true decision surface. This may not be the same as 'can do surprisingly well in classifying the points' since in many problems the Bayes error rate is high, so that no decision surface can separate the distributions of such problems very well. However, it means that the dramatic steps in improvement in classifier accuracy are made in the simple first steps. This is a phenomenon which has been noticed by others (e.g. Rendell and Seshu, 1990, p256; Shavlik et al., 1991; Mingers, 1989; Weiss et al., 1990; Holte, 1993). Holte (1993) in particular, carried out an investigation of this phenomenon. His 'simple classifier' (called 1R) consists of a partition of a single variable, with each cell of the partition possibly being assigned to a different class: it is a multiple-split single-level tree classifier. A search through the variables is used to find that which yields the best predictive accuracy. Holte compared this simple rule with C4.5, a more sophisticated tree algorithm, finding that 'on most of the datasets studied, 1R's accuracy is about 3 percentage points lower than C4's.'

We carried out a similar analysis. Perhaps the earliest classification method formally developed is Fisher's linear discriminant analysis (Fisher, 1936). Table 1 shows misclassification rates for this method and for the best performing method we could find in a search of the literature (these data were abstracted from the data accumulated by my PhD student Adrien Jamain, who is carrying out a major overview of comparative studies of classification rules) for a randomly selected sample of 10 datasets. The first numerical column shows the misclassification rate of the best method we found (m_T), the second that of linear discriminant analysis (m_L), the third the default rule of assigning every point to the majority class (m_0), and the final column shows the proportion of the difference between the default rule and the best rule which is achieved by linear discriminant analysis: $(m_0 - m_L)/(m_0 - m_T)$. It is likely that the best rules, being the best of many rules which researchers have applied, are producing results near the Bayes error rate.

The striking thing about this table are the large values of the percentages of classification accuracy gained by simple linear discriminant analysis. The lowest percentage is 85% and in most cases over ninety percent of the achievable improvement in predictive accuracy, over the simple baseline model, is achieved by the simple linear classifier.

Table 1. Performance of linear discriminant analysis and the best result we found on ten randomly selected data sets.

Dataset	Best method	Lindisc	Default	Prop.
Dataset	e.r.	e.r.	Rule	Linear
Segmentation	0.0140	0.083	0.760	0.907
Pima	0.1979	0.221	0.350	0.848
House-votes16	0.0270	0.046	0.386	0.948
Vehicle	0.1450	0.216	0.750	0.883
Satimage	0.0850	0.160	0.758	0.889
Heart Cleveland	0.1410	0.141	0.560	1.000
Splice	0.0330	0.057	0.475	0.945
Waveform21	0.0035	0.004	0.667	0.999
Led7	0.2650	0.265	0.900	1.000
Breast Wisconsin	0.0260	0.038	0.345	0.963

2.3 An Example

The complexity of the first forms of classifier to be developed, such as linear classifiers, could only be increased by increasing the number of variables in x, either by measuring more attributes, or by adding transformed versions of the existing ones. In fact, this led to a substantial early literature on 'feature extraction' from the pattern recognition community in which, essentially because computational power was limited, the variable selection process was separated from the estimation of the decision surface. Later, more advanced developments integrated the two steps: neural networks provide an obvious illustration of this. We can use the integration provided by more modern methods to illustrate how the substantial early gains in predictive accuracy are given by simpler methods. To do this, we progressively fit more complex models.

We illustrate on the sonar data from the UCI database. This data set consists of 208 observations, 111 of which belong to the class 'metal' and 97 of which belong to the class 'rock'. There are 60 predictor variables. The data were randomly divided into two parts, and a succession of neural networks with increasing numbers of hidden nodes to half of the data. The other half were used as a test set, and the error rates are shown in Figure 2. The left hand point, corresponding to 0 nodes, is the baseline misclassification rate achieved by assigning everyone in the test set to the larger class. The error bars are 95% confidence intervals calculated from 100 networks in each case. Figure 3 below shows a similar plot, but this time for a recursive partitioning tree classifier applied to the same data. The horizontal axis shows increasing numbers of leaf nodes. Standard methods of tree construction are used, in which a large tree is pruned back to the requisite number of nodes. In both of these figures we see the dramatic improvement arising from fitting the first non-trivial model. This far exceeds the subsequent improvement obtained in any later step.

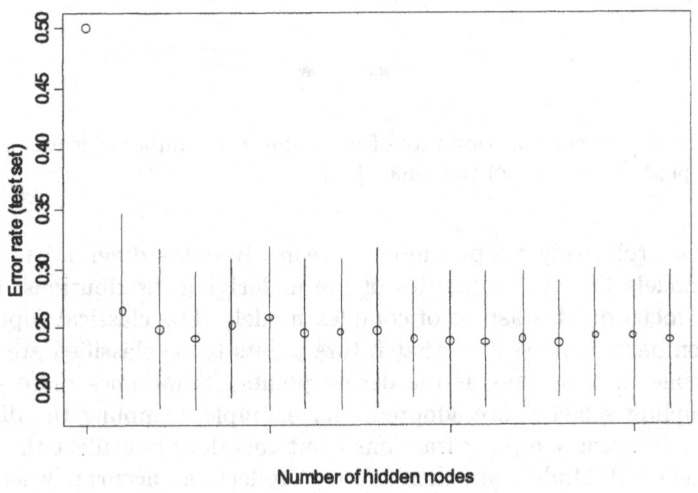

Fig. 2. Effect on misclassification rate of increasing the number of hidden nodes in a neural network to predict the class of the sonar data.

3 Overmodelling

In Section 2 we saw that, when building predictive models of increasing complexity, the simple (early) models typically provide the largest gains. In many cases, 'largest' can be very substantial, accounting for over 90% of the predictive power that can be achieved. The simple models also have the merit of being less likely to overfit the data, purely by virtue of the fact that they are less flexible.

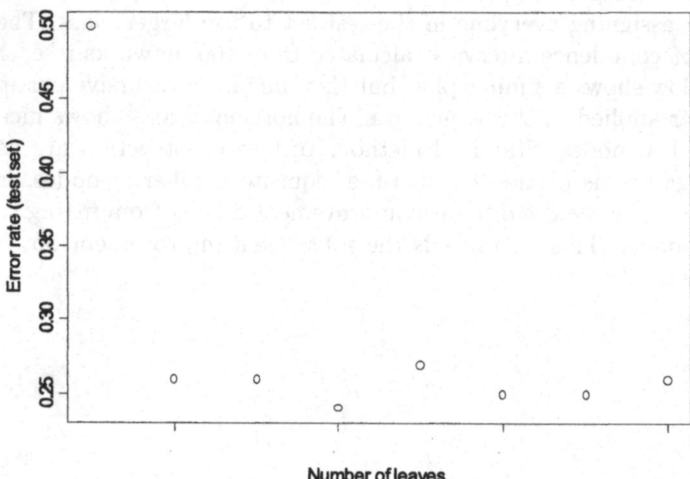

Fig. 3. Effect on misclassification rate of increasing the number of leaves in a tree classifier to predict the class of the sonar data.

Now, when relatively complex models are involved, the differences between two such models fit small subtleties of the underlying distributions. In this section, we focus on this aspect of complex models. The classical supervised classification paradigm assumes that future points to be classified are drawn from the same distributions as the design points. (Sometimes more sophisticated sampling schemes are adopted - for example, sampling the different classes with different sampling fractions - but this does not affect the thrust of the argument.) Models are then built to reflect, as accurately as possible, those distributions, and these are then used to make predictions for new points. However, in many practical situations, certain aspects of these basic assumptions of the classical supervised classification paradigm are untenable.

3.1 Population Drift

Intrinsic to the classical supervised classification paradigm is the assumption that the various distributions involved do not change over time. In fact, in many applications, this is unrealistic, and the population distributions do drift over time. For example, in most commercial applications concerned with human behaviour this will be unrealistic: customers will change their behaviour with price changes, with changes to products, with changing competition, and with changing economic conditions. One of the most important reasons for changes to the distribution of applicants is a change in marketing and advertising practice. Changes to these distributions are why, in the credit scoring and banking industries (Rosenberg and Gleit, 1994; Hand and Henley, 1997; Thomas, 2000; Hand, 2001b), the classification rules used for predicting which applicants are likely to default on loans are updated every few months: their performance degrades, not because the rules themselves change, but because the distributions to which they are being applied change.

An example of such drift is given in Figure 4. The available data consisted of the true classes ('bad' or 'good') and the values of 17 predictor variables for 92,258 customers taking out unsecured personal loans with a 24 month term given by a major UK bank during the period 1st January 1993 to 30th November 1997. 8.86% of the customers belonged to the 'bad' class. A linear discriminant analysis classifier and a tree classifier were built, using as the design set alternate customers, beginning with the first, up to the 4999th customer. The classifiers were then applied to alternate customers, beginning with the second, up to the 60,000th customer. This meant that different customers were used for designing and testing, even during the initial period, so that there would be no overfitting in the reported results. Figure 4 shows lowess smooths of the misclassification cost (that is, misclassification rate, with customers from each class weighted so that $c_0/c_1 = \pi_1/\pi_0$, where c_i is the cost of misclassifying a customer from class i and π_i is the prior (class size) of class i). As can be seen from the figure, The tree classifier is initially superior, but after a time its superiority begins to fade. This issue is particularly important in such applications because here the data are *always retrospective.* In the present case one cannot be sure that a customer is good until the entire 24 month loan term has elapsed. The fact that one has to wait until the end of the loan term means that the design data are always out of date: in the case of the present example, the design data must be at least two years old. Figure 5 shows a similar phenomenon using a different measure of separability between the predicted class distributions. Here points 1, 4, 7, 10,...,12000 were used as the design set, and the resulting classifiers were applied to points 2, 5, 8, 11, ..., 39998. The vertical axis shows a lowess smooth of the estimated probability of belonging to the true class, as estimated by a tree classifier and linear discriminant analysis. The tree classifier initially gives larger estimates, but this superiority is beginning to be lost towards the right hand side of the plot. This plot also shows that the estimates are gradually deteriorating over time: both classifiers are getting worse as the populations change.

In summary, the apparent superiority of the more sophisticated tree classifier over the very simple linear discriminant classifier is seen to fade when we take into account the fact that the classifiers must necessarily be applied in the future, to distributions which are likely to have changed from those which produced the design set. Since, as demonstrated in Section 2, the simple linear classifier captures most of the separation between the classes, the additional distributional subtleties captured by the tree method becomes less and less relevant when the distributions drift. Only the major aspects are still likely to hold.

In general, if the populations drift such that the joint distribution $p(j, \mathbf{x})$ changes in such a way that the conditional probabilities $p(j|\mathbf{x})$, $j = 1, ...c$, with c the number of classes, do not change, then the performance of the classification rule will not be affected. There are also other special cases in which the performance of the rule will not be affected, such as two-class cases in which regions of $\mathbf{x}$ where $p(1|\mathbf{x}) > t$ remain as regions with $p(1|\mathbf{x}) > t$, even if the actual value of $p(1|\mathbf{x})$ changes. Here t is the classification threshold: assign a point $\mathbf{x}$ to class 1, if the estimate of $p(1|\mathbf{x})$ is larger than t. This is equivalent to letting the probability distributions change subject to keeping the decision surface fixed. A simple artificial example arises with two multivariate normal distributions, with different mean vectors, but equal priors and equal covariance matrices of the form $\sigma^2\mathbf{I}$, when σ varies. Here $t = 0.5$.

Situations in which $p(j, \mathbf{x})$ changes, but $p(j|\mathbf{x})$ does not, do occur. For example, in the banking example it is entirely possible that the numbers of people with attribute vector $\mathbf{x}$ may change over time, while the propensity of people with attribute vector x to default may not change. In general, if the $\mathbf{x}$ variables capture all the information about class membership that can be captured then $p(j|\mathbf{x})$ will be unaffected by changes in the $\mathbf{x}$ distribution. Often, however, the true $p(j|\mathbf{x})$ are also functions of other variables (which may be precisely why the $p(j|\mathbf{x})$ take values other than 1 and 2) and these may change over time. These issues are also discussed in Kelly et al., (1999).

The impact of population drift on supervised classification rules is nicely described by the American philosopher Eric Hoffer, who said *'In times of change, learners inherit the Earth, while the learned find themselves beautifully equipped to deal with a world that no longer exists'.*

3.2 Sample Selectivity Bias

The previous subsection considered the impact, on classification rules, of distributions which changed over time. There is little point in optimising the rule to the extent that it models aspects of the distributions and decision surface which are likely to have changed by the time the rule is applied. In this section, we look at a similar issue, but one where the distortion in the distribution arises from other causes.

An important example of this phenomenon occurs in classifiers used for customer selection (for example, the banking context illustrated in the previous section)—see Hand (2001c). Essentially the aim is to predict, for example on the basis of application and other background variables, whether or not an applicant is likely to be a good customer. Those expected to be good are accepted, and those expected to be bad are rejected. For those which have been accepted we subsequently discover their true 'good' or 'bad' class. For the rejected applicants, however, we never know whether they are good or bad. The consequence is that the resulting sample is distorted as a sample from the population of applicants, which is our real interest for the future. Statistical models based on the available sample could be quite misleading as models of

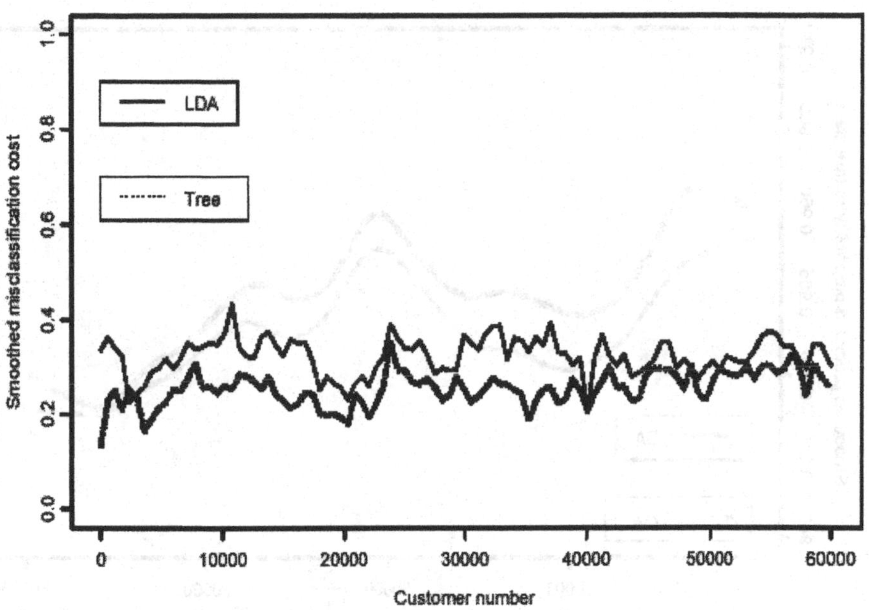

Fig. 4. Lowess smooths of cost weighted misclassification rate for tree and LDA applied to customers 2, 4, 6, ..., 60,000.

the entire applicant population. In particular, in the present context, using highly sophisticated methods to squeeze information from the design data is pointless if that data has been generated by a distribution which does not match the distribution of interest.

This problem has been the subject of intensive research in economics and social sciences. A classic model is that due to Heckman (1976). Suppose that y_1 is an incompletely observed response variable, y_2 is (a hidden variable which is) never observed, X are fully observed covariates, and

$$\binom{y_1}{y_2} = N\left(\binom{x^T\beta_1}{x^T\beta_2}, \begin{pmatrix}\sigma_1^2 & \rho\sigma_1\\ \rho\sigma_1 & 1\end{pmatrix}\right), \tag{8}$$

with $f(R|X,Y,\Psi)$ given by $r = I_{\{x>0\}}(y_2)$, an indicator function, where $r = 1$ means y_1 is missing and $r = 0$ means it is observed. Then it follows that

$$P(r = 1|y,x) = \Phi\left(\frac{x^T\beta_2 + \rho(y_1 - x^T\beta_1)/\sigma_1}{\sqrt{1-\rho^2}}\right), \tag{9}$$

so that, when $\rho \neq 0$, the probability that y_1 is missing depends on $y_1$beyond the information given in x. This model thus constructs a model for the re-

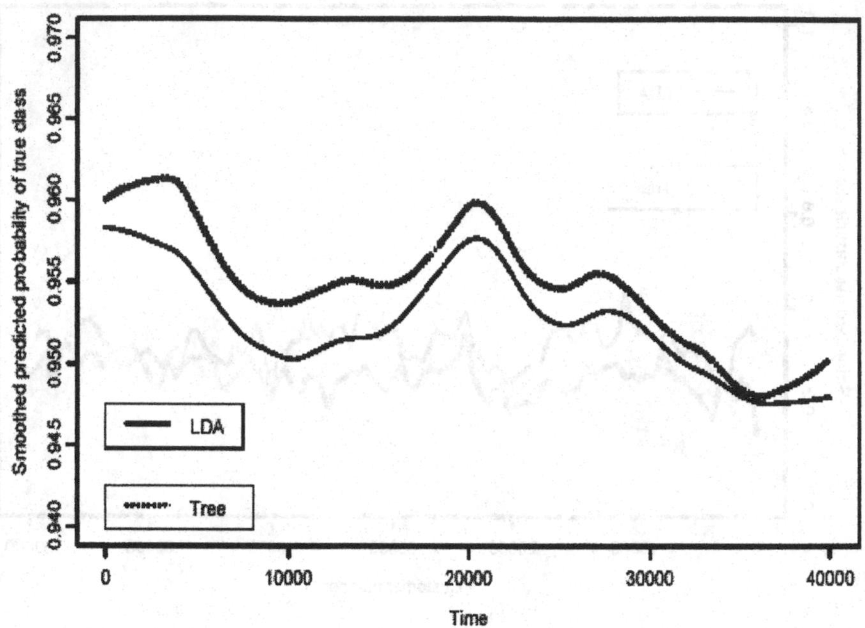

Fig. 5. Lowess smooth of estimated probability of belonging to the true class.

sponse of interest, and also a model for the probability that an observation will be missing. As one might expect, it turns out that the performance of the model is very sensitive to the validity of the structures assumed by the model.

3.3 Errors in Class Labels

The classical supervised classification paradigm is based on the assumption that there is no error in the true class labels. If one expects error in the class labels, then one can build models which explicitly allow for this, and there has been work developing such models. Difficulties arise, however, when one does not expect such errors, but they nevertheless occur.

Suppose that, with two classes, the true posterior class probabilities are $p(1|\mathbf{x})$ and $p(2|\mathbf{x})$ and that a (small) proportion of δ each class are incorrectly believed to come from the other class at each $\mathbf{x}$. Denoting the apparent posterior probability of class 1 by $p^*(1|\mathbf{x})$, we have

$$p^*(1|\mathbf{x}) = (1-\delta)p(1|\mathbf{x}) + \delta p(2|\mathbf{x}).$$

It follows that, if we let $r(\mathbf{x}) = p(1|\mathbf{x})/p(2|\mathbf{x})$ denote the true odds, and $r^*(\mathbf{x}) = p^*(1|\mathbf{x})/p^*(2|\mathbf{x})$ the apparent odds, then

$$r^*(\mathbf{x}) = \frac{r(\mathbf{x}) + c}{cr(\mathbf{x} + 1)} \tag{10}$$

with $c = \delta/(1 - \delta)$.

With small c, (10) is monotonic increasing in $r(\mathbf{x})$, so that contours of $r(\mathbf{x})$ map to corresponding contours of $r^*(\mathbf{x})$. In particular, the decision surface, $r(\mathbf{x}) = k$, will map to an identically shaped decision surface, $r^*(\mathbf{x}) = k^*$. However, it is easy to show that $r^*(\mathbf{x}) > r(\mathbf{x})$ whenever $r(\mathbf{x}) < 1$ and $r^*(\mathbf{x}) < r(\mathbf{x})$ whenever $r(\mathbf{x}) > 1$. That is, the effect of the errors in class labels is to shrink the posterior class odds towards 1. If the classification threshold is at 1, then such shrinkage can be advantageous (see Friedman, 1997), but with other classification thresholds, loss of accuracy is to be expected. More generally, however, the shrinkage will make it less easy to estimate the decision surface accurately. Put another way, there is less information in the data about the separation between the classes, so that the parameters are estimated less accurately and the danger of overfitting is enhanced. In such circumstances, there are clear advantages in sticking to simple models, and avoiding models yielding complicated decision surfaces.

3.4 Arbitrariness in the Class Definition

The classical supervised classification paradigm also takes as fundamental the fact that the classes are well-defined. That is, it takes as fundamental that there is some clear external criterion which is used to produce the class labels. In many situations, however, this is not the case. Sometimes, for example, the definition of the classes used to label the design set points may not be the same as the definition used when the classifier is applied to new data. Once again an example of this arises in consumer credit, where a customer may be defined as 'bad' if they fall three months in arrears with repayments. This definition, however, is not a qualitative one (such as 'has a tumour', 'does not have a tumour') but is very much a quantitative one. It is entirely reasonable that alternative definitions (e.g. four months in arrears) might be more useful if economic conditions were to change. This is a simple example, but in many situations much more complex class definitions based on logical combinations of numerical attributes split at fairly arbitrary thresholds are used. For example, student grades are often based on levels of performance in continuous assessment and examinations. Another example occurs in detecting vertebral deformities (in studies of osteoporosis, for example), where various ranges are specified for the anterior, posterior, and mid heights of the vertebra, as well as functions of these, such as ratios. Sometimes quite complicated Boolean combinations of conditions on these ranges provide the definition (e.g. Gallagher et al., 1988). Definitions formed in this sort of way are particularly common in situations involving customer management. For example, Lewis (1994, p36) defines a 'good' account in a revolving credit operation (such as a credit card) as someone whose billing account shows: (On the books for a minimum of 10 months) and (Activity in six of the most recent 10 months) and (Purchases of more than \$50 in at least three of the past 24 months) and (Not more than once 30 days delinquent in the past 24 months). A 'bad' account is defined as: (Delinquent for 90 days or more at any time with an outstanding undisputed balance of \$50 or more) or (Delinquent three times for 60 days in the past 12 months with an outstanding undisputed balance on each occasion of \$50 or more) or (Bankrupt while account was open). Li and Hand (2002) give an even more complicated example from retail banking.

The point about these complicated definitions is that they are fairly arbitrary: the thresholds used to partition the various continua are not 'natural' thresholds, but are imposed by humans. It is entirely possible that, retrospectively, one might decide that other thresholds would have been better. Ideally, under such circumstances, one would go back to the design data, redefine the classes, and recompute the classification rule. However, this requires that the raw data has been retained, at the level of the underlying continua used in the definitions. This is often not the case. The term *concept drift* is sometimes used to describe changes to the definitions of the classes. See, for example, the special issue of *Machine Learning* (1998, Vol. 32, No. 2), Widmer and Kubat (1996), and Lane and Brodley (1998). The problem of changing class definitions has been examined in Kelly and Hand (1999) and Kelly et al., (1998, 1999b).

If the very definitions of the classes are likely to change between designing the classification rule and applying it, then clearly there is little point in developing an over-refined model for the class definition which is no longer appropriate. Such models fail to take account of all sources of uncertainty in the problem. Of course, this does not necessarily imply that simple models will yield better classification results: this will depend on the nature of the difference between the design and application class definitions. However, there are similarities to the overfitting issue. Overfitting arises when a complicated model faithfully reflects aspects of the design data, to the extent that idiosyncrasies of that data, rather than merely of the distribution from which the data arose, are included in the model. Then simple models, which fit the design data less well, lead to superior classification. Likewise, in the present context, a model optimised on the design data class definition is reflecting idiosyncrasies of the design data which may not occur in application data, not because of random variation, but because of the different definitions of the classes. Thus it is possible that models that fit the design data less well will do better in future classification tasks.

3.5 Optimisation Criteria and Performance Assessment

When fitting a model to a design data set, one optimises some criterion of goodness of fit (perhaps modified by a penalisation term to avoid overfitting). However, it is not difficult to contrive data sets for which different optimisation criteria, each perfectly reasonable, lead to (for example) linear decision surfaces with very different orientations. Indeed, Figure 6 below, from the PhD thesis of one of my students (Benton, 2002, Chapter 4) illustrates this for the ionosphere data from the UCI data repository (Blake and Merz, 1998), and Hand (2003b) presents several examples of how different criteria can lead to contrary conclusions.

If the use to which the model will be put is well-specified, to the extent that a measure of performance can be precisely defined, then clearly this measure should determine the criterion of goodness of fit. For example, if one knew that one wished to minimise the proportion of class 1 points that were misclassified, subject to having no more than 5% of class 2 points misclassified, then an appropriate criterion would simply be the proportion of class 1 points misclassified when (no more than) 5% of class 2 points were misclassified. This seems so obvious as to make its statement almost an insult, but it is rarely applied in practice. There are several reasons for this, of which perhaps the most important is that one rarely actually knows precisely what one should regard as a good classifier, or how its performance should ideally be measured. Instead, as a consequence, the tendency is to adopt one of the widely used measures, such as misclassification rate, area under the ROC curve, or likelihood. We briefly examine these measures.

Many sophisticated estimates of the likely future misclassification rate of a classification rule have been developed (for reviews see Hand, 1986, and Schiavo and Hand, 2000) but this criterion assumes that all types of misclassification (from class i to class j, for $i \neq j$) are equally serious. This is seldom an appropriate assumption (Hand, 2001). More usually some types of misclassification are known to be more serious than other types, but it is difficult to quantify the relative severity precisely. This is true even for the two class case, let alone multiple class problems. If the relative misclassification severities are known, then weighted misclassification rate can be used as the optimisation criterion and performance measure. If they are not known, then, for the two class case, a common strategy is to integrate over all possible values of the misclassification cost ratio, using a given probability measure (for details see Hand, 2003b). This produces a measure equivalent to the area under the ROC curve. However, this does not really solve the problem, simply giving a weight to each possible misclassification cost ratio (whereas choosing one ratio weights all the others as zero). Adams and Hand (1999) propose an intermediate strategy, in which the analyst supplies an explicit weight function.

Measures such as misclassification rate and area under the ROC curve do, at least, explicitly recognise that the aim is classification. Measures such as likelihood are concerned with model fitting, and ignore the ultimate objective (to classify new points). One way of looking at such measures is that they are a recognition of the fact that the ideal criterion is unknown, so one optimises a criterion which is good in the general sense that it provides an overall good fit. This is fine if the true distributions from which the data arise are included in the family $p(y|\mathbf{x};\Theta)$ of distributions from which the maximum

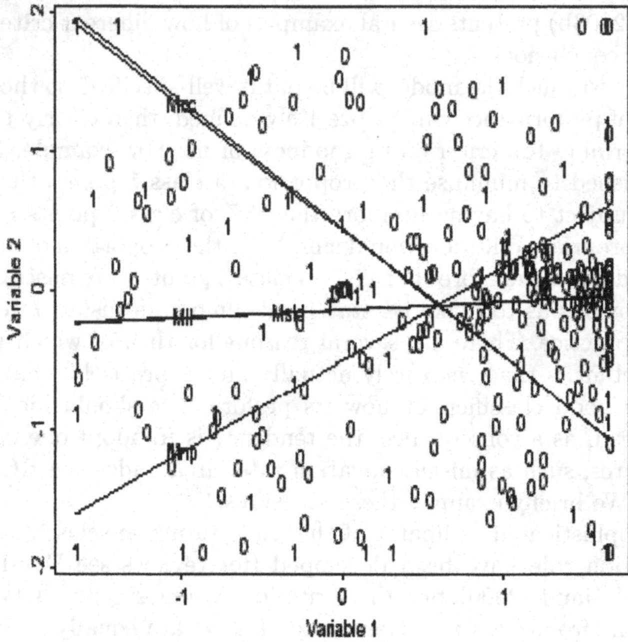

Fig. 6. The direction of maximally increasing error rate is indicated by the line starting at the top left, while the direction of maximally increasing Gini coefficient is indicated by the line starting at the bottom left.

likelihood estimate is sought. However, if the family does not include the true distribution, then difficulties can arise. In these circumstances, changes to the distribution of predictor variables, $p(\mathbf{x}$, can substantially alter the predictions of the model. Hand and Vinciotti (2003) have developed improved classification rules based on this fact—but they again rely on knowledge of the relative misclassification severities.

In the context of this paper, if there is uncertainty over the appropriate criterion to optimise to estimate the parameters of a model, then there is little point in fitting a highly sophisticated model which squeezes the last drop of accuracy of predictive fit to the data. For example, while one might improve a measure of the penalised likelihood by a small percentage, if misclassification rate is the real object of interest then this small percentage improvement is hardly relevant.

3.6 Lack of Improvement Over Time

Research and progress are, in certain contexts, almost synonymous. In particular, if research in classifier technology is useful, it is presumed to lead to more accurate classifiers. Ideally, researchers publish their work because they feel that their methods do better than existing methods. If all this is true, it should manifest itself in the literature. In particular, for any of the traditional test-bed datasets, such as those found in the UCI database (Blake and Merz, 1998), one might expect to see a gradual reduction in the best error rate attained, over time, as more and more sophisticated classification tools were developed. Of course, in theory, the minimum is bounded below by the Bayes error rate, so one might expect to see an asymptotic effect as this value is approached.. In practice, however, there will be a degree of overfitting—even to the test data—merely because so many models have been explored. This will introduce some randomness.

As part of a major study on comparative performance of classification rules, Adrien Jamain and myself plotted the published misclassification rates for a wide variety of methods on wide variety of familiar data sets. The plot in Figure 7 is typical of the results we obtained. This is a plot for the Pima Indian data from the UCI database. Most of the other datasets have similar patterns. The key aspect of the distribution for our purposes is that it shows little or no improvement over time. There appears to be no trend showing the expected gradual improvement over time. The value of the minima vary essentially randomly with time.

One possible explanation for the lack of a trend in the minimum error rate is that the graph covers an insufficient time scale: it might be argued that the technology has not changed much over the period covered by the graph. On the other hand, this plot does cover 10 years, so that presumably the later publications knew well what sort of results had appeared in the earlier ones. However, another possible explanation for the lack of downward trend for the minimum error rate is simply that the less powerful models (presumably those applied towards the left of the graph) have already eaten up most of the predictive power in the available predictor variables. That is, the big gains have already been taken, reducing the error rate to near the Bayes error rate, leaving only slight extra improvements to be made, and these slight extra possibilities are swamped by random aspects of the problem.

4 Discussion

The aim of this paper has been to demonstrate that the largest gains in classification accuracy are made by relatively simple models, and that real classification problems include elements of uncertainty, to the extent that more complex models often fail to improve things. We have discussed several important causes of such uncertainty in real problems, but there are many others. For example:

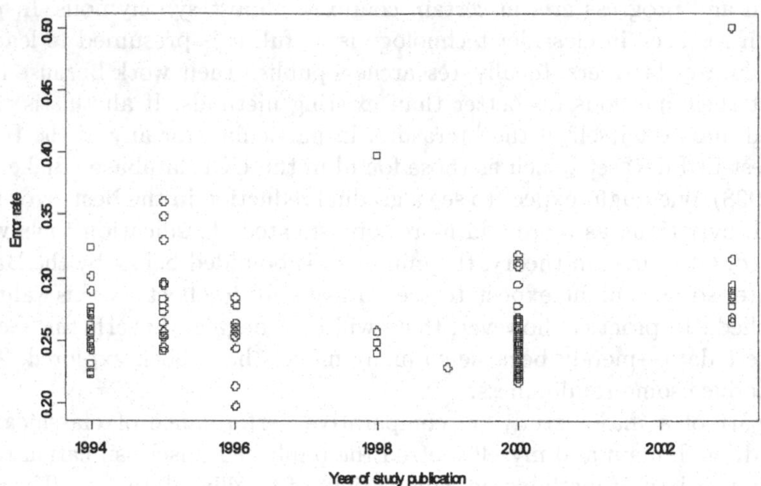

Fig. 7. Misclassification rates against publication date for a variety of classification rules applied to the Pima Indians data.

- more complicated models often require tuning of the parameters (e.g. the number of hidden nodes in a neural network) and, in general, experts are more able to obtain good results than are inexperienced users. On the other hand, simple models (e.g. perceptrons) can often be applied successfully by inexperienced users. The superiority of advanced and sophisticated tools may only be true if and when these tools are used by experts.

- since the improvements to be gained by advanced methods are relatively small, they may well be subject to large amounts of dataset bias. That is, data sets with different distributional structures may not respond as well to the advantages of the methods as the datasets used to illustrate the superiority of different approaches to supervised classification.

- many of the comparative studies between classification rules draw their conclusions from a very small number of points correctly classified by one method but not by another (the present author has not been immune from such inferences). This is to be expected, given our conclusion from Section 2 that most of the big gains come from the simple first steps of the models. However, it means that doubt must be cast on the generalisability of the conclusions to other data sets, and especially to other data sets from different kinds of source, even if a statistically significant difference has been established within the context of one data set.

- this entire paper has focused on classification performance as a goal, however that is defined. But classification rules are used in other ways. For example, Hand (1987, 1996) compares the use of classification rules for diagnosis, screening, and prevalence estimation. A rule which is good for one task may not be good for another.

The fact that simple models will often correctly classify most of the points has been implicitly used in classifier design in the past. For example, in the 'reject option', a simple classifier is used to filter out those points which are easy to classify, leaving the remainder to be classified by a more complicated model, typically based on more data.

Finally, we should note that there are other reasons for favouring simple models. Interpretability, in particular, is often an important requirement of a classification rule. Sometimes it is even a legal requirement (e.g. in credit scoring). This leads us to the observation that what is 'simple' may depend on the observer. In this paper we have taken a linear combination of the predictor variables, as used in linear discriminant analysis, the perceptron, and logistic discrimination, as embodying 'simple', but other perspectives could be taken. Tree classifiers—at least, shallow trees without too may internal nodes—are taken as simple in some contexts. Likewise, nearest neighbour methods have a very simple explanation ("most of the similar objects were class 1, so we assigned this object to class 1").

The literature of supervised classification is a literature of impressive theoretical and practical development. It is a literature in which deep advances have led to the creation of powerful computational tools. Furthermore, these tools have been applied to an immensely wide variety of real problems. However, the theories and methods of supervised classification are based on an abstracted general description of the supervised classification problem. Such a general description necessarily sacrifices details of each particular problem. These details—the differences between the different problems—become relatively more important as the general models are refined. At some point, the inaccuracies arising from sacrificing these details outweigh the inaccuracies arising from poorness of the fit of the model to the abstracted general problem. At this point there is no merit in developing solutions to the general problem any further. Rather, one should develop particular solutions, which take account of the special aspects of each problem. This paper has argued that there is evidence that this point has already often been reached. This raises the possibility that simpler classification methods, which do not over-refine the general model, might be more effective than more complex models, which model irrelevant aspects of the general problem with great accuracy. The paper produces some evidence to suggest that, at least in certain problems, this is the case.

References

1. Adams, N. M., and Hand, D. J. (1999). "Comparing Classifiers When the Misallocation Costs are Uncertain," *Pattern Recognition*, **32**, 1139–1147.
2. Benton, T. C. (2002). "Theoretical and Empirical Models," Ph.D. dissertation, Department of Mathematics, Imperial College London, UK.
3. Blake, C., and Merz, C. J. (1998). *UCI Repository of Machine Learning Databases* [www.ics.uci.edu/ mlearn/MLRepository.html], Irvine, CA: University of California, Department of Information and Computer Science.
4. Brodley, C. E., and Smyth, P. (1997). "Applying Classification Algorithms in Practice," *Statistics and Computing*, **7**, 45–56.
5. Cannan, E. (1892). "The Origin of the Law of Diminishing Returns," *Economic Journal*, **2**, 1813–1815.
6. Fisher, R. A. (1936). "The Use of Multiple Measurements in Taxonomic Problems," *Annals of Eugenics*, **7**, 179–184.
7. Friedman, J. H. (1997). On Bias, Variance, 0/1 Loss, and the Curse of Dimensionality," *Data Mining and Knowledge Discovery*, **1**, 55-77.
8. Gallagher, J. C., Hedlund, L. R., Stoner, S., and Meeger, C. (1988). "Vertebral Morphometry: Normative Data," *Bone and Mineral*, **4**, 189–196.
9. Hand, D. J. (1981). *Discrimination and Classification.* Chichester: Wiley.
10. Hand, D. J. (1986). "Recent Advances in Error Rate Estimation," *Pattern Recognition Letters*, **4**, 335–346.
11. Hand, D. J. (1987). "Screening Versus Prevalence Estimation," *Applied Statistics*, **36**, 1–7.
12. Hand, D. J. (1996). "Classification and Computers: Shifting the Focus," in *COMPSTAT - Proceedings in Computational Statistics, 1996,* ed. A. Prat, Physica-Verlag, pp. 77-88.
13. Hand, D. J. (1997). *Construction and Assessment of Classification Rules.* Chichester: Wiley.
14. Hand, D. J. (1998). "Strategy, Methods, and Solving the Right Problem," *Computational Statistics*, **13**, 5–14.
15. Hand, D. J., (1999). "Intelligent Data Analysis and Deep Understanding," in *Causal Models and Intelligent Data Management*, ed. A. Gammerman, Springer-Verlag, pp. 67–80.
16. Hand, D. J. (2001). "Measuring Diagnostic Accuracy of Statistical Prediction Rules," *Statistica Neerlandica*, **53**, 3–16.
17. Hand, D. J. (2001b). "Modelling Consumer Credit Risk," *IMA Journal of Management Mathematics*, **12**, 139–155.
18. Hand, D. J. (2001c). "Reject Inference in Credit Operations," in it Handbook of Credit Scoring, ed. E. Mays, Chicago: Glenlake Publishing, pp. 225–240.
19. Hand, D. J. (2003). "Supervised Classification and Tunnel Vision," Technical Report, Department of Mathematics, Imperial College London.
20. Hand, D. J. (2003b). "Good Practice in Retail Credit Scorecard Assessment," Technical Report, Department of Mathematics, Imperial College London.
21. Hand, D. J. (2003c). "Pattern Recognition," to appear in Handbook of Statistics, ed. E. Wegman.
22. Hand D. J. and Henley W.E. (1997). "Statistical Classification Methods in Consumer Credit Scoring: A Review," *Journal of the Royal Statistical Society, Series A*, **160**, 523–541.

23. Hand, D. J. and Vinciotti, V. (2003). "Local Versus Global Models for Classification Problems: Fitting Models Where It Matters," *The American Statistician*, **57**, 124–131.
24. Heckman, J. (1976). "The Common Structure of Statistical Models of Truncation, Sample Selection and Limited Dependent Variables, and a Simple Estimator for Such Models," *Annals of Economic and Social Measurement*, **5**, 475–492.
25. Holte, R. C. (1993). "Very Simple Classification Rules Perform Well on Most Commonly Used Datasets," *Machine Learning*, **11**, 63–91.
26. Kelly, M. G, and Hand, D. J. (1999). "Credit Scoring with Uncertain Class Definitions," *IMA Journal of Mathematics Applied in Business and Industry*, **10**, 331–345.
27. Kelly, M. G., Hand, D. J., and Adams, N. M. (1998). "Defining the Goals to Optimise Data Mining Performance," in *Proceedings of the Fourth International Conference on Knowledge Discovery and Data Mining*, ed. R. Agrawal, P. Stolorz, and G. Piatetsky-Shapiro, Menlo Park: AAAI Press, pp. 234–238.
28. Kelly, M. G., Hand, D. J., and Adams, N. M. (1999). "The Impact of Changing Populations on Classifier Performance," *Proceedings of the Fifth ACM SIGKDD International Conference on Knowledge Discovery and Data Mining*, ed. S. Chaudhuri and D. Madigan, Association for Computing Machinery, New York, pp. 367–371.
29. Kelly, M. G., Hand, D. J., and Adams, N. M. (1999b). "Supervised Classification Problems: How to be Both Judge and Jury," in *Advances in Intelligent Data Analysis*, ed. D. J. Hand, J. N. Kok, and M. R. Berthold, Springer, Berlin, pp. 235–244.
30. Lane, T. and Brodley, C. E. (1998). "Approaches to Online Learning and Concept Drift for User Identification in Computer Security," in *Proceedings of the Fourth International Conference on Knowledge Discovery and Data Mining*, ed. R. A. Agrawal, P. Stolorz, and G. Piatetsky-Shapiro, AAAI Press, Menlo Park, California, pp. 259–263.
31. Lewis, E. M. (1994). *An Introduction to Credit Scoring*, San Rafael, California: Athena Press.
32. Li, H. G. and Hand, D. J. (2002). "Direct Versus Indirect Credit Scoring Classifications," *Journal of the Operational Research Society*, **53**, 1-8.
33. Mingers, J. (1989). "An Empirical Comparison of Pruning Methods for Decision Tree Induction," *Machine Learning*, **4**, 227–243.
34. Rendell, L. and Sechu, R. (1990). "Learning Hard Concepts Through Constructive Induction," *Computational Intelligence*, **6**, 247–270.
35. Ripley, B. D. (1996). *Pattern Recognition and Neural Networks*, Cambridge University Press, Cambridge.
36. Rosenberg, E. and Gleit, A. (1994). "Quantitative Methods in Credit Management: A Survey," *Operations Research*, **42**, 589–613.
37. Schiavo, R. and Hand, D. J. (2000). "Ten More Years of Error Rate Research," *International Statistical Review*, **68**, 295–310.
38. Shavlik, J., Mooney, R. J., and Towell, G. (1991). "Symbolic and Neural Learning Algorithms: An Experimental Comparison," *Machine Learning*, **6**, 111-143.
39. Thomas, L. C. (2000). "A Survey of Credit and Behavioural Scoring: Forecasting Financial Risk of Lending to Consumers," *International Journal of Forecasting*, **16**, 149–172.
40. Webb, A. (2002). *Statistical Pattern Recognition*, 2nd ed. Chichester: Wiley.

41. Weiss, S. M., Galen, R. S., and Tadepalli, P. V. (1990). "Maximizing the Predictive Value of Production Rules," *Artificial Intelligence*, **45**, 47–71.
42. Widmer, G. and Kubat, M. (1996). "Learning in the Presence of Concept Drift and Hidden Contexts," *Machine Learning*, **23**, 69–101.

Modified Biplots for Enhancing Two-Class Discriminant Analysis

Sugnet Gardner and Niel le Roux

University of Stellenbosch, South Africa
njlr@sun.ac.za, Sugnet_Gardner@BAT.com

Abstract: When applied to discriminant analysis (DA) biplot methodology leads to useful graphical displays for describing and quantifying multidimensional separation and overlap among classes. The principles of ordinary scatterplots are extended in these plots by adding information of all variables on the plot. However, we show that there are fundamental differences between two-class DA problems and the case $J > 2$: describing overlap in the two-class situation is relatively straightforward using density estimates but adding information by way of multiple axes to the plot can be ambiguous unless care is taken. Contrary to this, describing overlap for $J > 2$ classes is relatively more complicated but the fitting of multiple calibrated axes to biplots is well defined.

We propose modifications to existing biplot methodology leading to useful biplots for use in the important case of two-class DA problems.

1 Introduction

The value of graphical displays to accompany formal statistical classification procedures can hardly be overrated. Indeed, it can be questioned if a complete understanding is possible of class structure, overlap and separation of classes and importantly, the role of the respective feature variables in separating the different classes, relying solely on the formal statistics. Although the biplot was originally proposed by Gabriel (1971) for displaying simultaneously the rows and columns of an $n \times p$ data matrix X in a single graph, the unified biplot methodology proposed by Gower (1995) and discussed in detail by Gower and Hand (1996) allows biplots to be viewed as multivariate extensions of scatterplots. The concept of inter-sample distance is central to this modern approach to biplots and forms the unifying concept. Gardner (2001) argued that this philosophy provides the infrastructure for constructing novel visual displays for unravelling the multidimensional relationships found in statistical classification problems.

Let us consider the following example where the aim is to optimally separate three classes of wood from the genus *Ocotea* from the family *Lauraceae.* Stinkwood (*O. bullata*) furniture items manufactured in the Cape region of South Africa between 1652-1900 are much more valuable than the old Cape furniture manufactured from imported imbuia (*O. porosa*). For both furniture dealers and historians it is extremely important to distinguish between the two types of wood. Traditional classification techniques between the two types and *O. kenyensis*, a third member of the family found in the eastern parts of South Africa but not used for furniture manufacturing, are generally based on subjective judgements of qualitative differences in colour, texture and smell. The following quantitative wood anatomical features were obtained for 20 *O. bullata*, 10 *O. porosa* and 7 *O. kenyensis* samples: tangential vessel diameter (VesD), vessel element length (VesL) and fibre length (FibL). A principal component analysis (PCA) biplot can be constructed to optimally represent the multidimensional variation in the data. The PCA biplot of the *Ocotea* data set in Fig. 1 is a multidimensional scatterplot with a biplot axis for each variable. It is constructed from the first two eigenvectors obtained from a singular value decomposition of the data matrix X but unlike the classical Gabriel biplot these eigenvectors are not shown. In accordance with the Gower and Hand philosophy these two eigenvectors provide the scaffolding for representing all samples together with p axes representing the original variables. Gower and Hand (1996) introduce the terms *interpolation* and *prediction* for the relationships between the scaffolding and the original variables. Interpolation is defined as the process of finding the representation of a given (new) sample point in the biplot space in terms of the biplot scaffolding. On the other hand, prediction is inferring the values of the original variables for a point given in the biplot space in terms of the biplot scaffolding. Generally different sets of axes are needed for interpolation and prediction. All biplots in this paper are equipped with prediction axes.

Each axis in the biplot of Fig. 1 is calibrated in the original measurements of the variables and can be used for inferring the values of the p original variables for any point in the biplot space. Although the three classes can be distinguished in this biplot, they are not optimally separated.

2 Optimal Separation of Classes

Linear discriminant analysis (LDA) is concerned with the optimal separation of classes. This is achieved by finding linear combinations of the predictor variables that maximise the between-class to within class variance ratio

$$\frac{\underline{\beta}' \Sigma_B \underline{\beta}}{\underline{\beta}' \Sigma_W \underline{\beta}.} \tag{1}$$

The solution to expression (1) can be formulated in terms of the two-sided eigenvalue problem

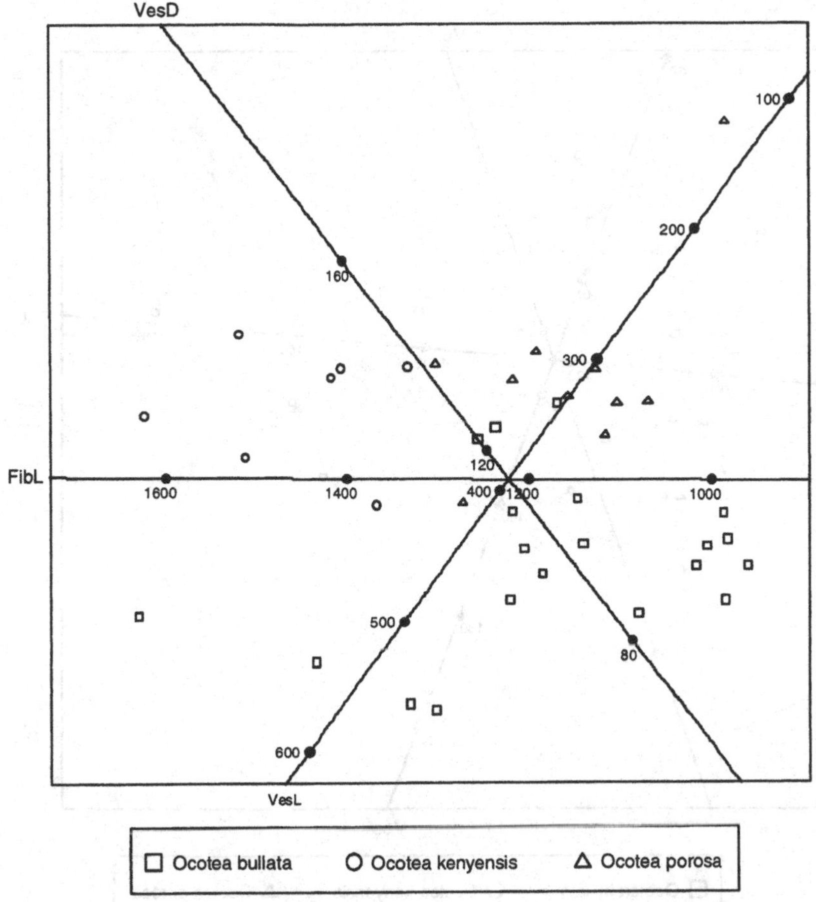

Fig. 1. PCA biplot of *Ocotea* data set.

$$\Sigma_B B = \Sigma_W B \Lambda \tag{2}$$

where the $p \times p$ matrix B contains $p-1$ sub-optimal solutions.

The matrix B defines the transformation XB from the original observation space to the canonical space $\mathbb{R}^p$. Since it follows from equation (2) that $BB' = \Sigma_W^{-1}$ the transformation to the canonical space results in Mahalanobis distances in the original space to be equivalent to Pythagorean distances in the canonical space.

The CVA biplot of the *Ocotea* data, in Fig. 2, shows very good separation between the classes. Since distances in the canonical space are interpreted in terms of Pythagorean distance, a new sample will be classified to the nearest class mean. Of importance is that the biplot also shows the role of all three variables in separating the classes.

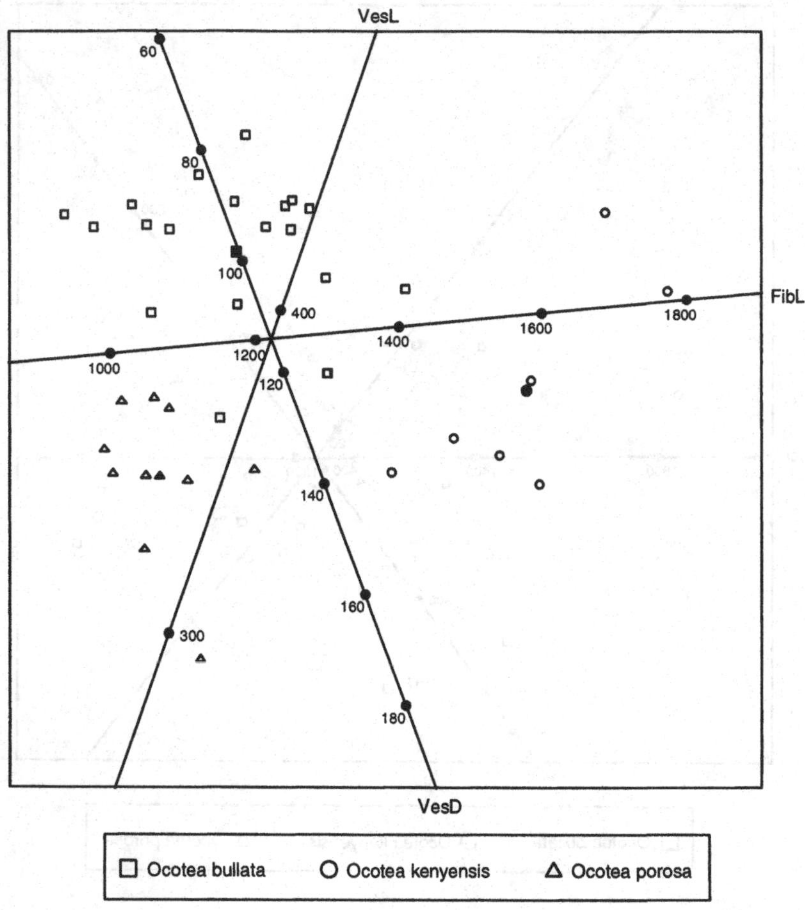

Fig. 2. CVA biplot of *Ocotea* data set.

3 Dimension of the Canonical Space

Let $\overline{x}_j$ denote the j-th class mean in the original observation space. Flury (1997), among others, proves that only the first $K = \min\{p, J-1\}$ elements of the vectors $\overline{z}_j$ differ, with the last $(p-K)$ elements being identical for all $j = 1, 2, \ldots, J$ where $\overline{z}_j' = \overline{x}_j' B$ is the j-th canonical mean and J denotes the number of classes.

In the example above we have $p = 3$ variables and $J = 3$ classes. The dimension of the canonical space is therefore $K = 2$. This results in no approximation and the class means in Fig. 2 are exactly represented. For $K > 2$ separating the classes and classifying new samples to the nearest class mean can be performed in K dimensions. However, the 2-dimensional CVA biplot will be an approximate representation. This biplot can be equipped with classification regions and the position of any new interpolated sample can be evaluated in terms of its relative (Pythagorean) distances to the different class means. It has been shown (see Gardner, 2001) that better classification performance can sometimes be obtained through dimension reduction and performing the DA in $k < K$ dimensions. Apart from supplying a visual representation of the classification of observations, biplot methodology has the advantage of a reduction in dimension. Hastie, Tibshirani and Buja (1994) remark that the reduced space can be more stable and therefore the dimension reduction could yield better classification performance.

Although DA for $J = 2$ classes is straightforward and is routinely performed, the CVA biplot procedure breaks down to a rather uninteresting one-dimensional 'biplot' $[K = \min\{p, 2-1\}]$ as shown in Fig. 3(a).

In a one-dimensional 'biplot' such as Fig. 3(a), it is often difficult to assess the overlap and separation between the classes, especially if many samples are present. Fitting a density estimate to the representation of each of the classes allows for visual appraisal of the overlap and separation between the classes. In Fig. 3(b) a Gaussian kernel density estimate has been fitted to each of the classes.

4 CVA Biplots for $J = 2$ Classes

The data set represented in Fig. 3 consist of 60 samples of a product representing the required quality level. This class is used as a control group to compare a new sample of 6 observations for quality purposes. Perusal of Fig. 3 shows that five out of the six samples do not meet the required quality criteria. It is however impossible to assess from Fig. 3 the reason for non-conformity. It is easy to construct a two-dimensional plot routinely using the first two eigenvectors. Although the procedure below might seem unnecessary complex it is essential for constructing a well-defined biplot providing information on the variables.

The two-sided eigenvalue solution for this data set illustrates why the CVA 'biplot' can only be one-dimensional: Equation (2) becomes

$$\Sigma_B \left[\underline{b}_1 \, \underline{b}_2 \, \underline{b}_3 \right] = \Sigma_W \left[\underline{b}_1 \, \underline{b}_2 \, \underline{b}_3 \right] \begin{bmatrix} 1.6 & 0 & 0 \\ 0 & 0 & 0 \\ 0 & 0 & 0 \end{bmatrix} . \tag{3}$$

Only one eigenvalue is non-zero. The vectors $\underline{b}_2$ and $\underline{b}_3$ span the vector space orthogonal to $\underline{b}_1$. The vector $\underline{b}_2$ is not uniquely defined and could be replaced with $\underline{b}_3$ or a linear combination of $\underline{b}_2$ and $\underline{b}_3$ orthogonal to $\underline{b}_3$. This non-uniqueness of the second column vector of B implies that a CVA biplot should not be constructed using the first two column vectors of B. In order to add information about the variables to the plot in Fig. 3, some matrix B_r is required for the formula

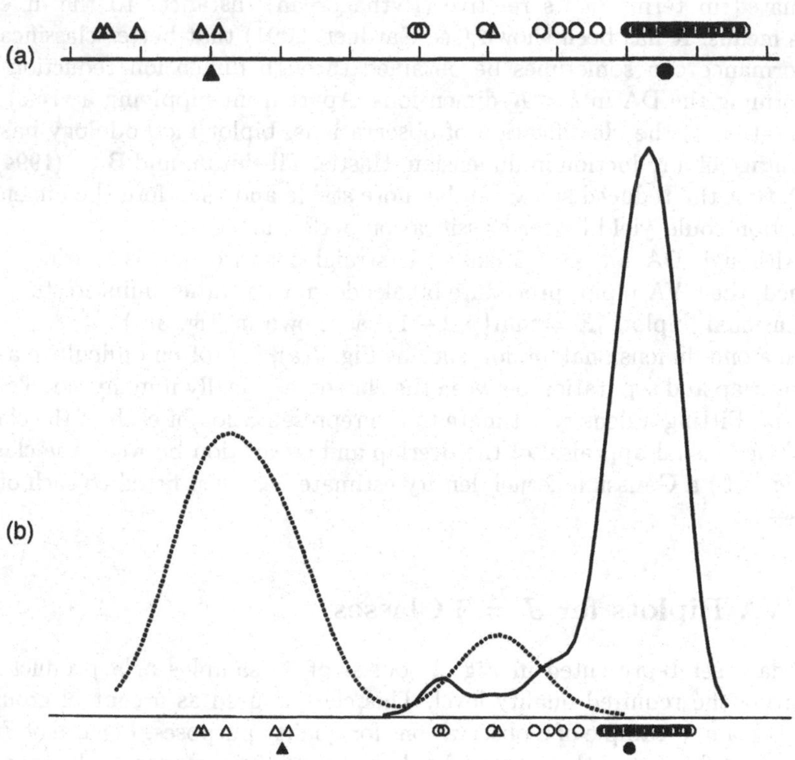

Fig. 3. (a) One dimensional 'biplot' and (b) density estimate superimposed on one dimensional 'biplot'.

$$Z = XB_r = X\left[\underline{b}_1\ \underline{b}^*\right]. \tag{4}$$

Strictly speaking, Fig. 3 is not a *bi*plot since it contains information of the samples only and not of the variables.

The vector $\underline{b}^*$ is defined in a PCA type context to represent the optimal variation in the orthogonal complement of $\underline{b}_1$. This is described in the following algorithm:

- Since the $p \times p$ matrix B is not orthogonal but is non-singular, then the vectors $\underline{b}_2, \ldots, \underline{b}_p$ are linearly independent but not necessarily orthogonal. Therefore, find an orthogonal basis for the vector space spanned by $\underline{b}_2, \cdots, \underline{b}_p$, given by the columns of the $p \times p - 1$ matrix V^*;
- $X^* = XV^*$ gives the representation of the sample points in the orthogonal complement of $\underline{b}_1$;

- Perform a PCA on X^*, solving the eigen-equation

$$(X^* - \frac{1}{n}\underline{1}\underline{1}'X^*)'(X^* - \frac{1}{n}\underline{1}\underline{1}'X^*) = V'\Delta V$$

to obtain the first principal component scores given by the first column $\underline{v}_1$ of the $p-1 \times p-1$ matrix V;
- Let $\underline{b}^* = V^*\underline{v}_1$.

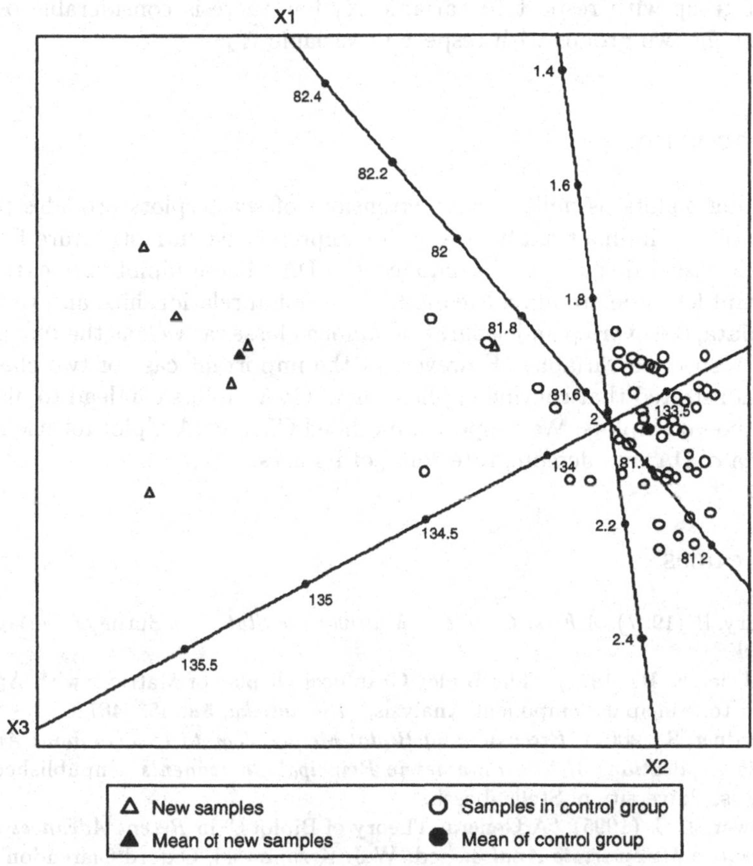

Fig. 4. Proposed biplot for a two-class DA.

Since the CVA biplot is based upon minimising the ratio (1) it is invariant with respect to standardising the original variables to unit variances. It is well-known that a PCA is not invariant with respect to such transformations. Therefore, although CVA biplots obtained from standardised and non-standardised observations are identical such scaling does affect the PCA-based CVA biplot proposal considered here for two-class DA problems. The above algorithm can easily be adapted to incorporate such standardisations when needed in practice.

Now this newly defined matrix $B_r = \left[\underline{b}_1 \; \underline{b}^* \right]$ can be used to construct a two-dimensional CVA biplot as shown in Fig. 4.

Note that projecting the samples in this biplot onto a horizontal line results in exactly the representation obtained in Fig. 3(a). It is now clear from Fig. 4 that variable X_3 separates five of the six samples in the new group from the control group. The samples in the new group are also well separated from the control group with respect to variable X_1 but there is considerable overlap between the two groups with respect to variable X_2.

5 Conclusion

Regarding biplots as multivariate extensions of scatterplots provides practitioners of discriminant analysis with a comprehensive infrastructure for constructing visual displays to accompany the DA. These biplots are extremely important for understanding the multidimensional relationships and variation in the data, the overlap and separation among classes as well as the role played by the respective variables. However, in the important case of two-class DA we demonstrated that routine application of CVA biplots can lead to nice but wrong axes on biplots. We propose a modified CVA-PCA biplot for use in this key area of DA and demonstrate some of its uses.

References

1. Flury, B. (1997). *A First Course in Multivariate Statistics.* Springer-Verlag, New York.
2. Gabriel, K. R. (1971). "The Biplot Graphical Display of Matrices with Application to Principal Component Analysis," *Biometrika*, **58**, 453–467.
3. Gardner, S. (2001). *Extensions of Biplot Methodology to Discriminant Analysis with Applications of Non-Parametric Principal Components.* Unpublished PhD thesis, University of Stellenbosch.
4. Gower, J. C. (1995). "A General Theory of Biplots," in *Recent Advances in Descriptive Multivariate Analysis*, ed. W.J. Krzanowski, Oxford:Clarendon Press, pp. 283–303.
5. Gower, J. C. and Hand, D. J. (1996). *Biplots.* Chapman and Hall, London.
6. Hastie, T., Tibshirani, R., and Buja, A. (1994). "Flexible Discriminant Analysis by Optimal Scoring," *Journal of the American Statistical Association*, **89**, 1255–1270.

Weighted Likelihood Estimation of Person Locations in an Unfolding Model for Polytomous Responses

Guanzhong Luo and David Andrich

Murdoch University, Australia
{g.luo,d.andrich}@murdoch.edu.au

Abstract: It is well known that there are no meaningful sufficient statistics for the person locations in a single peaked unfolding response model. The bias in the estimates of person locations of the general unfolding model for polytomous responses (Luo 2001) with conventional Maximum Likelihood Estimation (MLE) is likely to accumulate with various algorithms proposed in the literature. With the main aim of preventing the bias in the estimates of person locations in the equi-distant unfolding model when the values of item parameters are given, this paper derives the Weighted Likelihood Estimation (WLE) equations, following the approach of Warm (1989). A preliminary simulation study is also included.

In a general context, Samejima (1993) derived an approximation of the bias function of the MLE for person locations where the item responses are discrete as

$$Bias[MLE(\beta_n, \hat{\beta_n})] \cong E[\hat{\beta_n} - \beta_n | \beta_n] \tag{1}$$

$$\cong -\frac{1}{2[I(\beta_n)]^2} \sum_{i=1}^{I} \sum_{k=0}^{m_i} \frac{\frac{\partial P_{ni}(k)}{\partial \beta_n} \frac{\partial^2 P_{ni}(k)}{\partial \beta_n^2}}{P_{ni}(k)},$$

where $P_{ni}(k)$ is the probability that person n gives response category k on item i, $k = 0, 1, ...m_i; i = 1, ..., I$. The $I(\beta_n)$ is the information function of the person location parameter β_n.

To prevent the bias, Warm (1989) and Wang and Wang (2001) proposed that the solution equation for the person location β_n be modified with an additional term to

$$\frac{\partial \log L}{\partial \beta_n} - I(\beta_n) Bias(\beta_n); \tag{2}$$

where L is the likelihood function of β_n with given responses $\{X_{ni}, i = 1, ..., I\}$.The estimate of the person location β_n obtained by solving (2) is termed the weighted likelihood estimate (WLE).

This paper considers the situation when $P_{ni}(k)$ is defined by the general single peaked unfolding response model for polytomous responses (Luo 2001) and the distances between the thresholds are equal:

$$\Pr\{X_{ni} = k\} = \frac{\prod_{l=1}^{k} \Psi(\rho_{il}) \prod_{l=k+1}^{m_i} \Psi(\beta_n - \delta_i)}{\lambda_{ni}}, \quad k = 0, ..., m_i;$$
$$\rho_{il} = (m_i + 1 - l)\zeta_i, \quad l = 1, ..., m_i; \qquad (3)$$

where β_n is the location parameter for person n, δ_i is the location parameter and ρ_{ik} ($\geq$0) is the k-th threshold for item i. $\zeta > 0$ is termed the *item unit*. The function Ψ, termed the *operational function*, has the following properties:

(P1) *Non-negative:* $\Psi(t) \geq 0$ for any real t;
(P2) *Monotonic in the positive domain:* $\Psi(t_1) > \Psi(t_2)$ for any $t_1 > t_2 > 0$; and
(P3) *Ψ is an even function (symmetric about the origin)*: $\Psi(t) = \Psi(-t)$ for any real t.

The normalization factor in model (1) is

$$\lambda_{ni} = \sum_{k=0}^{m_i} \prod_{l=1}^{k} \Psi(\rho_{il}) \prod_{l=k+1}^{m_i} \Psi(\beta_n - \delta_i). \qquad (4)$$

In the rest of this paper, the model of Eq. (3) is termed the *equi-distant unfolding model*. As in the case of any unfolding model, there are no meaningful sufficient statistics for the person locations in the equi-distant unfolding model. In estimating the item parameters, therefore, the person parameters can not be "conditioned out" by the values of their sufficient statistics as in the case of the Rasch models (Andersen, 19070; Andrich and Luo, 2003). Two algorithms, namely the Joint Maximum Likelihood (JML) and the Marginal Maximum Likelihood (MML), have been proposed for the parameter estimation of probabilistic unfolding models (Luo, 1999; Roberts, Donoghue, and Laughlin, 2000; Luo and Andrich, 2003). Both involve iterations in solving the equation for estimating the person parameters. In doing so, the bias in the estimates of person locations using the MLE is likely to accumulate, affecting the quality of the final estimation of the item and person parameters.

This paper uses the WLE in estimating person locations with the values of item parameters are given. The full estimation algorithm for the parameters of the equi-distant unfolding model, which employs the estimation of person locations proposed in this paper, is provided in Luo and Andrich (2003).

According to (3), the likelihood function takes the form as

$$L = \prod_{i=1} \Pr\{X_{ni} = x_{ni}\} = \prod_{i=1}^{I} \frac{[\Psi(\beta_n - \delta_i)]^{m_i - x_{ni}} \prod_{l=1}^{x_{ni}} \Psi((m_i + 1 - l)\zeta_i)}{\lambda_{ni}}.$$

Then

$$\log L = \sum_{i=1} \Big\{(m_i - x_{ni})\log\Psi(\beta_n - \delta_i) + [\sum_{l=1}^{x_{ni}} log\Psi((m_i + 1 - l)\zeta_i)] - log\lambda_{ni}\Big\}.$$

The first derivative of log L with respect to β_n is

$$\varphi_{\beta_n} = \frac{\partial \log L}{\partial \beta_n} = \sum_{i=1}^{I} \Big\{ - x_{ni} + E[X_{ni}]\Big\} \frac{\partial \log\Psi(\beta_n - \delta_i)}{\partial \beta_n}. \tag{5}$$

The first derivative of $\Pr\{X_{ni} = k\}$ with respect to β_n is

$$\frac{\partial \Pr\{X_{ni} = k\}}{\partial \beta_n} = \Pr\{X_{ni} = k\} \cdot \{k - E_{ni}(\beta_n)\} \cdot \frac{\partial \log\Psi(\beta_n - \delta_i)}{\partial \beta_n}; \tag{6}$$

where

$$E_{ni}(\beta_n) \equiv E(X_{ni}|\beta_n) = \sum_{k=0}^{m_i} kP_{ni}(k). \tag{7}$$

In this situation, the *test information function* is defined as the expectation of the second derivative of Log L with respect to β_n, which is given by

$$I(\beta_n) \equiv E(\frac{\partial^2 \log L}{\partial \beta_n^2}) = E(\frac{\partial}{\partial \beta_n}\frac{\partial \log L}{\partial \beta_n}) \tag{8}$$

$$= \sum_{i=1}^{I} [\frac{\partial \log\Psi(\beta_n - \delta_i)}{\partial \beta_n}]^2 \cdot V_{ni}^2(\beta_n);$$

where

$$V_{ni}^2(\beta_n) \equiv \sum_{k=0}^{m_I} [k - E_{ni}(\beta_n)]^2 \cdot \Pr\{X_{ni} = k\} \tag{9}$$

Denote the information function component on item i as

$$I_i(\beta_n) = [\frac{\partial \log\Psi(\beta_n - \delta_i)}{\partial \beta_n}]^2 \cdot V_{ni}^2(\beta_n). \tag{10}$$

Now that the second derivative of $\Pr\{X_{ni} = k\}$ with respect to β_n is

$$\frac{\partial^2 P_{ni}(k)}{\partial\beta_n^2} = \frac{\partial}{\partial\beta_n}[\Pr\{X_{ni}=k\}\cdot\{k-E_{ni}(\beta_n)\}\cdot\frac{\partial\log\Psi(\beta_n-\delta_i)}{\partial\beta_n}]$$
$$= \frac{\partial\Pr\{X_{ni}=k\}}{\partial\beta_n^2}\cdot\{k-E_{ni}(\beta_n)\}\frac{\partial\log\Psi(\beta_n-\delta_i)}{\partial\beta_n}$$
$$+\Pr\{X_{ni}=k\}\cdot\frac{\partial\{k-E_{ni}(\beta_n)\}}{\partial\beta_n}\cdot\frac{\partial\log\Psi(\beta_n-\delta_i)}{\partial\beta_n} \tag{11}$$
$$+\Pr\{X_{ni}=k\}\cdot\{k-E_{ni}(\beta_n)\}\frac{\partial^2\log\Psi(\beta_n-\delta_i)}{\partial\beta_n^2};$$

it is evident that

$$\frac{\partial\{k-E_{ni}(\beta_n)\}}{\partial\beta_n} = -\frac{\partial\log\Psi(\beta_n-\delta_i)}{\partial\beta_n}\cdot V_{ni}^2(\beta_n). \tag{12}$$

Therefore,

$$\frac{\partial^2 P_{ni}(k)}{\partial\beta_n^2} = \Pr\{X_{ni}=k\}\cdot\{[\frac{\partial\log\Psi(\beta_n-\delta_i)}{\partial\beta_n}]^2\cdot \tag{13}$$
$$\{[k-E_{ni}(\beta_n)]^2-V_{ni}^2(\beta_n)\}+[k-E_{ni}(\beta_n)]\cdot\frac{\partial^2\log\Psi(\beta_n-\delta_i)}{\partial\beta_n^2}\}.$$

As a result,

$$\frac{\frac{\partial P_{ni}(k)}{\partial\beta_n}\frac{\partial^2 P_{ni}(k)}{\partial\beta_n^2}}{P_{ni}(k)} = [k-E_{ni}(\beta_n)]^3[\frac{\partial\log\Psi(\beta_n-\delta_i)}{\partial\beta_n}]^3\Pr\{X_{ni}=k\} \tag{14}$$
$$-[k-E_{ni}(\beta_n)][\frac{\partial\log\Psi(\beta_n-\delta_i)}{\partial\beta_n}]^3V_{ni}^2(\beta_n)\cdot\Pr\{X_{ni}=k\}$$
$$+[k-E_{ni}(\beta_n)]^2\frac{\partial\log\Psi(\beta_n-\delta_i)}{\partial\beta_n}\frac{\partial^2\log\Psi(\beta_n-\delta_i)}{\partial\beta_n^2}\cdot\Pr\{X_{ni}=k\}.$$

It is evident that

$$\sum_{k=0}^{m_I}[k-E_{ni}(\beta_n)]^3[\frac{\partial\log\Psi(\beta_n-\delta_i)}{\partial\beta_n}]^3\Pr\{X_{ni}=k\} \tag{15}$$
$$=[\frac{\partial\log\Psi(\beta_n-\delta_i)}{\partial\beta_n}]^3\sum_{k=0}^{m_I}[k-E_{ni}(\beta_n)]^3\Pr\{X_{ni}=k\},$$

and because of that

$$\sum_{k=0}^{m_I}P_{ni}(k)[k-E_{ni}(\beta_n)]=0. \tag{16}$$

We have

$$\sum_{k=0}^{m_I}[k-E_{ni}(\beta_n)][\frac{\partial\log\Psi(\beta_n-\delta_i)}{\partial\beta_n}]^3V_{ni}^3(\beta_n)\cdot\Pr\{X_{ni}=k\}=0. \tag{17}$$

Besides,

$$\sum_{k=0}^{m_i}[k-E_{ni}(\beta_n)]^2\frac{\partial\text{log}\Psi(\beta_n-\delta_i)}{\partial\beta_n}\frac{\partial^2\text{log}\Psi(\beta_n-\delta_i)}{\partial\beta_n^2}\cdot\Pr\{X_{ni}=k\}$$
$$=\frac{\partial\text{log}\Psi(\beta_n-\delta_i)}{\partial\beta_n}\frac{\partial^2\text{log}\Psi(\beta_n-\delta_i)}{\partial\beta_n^2}V_{ni}^2(\beta_n). \tag{18}$$

Therefore,

$$\sum_{k=0}^{m_i}\frac{\frac{\partial P_{ni}(k)}{\partial\beta_n}\frac{\partial P_{ni}^2(k)}{\partial\beta_n^2}}{P_{ni}(k)}=\frac{\partial\text{log}\Psi(\beta_n-\delta_i)}{\partial\beta_n}\{[\frac{\partial\text{log}\Psi(\beta_n-\delta_i)}{\partial\beta_n}]^2C_{ni}^3(\beta_n)$$
$$+\frac{\partial^2\text{log}\Psi(\beta_n-\delta_i)}{\partial\beta_n^2}V_{ni}^2(\beta_n)\},$$

where

$$C_{ni}^3(\beta_n)\equiv\sum_{k=0}^{m_i}[k-E_{ni}(\beta_n)]^3\Pr\{X_{ni}=k\}. \tag{19}$$

Finally, the MLE bias function is obtained as

$$Bias[MLE(\beta_n,\hat{\beta_n}]\cong E[\hat{\beta_n}-\beta_n|\beta_n]$$

which is

$$-\frac{\sum_{i=1}^{I}\frac{\partial\text{log}\Psi(\beta_n-\delta_i)}{\partial\beta_n}\{[\frac{\partial\text{log}\Psi(\beta_n-\delta_i)}{\partial\beta_n}]^2C_{ni}^3(\beta_n)+\frac{\partial^2\text{log}\Psi(\beta_n-\delta_i)}{\partial\beta_n^2}V_{ni}^2(\beta_n)\}}{2[\sum_{i=1}^{I}[\frac{\partial\text{log}\Psi(\beta_n-\delta_i)}{\partial\beta_n}]^2\cdot V_{ni}^2(\beta_n)]^2}.$$

The solution equation of the WLE for person location β_n with given values of item parameters is

$$\frac{\partial\text{log}L}{\partial\beta_n}-I(\beta_n)Bias(\beta_n)$$
$$=\sum_{i=1}^{I}\Big\{-x_{ni}+E[X_{ni}]\Big\}\frac{\partial\text{log}\Psi(\beta_n-\delta_n)}{\partial\beta_n}-I(\beta_n)Bias(\beta_n) \tag{20}$$
$$=0.$$

The following three specific models were investigated in Luo (2001) as special cases of the model of Eq. (3). The dichotomous counterparts of them were introduced in Andrich (1988), Andrich and Luo (1993), and (Hoijtink, 1990) respectively. Some of the mathematical details are omitted in order to reduce space.

Special case (I)-Simple Square Logistic Model for Polytomous responses.

$$\psi(t) = \exp(t^2).$$
$$\frac{\partial \log\Psi(\beta_n - \delta_i)}{\partial \beta_n} = 2(\beta_n - \delta_i);$$
$$\frac{\partial^2 \log\Psi(\beta_n - \delta_i)}{\partial \beta_n^2} = 2,$$

and

$$Bias[MLE(\beta_n, \hat{\beta_n}) \cong -\frac{4\sum_{i=1}^{I}(\beta_n - \delta_i)^3 C_{ni}^3(\beta_n) + \sum_{i=1}^{I}(\beta_n - \delta_i)V_{ni}^2(\beta_n)}{[\sum_{i=1}^{I}[2(\beta_n - \delta_i)]^2 \cdot V_{ni}^2(\beta_n)]^2}.$$

Special case (II)-Cosh Model for Polytomous Responses.

$$\psi(t) = \cosh(t);$$
$$\frac{\partial \log\Psi(\beta_n - \delta_i)}{\partial \beta_n} = \tanh(\beta_n - \delta_i);$$
$$\frac{\partial^2 \log\Psi(\beta_n - \delta_i)}{\partial \beta_n^2} = \frac{\partial(\beta_n - \delta_i)}{\partial \beta_n} = \frac{1}{[\cosh(\beta_n - \delta_i)]^2};$$

and

$$Bias[MLE(\beta_n, \hat{\beta_n}) \cong -\frac{\sum_{i=1}^{I}[\tanh(\beta_n - \delta_i)]^3 C_{ni}^3(\beta_n) + \sum_{i=1}^{I}\frac{\tanh(\beta_n - \delta_i)}{[\cosh(\beta_n - \delta_i)]^2}V_{ni}^2(\beta_n)}{s[\sum_{i=1}^{I}[\tanh(\beta_n - \delta_i)]^2 \cdot V_{ni}^2(\beta_n)]^2}.$$

Special case (III)-PARALLA model for Polytomous responses.

$$\psi(t) = t^2;$$
$$\frac{\partial \log\Psi(\beta_n - \delta_i)}{\partial \beta_n} = \frac{2}{(\beta_n - \delta_i)};$$
$$\frac{\partial^2 \log\Psi(\beta_n - \delta_i)}{\partial \beta_n^2} = 2\frac{\partial}{\partial \beta_n}\frac{1}{\beta_n - \delta_i} = \frac{-2}{(\beta_n - \delta_i)^2};$$

and

$$Bias[MLE(\beta_n, \hat{\beta_n}) \cong -\frac{2\sum_{i=1}^{I}(\beta_n - \delta_i)^{-3}\left[2C_{ni}^3(\beta_n - V_{ni}^2(\beta_n)\right]}{[\sum_{i=1}^{I}4(\beta_n - \delta_i)^{-2} \cdot V_{ni}^2(\beta_n)]^2}.$$

Simulation Studies

To show the efficiency the WLE procedures described above in preventing the accumulation of bias, preliminary simulation studies reported in this section provide comparisons of estimates of item parameters between the MLE and the WLE in estimating person locations. To save space, only the situation where the operational function is the hyperbolic cosine is reported. In each simulation, responses on 10 items with locations in the range [-2.0,2.0] were simulated. The item units were randomly generated in the interval [0.6, 1.0]. Five hundred person locations normally distributed with mean of 0.0 and variance of 2.0 were used in each simulatin. Each simulation had 10 replications. All the items involved had four categories, e.g., *0 -strongly disagree; 1 - disagree; 2 - agree and 3 - strongly agree.* The convergence criterion for all iterations was set as 0.001. In all estimations, the initial signs of the item locations were obtained using the Sign Analysis procedure (Luo, 1999). As described in Luo (1999) and Luo and Andrich (2003), the estimation procedure includes the following two steps:

Cycle 1. The value of mean unit parameter ζ is estimated together with all the person and statement location parameters.

Cycle 2. The parameters are re-estimated with the item unit parameter free to vary among items but with the constraint

$$\sqrt[I]{\prod_{i=1}^{I} \zeta_i} = \hat{\zeta}$$

using the estimate in Cycle 1.

Within each cycle, there are two steps: (i) item parameters are estimated while the person parameters are treated as known or fixed at their provisional values; (ii) person parameters are estimated while the item parameters are fixed at their estimated values in the first step. Then steps (i) and (ii) are repeated until the convergence is achieved. The MLE or WLE can be used in the step of estimating person parameters. Table 1 shows the estimation results of item locations with these two procedures. The standard errors reported in Table 1 were the means of the standard errors of the item over the ten repetitions.

The root mean squared error (RMSE) is calculated according to

$$MSRE_\delta = \sqrt{\sum_{i=1}^{I} (\hat{\delta}_i - \delta_i)^2 / I}. \quad (21)$$

Also in Table 1, the RMSE and correlation coefficients between the generated and estimated person locations for the two procedures are the average over the 10 repetitions.

Table 1 shows that while the MLE leads to inflated estimates for item locations, the estimates of item locations produced by the WLE are much closer to their corresponding generating values for most of the items. Similar results are also obtained when the operational function is the SSLM. Luo

Table 1. Recovery of item locations

Item	Generating	MLE	StdErr	WLE	StdErr
1	-2.000	-2.211	0.033	-2.149	0.032
2	-1.556	-1.721	0.034	-1.589	0.033
3	-1.111	-1.333	0.035	-1.134	0.034
4	-0.667	-0.789	0.034	-0.695	0.034
5	-0.222	-0.280	0.036	-0.275	0.035
6	0.222	0.268	0.036	0.249	0.036
7	0.667	0.747	0.036	0.692	0.036
8	1.111	1.282	0.034	1.153	0.034
9	1.556	1.748	0.034	1.645	0.033
10	2.000	2.290	0.033	2.103	0.032
Person correlation		0.933		0.940	
RMSE		0.172		0.116	

and Andrich (2003) also show that the results with a correction procedure on the item units are very close to those produced with the WLE. However, the WLE procedure is considered more tenable than the correction procedure because the latter is based on the combination of a heuristic rationale and the behaviour of the inconsistency of estimates in simulation studies.

References

1. Andersen, E. B. (1970). "Asymptotic Properties of Conditional Maximum-Likelihood Estimators," *Journal of the Royal Statistical Society, Series B*, **32**, 283-301.
2. Andrich, D. (1988). "The Application of an Unfolding Model of the PIRT Type to the Measurement of Attitude," *Applied Psychological Measurement*, **12**, 33–51.
3. Andrich, D., and Luo, G. (1993). "A Hyperbolic Cosine Latent Trait Model for Unfolding Dichotomous Single-Stimulus Responses," *Applied Psychological Measurement*, **17**, 253–276.
4. Andrich, D., and Luo, G. (2003). "Conditional Pairwise Estimation in the Rasch Model for Ordered Response Categories Using Principal Components," *Journal of Applied Measurement,* **4**, 205–221.
5. Hoijtink, H. (1990). "A Latent Trait Model for Dichotomous Choice Data," *Psychometrika*, **55**, 641–656.
6. Luo, G. (1999). "A Joint Maximum Likelihood Estimation Procedure for the Hyperbolic Cosine Model for Single Stimulus Responses, *Applied Psychological Measurement*, **24**, 33–49.
7. Luo, G. (2001). "A Class of Probabilistic Unfolding Models for Polytomous Responses," *Journal of Mathematical Psychology*, **45**, 224–248.
8. Luo, G., and Andrich, D. (2003). "The JML Estimation in the Equi-Distant Unfolding Model for Polytomous Responses," unpublished manuscript.

9. Roberts, J. S., Donoghue, J. R. and Laughlin, J. E. (2000). "A General Item Response Theory Model for Unfolding Unidimensional Polytomous Responses," *Applied Psychological Measurement*, **24**, 3–32.
10. Samejima, F. (1993). "An Approximation for the Bias Function of the Maximum Likelihood Estimates of a Latent Variable for the General Case Where the Item Responses are Discrete. *Psychometrika*, **58**, 119–138.
11. Wang, S., and Wang, T. (2001). "Precision of Warm's Weighted Likelihood Estimates for a Polytomous Model in Computerized Adaptive Testing, *Applied Psychological Measurement*, **12**, 307–314.
12. Warm, T. A. (1989). "Weighted Likelihood Estimation of Ability in Item Response Theory," *Psychometrika*, **54**, 427–450.

Classification of Geospatial Lattice Data and their Graphical Representation

Koji Kurihara

Okayama University, Japan
kurihara@ems.okayama-u.ac.jp

Abstract: Statistical analyses for spatial data are important problems in various types of fields. Lattice data are synoptic observations covering an entire spatial region, like cancer rates broken out by each county in a state. There are few approaches for cluster analysis of spatial data. But echelons are useful techniques to study the topological structure of such spatial data. In this paper, we explore cluster analysis for geospatial lattice data based on echelon analysis. We also provide new definitions of the neighbors and families of spatial data in order to support the clustering procedure. In addition, the spatial cluster structure is demonstrated by hierarchical graphical representation with several examples. Regional features are also shown in this dendrogram.

1 Introduction

Statistical analyses for spatial data are important problem for many types of fields. Spatial data are taken at specific locations or within specific regions and their relative positions are recorded. Lattice data are synoptic observation covering an entire spatial region, like cancer rates corresponding to each county in a state. There are few approaches for cluster analysis of such spatial data. Statistical map with shading are used to show how quantitative information varies geographically. But we can only find contiguous clusters in this map with the low accuracy of the visual decoding.

Echelon analysis (Myers et al., 1997) is a useful technique to study the topological structure of a surface in a systematic and objective manner. The echelons are derived from the changes in topological connectivity. Some approaches are designed for the comparative changes of remote sensing data and image data (Kurihara et al., 2000; Myers et al., 1999). In this paper, we explore the cluster analysis of geospatial lattice data based on echelon analysis. We also newly define the neighbors and families of spatial data to enable the clustering procedure. In addition, their spatial structure is demonstrated by hierarchical graphical representation with several examples. Regional features are also shown in this dendrogram.

2 Classification of One-Dimensional Spatial Data

One-dimensional spatial data has the position x and the value $h(x)$ on the horizontal and vertical axes, respectively. For k divided lattice (interval) data, data are taken at the interval $l_1(i) = (i-1, i]$, $i = 1, \ldots, k$. Table 1 shows the 25 intervals named from A to Y in order and their values. In order to use the information of spatial positions, we make the cross sectional view of topographical map like Figure 1.

Table 1. One-dimensional spatial interval data.

i	1	2	3	4	5	6	7	8	9	10	11	12	13	14	15	16	17	18	19	20	21	22	23	24	25
ID	A	B	C	D	E	F	G	H	I	J	K	L	M	N	O	P	Q	R	S	T	U	V	W	X	Y
$h(i)$	1	2	3	4	3	4	5	4	3	2	3	4	5	6	5	6	7	6	5	4	3	2	1	2	1

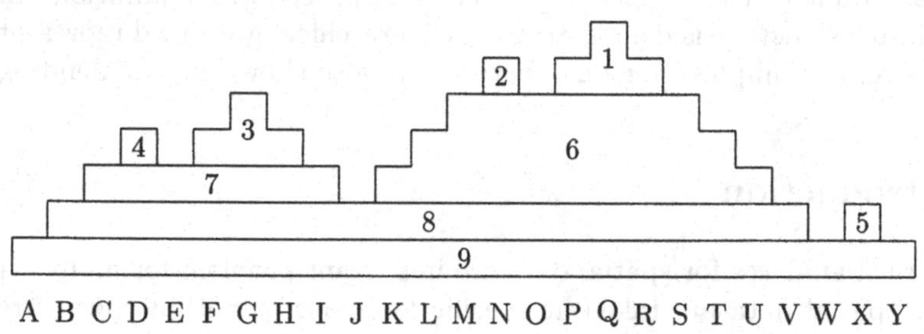

Fig. 1. The hypothetical set of hillforms in one-dimensional spatial data.

There are nine numbered parts with same topological structure in these hillforms. These parts are called echelons. These echelons consist of peaks, foundations of peaks, and foundations of foundations. The numbers 1, 2, 3, 4 and 5 are the peaks of hillforms. The numbers 6 and 7 are the foundations of two peaks. The number 8 is the foundation of two foundations. The number 9 is the foundation of a foundation and peaks and is also called the root. Thus we have nine clusters $G(i)$, $i = 1, \ldots, 9$ for specified intervals based on these echelons. These are following clusters of the five peaks:

$$G(1) = \{Q, P, R\},\ G(2) = \{N\},\ G(3) = \{G, F, H\}$$
$$G(4) = \{D\}, \quad G(5) = \{X\}$$

and these are the clusters of foundations:

$$G(6) = \{M, O, S, L, T, K, U\},\ G(7) = \{C, E, I\},\ G(8) = \{B, J, V\}$$

and this is the root cluster.

$$G(9) = \{A, W, Y\}.$$

The relationship among the clusters can be expressed as

$$9(8(7(43)6(21))5)$$

by use of the numbers of cluster.

The cluster $G(6)$ is a parent of $G(2)$ and $G(1)$, and $G(6)$ has two children of $G(2)$ and $G(1)$. Thus we define the children $CH(G(i))$ and family $FM(G(i))$ for the cluster $G(i)$ by:

$$CH(G(8)) = G(7) \cup G(4) \cup G(3) \cup G(6) \cup G(2) \cup G(1)$$
$$FM(G(8)) = G(8) \cup CH(G(8))$$

The graphical representation for these relationships is given by the dendrogram shown in Figure 2.

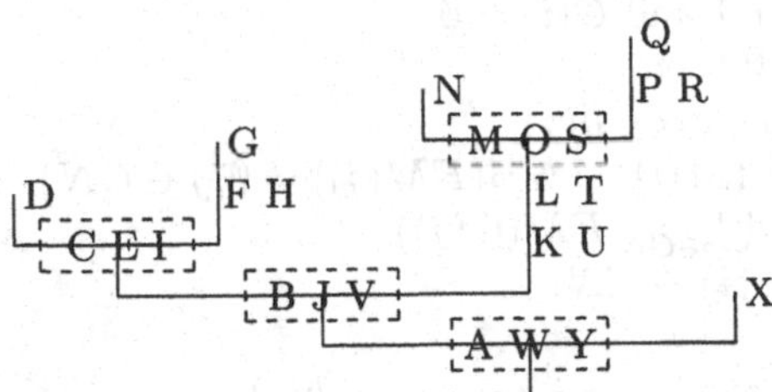

Fig. 2. The relation of clusters in the dendrogram.

2.1 Making Clusters from Spatial Lattice Data

In this section we describe the procedure for clustering spatial lattice data. At first, we define the neighbors of spatial data $l_1(i)$, say $NB(i)$. For $l_1(i) = (i-1, i]$, $i = 1, \ldots, k$, the neighbor $NB(i)$ is given by

$$NB(i) = \begin{cases} \{i+1\}, & i = 1 \\ \{i-1,\ i+1\}, & 1 < i < k \\ \{i-1\}, & i = k \end{cases} \tag{1}$$

The neighbor the jth cluster $G(j)$, $NB(G(j))$, is also given by

$$NB(G(j)) = \bigcup_{i \in FM(G(j))} NB(i) - \bigcup_{i \in FM(G(j))} \{i\} \qquad (2)$$

where $A - B = A \cap \{B^C\}$ for the sets of A and B and $NB(\emptyset) = \emptyset$.

In order to make the clusters $G(i)$, we find the peaks and the foundations using the following steps in Stages 1 and 2. To simplify the procedure, we assume there are no ties.

Stage 1. Find the peaks.
 Step 1: Set $i = 0$ and $RN = \{i|1 \le i \le k\}$.
 Step 2: Set $i = i + 1$ and $G(i) = \emptyset$.
 Step 3: If $G(i) = \emptyset$ then $h(M(i)) = \max_{j \in RN} h(j)$.
  Else $h(M(i)) = \max_{j \in NB(G(i))} h(j)$.
  End If.
 Step 4: Set $RN = RN - \{M(i)\}$. If $RN = \emptyset$ then END.
  If $h(M(i)) > \max_{j \in NB(M(i)) - G(i)} h(j)$ then $G(i) = G(i) \cup \{M(i)\}$ and go to Step 3.
  Else if $G(i) = \emptyset$ then $i = i - 1$ and go to Step 2.
  End If.
Stage 2. Find the foundations. Let l be the number of peaks.
 Step 1: Set $i = l$ and $RN = \{i|1 \le i \le k\} - \bigcup_{j=1}^{l} G(j)$. If $RN = \emptyset$ then END.
  Else $GN = \{i|1 \le i \le l\}$ and $FM(G(j)) = G(j)$, $j = 1, \ldots, l$.
 Step 2: Set $i = i + 1$ and $G(i) = \emptyset$.
 Step 3: If $G(i) = \emptyset$ then
   $h(M(i)) = \max_{j \in RN} h(j)$
   $CN = \{j|NB(M(i)) \cup NB(FM(j)) \neq \emptyset, j \in GN\}$
   $FM(G(i)) = \bigcup_{j \in CN} FM(G(j))$
   $GN = GN \cup \{i\} - CN$.
  Else
   $h(M(i)) = \max_{j \in NB(FM(G(i))) \cap RN} h(j)$.
  End If.
 Step 4: Set $RN = RN - \{M(i)\}$. If $RN = \emptyset$ then END.
  If $h(M(i)) > \max_{j \in NB(FM(G(i)) \cup M(i)) \cap RN} h(j)$ then
   $G(i) = G(i) \cup \{M(i)\}$
   $FM(G(i)) = FM(G(i)) \cup \{M(i)\}$
   Go to Step 3.
  Else $RN = RN \cup \{M(i)\}$; go to Step 2.
  End If.

3 Classification of Two-Dimensional Spatial Data

Two-dimensional spatial data has the value $h(x, y)$ for response variable at the position (x, y). In applications such as remote sensing the data are given as pixels of digital values over the $M \times N$ lattice area $l_2(i,j) = \{(x,y) : x_{i-1} < x < x_i, y_{j-1} < y < y_j\}$, $i = 1, \ldots, N$, $j = 1, \ldots, M$. For the lattice shown in Table 2, the neighbors of cell $l_2(i,j)$ are

$$NB(l_2(i,j)) = \{(k,l) | i-1 \leq k \leq i+1, \quad j-1 \leq l \leq j+1\} \\ \cap \{(k,l) | 1 \leq k \leq N, \quad 1 \leq l \leq M\} - \{(i,j)\}.$$

Table 2. The neighbor structure in a lattice.

	j		
	$i-1, j-1$	$i-1, j$	$i-1, j+1$
i	$i, j-1$	i, j	$i, j+1$
	$i+1, j-1$	$i+1, j$	$i+1, j+1$

If we make the correspondence from $l_2(i,j)$ to $l_1((i-1) * N + j)$, we can also form clusters for the two-dimensional spatial data in the same way as shown in Section 2 for one-dimensional data.

Table 3. The digital values over a 5×5 array.

	A	B	C	D	E
1	10	24	10	15	10
2	10	10	14	22	10
3	10	13	19	23	25
4	20	21	12	11	17
5	16	10	10	18	10

For illustration, we shall apply the digital values in the 5×5 array shown in Table 3. By use of Stages 1 and 2, the posterity $CH(G(i))$ and the families $FM(G(i))$ for $G(i)$ are calculated in Table 4. The graphical representation for these array data is shown as the dendrogram in Figure 3.

Table 4. The clusters of the 5×5 array.

Stage	i	$G(i)$	$CH(G(i))$	$FM(G(i))$
1	1	E3 D3 D2	ϕ	$G(1)$
1	2	B1	ϕ	$G(2)$
1	3	B4 A4	ϕ	$G(3)$
1	4	D5	ϕ	$G(4)$
2	5	C3	$G(j)\ j = 1,3$	$G(j)\ j = 1,3,5$
2	6	E4 A5 D1	$G(j)\ j = 1,3,4,5$	$G(j)\ j = 1,3,4,5,6$
2	7	C2 B3 C4 D4 and others	$G(j)\ j = 1,2,3,4,5,6$	$G(j)\ j = 1,2,3,4,5,6,7$

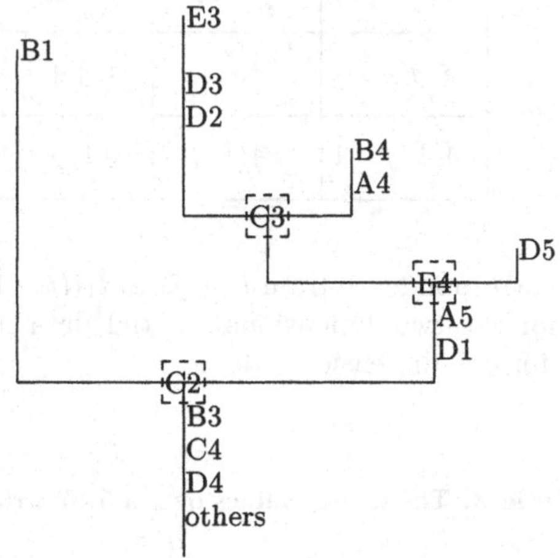

Fig. 3. The relation of clusters for 5-by-5 array.

4 Classification of Geospatial Lattice Data

Geospatial lattice data are areal-referenced values $h(D_i)$ within spatial regions $D_i\ i = 1, \ldots, n$. The regional features are mainly investigated over lattice regions like the watersheds in the state, the counties in the state, the states in the USA and so on. If we have the neighbors $NB(D_i)$ for each spatial regions, we can also make clusters for geospatial lattice data based on Stages 1 and 2.

Table 5 shows the rates of unemployment in 1997 corresponding to 50 states in the USA [Editor's Note: For reasons of space, Table 5 has been shortened; the full data are available from the author upon request]. These data are quoted from the Statistical Abstract of the United States 1998. The USA is divided into irregular states, so the lattice is irregular. The neighborhood information is also shown in this table; neighbors are defined by shared borders. Although the states of Alaska and Hawaii are isolated states, we assume that the states of Alaska and Hawaii are connected to the states of Washington and California, respectively.

Figure 4 shows the dendrogram of the rates of unemployment for the states in 1997. There are two large peaks in the unemployment rates of the USA. The first peak of western regions consists of the states of Alaska, Hawaii, California, Oregon, Montana and Idaho. These states mainly belong to the Pacific division. The second peak of eastern and southern regions consists of the states of West Virginia, Louisiana, Mississippi New Mexico and New York. The root consists of the state of North Dakota, Nebraska, South Dakota, Utah and New Hampshire. The main states of the root belong to the West North Central division. By use of this graphical representation, we gain a better understanding of regional unemployment patterns.

Table 5. States in USA, their neighbors, and unemployment rates (incomplete).

State name		neighbors of the states	rates	$G(i)$
Alabama	AL	FL GA MS TN	51	13
Alaska	AK	(WA)	79	1
Arizona	AZ	CA CO NM NV UT	46	15
Arkansas	AR	LA MS MO OK TN TX	53	10
California	CA	AZ NV OR (HI)	63	4
Colorado	CO	AZ KS NE NM OK UT WY	33	15
Connecticut	CT	MA NY RI	51	13
Delaware	DE	MD NJ PA	40	15
Florida	FL	AL GA	48	13
Georgia	GA	AL FL NC SC TN	45	15
Hawaii	HI	(CA)	64	4
Idaho	ID	MT NV OR UT WA WY	53	11
Illinois	IL	IA IN KY MO WI	47	13
Indiana	IN	IL KY MI OH	35	15
Iowa	IA	IL MN MO NE SD WI	33	15
Kansas	KS	CO MO NE OK	38	15
Kentucky	KY	IL IN MO OH TN VA WV	54	10
Louisiana	LA	AR MS TX	61	6

5 Conclusions

We dealt with cluster analysis for geospatial lattice data. Our method provides a unified framework for handling other types of lattice data. For point-referenced data, one needs to interpolate the surface value by some kind of kriging technique and make contour plots within the whole region. If we can make the contour map based on the interpolation of the values, this method is applied for the contour map as in the case of two-dimensional spatial data.

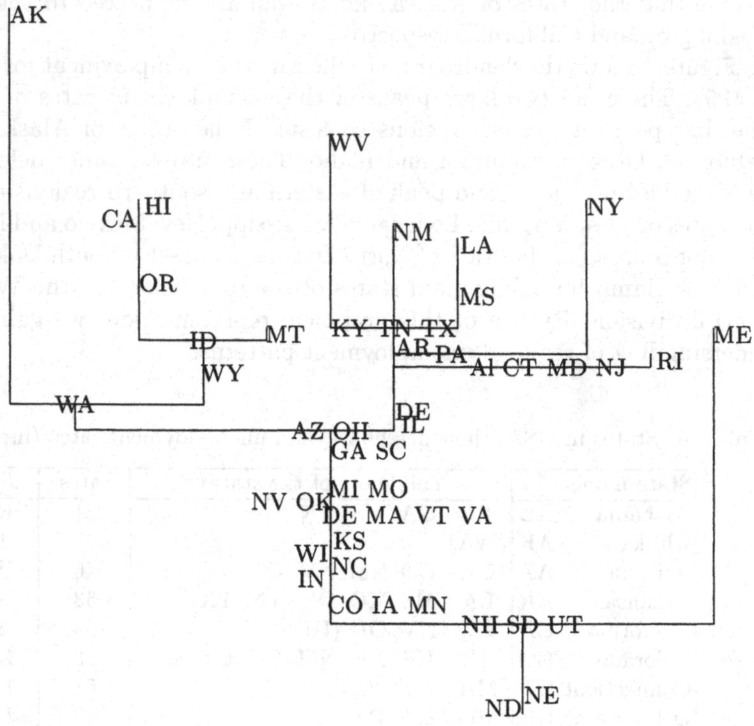

Fig. 4. The dendrogram of the unemployment rates in 1997.

References

1. Cressie, N., and Chan, N. H. (1989). "Spatial Modelling of Regional Variables," *Journal of the American Statistical Association*, **84**, 393–401.
2. Kurihara, K., Myers, W. L., and Patil, G. P. (2000). "Echelon Analysis of the Relationship Between Population and Land Cover Patterns Based on Remote Sensing Data," *Community Ecology*, **1**, 103–122.
3. Myers, W. M., Patil, G. P., and Joly, K. (1997). "Echelon Approach to Areas of Concern in Synoptic Regional Monitoring," *Environmental and Ecological Statistics*, **4**, 131–152.
4. Myers, W. M., Patil, G. P. and Taillie, C. (1999). "Conceptualizing Pattern Analysis of Spectral Change Relative to Ecosystem Status," *Ecosystem Health*, **5**, 285–293.

Degenerate Expectation-Maximization Algorithm for Local Dimension Reduction

Xiaodong Lin[1] and Yu Zhu[2]

[1] Statistical and Applied Mathematical Science Institute, U.S.A.
linxd@samsi.info
[2] Purdue University, U.S.A.
yuzhu@stat.purdue.edu

Abstract: Dimension reduction techniques based on principal component analysis (PCA) and factor analysis are commonly used in statistical data analysis. The effectiveness of these methods is limited by their global nature. Recent efforts have focused on relaxing global restrictions in order to identify subsets of data that are concentrated on lower dimensional subspaces. In this paper, we propose an adaptive local dimension reduction method, called the Degenerate Expectation-Maximization Algorithm (DEM). This method is based on the finite mixture model. We demonstrate that the DEM yields significantly better results than the local PCA (LPCA) and other related methods in a variety of synthetic and real datasets. The DEM algorithm can be used in various applications ranging from clustering to information retrieval.

1 Introduction

Dimension reduction is commonly used for analyzing large datasets. Over the years, several methods have been proposed for dimension reduction, among which are Principal Component Analysis, Factor Analysis, Self Organizing Map (Kohonen, 1989, 1990) and Principal Curve (Hastie and Stuetzle, 1989). One important assumption for these methods is the existence of a global low dimensional structure. However, this does not hold in general. For a high dimensional data set, different subsets of the data may concentrate on different subspaces. Thus it is important to develop methods that can identify low dimensional structures locally.

As an early effort to solve this problem, Kambhatla and Leen (1997) and Archer(1999) proposed Local Principal Component Analysis (LPCA). The high dimensional data is assumed to consist of a number of clustered subsets. Starting from an initial assignment of cluster membership to the data points, the LPCA determine a principal subspace for each cluster. Then it allocates data points, one by one, to the clusters whose principal subspaces are the closest to them. This iterative procedure continues until a stopping criterion is met. It has been shown that the LPCA has many advantages over the popular classical dimension reduction techniques.

In this paper we propose the DEM algorithm based on the finite mixture model for local dimension reduction. In a finite mixture model, each component is modelled by a probability density belonging to a parametric family $f_j(x;\theta_j)$ and the mixture density is

$$f(x;\theta) = \sum_{j=1}^{m} \pi_j f_j(x;\theta_j), \tag{1}$$

where $\pi_j > 0$ and $\sum_{j=1}^{m} \pi_j = 1$. When $f_j(x;\theta_j)$ are multivariate Gaussian distributions with parameters μ_j and Σ_j for $1 \leq j \leq m$, (1) is a typical Gaussian mixture model. The Gaussian mixture model has been used for model based clustering and the EM algorithm is usually used for parameter estimation. Note that the covariance matrices for the Gaussian mixture model contain the information regarding the shape of the components. When some of the covariance matrices become singular or near singular, it implies that the corresponding components are concentrated on low dimensional subspaces. Thus the finite mixture model can also be used as a device for local dimension reduction.

The existing methods for finite mixture model cannot be directly applied to achieve our goal. First, the likelihood function for the Gaussian mixture density with unequal covariance matrices is unbounded (Kiefer and Wolfowitz (1956)), so many numerical methods for computing the MLE may not work well. Hathaway (1985) and Ciuperea et. al. (2003) proposed the constrained and the penalized methods respectively to address this problem. They avoided the likelihood unboundedness problem by discarding the degenerate components, genuine or spurious. Their methods are quite unstable when the true parameters are close to the boundary of the parameter space. Secondly, in computation, when some parameter estimates get close to degeneration which causes the likelihood function to be infinity, the computing has to stop. However, other parameter estimates may not have converged yet. Therefore, the resulted parameter estimates cannot be used. The DEM algorithm described below solves these two problems by adaptively adding perturbations to the singular covariance matrices of the corresponding components. It will be demonstrated later that the DEM can also distinguish genuine degenerate components from the spurious ones and achieve the goal of local dimension reduction.

This paper is organized as follows. In Section 2, we discuss the likelihood unboundedness problem and the breakdown of the EM algorithm, then propose the DEM algorithm to address these issues. Simulation results are presented in Section 3. Section 4 contains the conclusions and future work.

2 Degenerate EM Algorithm (DEM)

In the Gaussian mixture model, both spurious and genuine degeneration can lead to likelihood unboundedness. Spurious degeneration occurs when a cluster with a small number of points lies on a lower dimensional subspace. Genuine degeneration, on the other hand, occurs when a large portion of the data are concentrated on a lower dimensional subspace. Traditional approaches avoid degeneracy by confining the parameters to the interior of the parameter space. In high dimensional data analysis, however, it is likely that one or more components can be genuinely degenerate. New methods are needed to distinguish between these two cases.

2.1 Infinite Likelihood and Breakdown Point

It is known that the likelihood function of a Gaussian mixture model goes to infinity when certain parameters reach the boundary of the parameter space. In the EM algorithm, it is important to find out when the breakdown occurs. Given the observed data $\mathbf{x}$, at the E-step of the (k)th iteration, expected value of the complete data likelihood is

$$E_{\theta^{(k)}}(l_c(\theta)|\mathbf{x}) = \sum_{j=1}^{m}\sum_{i=1}^{n} E_{\theta^{(k)}}(Z_{ij}|\mathbf{x})\{\log \pi_j + \log f_j(x_i;\theta_j)\}, \tag{2}$$

where Z_{ij} is the usual missing value and $\theta^{(k)}$ is the parameter estimate after (k)th iteration. Define

$$z_{ij}^{(k)} \doteq E_{\theta^{(k)}}(Z_{ij}|\mathbf{x}). \tag{3}$$

It can be shown that $E_{\theta^{(k)}}(l_c(\theta)|\mathbf{x})$ reaches infinity only when z_{ij} are strictly 0 or 1 for some components, i.e., when

$$z_{ij}^{(k)} = \begin{cases} 1 & \text{while } x_i \in \text{the degenerate component j} \\ 0 & \text{else} \end{cases} . \tag{4}$$

Before this point is reached, maximizing $E_{\theta^{(k)}}(l_c(\theta)|\mathbf{x})$ ensures the increase of the observed data log likelihood. When $E_{\theta^{(k)}}(l_c(\theta)|\mathbf{x})$ reaches infinity, we can detect the degenerate components with singular covariance matrices.

The first goal of the DEM algorithm is to prevent the iterative procedure from breaking down. To achieve this goal, artificial perturbations are applied to the detected singular covariance matrices. This can force the covariance matrices to become non-singular, thus assures the likelihood function to be bounded. The second goal of the DEM algorithm is to discriminate between spurious and genuine degeneration. The points trapped in spurious degenerate components should be reassigned. This is done by adjusting their corresponding z_{ij} values: the probability that the datum x_i is assigned to component j.

For a spuriously degenerate component, a large perturbation needs to be applied on the covariance matrix in order to deviate the component from degeneration. Meanwhile, for a genuine degenerate components, the perturbation on the covariance matrix should be relatively small so that the degeneracy can be retained. The proper level of perturbation depends on the size of the degenerate component and its relative distance from the other components.

2.2 The DEM Algorithm

The key steps of the proposed DEM algorithm include the identification of the degenerate components and directions and the perturbation of the singular covariance matrices. When a degenerate component, e.g., component j, is identified, its covariance matrix will be decomposed into $D_j' \Lambda_j D_j$, with $\Lambda_j = \text{diag}\{\lambda_1, \cdots, \lambda_d\}$. Here, $\lambda_1, \cdots, \lambda_d$ are the sorted eigenvalues of Σ_j in a decreasing order and the columns of D_j consist of the corresponding eigenvectors. Should this matrix be singular, there exists an s such that when $p \geq s$, $\lambda_p = 0$. For the identification of a nearly singular covariance matrix, the criterion can be defined as: $\lambda_p \leq \alpha$, where α is a pre-specified threshold.

Assume an m-component Gaussian mixture model. Without loss of generality, assume further that component 1 is degenerate at a breakdown point. The observed data log likelihood and the complete data log likelihood are

$$l = \sum_{i=1}^{n} \log(\sum_{j=1}^{m} \pi_j f_j(x_i; \theta_j)), \tag{5}$$

and

$$l_c = \sum_{i=1}^{n} \sum_{j=1}^{m} Z_{ij} \{\log \pi_j + \log f_j(x_i; \theta_j)\}, \tag{6}$$

respectively, where

$$f_1(x_i, \theta_1) = \frac{\delta(\mathbf{NX} = \mathbf{B})}{\sqrt{\lambda_1 \cdots \lambda_{s-1}}} \exp\{-\frac{1}{2}(x_i - \mu_1)' \Sigma_1^- (x_i - \mu_1)\},$$

and

$$\Sigma_1^- = D' \cdot \text{diag}\{\lambda_1^{-1}, \cdots, \lambda_{s-1}^{-1}, 0, \cdots, 0\} \cdot D.$$

The $\mathbf{NX} = \mathbf{B}$ is a set of $d - s$ linear equations representing the subspace spanned by the non-degenerate eigen-directions. Σ_1^- is the generalized inverse of Σ_1 and δ is the usual delta function.

In order to achieve the goals discussed in the previous subsection, we substitute $\delta(.)$ with a bounded regular density function. With an artificial perturbation added, the proposed substituting function $K(x)$ is

$$K(x) = \frac{1}{\sqrt{\lambda_s \cdots \lambda_d}} \exp\{-\frac{1}{2}(x - \mu_1)'(\Sigma_1^* - \Sigma_1^-)(x - \mu_1)\}, \tag{7}$$

where

$$\Sigma_1^* = D'\Lambda^* D \tag{8}$$

and

$$\Lambda^* = \text{diag}\{\lambda_1^{-1}, \cdots, \lambda_{s-1}^{-1}, \lambda_s^{-1}, \cdots, \lambda_d^{-1}\}. \tag{9}$$

For simplicity, we assume $\lambda_s = \cdots = \lambda_d = \lambda^*$. Clearly λ^* controls the level of perturbation applied to the covariance matrix, and using a proper λ^* value is essential for the success of the algorithm. For spurious degeneration, λ^* should be large so that it is difficult for the algorithm to return to the same spurious solution. For genuine degeneration, this value should be small so that the true degenerate components can be preserved. adaptiveness of λ^* to data

The values of $z_{ij}^{(k)}$ determine the assignment of each data point to certain component. After the perturbation, Σ_1 in $\theta^{(k)}$ is replaced by Σ_1^*, and the corresponding $z_{i1}^{(k)}$ becomes z_{i1}^*, where

$$z_{i1}^{(k)} = \frac{\pi_1^{(k)} f_1(x_i, \theta^{(k)})}{\sum_{j=1}^m \pi_j^{(k)} f_j(x_i, \theta^{(k)})},$$

$$z_{i1}^* = \frac{\pi_1^{(k)} f_1(x_i, \theta^*)}{\pi_1^{(k)} f_1(x_i, \theta^*) + \sum_{j=2}^m \pi_j^{(k)} f_j(x_i, \theta^{(k)})},$$

and θ^* denotes the new parameter estimates. The i is the index for the data points in the degenerate component only. Define

$$U_1 = \sum_{i=1}^{n_1} z_{i1}^{(k)}, \quad U_1^* = \sum_{i=1}^{n_1} z_{i1}^*,$$

$$D_U = |U_1 - U_1^*|,$$

where n_1 is the number of points in component 1. D_U indicates the effect of perturbation on the degenerate component. the data points belonging to Finally, the perturbation λ_{DEM}^* is defined as

$$\lambda_{DEM}^* = \max\{\lambda^* | D_U \leq \beta\}, \tag{10}$$

where β is a pre-specified threshold. Let us discuss two properties of D_U which are related to the size of the degenerate component and the relative distance between components.

(1) D_U is positively associated with the size of the degenerate component. For a fixed β, a spurious degenerate component with small size gives a large λ_{DEM}^* value. After applying the perturbation with λ_{DEM}^*, the nearby data points will be absorbed into the degenerate component so that the DEM algorithm can divert from breakdown.

(2) Let the distance between components j and k be the usual Kullback-Leibler distance between $f_j(x|\theta_j)$ and $f_k(x|\theta_k)$. Then D_U depends on the relative distance between the degenerate component and the other components. When a degenerate component is far away from the others, a large λ^*_{DEM} is needed to reach a certain β level.

In practice, if a component is found to be degenerate repeatedly, the degeneration is likely to be genuine. In order for the algorithm to converge, it is necessary to have the perturbation level decrease to zero. To achieve this, every time when the same degeneration is repeated, β will be decreased by a certain ratio. A value s is used to count the number of reoccurrence of the same degeneration. Once this value exceeds a threshold (in the algorithm we set to 10), the DEM algorithm declares that a genuine degenerate component has been founded and stop the iteration.

The DEM algorithm is summarized in Algorithm 1. For simplicity and the clarity of presentation, we assume there exists only one degenerate component at a time. The α is used as a threshold to identify the nearly degenerate components. If we care looking for complete degeneration, α is set to be 0. Usually α is a value specified by the user.

Table 1. The three components detected by DEM for Synthetic Dataset 1 and the corresponding eigenvalues.

Comp.	Corresponding Eigenvalues		
1	1.0722954	0.9034532	0.8311285
2	0.9034483	0.9023349	0
3	0.8713843	1.2013586e-03	1.6785237e-05

3 Experimental Results

A number of simulations are performed to compare the DEM with the LPCA algorithm. We show that the DEM gives significantly better results in various datasets. In the following experiments, we set $\beta = 1$ and $\alpha = 0.01$.

Synthetic Dataset 1.

This dataset is comprised of three components, one component is a three-dimensional sphere with 120 points, another is a two-dimensional plane with 80 points, and the third, a one-dimensional line with 80 points. The means of these three components are (0,0,0), (0,0,1), and (0,0,-1), respectively. We report the eigenvalues of the three component covariance matrices given by the DEM in Table (1).

Algorithm 1 The Degenerate EM algorithm

For each component j, set counters $\beta_j = \beta_0$ and $s_j = 0$.

Run the EM algorithm until a degenerate component is found, say the (l)th component.

Decompose Σ_l into $D_l' \Lambda_l D_l$ as described in Section (2.2).

Identify zero (close to zero for $\alpha > 0$) eigenvalues $\lambda_s, \cdots, \lambda_d$ for those $\lambda \leq \alpha$.

while (zero (close to zero for $\alpha > 0$) eigenvalues exist) and $s_l < 10$ **do**

Calculate:

$$\lambda^*_{DEM} = \max\{\lambda^* : \ D_U < \beta\}.$$

Modify Σ_l by

$$\Sigma_l^* = D' Diag\{\lambda_1^{-1}, \cdots, \lambda_{s-1}^{-1}, \lambda_{DEM}^{*-1}, \cdots, \lambda_{DEM}^{*-1}\} D. \tag{11}$$

Update z_{il} by setting

$$z_{il} = z_{il}^* = \frac{\pi_l f_l^*(x_i)}{\sum_{k \neq l} \pi_k f_k(x_i, \mu_k, \Sigma_k) + \pi_l f_l^*(x_i, \mu_l, \Sigma_l^*)}. \tag{12}$$

The probabilities for the point allocations z_{ij} become z_{ij}^*, where $1 \leq i \leq n$ and $1 \leq j \leq m$.

Update parameters for all the components: $j \in \{1 : m\}$ by:

$$\mu_j = \sum_{i=1}^{n} z_{ij}^* x_i / \sum_{i=1}^{n} z_{ij}^*,$$

$$\Sigma_j = \sum_{j=1}^{m} \sum_{i=1}^{n} z_{ij}^* (x_i - \mu_j)(x_i - \mu_j)'/n,$$

$$\pi_j = \sum_{i=1}^{n} z_{ij}^* / n.$$

$\beta_l = \beta_l / 5$; $s_l = s_l + 1$.

end while

Judging from the strength of their eigenvalues, It is evident from this table that the three components have been clearly identified, with component 1 being the sphere, component 2 the plane and component 3 the line.

Synthetic Dataset 2.

We further validate these results on a 50 dimensional dataset with three components. Each component has 500 data points generated from $\mathcal{N}(0, \Sigma_j)$, $1 \leq j \leq 3$. The component covariance matrices Σ_1, Σ_2 and Σ_3 are of ranks 50, 30 and 20 respectively. Because all the three components are centered at the origin, distance based clustering methods such as K-means will perform poorly. Judging from the mis-allocation rate in Table (2), the LPCA does not work well either. However, the DEM algorithm has identified all the components and has achieved very low error rates.

Table 2. Comparison of the errors and the error rates of DEM and LPCA for Synthetic Dataset 2.

Data	Error		Error Rate	
Set	DEM	LPCA	DEM	LPCA
1	0	513.2	0	34.2 %
2	1.2	488.4	0.08 %	32.6 %
3	0.8	396.1	0.053 %	26.4 %

Synthetic Dataset 3.

The DEM algorithm is designed to distinguish spurious degeneration from genuine degeneration. In Figure 1, all the plots contain two components: one line and one two-dimensional plane. For the two plots in the upper panel, Plot (A) indicate the initial allocation of data points to components 1 and 2. Clearly, component 1 is degenerate and spurious, because it contains only a small portion of the genuine degenerate component. Plot (B) indicates the result of the DEM algorithm, in which we can see that the one-dimensional and two-dimensional structures have been identified. For the two plots in the lower panel, Plot (C) indicates the initial allocation of the data with a spurious degenerate component around the center of the data. After running the DEM, the genuine degenerate component as well as the two-dimensional plane have been clearly recovered, as shown in plot (D).

Iris data.

The Iris data consist of measurements of the length and width of both sepals and petals of 50 plants for each of the three types of Iris species – Setosa, Versicolor, and Virginica. The objective is to demonstrate the ability of the DEM algorithm for identifying subsets of data that are degenerate. The simulation result of the DEM is compared with that of the LPCA algorithm, with the first two eigen-directions retained.

All but 4 points (69, 71, 73 and 84th data points) are classified accurately by the DEM algorithm. In contrast, the LPCA algorithm misclassifies 58 points. The superior performance of the DEM algorithm on the Iris data is attributed to its ability to detect degeneracy effectively. In Table (3), we include the eigenvalues corresponding to the component covariance matrices respectively. Clearly there is a sharp drop between the third and the fourth eigenvalues in components 1 and 2, while the change is moderate in component 3. This implies that components 1 and 2 are in fact degenerate.

4 Conclusions

In high dimensional data analysis, it is often the case that subsets of data lie on different low dimensional subspaces. In this paper, we have proposed

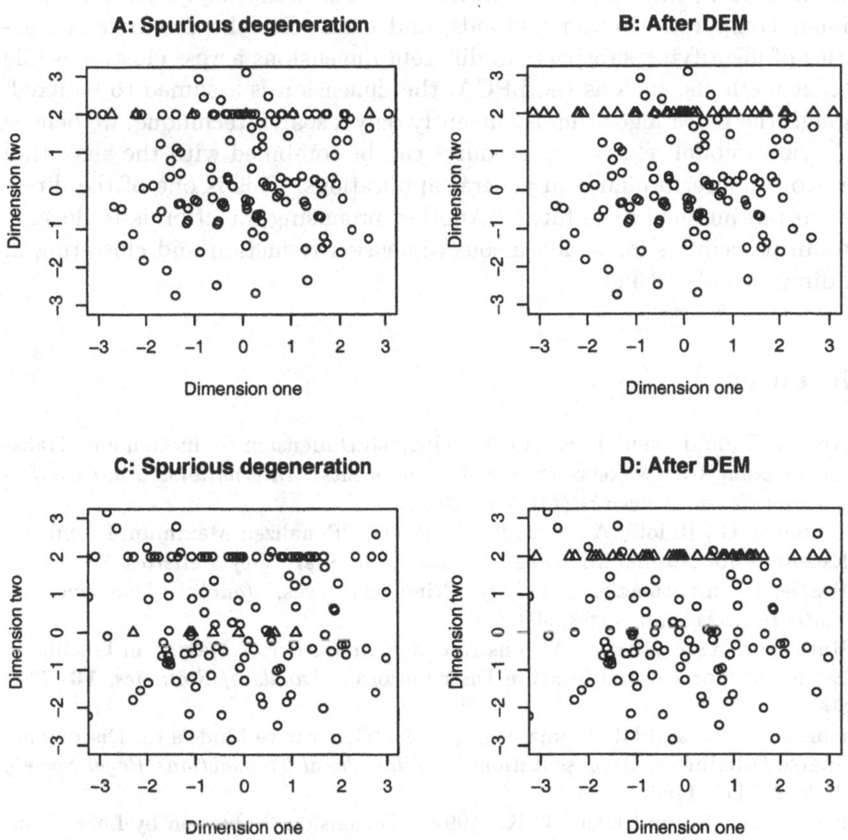

Fig. 1. Dataset A and B used to demonstrate the ability of DEM in deviating from spurious degeneracies. △ denotes component 1 and ○ denotes component 2.

Table 3. Eigenvalues of Iris data after running DEM.

Comp.	1st Eigen	2nd Eigen	3rd Eigen	4th Eigen
1	0.23645569	0.03691873	0.02679643	0.00903326
2	0.48787394	0.07238410	0.05477608	0.00979036
3	0.69525484	0.10655123	0.05229543	0.03426585

the DEM algorithm to address this problem. The DEM enjoys superior performance compared to other methods, and it also has the desirable characteristics of identifying subspaces of different dimensions across clusters, while for other methods, such as the LPCA, the dimension is assumed to be fixed. Although the DEM algorithm is currently only a search technique, we believe that various model selection procedures can be combined with the algorithm to improve its performance in general applications. This is one of the directions we will pursue in the future. Another promising direction is to develop Bayesian procedures for simultaneous dimension reduction and clustering in high dimensional settings.

References

1. Archer, C., and Leen, T. K. (1999). "Optimal Dimension Reduction and Transform Coding with Mixture Principal Components," *International Joint Conference on Neural Networks (IJCNN)*, IEEE.
2. Ciuperca, G., Ridolfi, A., and Idier, J. (2003). "Penalized Maximum Likelihood Estimator for Normal Mixtures," *Scandinavian Journal of Statistics*, **30**, 45–59.
3. Hastie, T., and Stuetzle, W. (1989). "Principal Curves," *Journal of the American Statistical Association*, **84**, 502–516.
4. Hathaway, R. J. (1985). "A Constrained Formulation of Maximum-Likelihood Estimation for Normal Mixture Distributions," *Annals of Statistics*, **13**, 795–800.
5. Hinton, G. E., and Ghahramani, Z. (1997). "Generative Models for Discovering Sparse Distributed Representations," *Philosophical Transactions Royal Society B*, **352**, 1177–1190.
6. Kambhatla, N., and Leen, T. K. (1997). "Dimension Reduction by Local Principal Component Analysis," *Neural Computation*, **9**, 1793–1516.
7. Kiefer, J., and Wolfowitz, J. (1956). "Consistency of the Maximum Likelihood Estimates in the Presence of Infinitely Many Incidental Parameters," *Annals of Mathematical Statistics*, **27**, 887–906.
8. Kohonen, T. (1989). *Self-Organization and Associative Memory* (3rd ed.), Springer- Verlag, Berlin.
9. Kohonen, T. (1990). "The Self-Organizing Map," in *Proceedings of the IEEE*, **78**, pp. 1464–1479.
10. Lin, X. (2003). *Finite Mixture Models for Clustering, Dimension Reduction and Privacy Preserving Data Mining*, Ph.D. Thesis, Purdue University.

A Dimension Reduction Technique for Local Linear Regression

Joseph Lucas

Duke University, U.S.A.
joe@stat.duke.edu

Abstract: We offer a refinement to the technique of loca regression which allows for dimension reduction and data compression.

1 Introduction

Partition of Unity Local Regression (PULR) is a technique by which a data set is modeled by fitting some parametric family of functions to it locally, and then patching the fitted functions together on the areas in which they intersect. As a general description, one starts with a covering of the data set by some collection of sets, and a collection of functions subordinate to these sets which satisfy the conditions for being a partition of unity. (That is, they sum to one at every point.) Local fitting is then done within each of these sets, and the final model is computed at any point as the weighted average of the local values from each set, the weights coming from the function values at that point.

This differs from what is typically called local regression. For standard local regression, one defines a weight function and, at each point, the response variable is computed as though it were the center of a neighborhood with the chosen weight function. That is, a regression line is fitted through the point which minimizes the weight sum of squares. The technique that I propose, PULR, requires a regression calculation at only a fixed, relatively small, number of points, and these results are averaged to compute the response variable between these points. Notice that our algorithm will produce results similar to local regression (it is exactly equal at the centers of the neighborhoods), but that it is computationally less demanding because a regression must be done at only a few places. Because of this, it scales to higher dimensions more easily. Additionally, the results from PULR at its simplest may be enumerated as a list of neighborhood centers, radii, and orthogonal directions. This opens up the possibility of using it for data compression. Finally, local regression will, by its nature, smooth corners, and create curves where there are step functions. If one is clever about the choice of neighborhoods, PULR does not suffer from this restriction.

There are evidently a number of choices to be made in the construction of such a PULR model. We must choose the covering collection of sets, the weight functions, the parametric family of functions to fit to the data locally, and the criterion by which we will fit this family.

Perhaps the most difficult of these choices is the choice of covering sets. Some simple solutions are to choose a fixed set of "centers", each the center of a ball of fixed radius. Another choice is to fix not the radius, but rather fix the number of points in the ball (varying the radius accordingly). The choice of these neighborhoods is, in some sense, crucial because choosing poorly can lead to bias at sharp corners, and smoothing of edges in the data set.

Having chosen the covering for the space, the construction of the weight functions is not difficult. Let $g_i(x)$ be any function supported by set U_i. Then $\forall x$, define $w_i(x) = g_i(x)/\sum_i g_i(x)$. This is the weight function associated with U_i. Clearly, then, $\forall x$, $\sum_i w_i(x) = 1$.

We are now left to decide the shape of g_i. The simplest choice would be I_{U_i} (the index function on U_i), however, this gives results in a model that is essentially equivalent to PULR in neighborhoods that don't overlap (the resulting model has distinct faces and angles). For our experiments, we chose g_i to be a pyramid. That is, if c_i is the center of our set and r_i the radius, then $g_i(x) = \max\{r - abs(c_i - x), 0\}$. If one is interested in a smooth ($\mathbf{C}^\infty$) final solution, then each g_i may be chosen to be smooth.

The choice of parametric families should rely on prior knowledge regarding the data. For example, if it is expected that the data is harmonic, then one can expect a better convergence to the "true" function if harmonic functions or harmonic polynomials are used (cf. Melenk and Babuska, 1996). For our purposes, simple linear regression will be used, but our results apply to any choice of parametric families.

We use least squares to fit our regression hyper-planes, but in general the choice of fitting should be based on assumptions about the distribution of the data.

2 Previous Work

All previous work on using regression locally to model or smooth data differs from the algorithm proposed here as described above. However, because of the similarities between the two methods, PULR may draw from results concerning selection of weight functions, selection of neighborhood sizes, and selection of parametric families from local regression. These results are outlined nicely in a survey paper by Cleveland and Loader (1995).

3 Methods

Definition 1. *Let $S \subset \mathbb{R}^n$. A Partition of Unity on S, is a collection of pairs, $\{(U_i, f_i)\}_{i=1}^K$, such that:*

i) U_i form an open cover of S
ii) $f_i : S \to \mathbb{R}$ are functions with support contained in the closure of U_i $\forall i$
iii) $S \subset \cup Support(f_i)$
iv) $\forall x \in S$, $\sum_{i=1}^n f_i = 1$

Definition 2. *Given Partition of Unity, $\{(U_i, f_i)\}_{i=1}^K$, on a set S, and a collection of functions $g_i : U_i \to \mathbb{R}$, a Partition of Unity Local Regression is the map defined by $\sum_{i=1}^K f_i g_i$.*

In this paper, we explore a specific case of PULR. We choose S to be a region containing some data set of interest. From this data set, we create U_i by choosing a point in the data set and finding its n closest neighbors (including the point). We find the center, c_i, of these points (found by averaging coordinates) and define $f_i(x) = \max(0, r_i - ||c_i - x||)$ where r_i is the radius of the neighborhood. Finally, the g_i are the least squares hyperplanes fitted to the data points in U_i.

These choices are made for simplicity and to show proof of concept. Work in the field of local regression provides many interesting alternatives for all of these choices. In particular, there are adaptive procedures for choosing neighborhood sizes which may perform better, the weight functions, f_i, may be chosen to be smooth, and any sort of local fitting function may be used (nth order splines, kernel smoothers, etc.).

We use simulated annealing to make an intellegent choice of covering sets. The technique provides a method for minimizing the energy of a system (Kirkpatrick et al., 1983). To use simulated annealing, we need to assign an energy function to the space of such models which may be minimized. The choices are many. Some obvious ones are the maximum distance between the data set and the model and the sum of squared distances between data set and model. If we think of a picture as a data set, and we are using this technique to compress the image, then the former is an excellent candidate to avoid significant distortion at any one place. On the other hand, if we are looking for a statistical model of some data, and want to place more weight on groups of points than individual points, then the latter is the appropriate choice. For a model that is even more robust to outliers, one would choose the sum of absolute distances as the energy.

However, we use none of these. In our attempts to model our data with local linear regression, we would like to choose the neighborhoods in such a way as to ensure that the points within those neighborhoods as close to linear as possible.

Every linear transformation can be broken down into a combination of "stretching" in various directions and "rotation". If we have a matrix A which

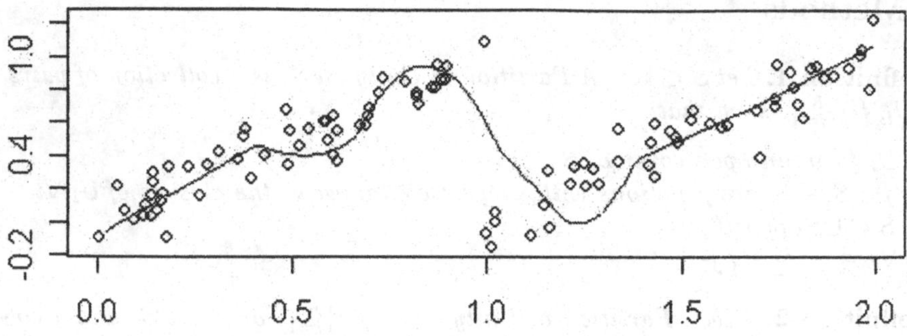

Fig. 1. Result obtained by simply choosing the centers at random. The data was generated from $y = x \bmod(1)$

represents a linear transformation, then singular value decomposition (SVD) provides a very efficient way to break A down into its components, usually labeled UDV^T. If A is square, then U and V are orthogonal matrices, and D is a diagonal matrix of decreasing eigenvalues. U represents a rotation sending the directions of "stretching" into the basis vectors, D actually accomplishing the stretching, and V^T returning the space to the original basis vectors and applying the "rotation". The matrix A need not be square to perform singular value decomposition, and in fact it is a well known fact that if one performs singular value decomposition on a set of points in $\mathbf{R}^n$, then the resulting rotation sends the least squares hyper-plane (from multiple linear regression) into the first $n-1$ basis vectors. Thus SVD provides a computationally efficient technique for performing linear regression on an arbitrary number of points in a high dimensional space. In addition, the magnitude of the last value in the diagonal matrix provides a measure of the fit of the hyper-plane to the data points. Thus SVD gives us, in one step, a technique for performing the linear regression and measuring the validity of our regression. The last value in the diagonal matrix will function as the "energy" contribution from its neighborhood. If we then sum these values for all of the neighborhoods in our PULR, we obtain an energy function that measures the "fit" of our choice of neighborhood centers.

Our algorithm proceeds as follows. First, neighborhood centers are chosen until their corresponding order K neighborhoods cover the space. Then SVD is performed on the set of points in each neighborhood and an energy is calculated. If E_n is the energy of the new state, and E_o that of the old, then we accept this new state with probability $= \exp[(E_o - E_n)/T]$ (which is the ratio of the probabilities as prescribed by MCMC). We generate a new state from an old one by first choosing a random number of centers to fix, k, and then choosing which k neighborhoods to keep based on their individual

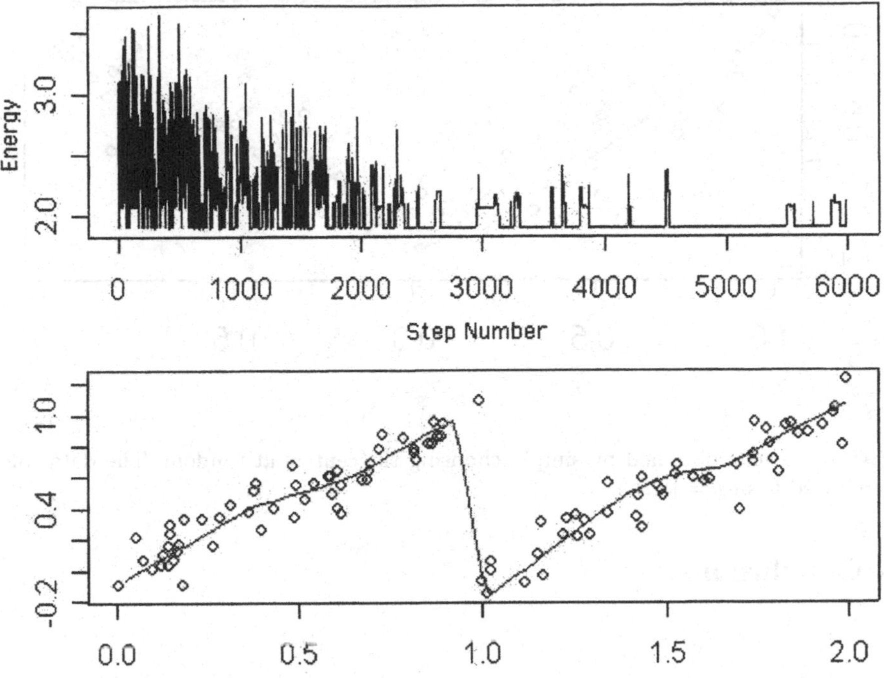

Fig. 2. Results of PULR after model selection by simulated annealing. The energy at each step is plotted above. There were 500 steps taken at each temperature from 10 to 1, and 500 steps at each of .5 and .1. The data was generated from $y = x \bmod(1)$

contributions to the total energy. We find that this increases the acceptance rate anywhere from 20-50 percent over simply re-randomizing.

4 Results

In general, simply choosing the center points for our PULR at random performs quite well if the data is smooth (figure 5). The difficulty with this is that the technique will usually smooth corners if they are sharp, and it will place curves where there are step functions (figures 1 and 3). We find that our algorithm performs excellently in these situations (figures 2 and 4). An additional benefit to our algorithm is that it generalizes immediately to higher dimensions. Figure 5 shows its application to the function $\sin(x)\sin(y)$, and figure 6 shows $|x| + |y|$. The algorithm also works well in higher dimensions, but the difficulties of presenting results on a two dimensional piece of paper preclude figures.

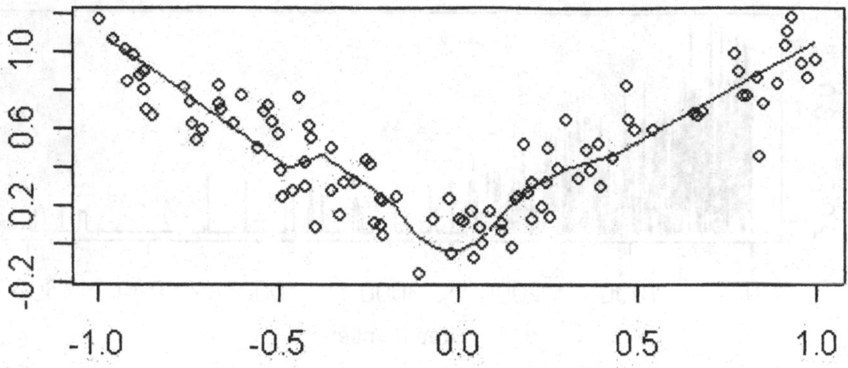

Fig. 3. Results obtained by simply choosing the centers at random. The data was generated from $y = |x|$.

5 Conclusions

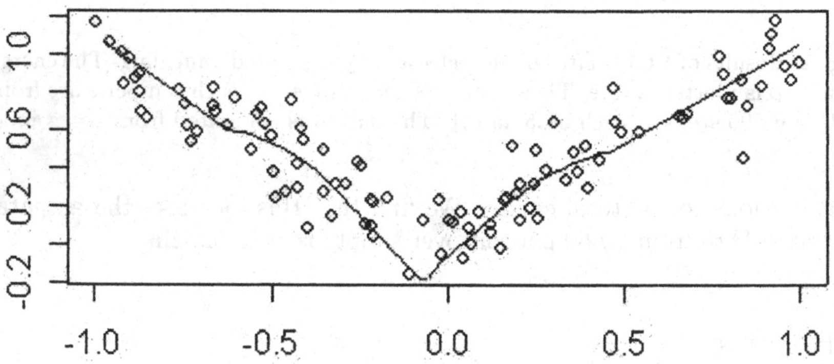

Fig. 4. Results after simulated annealing. There were 1000 steps taken at each temperature from 10 to 1, and 1000 steps at each of .5 and .1. The data was generated from $y = |x|$.

One application of our algorithm worth exploring is in the compression of video. Each pixel can be located in three-space (two dimensions on the screen and one corresponding to frame number). The red, yellow and blue color levels can be modeled separately, and the final product can be reconstructed from just the list of neighborhood centers and sizes.

Our algorithm forms an excellent basis for modeling, smoothing, and even compression of data. Most any shape can be modeled well with PULR if the choice of model is made carefully. This paper only begins to look at the application of MCMC and simulated annealing to this task. Our algorithm assumes a fixed neighborhood size for all neighborhoods, and this is certainly not required.

Notice that this assumption means that, at the corners of our data set we will find an almost identical neighborhood no matter what the choice of PULR. One solution to this difficulty would be to add a size as well as a center and direction to each neighborhood and searching in this enlarged parameter space. There is a difficulty here because the energy we have used increases with the number of points that are in overlapping neighborhoods. Thus, some technique must be devised to compensate for the bias towards large neighborhoods, or one of the other energy functions mentioned must be used.

Additionally, improvements can be had by including more functions in the family that is used to model locally, allowing the neighborhood radius to extend beyond the farthest points included in the regression, or modifying the weight functions dynamically based on some measure of certainty of the model locally.

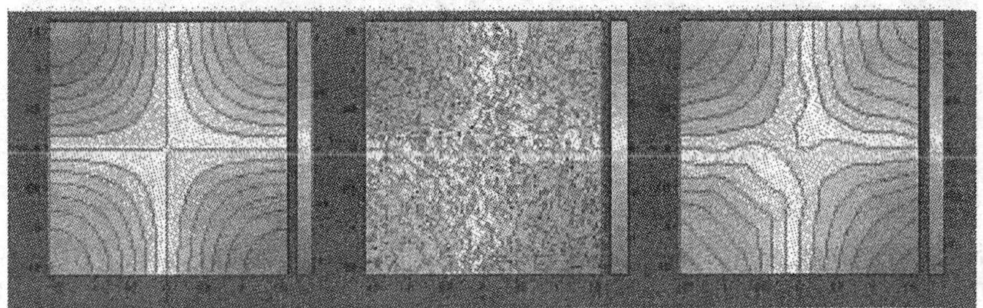

Fig. 5. The original function, $z = \sin(x)\sin(y)$, the function after some random noise has been added, and the results of local linear regression on the noisy data.

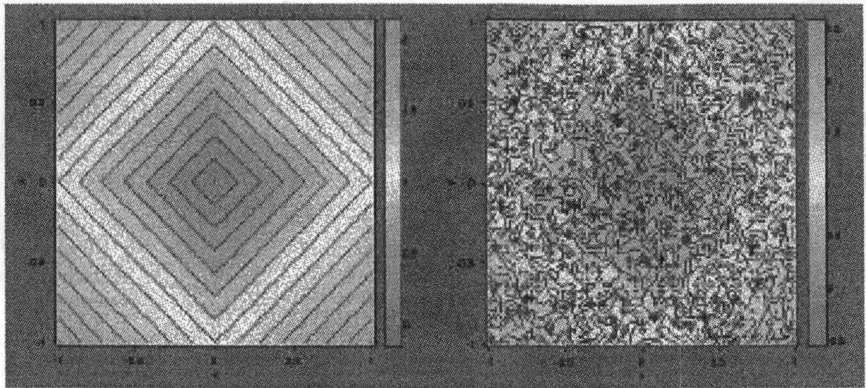

Fig. 6. The function $z = |x| + |y|$ before and after random noise has been added.

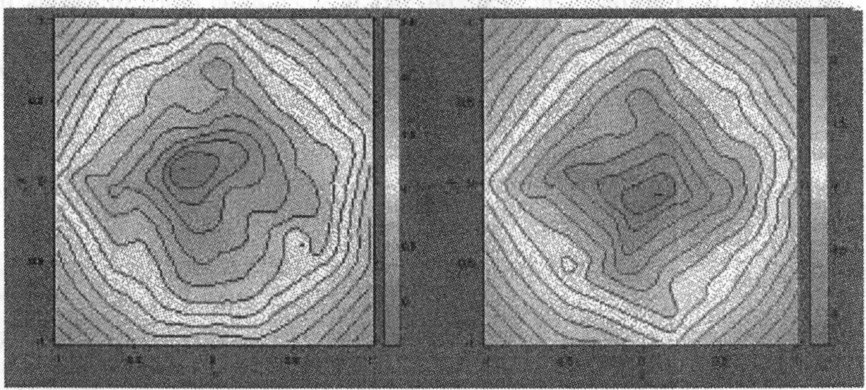

Fig. 7. Left: The function $z = |x|+|y|$ after smoothing by a random PULR. **Right:** The same function after smoothing by PULR with model selection by simulated annealing. Notice that the model chosen by simulated annealing exhibits straight edges much closer to the center of the data set.

References

1. Cleveland, W., and Loader, C. (1995). "Smoothing by Local Regression: Principles and Methods," in *Statistical Theory and Computational Aspects of Smoothing*, eds. W. Haerdle and M. G. Schimek, New York:Springer, pp. 10–49.
2. Melenk, J.M., and Babuska, I. (1996). "The Partition of Unity Finite Element Method: Basic Theory and Applications. *Computational Methods in Applied Mechanical Engineering*, **139**, 289–314
3. Kirkpatrick, S., Gelatt, C. D., and Vecchi, M. P. (1983). "Optimization by Simulated Annealing," *Science*, **220**, 671–681

Reducing the Number of Variables Using Implicative Analysis

Raphaël Couturier[1], Régis Gras[2], and Fabrice Guillet[2]

[1] LIFC - IUT Belfort-Montbéliard, France
couturie@iut-bm.univ-fcomte.fr
[2] École Polytechnique de l'Université de Nantes, France
regisgra@club-internet.fr, fabrice.guillet@polytech.univ-nantes.fr

Abstract: The interpretation of complex data with data mining techniques is often a difficult task. Nevertheless, this task may be simplified by reducing the variables which could be considered as equivalent. The aim of this paper is to describe a new method for reducing the number of variables in a large set of data. Implicative analysis, which builds association rules with a measure more powerful than conditional probability, is used to detect quasi-equivalent variables. This technique has some advantages over traditional similarity analysis.

1 Introduction

One of the main data mining challenge is to provide a way of discovering new information in the data (Agrawal and al., 1993). There are several methods and techniques to complete this task. But when a human expert needs to make a decision based on the information provided by data mining tools, he is often confronted with a large number of rules that may be very difficult to analyze. In large data sets, a lot of variables can be considered as equivalent, depending on the problem (Gras and al., 2002). In this case, an automatic way to detect quasi-equivalent data is preferred to other techniques because this detection can be time-consuming.

The notion of quasi-equivalence is related to a given problem and the detection process is strongly dependent on several parameters. For example, the origin of the data may allow us to definitively conclude whether some variables are equivalent or not. The presence of important noise has an impact on the complexity of this detection. The number of variables and the size of data are likewise important clues which have to be taken into account. Another interesting point concerns the sensitivity of the detection process; indeed an expert often wants to interact with the tool implementing the method in order to get more accurate results. Thus the method used to compute quasi-equivalent variables has to integrate all those parameters.

In this article, our aim is to provide a solution in order to automatically detect quasi-equivalent variables, thus allowing the generation of a smaller new set of data without the equivalent variables in which the semantic should be globally conserved. Therefore this smaller new set should be easier to be analysed. Nevertheless, this reduction introduces another problem. Indeed, once the set of equivalent variables is detected, only one of them (or a new one) should be used to replace the initial set. Either the expert has to decide how to proceed or the most representative variable has to be automatically detected. In the latter case, the problem of representativeness should be considered.

Several indexes have been defined to measure the similarities. For example, Jaccard's index, Russel and Rao's index, and Rogers and Tanimoto's index (presented in Section 4) define three different similarities indexes. Aggarwal (2001) gives an example in which data are transformed into a lower dimensional space by using similarity. We choose to define a new similarity measure based on the implicative analysis introduced by Gras, which selects rules having the form $A \Rightarrow B$. This measure is asymmetric, which guarantees that when symmetry is obtained between $A \Rightarrow B$ and $B \Rightarrow A$, it is very informative. Moreover, the implicative analysis is noise-resistant and depends on the data size.

The following section recalls the principle of implicative analysis. In Section 3, our new method for detecting quasi-equivalent variables is described. Section 4 is devoted to comparing our method with related works. Next, in Section 5, we propose a way to determine the leader of each class. Finally, Section 6 gives a test on a synthetic sample.

2 Implicative Analysis

Implicative analysis uses a measure that selects association rules. Implication intensity measures the degree of surprise inherent in a rule. Hence, trivial rules that are potentially well known to the expert are discarded. This implication intensity is reinforced by the degree of validity that is based on Shannon's entropy. This measure does not only take into account the validity of a rule itself, but its counterpart too. Indeed, when an association rule is estimated as valid, i.e., the set of items A is strongly associated with the set of items B, then, it is legitimate and intuitive to expect that its counterpart is also valid, i.e., the set of non-B items is strongly associated with the set of non-A items. Both of these original measures are completed by a classical utility measure based on the size of the support rule and are combined to define a final relevance measure that inherits the qualities of the three measures, i.e., it is noise-resistant as the rule counterpart is taken into account, and it only selects non trivial rules. For further information the reader is invited to consult (Gras et al., 2001). In the following, the classical statistics framework is considered and definitions of implication intensity, validity, and usefulness are given.

Let us introduce the notation that will be used in this paper. Let $A \Rightarrow B$ be an association rule over two sets of items A and B (these items can be single items or conjonctions of items), included in a global data set I. Let I_A represent individuals described by the properties A, and let I_B represents individuals described by the properties B. So $I_{A \wedge B}$ represents individuals described by the properties A and B. And $I_{A \wedge \overline{B}}$ represents individuals described by the properties A without being described by the properties B; those individuals are the counter-examples of the rules $A \Rightarrow B$. The implication intensity of a rule is defined by the number of times this rule is denied by a small number of counter-examples. In other words, we measure the astonishment to discover that the cardinality of $I_{A \wedge \overline{B}}$ is small compared to the expected cardinality of $I_{A \wedge \overline{B}}$ when I_A and I_B are randomly selected in I.

Definition 1 (Implication intensity) *The implication intensity of an association rule $A \Rightarrow B$ which is obtained on a set I of n individuals is measured by a coefficient is denoted by $ImpInt$ $(A \Rightarrow B)$, where $ImpInt$ $(A \Rightarrow B)$ takes its values in* $[0,\ 1]$ *such that the intensity is maximum when $ImpInt$ $(A \Rightarrow B) = 1$ and minimum when $ImpInt$ $(A \Rightarrow B) = 0$. The $ImpInt$ $(A \Rightarrow B)$ is defined as follows:*

$$ImpInt\ (A \Rightarrow B) = \frac{1}{\sqrt{2\pi}} \int_q^{\infty} \exp[-t^2/2]\, dt$$

where

$$q = \left[\mid I_{A \wedge \overline{B}} \mid - \frac{\mid I_A \mid \times \mid \overline{I_B} \mid}{n} \right] \left[\sqrt{\frac{\mid I_A \mid \times \mid \overline{I_B} \mid}{n} (1 - \frac{\mid I_A \mid \times \mid \overline{I_B} \mid}{n^2})} \right]^{-1} .$$

This index has an advantage compared to the linear correlation coefficient which is not resistant to some trivial situations and which is unstable. For instance, the correlation coefficient is equal to 1 if $\mid I \mid = 1000$, $\mid I_{A \wedge B} \mid = 1$ and $\mid I_{\overline{A} \wedge \overline{B}} \mid = 999$ whereas $ImpInt(A \Rightarrow B) \simeq 0.65$. Intuitively, a rule is valid when there is a large proportion of individuals described by the properties A that are also described by the properties B. In other words, the more I_A is included in I_B, the more the rule $A \Rightarrow B$ is valid. To follow this intuitive definition, we propose to measure the *validity coefficient* associated with an association rule $A \Rightarrow B$ as the degree of inclusion of I_A in I_B. According to the Shannon's information theory, the disorder in the population I_A is the *entropy*, defined by $E(f) = -f \log_2(f) - (1-f) \log_2(1-f)$.

Definition 2 (Validity) *The validity of an association rule $A \Rightarrow B$ which is obtained on a set I of n individuals is measured by the validity coefficient $Validity(A \Rightarrow B)$, defined as follows: $Validity(A \Rightarrow B) = 1 - E(f_1)^2$ if $f_1 \in [0,\ 0.5]$ and 0 if $f_1 \in [0.5,\ 1]$. Here $f_1 = \mid I_{A \wedge \overline{B}} \mid / \mid I_A \mid$ is the relative frequency of $I_{A \wedge \overline{B}}$ within I_A and $E(f)$ is the entropy function.*

In bivalent logic theory, the rule $A \Rightarrow B$ is equivalent to its counterpart $\neg B \Rightarrow \neg A$, where "$\neg$" is used as the negation symbol. By way of consequence, the validity of an association rule $A \Rightarrow B$ is strongly linked to the validity of its counterpart $\neg B \Rightarrow \neg A$. A rule cannot be viewed as valid if its counterpart is not also valid, and reciprocally. That is why we introduce the notion of *global validity* of a rule $A \Rightarrow B$ that depends, on one hand, on the validity of the rule and, on the other hand, on the validity of the rule counterpart.

Definition 3 (global validity) *The global validity of an association rule $A \Rightarrow B$ which is obtained on a set I of n individuals is measured by the coefficient $GloVal$ $(A \Rightarrow B)$ defined as follows:*

$$GloVal\ (A \Rightarrow B) = \left[Validity\ (A \Rightarrow B) \times Validity\ (\neg B \Rightarrow \neg A)\right]^{1/4}.$$

One can notice that the rules $A \Rightarrow B$ and $\neg B \Rightarrow \neg A$ have the same set of counter-examples which is noted $I_{A \wedge \overline{B}}$. Then, the validity coefficient of $\neg B \Rightarrow \neg A$ that characterizes the inclusion of $\overline{I_B}$ into $\overline{I_A}$ depends on the relative frequency of $I_{A \wedge \overline{B}}$ within $\overline{I_B}$. Because $\overline{I_B}$ is the complementary of I_B, its cardinality is equal to $\mid I \mid - \mid I_B \mid = n - \mid I_B \mid$. In other words, the validity coefficient of $\neg B \Rightarrow \neg A$ is obtained by taking $f_2 = \mid I_{A \wedge \overline{B}} \mid / [n - \mid I_B \mid]$ in place of f_1 in the previous definition. An association rule is useful when it helps to characterize enough individuals of the studied set I.

Definition 4 (Usefulness) *The usefulness of an association rule $A \Rightarrow B$ is measured by the coefficient $Use(A \Rightarrow B)$ defined as follows:*

$$Use(A \Rightarrow B) = \begin{cases} 1 & \text{if } \mid I_A \cap I_B \mid \geq MinSup \\ 0 & \text{otherwise} \end{cases}$$

where $MinSup$ is the minimum number of individuals that are needed to verify the rule, and $MinSup$ is defined by the analyst.

As previously mentioned, the degree of relevance associated to a rule needs to integrate the notions of implication intensity, validity and usefulness. The following definition is adopted:

Definition 5 (Relevance) *The relevance of an association rule $A \Rightarrow B$ is measured by the coefficient $Rel(A \Rightarrow B)$, defined as follows:*

$$Rel(A \Rightarrow B) = \sqrt{ImpInt(A \Rightarrow B) \times GloVal(A \Rightarrow B)} \times Use(A \Rightarrow B).$$

3 Detection of Quasi-Equivalent Variables

Once the principles of the implicative analysis are given, we shall see how to use it in order to define a method to detect quasi-equivalent variables. Logically, two variables A and B are equivalent if and only if $A \Rightarrow B$ and $B \Rightarrow A$. Thus, based on the logical definition of the equivalence, the quasi-equivalence is defined as:

Definition 6 (quasi-equivalence) *The quasi-equivalence of two variables A and B is measured by the coefficient Quasi(A, B), defined as follows:*

$$Quasi(A,B) = \sqrt{Rel(A \Rightarrow B) * Rel(B \Rightarrow A)}.$$

Given a threshold and using this formula for the quasi-equivalence, a list L of couples of variables having a coefficient of quasi-equivalence greater or equal to the threshold is obtained. Depending on the studied data set and according to the users' criteria, a threshold and an appropriate value of $MinSup$ for the usefulness coefficient are defined. Then we define a quasi-equivalence class as:

Definition 7 (quasi-equivalence class) *The quasi-equivalence class of n variables $A_1, \ldots, A_n$ is measured by the quasi-equivalence coefficient of this class defined as follows:*

$$Quasi - equivalence\ class(A) = \min_{\substack{i=1,\ldots,n-1 \\ j=i+1,\ldots,n}} (Quasi(A_i, A_j)).$$

4 Related Work

There are several other similarity indexes, among which we choose to present only four that are commonly used in the literature. Let us add the following notation as a complement to the previous ones. First, $I_{\overline{A} \wedge B}$ represents individuals described by the property B without being described by the property A. And $I_{\overline{A} \wedge \overline{B}}$ represents individuals not described by the property A and not described by the property B.

Jaccard's index is

$$I_{A \wedge B}/[I_{A \wedge B} + I_{A \wedge \overline{B}} + I_{\overline{A} \wedge B}].$$

Russel and Rao's index is

$$I_{A \wedge B}[I_{A \wedge B} + I_{A \wedge \overline{B}} + I_{\overline{A} \wedge B} + I_{\overline{A} \wedge \overline{B}}].$$

Rogers and Tanimoto's index

$$[I_{A \wedge B} + I_{\overline{A} \wedge \overline{B}}][I_{A \wedge B} + I_{\overline{A} \wedge \overline{B}} + 2 * (I_{A \wedge \overline{B}} + I_{\overline{A} \wedge B})].$$

Piatetsky-Shapiro's index is

$$[I_{A \wedge B}/I] - [I_A I * \frac{I_B}{I}].$$

These four indexes and all the similar ones are simple linear combinations of the four different sets $I_{A \wedge B}$, $I_{A \wedge \overline{B}}$, $I_{A \wedge \overline{B}}$ and $I_{\overline{A} \wedge \overline{B}}$. As a consequence, these indexes do not have the properties that interest us: noise resistance, only non-trivial rules selection, and suppression of useless rules. So we are interested in simulating the behavior of our index, the quasi-equivalence, compared to these three indexes. For all these simulations, we consider a constant size of $| I |= 100$. Then we choose three configurations in which the cardinals of A and B sets are relatively close and for each simulation we vary the cardinal of $| I_{A \wedge \overline{B}} |$, i.e., we increase the number of counter-examples of $I_A \wedge I_B$.

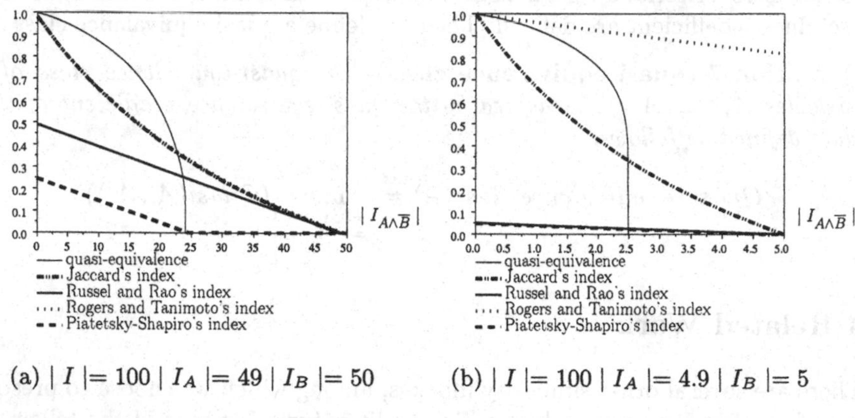

(a) $| I |= 100 \mid I_A |= 49 \mid I_B |= 50$ (b) $| I |= 100 \mid I_A |= 4.9 \mid I_B |= 5$

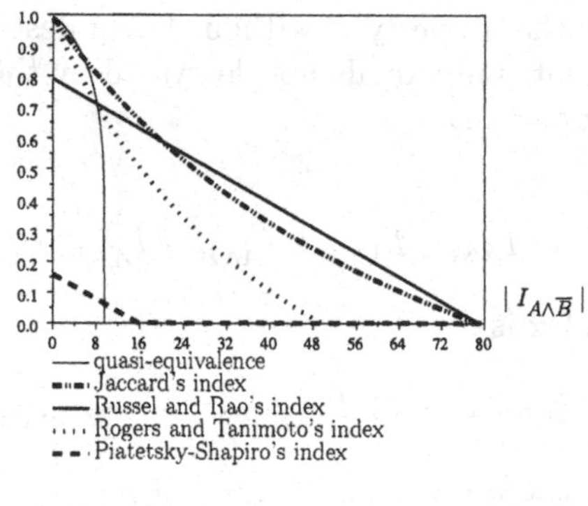

(c) $| I |= 100 \mid I_A |= 79 \mid I_B |= 80$

Fig. 1. Comparison of indexes.

Figure 1.a shows that Jaccard's index and Rogers and Tanimoto's index are very similar. Moreover we notice that Russel and Rao's index and Piatetsky-Shapiro's index (Matheus et al., 1996) are not satisfactory because even if $I_A \subset I_B$, i.e., if there is no counter-example of $| I_{A \wedge \overline{B}} |$, this index is below 0.5. On Figure 1.b, A and B sets keep the same ratio but they have a smaller cardinality and we can observe that Jaccard's index and ours have a behavior which is more similar than previously in Figure 1.a (however our index slightly changes with the size of data), whereas Rusell and Rao's index and Rogers, Tanimoto's and Piatetsky-Shapiro's index have completely changed and this is not an interesting property. Finally Figure 1.c clearly shows the advantage of our index. In this case, important values of $\mid I_A \mid$ and $\mid I_B \mid$ which are compared with $\mid I \mid$ do not bring new information since it is quite obvious that A and B tend to be equivalent. This is easier to understand with the following example. Let us suppose we have 100 individuals. The fact that 80 of them have glasses and 79 of them like wine tends to a similarity that is strongly correlated with the contingency table. In this case the correlation coefficient would inform us without taking into consideration the strong relationship between these two properties. On the contrary, the refusal of the similarity in presence of 10 counter-examples is reinforced by the fact that no necessary relation is required between these properties. So, the fact that our index quickly decreases as $\mid I_{A \wedge \overline{B}} \mid$ increases is a very interesting property that cannot be found in any other traditional similarity indexes.

5 Automatic Choice of a Class Leader

After having determined a quasi-equivalence class, an existing variable or a new one is selected to replace all the variables of the class. We call this variable a class leader. The choice of the class leader can either be made by the expert or automatically. An expert will probably choose the class leader by taking into consideration the class semantic; yet to include such a semantic in an automatic method is obviously very difficult. The method we decided to implement consists in defining a distance notion between the elements of the class and then in electing the class leader according to this measure. Thus, the class leader has effectively a leader role, in the sense that it represents the class better than any other variable. Moreover, the class leader is not a new variable. Our distance notion is defined as follows:

Definition 8 (distance between two variables) *The distance between A and B is defined as follows:*

$$dist(A,B) = \mid Rel(A,B) - Rel(B,A)) \mid .$$

With this distance, it is possible to know the distance between a variable and the other variables of the class.

Definition 9 (distance between a variable and the other variables) *The distance from a variable A_i to all other variables A_j in a class C with cardinality $\mid C \mid$ is:*

$$dist(A_i, C) = \mid C \mid^{-1} \sum_{A_j \in C; A_i \neq A_j} dist(A_i, A_j).$$

Then the leader of a class is the variable that minimizes this distance when compared to any other variables.

Definition 10 (class leader) *The leader A_i of the class C is:*

$$leader(C) = \min_{A_i \in C} dist(A_i, C).$$

We note that the leader of a class with only two elements cannot be determined since distances are equal. As a consequence, in this case we choose to define the leader as the variable with the greater relevance. Our reduction is based on a statistical criterion. Nevertheless, our measure ensures a similarity on the semantic point of view.

6 Experimentation

Within the framework of a student research project of the Polytechnic School of the University of Nantes (in France), a questionnaire is proposed to all the students of this School. Questions consist in making them quote 75 adjectives likely to be associated or not with 41 animals. Hence, a 75×41 matrix is considered. A matrix element contains 1 (respectively 0) if an adjective i characterizes (respectively does not characterize) the animal j. Our reduction algorithm provides the following quasi-equivalence classes:

{Crotale, Grass snake}, the leader is Grass snake; {Tiger, Shark} the leader is Shark; {Fox, Cat} the leader is Cat; {Vulture, Crow} the leader is Crow; {Hen, Sheep} the leader is Hen; {Lynx, Wolf} the leader is Wolf; {Rabbit, Dolphin} the leader is Dolphin. Hence, the reduction entails the suppression of 7 variables.

7 Conclusion

A new method to reduce the number of variables is introduced in this paper. It is based on an implicative analysis index that has already been shown to have good semantic and interesting properties compared to traditional indexes. With this implicative index that measures the validity of a rule $A \Rightarrow B$, the quasi-equivalence index is built by computing the geometric average of $A \Rightarrow B$ and $B \Rightarrow A$. Then, we define the method to find quasi-equivalent classes of variables (i.e., a class where each couple of variables is quasi-equivalent).

In this article, simulations have been done in order to compare the behavior of our index with some traditional indexes and the results clearly show that our index has interesting behavior such as its noise-resitance and its small variation with the size of data. Finally, an automatic method for selecting a variable that will replace a set of equivalent variables is defined. The elected variable minimizes a notion of distance with all the other variables. According to the nature of data and its knowledge, an expert can choose another variable (that could be a new one) or choose the elected variable. That is why we think that our method for reducing the number of variables should interest experts who are confronted to large sets of variables.

References

1. Agrawal, R., Imielinski, T., Swami, A. (1993). "Mining Association Rules between Sets of Items in Large Databases," in *International Conference on Management of Data*, eds. P. Buneman and S. Jajodia, ACM Press, pp. 207–216.
2. Aggarwal, C. (2001). "On the Effects of Dimensionality Reduction on High Dimensional Similarity Search," in *Symposium on Principles of Database Systems*, ACM Press, pp. 256–266.
3. Gras, Ré., Guillet, F., Gras, Ro., Philippé, J. (2002). "Réduction des Colonnes d'un Tableau de Données par Quasi-Équivalence Entre Variables," in *Extraction des Connaissances et Apprentissage*, Hermès Science Publication, **1**, 197–202.
4. Gras, R., Kuntz., P., Couturier, R., Guillet, F. (2001). "Une Version Entropique de l'Intensité d'Implication pour les Corpus de Volumineux," in *Extraction des Connaissances dans les Données*, Hermès Science Publication, **1**, 68–80.
5. Matheus, C. J., Piatetsky-Shapiro, G., McNeill, D. (1996). "Selecting and Reporting What Is Interesting," in *Advances in Knowledge Discovery and Data Mining*, AAAI Press/MIT Press, pp. 495–515.

Optimal Discretization of Quantitative Attributes for Association Rules

Stefan Born[1] and Lars Schmidt-Thieme[2]

[1] Liebig University, Germany
stefan.born@math.uni-giessen.de
[2] University of Freiburg, Germany
lst@informatik.uni-freiburg.de

Abstract: Association rules for objects with quantitative attributes require the discretization of these attributes to limit the size of the search space. As each such discretization might collapse attribute levels that need to be distinguished for finding association rules, optimal discretization strategies are of interest. In 1996 Srikant and Agrawal formulated an information loss measure called *measure of partial completeness* and claimed that equidepth partitioning (i.e. discretization based on base intervals of equal support) minimizes this measure. We prove that in many cases equidepth partitioning is not an optimal solution of the corresponding optimization problem. In simple cases an exact solution can be calculated, but in general optimization techniques have to be applied to find good solutions.

1 Introduction

Since its inception in 1993 and its first stable solution, the Apriori algorithm of Agrawal and Srikant (1994) has made association rule mining one of the most prominent tasks of machine learning. Though the recent decade has given birth to a vast literature on many aspects of the problem, association rules with quantitative attributes have received only little attention. Srikant and Agrawal have given a formulation of this problem in terms of association rules of non-interpreted items in Srikant and Agrawal (1996). They presented a variant of Apriori that could handle quantitative attributes after a discretization, formulated an information loss criterion called *measure of partial completeness*, and finally showed that a very simple discretization, the partition into intervals with equal support, optimizes this measure.

Later authors often changed the original problem by introducing additional constraints; e.g., Aumann and Lindell (1999) and Webb (2001) focus on rules with a quantitative variable in the consequent of a rule and circumvent discretization for this special case. Fukuda et al. (1999) and Rastogi and Shim

(2001) looked at rules with quantitative attributes in the precedent (called optimized association rules). In both cases the quantitative variable is discretized locally for a given rule template, so that the problem is transformed in a sort of supervised discretization scheme. See Dougherty et al. (1995) for a general survey on such methods.

Bay (2001) questioned the adequacy of the measure of partial completeness and developed a multivariate discretization method, which takes into account several variables at once, by consecutively joining intervals starting with the original discretization scheme of Srikant and Agrawal (1996).

Thus, Srikant's and Agrawal's (1996) method is still the most general approach, and consequently is prominent even in such recent survey literature on the topic as Adamo (2001). Surprisingly, though equi-volume partitions seem to be a natural candidate for a discretization that preserves maximal information, it is not treated.

We will start with an elegant reformulation of the mining task for association rules with quantitative attributes as mining partial objects in Section 2. In Section 3 we describe the task of minimizing the measure of partial completeness as a discrete optimization problem and formulate a corresponding continuous optimization problem that allows one to find good approximations to the solutions of the first problem.

2 Rules for Objects with Quantitative Attributes

Let $\mathcal{R} := \prod_{i \in I} A_i$ be a *space of objects* described by *attributes* A_i, where I is a finite set of indices, i.e., $I := \{1, \ldots, n\}$ and the A_i are arbitrary sets.

We distinguish three different types of attributes: An attribute A is called *nominal*, if A is a set of non-interpreted items that we can compare only for equality; however, we shall often number these items as $A := \{1, 2, 3, \ldots\}$. An attribute A is called *quantitative* if there is a total order $<$ defined on A; typically A are natural or real numbers. An attribute A is called *hierarchical* if there is a partial order $<$ defined on A. Let $I = I_O \cup I_Q \cup I_H$ be a partition of the attributes in these three types. Note that we do not distinguish between ordinal and interval-scaled attributes here, but only take the order structure on A into account.

We call

$$\mathcal{X} := \prod_{i \in I_O \cup I_H} (A_i \cup \{\emptyset\}) \times \prod_{i \in I_Q} \operatorname{Int}(A_i)$$

the *space of partial objects*, where $\operatorname{Int}(A_i)$ is the set of intervals in A_i. We call a partial object $x \in \mathcal{X}$ *unspecified in* A_i if $x_i = \emptyset$, and we use $\emptyset$ as shorthand for the completely unspecified partial object, i.e., the object x with $x_i = \emptyset$ for all $i \in I$.

For $x, y \in \mathcal{X}$ we define

$$\begin{aligned} x \leq y \;:\Leftrightarrow\; & x_i = \emptyset \text{ or } x_i = y_i \quad \forall i \in I_O \\ \text{and } & x_i = \emptyset \text{ or } x_i \leq y_i \quad \forall i \in I_H \\ \text{and } & x_i = \emptyset \text{ or } x_i \subseteq y_i \quad \forall i \in I_Q, \end{aligned}$$

a partial order on $\mathcal{X}$. If $x < y$, we call x *more general than* y (or a *generalization of* y) and y *more specific than* x (or a *specialization of* x).

For two partial objects x, y there always exists a common generalization and, if all hierarchical attributes are lattices, then there is exactly one most specific generalization that we call their *minimum* $x \vee y$. In contrast, it is quite common that partial objects do not have a common specialization, for example, two different objects. Therefore we say two partial objects x, y are *compatible* ($x \bowtie y$), if there exists such a common specialization. If all hierarchical attributes are lattices, there is at most one most general common specialization that we call their *maximum* $x \wedge y$. Let $\mathcal{X} \times_{\bowtie} \mathcal{X}$ denote the set of all compatible pairs of partial objects.

The space $\mathcal{R}$ of objects is a subspace of the space $\mathcal{X}$ of partial objects and all objects are maximal specific. We also say a partial object y *occurs* in an object x if x is a specialization of y. For a partial object x and a subset of attributes $J \subseteq I$ we define

$$x|_J := \begin{cases} x_i & \text{if } i \in J \\ \emptyset & \text{else} \end{cases}$$

as the *projection of* x *on* I. Obviously $x|_J$ is a generalization of x.

2.1 Frequent Partial Objects

Let $\mathcal{A} \subseteq \mathcal{R}$ be a fixed multiset of objects (called a *database*). For a partial object $x \in \mathcal{X}$ we call the relative frequency of objects $a \in \mathcal{A}$ that are specializations of x the *support of* x *w.r.t. to* $\mathcal{A}$:

$$\sup_{\mathcal{A}}(x) := \frac{|\{a \in \mathcal{A} \,|\, x \leq a\}|}{|\mathcal{A}|}.$$

A partial object x is *frequent* (w.r.t. $\mathcal{A}$ and minsup) if its support is at least as large as a fixed lower bound minsup $\in [0, 1]$ called the *minimal support.*

The task of mining all frequent partial objects of a database $\mathcal{A}$ relative to a minimal support describes the enumeration of all frequent partial objects. We measure the interestingness of a frequent partial object as quotient of its support and the expected support, if all attributes were independent:

$$\text{lift}(x) := \frac{\sup(x)}{\prod_{i \in I} \sup(x|_i)}.$$

Though we shall restrict ourselves in the following mainly to mining frequent partial objects and make only sporadic references to association rules, let us outline the context. An association rule is a pair of compatible frequent partial objects $(x, y) \in \mathcal{X} \times_{\bowtie} \mathcal{X}$, often written $x \to y$. By its support we mean the support of their maximum $x \wedge y$, by its confidence $\text{conf}(x, y) := \text{sup}(x \wedge y)/\text{sup}(x)$.

Classical association rules are defined in terms of sets of items. We can view this as a special case of our notation where all attributes are binary, i.e., nominal with only two different values 0 and 1, and the value 0 is identified with $\emptyset$. Then we can describe a partial object x by the set J of indices where $x_i = 1$. Two such partial objects are compatible if their index sets—called itemsets in the classical context—are disjoint, and if the index set of their maximum is the union of their index sets.

2.2 The Need for Discretization

To make use of solutions developed in the context of classical frequent set mining, as, e.g., the Apriori algorithm (see Agrawal and Srikant, 1994), attribute values have to be mapped to a manageable set of items that is by far exceeded by the number of different intervals.

Furthermore, as a frequent partial has only frequent generalizations, even classical frequent set and association rule mining tasks suffer from the problem that lots of frequent sets and rules are generated. Although this problem is mitigated by the use of interestingness measures like lift that restrict the resulting set to those frequent partial objects with at least a given minimal lift, it is still an obstacle for data with quantitative attributes, since with each interval each small shift has almost the same support and the same lift. Therefore a system of representatives of all intervals has to be found.

The approach originally presented in Srikant and Agrawal (1996) is to partition each quantitative attribute A into a set of intervals $B := \{b_1, \ldots, b_l\}$ (i.e. $b_i \in \text{Int}(A)$, $b_i \neq \emptyset$, $\bigcup_i b_i = A$, and $b_i \cap b_j = \emptyset$ for $i \neq j$). The intervals in B are called *base intervals*. Then all unions of chains of contiguous base intervals are used as representatives:

$$\text{Int}_B(A) := \{\bigcup_{i \in J} b_i \mid J \subseteq I \text{ with } \bigcup_{i \in J} b_i \text{ an interval}\}.$$

The set $\text{Int}_B(A)$ is a subset of $\text{Int}(A)$ and forms a hierarchy with the inherited subset relation. Thus the handling of quantitative attributes is reduced to the case of hierarchical attributes. Since this hierarchy contains many large intervals with normally high support but low information, one can reduce the hierachy by omitting all intervals that exceed a given upper support bound maxsup. As we shall only need superintervals of frequent intervals, we can also bound the support from below:

$$\begin{aligned}\text{Int}|_{B,\text{maxsup}}(A) := \{\bigcup_{i \in J} b_i \mid J \subseteq I \text{ with } \bigcup_{i \in J} b_i \text{ an interval}, \\ \text{and minsup} \leq \text{sup}(\bigcup_{i \in J} b_i) \leq \text{maxsup} \cup \{\emptyset\}.\end{aligned}$$

By abuse of language we call these intervals *discrete*.

For each (frequent) interval $x \in \mathrm{Int}(A)$ there exists a most specific discrete generalization $\hat{x} \in \mathrm{Int}_B(A)$ (i.e., a smallest superinterval). The maximal relative increase of support for discrete generalizations of frequent intervals is called the *measure of partial completeness* of the discretization B:

$$k(B) := \max\{\frac{\sup(\hat{x})}{\sup(x)} \,|\, x \in F\},$$

where F is the set of all frequent intervals. We simply say that B is *k-complete*. The following lemma is straightforward:

Lemma 1 (Srikant and Agrawal (1996)). *If* $\sup(b) \leq \frac{1}{2}(k-1)minsup$ *or* $|b| = 1$ *for all base intervals* $b \in B$*, then* B *is k-complete.*

Now let $\mathcal{R}$ be an object space and B_i a discretization for each quantitative attribute $i \in I_Q$. Then

$$\mathcal{X}|_{\mathcal{B}} := \prod_{i \in I_O \cup I_H} (A_i \cup \{\emptyset\}) \times \prod_{i \in I_Q} \mathrm{Int}_{B_i}(A_i)$$

is called the *space of discrete partial objects* for the discretization $\mathcal{B} := \{B_i \,|\, i \in I_Q\}$. Again, for each (frequent) partial object $x \in \mathcal{X}$ there exists a most specific discrete generalization $\hat{x} \in \mathcal{X}|_{\mathcal{B}}$. We sporadically call $\hat{x}$ the *approximation of* x. The maximal relative increase of support for discrete generalizations of frequent partial objects is called the *measure of partial completeness* of the discretization $\mathcal{B}$:

$$k(\mathcal{B}) := \max\left\{\frac{\sup(\hat{x})}{\sup(x)} \,|\, x \in \mathcal{F}\right\}$$

where $\mathcal{F}$ is the set of all frequent partial objects. Again we simply say that the discretization $\mathcal{B}$ is *k-complete*.

Lemma 2. *Let* $\mathcal{B}$ *be k-complete. Then for each frequent partial object* $x \in \mathcal{X}$ *the approximation* $\hat{x}$ *of* x *satisfies:*

$$\sup(x) \leq \sup(\hat{x}) \leq k \cdot \sup(x) \tag{1}$$

$$\frac{1}{k} \cdot \mathrm{lift}(x) \leq \mathrm{lift}(\hat{x}) \leq k \cdot \mathrm{lift}(\hat{x}). \tag{2}$$

For a pair (x, y) *of compatible partial objects, the pair* $(\hat{x}, \hat{y})$ *of their approximations is again compatible, and*

$$\frac{1}{k} \cdot \mathrm{conf}(x, y) \leq \mathrm{conf}(\hat{x}) \leq k \cdot \mathrm{conf}(\hat{x}). \tag{3}$$

For all inequalities stricter bounds depending on x *can be achieved, if* k *is replaced by* $k'(x) := \prod\{k_i \,|\, i \in I_Q, x_i \neq \emptyset\}$.

Basically, the lemma states that we have to lower the minimum lift threshold to minlift$/k$ to assure that the result set contains the approximations for all frequent partial objects with at least lift minlift. Obviously, a representation system is more accurate if k is small, and more manageable if its size $|\mathcal{X}|_{\mathcal{B}}|$ is small.

3 Optimal Discretizations

As we have seen it is desirable to find a partition in n intervals of a given quantitative attribute that minimizes the measure of partial completeness or to find the minimal number n of intervals that allows one to achieve a measure of partial completeness less than or equal to a given value. For the moment let us restrict ourselves to the first task and fix the number of intervals n as well as the minimal support minsup.

The upper bound for the measure of partial completeness given by Lemma 1 attains its smallest value for a so-called *equidepth partition*, which is characterized by the property that the maximal support of all base intervals that contain more than one point should be minimal. If the quantitative attribute realizes a random variable uniformly distributed over $[0,1]$, then this amounts to a partition into bins of almost equal support $\approx 1/n$ for large sample sizes, hence the name. The further claim of Srikant and Agrawal (1996) that *equidepth partitions* indeed minimize the measure of partial completeness is incorrect, though appealing. There exist quite simple counterexamples:

Example 1. Consider the attribute $A := \{1, 2, \dots, 12\}$ such that each value occurs with the same frequency. Thus the support of an interval $\{i, \dots, j\}, 1 \leq i \leq j \leq 12, i, j \in \mathbb{N}$ is exactly $j - i + 1/12$. We seek an optimal partition into three intervals with respect to minsup $= \frac{2}{12} = \frac{1}{6}$. The (in this case unique) *equidepth partition* is

$$\{\{1, \dots, 4\}, \{5, \dots, 8\}, \{9, \dots, 12\}\}.$$

An easy calculation shows that the measure of partial completeness is 4. Now consider the partition

$$\{\{1, \dots, 5\}, \{6, 7\}, \{8, \dots, 12\}\}.$$

Its measure of partial completeness is $7/2$.

An easy algorithm with complexity $\mathcal{O}(l^2)$ (if l is the cardinality of the partition) allows us to calculate the measure of partial completeness for a given partition of a quantitative attribute with respect to a database. We now could try to run a discrete optimization in order to find the *best partition*, i.e. the partition with minimal measure of partial completeness. However, for a large database $\mathcal{A}$ and a continuously distributed quantitative attribute A

the best partition can be approximated by the solution(s) of a corresponding continuous optimization problem.

After rescaling we can assume that $A = \{a_1, \ldots, a_k\}$, $a_1 < \ldots < a_k$, $a_i \in [0,1]$ for all $i \in \{1 \ldots k\}$ and $sup_{\mathcal{A}}(\{a_1, \ldots, a_i\}) = a_i$ for all $i \in \{1 \ldots k\}$. Let us further suppose that $|a_i - a_{i-1}| \leq \epsilon$ for all $i \in \{2 \ldots k\}$ and some $\epsilon > 0$. (For a continuously distributed attribute A that can be measured with arbitrary precision different objects in the database almost surely have different values, hence $a_i = i/k$ and $k = |\mathcal{A}|$. In this case we can choose $\epsilon = 1/|\mathcal{A}|$, which converges to zero as $|\mathcal{A}|$ increases. In many contexts the measurement is not arbitrarily precise, but already discrete, which yields a bound for ϵ from below, but let us have in mind the "continuous" case.) Now for any interval $[a,b] \subset [0,1]$ we have

$$|sup_{\mathcal{A}}([a,b]) - |b-a|| \leq 2\epsilon,$$

which means that the length of an interval is an approximation of its support with error at most 2ϵ.

All definitions of Section 2 extend easily to $A = [0,1]$ and to the length of an interval instead of its support. (We might as well consider infinite databases with a probability measure.) Intervals $x \subset [0,1]$ with $|x| \geq$ minsup are also called *frequent intervals*. For a partition $B = \{I_1, \ldots, I_l\}$ of $[0,1]$ and an interval $x \subset [0,1]$ we likewise define $\text{Int}_B(A) = \{\bigcup_{j \in J} I_j | \bigcup_{j \in J} I_j \text{ is an interval}\}$ and the *most specific generalization*

$$\hat{x} := \bigcap_{I \in \text{Int}_B(A), x \subset I} I.$$

For a partition B of $[0,1]$ into l intervals we define the (continuous) *measure of partial completeness* as the maximal relative increase of length for all frequent intervals, i. e.,

$$k(B) := \underset{x \in \text{Int}(A), |x| > \text{minsup}}{\text{supremum}} \frac{|\hat{x}|}{|x|}.$$

Whenever we mention partitions $\{I_1, \ldots, I_l\}$ let us suppose that the intervals are ordered so that $\forall i < j$, $\forall x \in I_i$ and $\forall y \in I_j$, we have $x < y$.

Lemma 3. *For a partition* $B = \{I_1, \ldots, I_l\}$ *and* minsup $\in (0,1)$ *the measure of partial completeness satisfies*

$$k(B) = \max_{1 \leq i \leq j \leq l} \frac{|I_1 \cup \cdots \cup I_j|}{\max(|I_1 \cup \cdots \cup I_j \backslash (I_i \cup I_j)|, \text{minsup})}.$$

Proof. We have

$$k(B) = \max_{x \text{ interval in } [0,1], |x| \geq \text{minsup}} \frac{|\hat{x}|}{|x|} = \max_{x \text{ interval in } [0,1]} \frac{|\hat{x}|}{\max(|x|, \text{minsup})}.$$

The set $\{I_i \cup \ldots \cup I_j \ |1 \leq i \leq j \leq l\}$ is the set of all numerators $\hat{x}$ that contribute to $k(B)$ in the second formula.

Now consider one of these numerators $y = I_0 \cup \ldots \cup I_j$. If $|y| <$ minsup it will not contribute to $k(B)$, as $k(B) \geq 1$ anyway. Suppose $|y| \geq$ minsup. If $|y \backslash (I_i \cup I_j)| \geq$ minsup, there are superintervals of $y \backslash (I_i \cup I_j)$ of length arbitrarily close to $|y \backslash (I_i \cup I_j)|$ whose most specific generalization is y, but no subintervals, thus the supremum of all occuring quotients with numerator y is $|y|/|y \backslash (I_i \cup I_j)|$. If $|y \backslash (I_i \cup I_j)| <$ minsup then there is a subinterval of y whose most specific generalization is y and whose length is minsup, hence the supremum of all quotients with numerator y is $|y|/\text{minsup}$. □

The endpoints are not relevant for the length (the measure) of an interval. Therefore any partition is determined up to the endpoints by $(x_1, \ldots, x_{l-1}) \in \mathbb{R}^{n-1}$ with $0 \leq x_i$ for all $1 \leq i \leq l$ and $x_1 + \cdots + x_{l-1} \leq 1$. The set C of these x is convex and compact, and the map

$$\begin{aligned} \phi: \quad C &\longrightarrow \mathcal{P}(\mathrm{Int}([0,1])) \\ x &\mapsto \{[x_1 + \cdots + x_i, x_1 + \cdots + x_{i+1}] | i = 1, \ldots, l-2\} \\ &\quad \cup \{[0, x_1), [x_1 + \cdots + x_{l-1}, 1]\} \end{aligned}$$

maps tuples to partitions. The following obviously holds:

Lemma 4. *The map* $C \to \mathbb{R}^+, \quad x \mapsto k(\phi(x))$ *is continuous.*

Now we can formulate the continuous optimization problem: *Find* $x \in C$, *so that* $k(\phi(x))$ *is minimal.* As C is compact the minimum is attained.

3.1 Solving the Continuous Problem

We did some numerical calculations by means of the Nelder-Mead algorithm, which converges rather slowly but behaves well with the non-differentiable function $x \mapsto k(\phi(x))$. (As the non-differentiability is of a harmless type, we could also successfully apply a descent method.) Let us consider three examples (with precision 0.001):

minsup	l	$\lvert I_1\rvert, \ldots, \lvert I_l\rvert$ for opt. part. B_{opt}	$k(B_{opt})$	$k(B_{equi})$
0.3	3	0.289, 0.422, 0.289	2.370	3.000
0.3	4	0.226, 0.101, 0.345, 0.327	2.241	2.500
0.08	3	0.4300.1400.430	7.127	8.333
0.08	10	0.111, 0.119, 0.111, 0.089, 0.052, 0.089, 0.111, 0.119, 0.111, 0.089	2.871	3.000

The results are rather surprising. For certain values of minsup and l the optimal numerical solution (in this paragraph: solution) is not the equidepth partition, nor even close to it. The second row shows a case where exactly two solutions exist, the one shown and its inverse order. However, for $2/(l \cdot \text{minsup}) = 3$ and l even, the equidepth partition is optimal, but not unique. Actually there is a continuum of solutions. For $2/(l \cdot \text{minsup}) = 3$ and l even, the equidepth partition is the only solution. For all other values of minsup and l, the equidepth partition is not optimal, and sometimes there is more than one optimal solution. A deeper analysis reveals that the solutions of the optimization problem satisfy certain sets of algebraic equations. For example we obtain the exact solution for $l = 3$ and minsup $= 0.08$ that corresponds to the third line:

$$|I_2| = -\frac{1}{2} + \frac{1}{10}\sqrt{41},\ |I_3| = |I_1| = \frac{3}{4} - \frac{1}{20}\sqrt{41},\ k(B) = \frac{25}{8} + \frac{5}{8}\sqrt{41}.$$

We want to understand this behaviour. For this purpose we analyse the expression for $k(B)$ in Lemma 3.

Consider a partition B with a measure of partial completeness $k(B)$ that is not minimal. All quotients that occur in the above formula have to be less than or equal to $k(B)$, and each defines (via ϕ) a half space in $\mathbb{R}^{l-1}$; e. g., $|I_1 \cup I_2|/\text{minsup} \leq k(B)$ yields the inequality $x_1 + x_2 \leq k \cdot \text{minsup}$. This system of inequalities defines a non-empty convex set in $\mathbb{R}^{l-1}$. The non-optimality implies that this polygon has a non-empty interior. If we lower the parameter k, the volume of the set decreases and becomes zero before the system ceases to be feasible. If, for $k = k_{\text{opt}}$, the set consists of one point, this point satisfies $l - 1$ equations corresponding to a selection of the inequalities. By means of the computer algebra system Maple 9 it was possible to collect these equations and to solve them symbolically for certain values of minsup and $l = 3, \ldots, 20$. The result of the numerical optimization was needed as an input for these calculations. Thus we performed a numerical-symbolical optimization.

4 Outlook

If the measure of partial completeness is adequate for an association rule mining setup one should expect a better performance with the optimal partitioning, at least in some cases. There might be, however, other measures with a different behaviour, e.g., the average relative increase of volume or the average absolute increase of volume. For each measure an optimzation ought to be possible. Numerical experiments yielded a solution quite close to equidepth paritioning for the task of finding the minimal mean relative volume increase. The consequences of different types of discretization ought to be compared.

Based on optimal discretization schemes for intervals, more sophisticated methods taking into account several variables at once could be approached as in Bay (2001).

Furthermore, for mining hierarchical sets of items the nested Apriori algorithm for complex patterns (cf. Schmidt-Thieme, 2003) could be used. Embedding quantitative attributes in complex patterns would allow a more general use in a much wider set of patterns, as e.g., sequential patterns.

References

1. Adamo, J.-M. (2001). *Data Mining for Association Rules and Sequential Patterns.* Springer, Berlin.
2. Agrawal, R., and Srikant, R. (1994). "Fast Algorithms for Mining Association Rules," in *Proceedings of the 20th International Conference on Very Large Data Bases (VLDB'94)*, Chile, pp. 487–499.
3. Aumann, Y., and Lindell, Y. (1999). "A Statistical Theory for Quantitative Association Rules," in *Proceedings of the Fifth ACM SIGKDD International Conference on Knowledge Discovery and Data Mining*, San Diego, pp. 261–270.
4. Bay, S. D. (2001). "Multivariate Discretization for Set Mining," *Knowledge and Information Systems*, **3**, 491–512.
5. Dougherty, J., Kohavi, R., and Sahami, M. (1995). "Supervised and Unsupervised Discretization of Continuous Features," in *Proceedings of the Twelfth International Conference on Machine Learning*, eds. A. Preiditis and S. Russell, San Mateo:Morgan Kaufmann, pp. 194–202.
6. Fukuda, T., Morimoto, Y., Morishita, S., and Tokuyama, T. (1999). "Mining Optimized Association Rules for Numeric Attributes," *Journal of Computer and System Sciences (JCSS)*, **58**, 1–12.
7. Rastogi, R., and Shim, K. (2001). "Mining Optimized Support Rules for Numeric Attributes," *Information Systems*, **26**, 425–444.
8. Schmidt-Thieme, L. (2003). *Assoziationsregel-Algorithmen fuer Daten mit komplexer Struktur*, Peter Lang-Verlag.
9. Srikant, R., and Agrawal, R. (1996). "Mining Quantitative Association Rules in Large Relational Tables," in *Proceedings of the 1996 ACM SIGMOD International Conference on Management of Data*, eds. H. Jagadish and I. S. Mumic, SIGMOD Record **25**, pp. 1–11.
10. Webb, G. I. (2001). "Discovering Associations with Numeric Variables," in *Proceedings of the Seventh ACM SIGKDD International Conference on Knowledge Discovery and Data Mining*, pp. 383–388.

Part IV

Symbolic Data Analysis

Clustering Methods in Symbolic Data Analysis

Rosanna Verde

Universitá di Napoli, Italy
rosanna.verde@unina2.it

Abstract: We present an overview of the clustering methods developed in Symbolic Data Analysis to partition a set of conceptual data into a fixed number of classes. The proposed algorithms are based on a generalization of the classical Dynamical Clustering Algorithm (DCA) (Nuées Dynamiques méthode). The criterion optimized in DCA is a measure of the fit between the partition and the representation of the classes. The prototype is a model of the representation of a class, and it can be an element of the same space of representation as the symbolic data to be clustered or, according to the nature of the data, the prototype is a higher-order object which generalizes the characteristics of the elements belonging to the class.
The allocation function for the assignment of the objects to the classes depends on the nature of the variables which describe the symbolic objects. The choice of such function must be related to the particular type of prototype preferred as the representation model of the classes.

1 Introduction to Symbolic Data Analysis

Symbolic Data Analysis was born as a new set of statistical methods able to analyze complex, structured, aggregated, relational and high-level data—called Symbolic Objects (Diday, 1987; Bock and Diday, 2000). Whatever complex units (aggregated data, group of individuals, or typology) are characterized by a set of properties, they can be referred to as a concept by defining suitable new statistical units able of keeping the most part of information. Therefore, Symbolic Object has been proposed as a suitable mathematical model of a concept, which is defined by its description, called intent, (e.g., multi-valued variables, logical rules, taxonomies) and a way to compute its extent. The symbolic object extent is based on a given set of individuals and on a mapping function allowing recognition of the membership of an individual in the concept if it satisfies its properties. It should be noted that it is infeasible to get all the properties (intent) of a concept as impossible to accommodate of an infinite set of individuals to compute its complete extent. That is why a symbolic object can be assumed just as a mathematical approximation of a concept which can be improved by a learning process. "The model concept holding in our mind is given only by its intent and by the way of finding its extent" (Diday, 2001). Thus, the definition of symbolic object is reminiscent of Aristotle's idea of a concept rather than the interpretation provided in logic formal concept where a concept is more properly interpreted according to both its intent and extent. In real life, symbolic data arise from many sources; for instance summarizing huge data bases by queries to get underlying descriptions of concepts, as well as modelling information given by experts, usually expressed in a form closer to natural language. As the description of each concept must accommodate its internal variation, symbolic objects' description is collected in a "symbolic data table," containing along each row the complete description of a concept and along the columns the symbolic descriptors of multi-valued variables. Then, each cell contains multi-values for each symbolic descriptor. These values can be intervals of continuous variables, different categories of nominal variables, empirical distribution or probability functions. Symbolic Data Analysis (SDA) consists of a collection of new techniques, mainly developed in the framework of European projects, aiming at comparing, classifying, representing, synthesizing, visualizing and interpreting symbolic data. The methodological issues under development generalize the classical exploratory data analysis techniques, like visualization, factorial methods, clustering, decision trees, regression, discrimination and classification. SDA are implemented in specialized software: SODAS (http://www.ceremade.dauphine.fr/ touati/sodas-pagegarde.htm), already at the second version, SODAS 2. We note that all the SDA methods require as input symbolic data tables. The implemented procedure uses both symbolic operators (generalization and specialization) and numerical criteria. Many SDA methods are symbolic-numerical-symbolic approaches. It should be highlighted that even if the symbolic data correspond to a numerical description of a conceptual model, to extend the most useful data analysis techniques to such kind of data, a numerical coding is quite often required. A symbolic interpretation of results, whether final or intermediate, is a benefit of the symbolic data techniques and further allows building a new or high-order conceptual model.

2 Principles of Symbolic Data Clustering

In the present work we propose an overview of the main clustering methods recently achieved in the context of Symbolic Data Analysis. Clustering problems assume in SDA a central relevance for the nature of the data and for their conceptual meaning. Therefore, comparison between objects, aggregation of objects in classes consistent with their conceptual implication, partitioning of set of objects in homogeneous typologies and so on, are surely the most consistent analyses which can be performed on such data.

In the recent years the partitioning of a set of symbolic data has been widely dealt with by many authors (Chavent, 1997; Lauro et Verde, 2000; De Carvalho et al., 1999; 2001; Verde and Lechevallier, 2003) and some proposals of new algorithms were born from collaborations being still in progress. The techniques will be presented hereafter, have been mostly achieved thanks to the activity of a group of research in the framework of the European SODAS and ASSO projects (http://www.info.fundp.ac.be/asso/). A long cooperation has been promoted by Yves Lechevallier at INRIA, which involved several colleagues, coming from different countries. Among them, Francisco T. de A. de Carvalho, from CIN/UFPE of Recife, should be of course acknowledged, as well as Marie Chavent of the University of Bordeaux 1 and Paula Brito of the University of Porto. Active participation and relevant scientific support has been given by Hans-Herman Bock, especially in the extension of Kohonen Maps to symbolic objects.

The symbolic partitioning algorithms are heavily based on an extension of a dynamic clustering method, such as "des nuées dynamiques" (Diday and Simon, 1976; Diday et al., 1980; Celeux et al, 1980). It represents a general reference for iterative clustering algorithms, not hierarchical, based on the best fit between the partition of a set of individuals and the way to represent the classes of the partition. The algorithm looks simultaneously for the partition and the best representation of the classes constituting such partition. The convergence of the algorithm is ensured by the consistency between the representation and the allocation function of the objects to the classes. Therefore, the suitable choice of the allocation and the representation functions is the crucial point. Dynamic clustering algorithm requires, in the first, to specify the elements (seeds) which allow to represent the clusters. According to "des nuées dynamiques" method, the seeds can be chosen, for instance, as barycenters, axes, probability distributions, groups of elements, thus extending the concept of representing a class by an element of a class to a wider choice than the usual "centroid" as in the k-means algorithms (MacQueen, 1967). Symbolic data are constituted by a set of values of the multi-valued descriptors (multi-categories, intervals). Moreover they can take into account also logical relationships between descriptors. In such a way, centroids, as well as the inertia and all the classical descriptive measures, cannot be easily defined for such data.

However, we introduce the concept of *prototype* to represent the SO clusters. Usually, a prototype is defined as an element able to summarize optimally all the characteristics of the set of objects belonging to the cluster. In this sense, the prototype of a set (a class) is generally one of its elements. In the extension of the dynamical clustering algorithm to the partitioning of a set of symbolic data, the prototype is a *concept of seed*, and it is a model of representation of a class. In this context the prototype could be both an element (object) of the set to be clustered as a model of a high order concept (g-prototype) that generalizes the characteristics of the elements belonging to the class (De Carvalho, Lechevallier and Verde, 2001).

Based on the choice of the prototypes, we also distinguish between two different cluster representations (Lauro and Verde, 2000): Cluster of Symbolic Objects (CSO) and Symbolic Objects Cluster (SOC). In particular, a CSO is constituted by a collection of the symbolic objects' membership of the cluster; while, a SOC is itself (of the same or high order) symbolic object, expressing the whole information of the symbolic objects belonging to the cluster. That last type of representation has been widely proposed in the context of Conceptual Clustering (CC) (Michalski et al., 1981; Kodratoff and Bisson, 1992), even if conceptual clustering algorithms aim mainly to aggregate the elements into a cluster "not because of their pair-wise similarity, but because together they represent a concept from a predefined set of concepts," that is also tied to the conceptual interpretation of the classes: "a clustering algorithm should not only to assemble elements, but also to provide descriptions of the obtained clusters" (Michalski, 1980).

The second main aspect in the dynamical clustering algorithms concerns the choice of the allocation function to assign the symbolic objects to the clusters at each iteration, according to the representation of the clusters.

In the SDA context, some alternative proximity functions have been proposed (e.g., Gowda and Diday, 1991; Ichino and Yaguchi, 1994; De Carvalho et al., 1994, 1998, 2000, 2001, 2002; Palumbo and Benedetto, 1997; Chavent 1997; Rizzi, 1998; Chavent et al. 2003) which could be suitably proposed as on allocation function in the dynamical clustering algorithm. However, the choice of the allocation function must be consistent with the type of representation function. Several approaches have been followed in the choice of the representation model and of the allocation function. Even if they clearly can be related to the particular kind of symbolic descriptors, however they originate from two different approaches to symbolic data clustering: in the first one, the prototype is a concept of the same space of representation of the objects to be clustered, then the elements are assigned to the classes according to a function which computes the proximity between pairs of symbolic data. An elements can be allocated to the class according to how well it presents the minimum average dissimilarity value from all the elements of this class. Otherwise, the "nearest" element (represented as the minimum value of the dissimilarity function) from all the others of the class can be chosen as prototype to represent such a class; in the second one, the prototype is in a different space of representation of the objects to be clustered, then the algorithm proceeds matching the objects descriptions to the prototype according suitable flexible matching functions proposed in this context of analysis. Moreover, the type of descriptors of the symbolic objects are strongly influential in selecting the allocation function.

- In the first approach, when the symbolic descriptors are interval variables, a possible choice is given by Hausdorff distance (Chavent et al., 2002, 2003). The advantage in using this dissimilarity measure is that the convergence of the algorithm has been demonstrated (Chavent and Lechevallier, 2002) when the prototype is the median interval. Whereas the descriptors are multi-categorical and the prototype is the object at the minimum distance by all the elements of the class, suitable dissimilarity function can be used (De Carvalho, 1998), based on a generalization of association measures between categorical variables. Finally, if the descriptors are modal variables (multi-categorical with distribution associated) and the prototypes are taken as marginal profiles of the classes, the ϕ^2 set as distance can be proposed. This approach is more consistent with the COS representation of the symbolic clusters.

In the second approach, the allocation function has to be a matching function because the prototypes are not in the same space of representation as the objects to be clustered. In particular the prototypes are modeled by distributions (or modal objects) that describe high-order symbolic objects, and their conceptual meaning is nearer to the SOC representation. Context dependent dissimilarity functions (De Carvalho et al., 1998) have been proposed to match objects described by different kind of descriptors (intervals, multi-categorical) with the description of the prototype. De Carvalho has proposed in the last year several "families" of proximities, more or less complex in their formulation, which improve the results of homogeneity of the final clusters and, from a computational point of view, the efficiency of the algorithm. The choice to represent the classes by prototypes associated with a context dependent allocation function makes this clustering algorithm able to compromise the numerical classical criteria to clustering, as in exploratory Data Analysis, and 'the Gestalt property of the objects, as in the conceptual clustering from Machine Learning. According to this property, a class is characterized by a certain configuration of elements considered as a whole, and not as a collection of independent elements. It is worth noting we cluster symbolic objects and not only symbolic data. In fact, the representation of each class by a prototype is a symbolic object too, having associated with its description "the way" to compute its extent, by the allocation function. Following the second approach, a mapping function and a threshold can be associated with the prototype of the class in order to recognize the elements as belonging to its extent.

Finally, it is particular interesting to observe, as a structure on the categories of symbolic objects, that descriptors can be achieved by a clustering strategy which performs cross classification along the rows (symbolic objects' descriptions) and along the columns (multi-valued variables) of the symbolic table.
As the basis of such algorithms, we propose the scheme of the dynamical clustering algorithm on symbolic data. Moreover, an extension of the cross-clustering algorithm (CCA) proposed by Govaert (1995) in the classification of a binary table can be suitably performed to cluster a set of symbolic objects described by multi-categorical descriptors. Generally, CCA can be suitably generalized to the cluster symbolic objects described by intervals or distributions according to the criteria optimized in DCA on such kind of data.

To find a structure on the symbolic descriptors is perfectly consistent with the conceptual modelling of the data. Taxonomies on the categories of the multi-categorical variables as well as logical relationships between descriptors are additional information in the definition of a symbolic object. Thus, this last approach proposed in the context of SDA place more relevance again on the rule of clustering procedures in symbolic objects' definition.

3 Notation for Symbolic Objects

In the classical dynamical algorithm it is necessary to specify: (*i.*) the set E of objects to be clustered in k classes; (*ii.*) the set of variables describing objects; (*iii.*) The prototypes representing the classes; (*iv.*) an allocation function based on proximity measure between objects and prototypes; (*v.*) a structure of object partitions; (*vi.*) the criterion of the best fitting between the structure of the partition in k classes and the k prototypes.

In the extension of the general dynamical clustering algorithm, let E be the set of symbolic objects, described by multi-valued variables y_j $(j = 1, \ldots, p)$ with domain in $D = (D_1, \ldots, D_p)$.

According to the standard definition (Diday, 1998; Bock and Diday, 2000) a symbolic object $x \in E$ is expressed by the triple (a, R, d), where: $d = (d_1, \ldots, d_p)$ and $y_j(x) = d_j \subseteq D_j$ is the representation set of x. The y_j $(j = 1, \ldots, p)$ can be *intervals* or multi-categorical variables whenever they are referred to the so called *Boolean* symbolic objects, whereas *modal* SO are characterized by distributions associated with the descriptors.
Furthermore $R = (R_1, \ldots, R_p)$ (e.g. $\leq, \in, \subseteq, \ldots$) is a set of relations.

Given a set Ω of individuals ω, characterized by y_j^* (j=1, ..., p) descriptors with the same support D_j (j=1,..., p) of the symbolic descriptors, the function a: $\Omega \rightarrow \{0, 1\}$ is a *mapping function* which allows computing the extent of x as the set of $\omega \in \Omega$ that respects the properties in d_x by means the relations in R, i.e. $a_x(\omega) = R(y^*(\omega), d_x) = 1$.

Similarly a *modal symbolic object* $s \in L$ is defined as the triple (b, M, d), where its description $d \in D$ (with $D = \times_{j=1}^{p} Q(D_j)$) is represented now by the distributions of its descriptor.

The measures associated to the categories of the p symbolic descriptors are computed by using the function Q defined on the domain D_j of each descriptors.

The function $b_s(x) : E \rightarrow [0, 1]$ allows deciding whether x belonging to the extent of the modal symbolic object s as: $b_s(x) = M(y(x), d_s)$, where M is a matching function when x is a Boolean symbolic object.

If we consider a suitable transformation of the description d_x of $x \in E$ in a modal description, the relation function defining the modal SO is more properly a comparison function, here denoted Φ, so that the mapping function is $b_s(x) = \Phi(\widehat{y}(x), d_s)$.

The set of elements ω constituting the extent of modal symbolic object $s \in L$ can be obtained as follows:

$$Ext_{\alpha}(s|\Omega) = a^{-1}(b_s^{-1}[\alpha, 1]).$$

The function b_s assumes values in the range $[0, 1]$. The relation $M(y(x), d_s))$ furnishes the *matching value* between the descriptions of the Boolean symbolic object x and the modal symbolic object s. A bound α can be fixed according to a fuzzy matching criterion to include an element x in the extent of s if the matching function assumes a value greater than α. When x and s are both modal symbolic objects, the function b_s is a comparison function. It measures the fitting between modal SO's descriptions. Similarly, a bound is fixed to include an element x in the extent of s when the normalized measure Φ is greater than α.

4 Dynamic Clustering Objects Algorithm

The clustering algorithm is performed in two steps: first, the description step, consists of describing the classes by prototypes; the second one, the allocation step, concerns the assignment of the objects to the classes, according to their proximity to the prototypes.

The novelty of the proposed approach consists of getting a class descriptions using modal SO's.
The convergence of the algorithm to a stationary value of the criterion function Δ is guaranteed by the optimal fit between the type of representation of the classes and the allocation function.

4.1 General Scheme of the DCA

As in the standard dynamic clustering algorithm (Celeux et al., 1989) we look for the partition $P \in P_k$ of E in k classes, among all the possible partitions P_k, and the vector $L \in L_k$ of k prototypes representing the classes in P, such that, a criterion Δ of fit between L and P is minimized:

$$\Delta(P^*, L^*) = \min\{\Delta(P, L) \mid P \in P_k, L \in L_k\}.$$

The dynamic algorithm proceeds iteratively by alternating the representation and the allocation steps until the convergence:

a) *Initialization*; a partition $P = (C_1, \ldots, C_k)$ of E is randomly chosen.

b) *representation step:*
   for j=1 to k, find G_h associated with C_h such that $\sum_{x_i \in C_h} \delta(x_i, G_h)$ is minimized.

c) *allocation step:*
test $\longleftarrow 0$
for all x_i do
find m such that C_m is the class of x_i;
find l such that: $l = \arg \min_{h=1,\ldots,k} \delta(x_i, G_h)$;
if $l \neq m$
test $\longleftarrow 1$
$C_l \longleftarrow C_l \cup \{x_i\}$ and $C_m \longleftarrow C_m - \{x_i\}$.

d) if *test* $= 0$ then stop, else go to b).

Then, using randomly initialized the partition P, the first choice concerns the representation structure by prototypes $(G_1, \ldots, G_k)$ for the classes $\{C_1, \ldots, C_k\} \in P$.

The criterion $\Delta(P, L)$, optimized in the dynamic clustering algorithm is usually defined as the sum of the measures $\delta(x_i, G_h)$ of fitting between each object x_i belonging to a class $C_h \in P$ and the class representation $G_h \in L$:

$$\Delta(P, L) = \sum_{i=1}^{k} \sum_{x_i \in C_h} \delta(x_i, G_h),$$

where δ is a suitable dissimilarity or distance function. Usually such criterion $\Delta(P, L)$ is additive with respect to the p SO's descriptors.

An alternative general scheme, even based on the optimization of the criterion $\Delta(P, L)$: sum of the distance or dissimilarity measures $\delta(x_i, G_h)$, can be a *K-means like* one (MacQueen, 1967). That approach performs the allocation step followed by the representation one:

a) *Initialization*: Choose a set of prototypes $(G_1, \ldots, G_k)$ of L.

b) test $\leftarrow 0$.

For every $x_i \in E$ the two following steps are performed alternatively:

b1) *allocation step:*
for all x_i do:
find l such that: $l = \arg \min_{h=1,\ldots,k} \delta(x_i, G_h)$
if $l \neq m$
test $\longleftarrow 1$
$C_l \longleftarrow C_l \cup \{x_i\}$ and $C_m \longleftarrow C_m - \{x_i\}$

b2) *representation step:*
find G_l, such that: $\sum_{x_i \in C_l} \delta(x_i, G_l)$ is minimized, and
find G_m, such that: $\sum_{x_i \in C_m} \delta(x_i, G_m)$ is minimized;

c) if *test* $= 0$ then stop, else go to b)

Then, having initialized the algorithm with a set of prototypes $(G_1, \ldots, G_k)$ of L to represent the k classes of an initial partition P, the first choice concerns the allocation of the x_i to the classes. Note that the choice of the prototypes can be even independent from an initial partition of set E. They can be taken either as a random set of k elements of E or as a function of the descriptions of k groups of elements of E, such that to be considered as representative elements of the k classes of the starting partition P.

As with all the partitioning procedures, the initial solution strongly influences the final partition reached by the algorithm. Thus, as a random initial partition and an initial set of prototypes is going to condition the results. However, in the second algorithm shown above, the initialization by k prototypes could be more influential on the final solution than the initial partition chosen as starting solution in the first algorithm. That result can happen especially whenever the prototypes are defined on the basis of subsets of elements of E while the initial partition involves all the elements of the set E. We have, in fact already said, that according to the nature of the data, the prototype should contain the most part of information of the elements belonging to the class.

5 Representation and Allocation Functions

5.1 Representation Stage

The first phase of the proposed algorithm consists of defining a suitable representation of the classes of objects. Similarly to dynamical clustering methods on individual data, we resort to suitable seeds to represent the clusters.

For reasons of brevity and having already exposed some of the main conceptual aspects applied to the representation of classes of SO's, we here make reference only to the two main representation of the classes of a SO's set partition: the former is related to the conceptual interpretation of the classes as *Cluster of Symbolic Objects* (CSO), that is a collection of SO's; the latter refers to the classes like *Symbolic Object Cluster* (SOC), that is to SO's of higher order with respect to the SO's of E.

The representation of the CSO's can be expressed by a single element of the class (e.g., the element that presents the minimum average value of the dissimilarity measure with respect to all the others belonging to the class), as well as by the element whose description minimizes the criterion function. Whereas the elements of the partition are interpreted as SOC's, the representation of each class is more suitably given by a prototype which summarizes the whole information of the SO's belonging to the class. A prototype can be modelled as a *modal SO* (Diday, 1998; Bock and Diday, 2000). The description of a modal SO is given by frequency (or probability) distributions associated with the p descriptors.

According to the nature of the descriptors of the set E of SO's we distinguish different cases:

i. all the SO descriptors are intervals;
ii. all the SO descriptors are multi-categorical variables;

iii. all the SO descriptors are *modal* variables;
iv. the SO's are described by mixed variables.

In case (i), Chavent (1997) and Chavent et al. (2001, 2003) demonstrated that is possible to represent a class by an interval chosen as the one at minimum average distance from all the others intervals which describe the elements of the class.

The optimal solution was found analytically, assuming as distance a suitable measure defined on intervals: the *Hausdorff distance*, and using some relations and theorems of the *interval algebra* (Moore, 1966).

Case (ii) can be considered according to two different approaches: the prototype is expressed by the most representative element of the class (or by a virtual element v_i) according to the *allocation* function; or the prototype is a high order SO, described by the distribution function associated with the multi-nominal variable domains.

In particular, in the first approach the prototype is selected as the neighbour of all the elements of the class. Given a suitable *allocation* function $d(x_i, G_h)$ the prototype G_h of the class C_h is chosen as the object x_i such that: $\min_{i \in C_h} d(x_i, x_i')$ with $x_i' \neq x_i \in C_h$. Similarly, a virtual prototype v_h of C_h can be constructed considering all the descriptions of the SO's $x_i \in C_h$ and associating with them a set of descriptions corresponding to the most representatives among the elements of C_h, such that $d(v_h, x_i) = \min! \; \forall x_i \in C_h$.

A similar criterion has been followed by Chavent et al. (2002, 2003) in the choice of the prototypes as interval data, according to the Hausdorff distance.

Nevertheless, we can point out the virtual prototype v_h is not a SO's of E and its description could be inconsistent with a conceptual meaning own of a symbolic object. So that, instead of taking v_h to represent the C_h it is more appropriate to choose the nearest SO $x_i \in C_h$, according to the allocation function value.

This choice is a generalization of the nearest neighbors algorithm criterion in the dynamical clustering. However, it respects the numerical criterion of the minimum dissimilarity measure and guarantees coherence with the allocation function. In fact, the elements are assigned to a cluster according to their minimum dissimilarity to the prototype. That is, a SO x_i is assigned to C_h if: $d(x_i, G_h) \leq d(x_i, G_{h'})$, where (G_h) and (G_h') are the prototypes of the clusters C_h and $C_{h'}$, respectively, with $h \neq h'$ ordered indices of the classes.

In the second approach, we can also assume to associate with multi-categorical variables a uniform distribution to transform SO descriptors in *modal* ones.

Different from the first two proposals, this choice concerns the case where the clusters are represented by SOC's. The SO G_h representing the cluster C_h is described by the minimum generalization of the descriptions d_{j,x_i}, for all the multi-categorical variables of the SO's belonging to the class C_h.

In case (iii), because SO's are described by all *modal* variables, the prototypes G_h associated with each class C_h, are defined in the same space of representation of the objects of E, and they are represented as the average profile, according to a suitable *allocation* function (ϕ^2 or *context dependent dissimilarity*, De Carvalho, 1998).

In the last case, (iv), a possible choice is given by transforming all the descriptors into *modal* variables. Another suggestion, which can be proposed in such a case, consists of taking different prototype models according to the nature of the SO descriptors. This choice needs simultaneously to define the criterion as a function of different dissimilarity measures, depending on the nature of each descriptor and the choice of the prototypes. Therefore, the dissimilarity between objects and prototypes is determined by a linear combination of the different measures.

That approach returns homogeneity in the clusters representation space. But, the criterion value could be more influenced by some dissimilarity functions than by others. For these reasons, in the following we prefer to follow the second approach by transforming SO descriptors in modal ones. Thus, the multi-categorical variables y_j (for $j = 1, \ldots, J_c$; where $J_c \leq p$ is the number of the multi-categorical variables in the set y of the SO's descriptors) are assumed to be uniformly distributed.

Given d_{j,x_i} the set of categories of a multi-categorical descriptor y_j presented in the description of the SO x_i. The distribution value q_{j,x_i}, associated with the category c_m ($m = 1, \ldots, |d_{j,x_i}|$) of y_j, is given by:

$$q_{j,x_i}(c_m) = \begin{cases} \dfrac{1}{|d_{j,x_i}|}, & \text{if } \{c_m\} \in d_{j,x_i} \\ 0 & \text{otherwise,} \end{cases}$$

with $|d_{j,x_i}|$ equal to the cardinality of (d_{j,x_i}).

The description of the prototype G_h, d_{j,G_h}, is defined by a linear combination of the distributions q_{j,x_i} of the $x_i \in C_h$. Therefore, for each j ($j = 1, \ldots, J_c$) the distribution associated with the descriptor y_j of G_h is: $g_{j,G_h} = f(q_{j,x_i} \mid x_i \in C_h)$.
The interval descriptors y'_j of the SO's of E (for $j = 1, \ldots, J_t$; where $J_t \leq p$ is the number of the interval variables in the set y of the SO's descriptors) present J_t sets of intervals $A_j = \{A_{1j}, \ldots, A_{ij}, \ldots, A_{nj}\}$ in the description of the elements of E. For each y'_j the domain D_j is shared in the minimum number H of non overlapping intervals: $I^j_u = [a^j_u, b^j_u]$ (for $u = 1, ..., H_j$), such that they sutisfy the following properties:

i. $\bigcup_{u=1}^{H_j} I^j_u = \bigcup_{i=1}^{nj} A_{ij}$;
ii. $I^j_u \cap I^j_{u'} = \emptyset$ for $u \neq u'$;
iii. $\forall u \; \exists i$ such that: $I^j_u \cap A_{ij} \neq \emptyset$;
iv. $\exists S_i$ such that: $\bigcup_{u \in S_i} I^j_u = A_{ij}$.

The intervals of the set I^j are called *elementary* if they constitute a base for the set of interval A_j. Every interval A_{ij} is then decomposed in a set of disjoint intervals I^j_u with $u \in S_i$ (see property (*iv*)). It is possible to define the *modal* description associate with the interval variable y'_j:

$$D(A_{ij}) = \{(I^j_u, q_{uj}) \mid u \in S_i;\ q_{uj} > 0\} \quad \text{with} \sum_h q_{uj} = 1.$$

That is a distribution on the set of *elementary* intervals I^j_u constituting A_{ij} $\forall i$. For every elementary interval $I^j_u \in A_{ij}$ the weight $q_{uj}(A_i) \in [0,1]$ is proportional to its length and dependent on A_{ij}:

$$q_{uj}(A_i) = \frac{b^i_u - a^i_u}{b^i - a^i},$$

where $(b^i_u - a^i_u)$ and $(b^i - a^i)$ are the lengths of general elementary interval $I^j_u \in A_{ij}$ and of the interval A_{ij}, respectively.

In this case, the representation space L is given by the distribution, in the description of the prototypes G_h associates to the classes C_h (for $h = 1, \ldots, k$), defined on the set of *elementary intervals* I^j (for $j = 1, \ldots, J_t$). For the interval variable y'_j, the class C_h is described by the set of $H_{jh} \subseteq H_j$ intervals that represent the descriptions of the symbolic objects belonging to the class C_h. The distribution of the variable y'_j on the H_{jh} *elementary intervals*, in the class C_h, can be estimated as the elements of the vector: $q_{uj}(C_h) = \{q^h_{1j}, \ldots, q^h_{H_h j}\}$. The distribution $q_j(C_h)$ with domain on the set I^j_h is the description of the prototype G_h associated with the class C_h. It is estimated by the average of the $q_{uj}(C_h)$ of each interval I^j_u (with $u = 1, \ldots, H_{jh}$) for the elements $x_i \in C_h$:

$$q^h_{uj} = \frac{1}{n_h} \sum_{i=1}^{n_h} q^i_{uj}.$$

The description d_{j,G_h} of the prototype G_h associated with class C_h, is given by the marginal profile (normalized to n_h) of the distributions q^h_j on the set of *elementary intervals* I^j for each j $(j = 1, \ldots, J_H)$: $d_{j,G_h} = \{I^j_h, q^h_{uj}\}$.

Whereas all the SO descriptors are *modal* variables, the prototypes representation space is the same of the SO's in E. In such case, none transformation on the descriptors is performed. The description d_{j,G_h} (for $j = 1, \ldots, J_m$; with J_m the number of the SO modal descriptors) of prototype G_h of the class C_h is given by a linear combination of the distributions which describe the objects belonging to C_h: $d_{j,G_h} = f(d_{j,x_i} \mid x_i \in C_h)$.

5.2 Allocation Stage

The other main aspect of this algorithm concerns the choice of the proximity function to assign SO's to the classes. This function must be coherent with the particular kind of prototype chosen to represent the classes to guarantee the convergence of the partitioning algorithm. Thus, we distinguish to different situations: *(i).* the description space of SO's $\in E$ and prototypes is the same; *(ii).* the prototypes are represented as modal SO's.

In the first case, both prototypes and SO's are modelled by vectors of intervals for interval descriptors as well as, by sets of categories for multi-categorical variables. Finally, they also occupy the same space of representation whenever both are described by *modal* variables.

The second case corresponds to situation where the prototypes are modelled by distributions, whereas the SO's are described by interval and/or multi-categorical variables.

According with the general scheme of DCA, SO's are assigned to the classes according to a dissimilarity measure, computed between each SO and the prototypes of the different classes.

In the SDA context, many proximities, dissimilarities and distance functions have been proposed to compare pairs of objects, expressed by the same set of descriptors. In the present work we mention only some dissimilarity measures, selected from the most used and implemented in SODAS software, issued by European projects (SODAS and ASSO) and including SDA techniques.

– *Hausdorff distance: a function to compare interval data*

As noted above, Chavent (1997) and Chavent et al. (2001, 2003) proposed the Hausdorff distance in SO's clustering procedure.
The *Hausdorff distance* is usually proposed as a distance between two sets A and B and it is defined as follows:

$$d_H(A,B) = \max\{\sup_{a\in A} \inf_{b\in B} d(a,b),\ \sup_{b\in B} \inf_{a\in A} d(a,b)\}.$$

where $d(A,B)$ is a distance between two elements a and b. When A and B are two intervals, $[\underline{a},\overline{a}]$, $[\underline{b},\overline{b}] \subset \mathbb{R}$, the Hausdroff distance is:

$$d_H(A,B) = \max\{|\underline{a}-\underline{b}|, |\overline{a}-\overline{b}|\},$$

which is a L_∞ distance.

A considerable contribution of those authors (Chavent et al., 2001, 2003) was to find the best representation clusters interval by minimizing the Hausdorff average distance between all the intervals describing the objects of the class and the more suitable interval $[\underline{\theta},\overline{\theta}]$ representing the class. Because the Hausdorff distance is additive, the criterion function (for all the class C_h; with $h = 1,\ldots,k$) is:

$$f(G_h) = \sum_{i \in C_h} d(x_i, G) = \sum_{i \in C_h} \sum_{j=1}^{J_t} d(x_i^j, G_h^j).$$

Thus, the interval "best" can be found for each interval variable y_j ($j = 1, \ldots, J_t$), minimizing:

$$f(G_h^j) = \sum_{i \in C_h} d(x_i^j, G_h^j) = \max \sum_{i \in C_h} \{|\underline{\theta^j} - \underline{a}_i^j|, |\overline{\theta^j} - \overline{a}_i^j|\},$$

where $d_{x_i,j}$ is the interval $A_i^j = [\underline{a}_i^j, \overline{a}_i^j]$ for each y_j'.

It is known that the Hausdorff distance $d(A, B)$ between two intervals can be decomposed as the sum of the distances between the middle points, μ_A and μ_B, and between the radius λ_A and λ_B (semi-length) of A and B:

$$d_H(A, B) = |\mu_A - \mu_B| + |\lambda_A - \lambda_B|.$$

Defining $R_{\mu^j,h} = [\underline{\mu_i^j}, \overline{\mu_i^j}]$ and $R_{\lambda^j,h} = [\underline{\lambda_i^j}, \overline{\lambda_i^j}]$ for $x_i \in C_h$, the interval $[\underline{\theta^j}, \overline{\theta^j}]$ (for each j) is estimated as a solution of the two minimization problems:

$$\min_{\mu \in R_{\mu^j,h}} = \sum_{i \in C_h} |\widehat{\mu}^j - \mu_i^j| \quad and \quad \min_{\lambda \in R_{\lambda^j,h}} = \sum_{i \in C_h} |\widehat{\lambda}^j - \lambda_i^j|$$

Then, $\widehat{\mu}^j$ and $\widehat{\lambda}^j$ correspond to the median values of the μ_i^j and λ_i^j distributions on the elements $x_i \in C_h$ (for each class C_h; $h = 1, \ldots, k$):

$$[\underline{\theta}^j, \overline{\theta}^j] = [\widehat{\mu}^j - \widehat{\lambda}^j, \widehat{\mu}^j + \widehat{\lambda}^j]$$

– *A context dependent dissimilarity function (Ichino-Yaguci's) to compare multi-nominal data*

Among the dissimilarity functions proposed in the SDA context to compare SO's we can assume as an *allocation function* in the clustering algorithm the most general *context dependent dissimilarity function* (Ichino-Yaguchi, 1994) when the SO's of E are described by all interval data or by all multi-categorical variables. In the case of interval descriptions, this measure is an alternative to the Hausdorff distance.

Ichino-Yaguchi proposed this measure as a suitable comparison function between pairs of objects. In our context of analysis, the measure consistent with the fitting criterion of the algorithm when the prototype is in the same space of representation of the elements of the class.

To define this *context dependent dissimilarity* we need to introduce the *potential descriptor* function $\eta(d_j, x_i)$, proposed by De Carvalho (1992): for each descriptor y_j of x_i, $\eta(d_{j,x_i})$ is the length of the interval $A_{j,i}$ in d_{j,x_i} if y_j is an interval variable, or $\eta(d_{j,x_i})$ is the cardinality of the set of values in d_{j,x_i} if y_j is multi-categorical.

Given two general SO's x_i and $x_{i'} \in E$ with description in $d_i = \{d_{1,i}, \ldots, d_{j,i}, \ldots, d_{p,i}\}$ and $d'_i = \{d_{1,i'}, \ldots, d_{j,i'}, \ldots, d_{p,i'}\}$, (for simplicity of notation, the description sets d_{j,x_i} have been replaced by $d_{j,i}$) this measure is expressed by the following formula:

$$\delta_j(x_i, x_{i'}) = \eta(d_{j,i}\_op\_d_{j,i'}) - \eta(d_{j,i} \cap d_{j,i'}) + \gamma(2\eta(d_{j,i} \cap d_{j,i'} - \eta(d_{j,i}) - \eta(d_{j,i'}))$$

for each $y_j = 1, \ldots, p$ (multi-categorical or interval variables).

where: $\_op\_$ can be the *join* or the *union* operator and γ is a parameter, fixed equal to 0.5 in Ichino-Yaguchi's function. In this way the function is transformed as follows:

$$\delta_j(x_i, x_{i'}) = \eta(d_{j,i}\_op\_d_{j,i'}) - \frac{\eta(d_{j,i}) + \eta(d_{j,i'})}{2}.$$

Starting from this measure De Carvalho (1994, 1998) proposed a different normalization of δ by: *potential descriptor* $\eta(D_j)$ of the domain D_j of y_j or the *potential descriptor* of the combination set of the two SO's descriptions, $\eta(d_{j,i}\_op\_d_{j,i'})$. Further values for the parameter γ in [0,0.5] were also considered. Then, the aggregation function is usually chosen according to a Minkowski metric (with parameter r):

$$\delta_j(x_i, x_{i'}) = p^{-1}\left[\sum_{j=1}^{J}(\delta_j(x_i, x_{i'}))^r\right]^{\frac{1}{r}} \qquad (r \geq 1).$$

We note that the prototype of the classes of objects (COS's), described by interval data, are chosen as the neighbours elements from all the other ones, according to this allocation function. In such context, the *virtual* intervals equal to the median intervals of the elements of each classes, if they are consistent for the Hausdorff distance, they are not consistent with respect to this different type of dissimilarity measure.

– *Classical ϕ^2 distance to compare modal data*

When both SO's and prototypes are modelled by distributions a classical ϕ^2 distance can be proposed as allocation function. As noted above, modal data can be derived by imposing a system of weights (pseudo-frequencies, probabilities, believes) on the domain of multi-categorical or interval SO's descriptors. These transformations of the SO's representation space are requested wherever prototypes have been chosen as modal SO's.

In this way, SO's $x_i \in E$ are allocated to the classes according to their minimum distance from the prototype. Because the ϕ^2 is also an additive measure, the distance of x_i to G_h can be expressed as follows:

$$d_{\phi^2}(x_i, G_h) = \sum_{j=1}^{J} \sum_{v=1}^{L_j} \frac{1}{q_{v\cdot}} (q_{vj}^i - q_{vj}^h)^2,$$

where $v = 1, \ldots, L_j$ is the set of the L_j categories constituting the domain of the variable y_j (e.g., multi-nominal, elementary intervals)

Recall that q_{j,G_h} was built as average profile of the distributions associated with the SO's x_i in the class C_h Thus, simple Euclidean distances between profiles too can be suitably used.

- *Two components distance as allocation matching function*

When SO's and prototype are represented in two different spaces, we consider a suitable *context dependent proximity function* δ (De Carvalho et al., 1998), as a matching function, to compare the objects to prototypes.

The representation space of the SO's $x_i \in E$ to be clustered and the representation space L associated with each partition P of E, are not homogeneous because the x_i are described by multi-nominal or interval variables, and the prototypes are described by *modal* ones. To retrieve the two configurations of data in the same representation space, we consider the transformation on the SO's description by a uniform distribution (as shown above) and we estimate the empirical distribution of the prototypes. Note that the distributions can be assumed non uniform on the basis of external information on the SO's descriptions.

Therefore, the *allocation function* δ can be considered as a suitable comparison function which measures the matching degree between the SO x_i and the prototype G_h $(\forall x_i, G_h)$, according to their description d_{G_h} and d_{x_i}. The particular allocation function that we consider is based on the following two additive components:

$$\delta(x_i, G_h) = \sum_{j=1}^{p} \sum_{s:\ c(s) \in D_j} (\gamma_s \cdot g_{j,G_h}(c_s) + \gamma_s' \cdot q_{j,x_i}(c_s)),$$

where γ_s and γ_s' can take values $\{0, 1\}$, under the following conditions:

$$\gamma_s = \begin{cases} 1 \text{ if } c_s \in d_{j,G_h} \ \& \ c_s \notin d_{j,x_i} \\ 0 \text{ otherwise }, \end{cases} \text{ and } \gamma_s' = \begin{cases} 1 \text{ if } c_s \in d_{j,x_i} \ \& \ c_s \notin d_{j,G_h} \\ 0 \text{ otherwise }. \end{cases}$$

6 Crossed Dynamical Clustering Algorithm

The general scheme of DCA described above can be suitably used to find a structure the symbolic data. In this context of analysis, we make reference only to a set of SO's described by multi-categorical variables. Assume a symbolic data table containing along its rows the SO's descriptions and along its columns the categories of the SO's descriptors.

The Crossed dynamical Clustering Algorithm (CCA) performs a partition of the rows of the symbolic data table into a set of homogeneous classes, representing typology of SO's or groups of categories. Therefore, the general scheme followed by the procedure is based on two iterative phases: the optimal clustering of the rows and columns, according to a criterion function.

In the classical approach to contingency table classification, some authors (Govaert, 1977, Govaert and Nadif, 2003) proposed the maximization of the χ^2 criterion between rows and columns.

In our context, a contingency table can be modelled by a modal symbolic variable where each component represent a category. Moreover, we extend the χ^2 criterion on symbolic modal variables and we assume the following additive criterion:

$$\Delta(P,(Q^1,\ldots,Q^p)) = \sum_{j=1}^{p} \chi^2(P,Q^j),$$

where Q^j is the partition associated to the modal variable y_j.

The cells of the crossed tables can be modelling by marginal distributions (or profiles) summarizing the classes descriptions of the rows and columns.

Because the criterion Δ is additive with respect to the data descriptors, the distance d is the sum of the distances d_j defined on each symbolic variable.

The criterion $\Delta(P,Q,G) = \chi^2(P,Q)$ optimized in the CCA is consistent with the clustering one. The algorithm optimizes iteratively the two partitions P and Q and the related representation $g_1,\ldots,g_k$.

The results of the CCA seem particularly appropriate for defining taxonomies and relationships among the categories of symbolic variables.

An extension to interval data could be easily proposed considering the elementary interval decomposition of the domain of such symbolic variables.

7 Conclusion

The DCA can be arguably considered as the most suitable compromise in SDA techniques, between a conceptual and numerical approach. By an automatic procedure it implements a partition of conceptual data without following the simple judgements of experts but optimizes a numerical criterion that allows however taking into account the expert information. The generalized dynamic algorithm on symbolic objects has been proposed in different contexts of analysis; for example, to cluster archaeological data described by multi-categorical variables, to look for typologies of waves characterized by intervals values, to analyze similarities between the different shapes of micro-organism described by both multi-categorical and intervals to compare socio-economic characteristics of different geographical areas with respect to the distributions of some variables (e.g., economic activities, income distributions, worked hours, etc.). The main advantage of using a symbolic cluster algorithm is to get a tool for comparing and clustering aggregated and structured data. From a generalization of the crossed clustering algorithm to symbolic data has also been proposed in Usage Web Mining (Arnoux et al., 2003) to detect typologies of Internet users and to identify recursive paths in the web navigation.

The main prospectives in the following developments of DCA are diverted toward an extension of such algorithms to the treatment of symbolic data characterized by different kind of variables, to take more into account logical relationships defined on the symbolic descriptors and to improve the conceptual meaning of the classes of the partition, according to suitable homogeneity measures defined on the symbolic descriptors of the clusters.

The implementation of new procedures and new parameters in the SODAS software will allow to testing the proposed clustering methods on real data.

References

1. Arnoux, M., Lechevallier, Y., Tanasa, D., Trousse, B., and Verde, R. (2003). "Automatic Clustering for Web Usage Mining," in *Proceeding of SYNASC-2003 - 5th International Workshop on Symbolic and Numeric Algorithms for Scientific Computing*, Timisoara, 1-4 October.
2. Bock, H.-H., and Diday, E. (eds.), (1999). *Analysis of Symbolic Data, Exploratory Methods for Extracting Statistical Information from Complex Data*, Springer-Verlag, Berlin.
3. Celeux, G., Diday, E., Govaert, G., Lechevallier, Y., and Ralambondrainy, H. (1989). *Classification Automatique des Données*, Bordas, Paris.
4. Chavent, M. (1997): *Analyse des Données Symboliques. Une Méthode Divisive de Classification.* Thèse de l'Université de PARIS-IX Dauphine.
5. Chavent, M., De Carvalho, F. A. T., and Lechevallier, Y. (2002): Dynamical Clustering of interval data. Optimization of an adequacy criterion based on Hausdorff distance, In: *Classification, Clustering and Data Analysis*, K. Jaguga et al. (Eds.), Springer, 53–60
6. Chavent, M., De Carvalho, F.A.T., Lechevallier, Y., Verde, R. (2003). "Trois Nouvelles Méthodes de Classification Automatique de Données Symboliques de Type Intervalle," *Revue de Statistique Appliquées*, **4**, 5–29.
7. De Carvalho, F. A. T. (1992). *Méthodes Descriptives en Analyse de Donnés Symbolique*, Thesis of Doctorate in Informatique des Organisations, Université de Paris IX Dauphine.
8. De Carvalho, F.A.T., Verde, R., and Lechevallier, Y. (1999). "A Dynamical Clustering of Symbolic Objects Based on a Context Dependent Proximity Measure," in *Proc. IX International Symposium - ASMDA'99*, eds H. Bacelar-Nicolau, F. C. Nicolau, and J. Janssen, J., Lisobon:LEAD, Universidade de Lisboa, pp. 237–242.

9. De Carvalho, F. A. T., Verde, R., and Lechevallier, Y. (2001). "Deux Nouvelles Méthodes de Classification Automatique d'Ensembles d'Objets Symboliques dÉcrits par des Variables Intervalles," *SFC'2001*, Guadeloupe.
10. De Carvalho, F. A. T., and Souza, R. M. C. (1998). "Statistical Proximity Functions of Boolean Symbolic Objects Based on Histograms," in *Advances in Data Science and Classification*, eds. A. Rizzi, M. Vichi, and H.-H. Bock, Heidelberg:Springer-Verlag, pp. 391–396.
11. Diday, E. (1971). "La méthode des Nuées Dynamiques," *Revue de Statistique Appliquée*, **19:2**, 19–34.
12. Diday, E., and Simon, J. C. (1976). "Clustering Analysis," in *Digital Pattern Recognition*, ed. K. S. Fu, Heidelberg:Springer-Verlag, pp. 47–94.
13. Diday, E. (1989). "Knowledge Representation and Symbolic Data Analysis," in *Proceeding of the 2nd International Workshop on Data, Expert Knowledge, and Decision*, Hamburg.
14. Diday, E. (2001). "An Introduction to Symbolic Data Analysis and SODAS Software," Tutorial on Symbolic Data Analysis, GfKl 2001, Munich.
15. Govaert, G. (1977). "Algorithme de Classification d'un Tableau de Contingence," in *Proceeding of First International Symposium on Data Analysis and Informatics*, INRIA, Versailles, pp. 487–500.
16. Govaert, G. (1995). "Simultaneous Clustering of Rows and Columns," *Control Cybernetics*, **24**, 437–458
17. Govaert, G., and Nadif, M. (2003). "Clustering with Block Mixture Models," *Pattern Recognition*, **36**, 463–473
18. Ichino, M., and Yaguchi, H. (1994). "Generalized Minkowski Metrics for Mixed Feature Type Data Analysis," *IEEE Transactions Systems, Man and Cybernetics*, **1**, 494–497.
19. Lechevallier, Y., Trousse, B., Verde, R., and Tanasa, D. (2003). "Classification Automatique: Applications au Web-Mining," in Proceedings of SFC2003, Neuchatel.
20. Michalski, R. S., Diday, E., and Stepp, R. E. (1981). "A Recent Advance in Data Analysis: Clustering Objects into Classes Characterized by Conjunctive Concepts," in *Progress in Pattern Recognition*, eds. L. N. Kanal and A. Rosendfeld, Amsterdam:North Holland, pp. 33-56.
21. MacQueen, J. (1967). "Some Methods for Classification and Analysis of Multivariate Observations," in *Proceedings of the Fifth Berkeley Symposium on Mathematical Statistics and Probability*, **1**, eds. J. Neyman et al., Berkeley: University of California Press, pp. 281–297.
22. Moore, R. E. (1966). *Interval Analysis*, Prentice-Hall, Englewood Cliffs N.J.
23. Sauberlich, F., and Huber K.-P. (2001). "A Framework for Web Usage Mining on Anonymous Logfile Data," in *Exploratory Data Analysis in Empirical Research*, eds. M. Schwaiger and O. Opitz, Heidelberg:Springer-Verlag, pp. 309–318.
24. Verde, R., De Carvalho, F. A. T., and Lechevallier, Y. (2000). "A Dynamical Clustering Algorithm for Multi-Nominal Data," in *Data Analysis, Classification, and Related Methods*, eds. H. A. L. Kiers et al., Heidelberg:Springer, pp. 387-394.

Dependencies in Bivariate Interval-Valued Symbolic Data

L. Billard

University of Georgia, U.S.A.
lynne@stat.uga.edu

Abstract: This paper looks at measures of dependence for symbolic interval-valued data. A method is given to calculate an empirical copula for a bivariate interval-valued variable. This copula is then used to determine an empirical formula for calculating Spearman's rho for such data. The methodology is illustrated from a set of hematocrit-hemoglobin data and the results compared with Pearson's product-moment correlation coefficient.

1 Introduction

Contemporary datasets can be too large for analysis via standard classical statistical methodologies. One approach for handling such situations is to aggregate the data according to some specific meaningful concept underlying the data. The resulting smaller dataset would then consist of data which are no longer (classical) single points but rather are symbolic data such as hypercubes in p-dimensional space. Analysis of these symbolic data requires symbolic methodologies; see Billard and Diday (2003) for a recent review.

The focus of this paper is on dependence relations for bivariate interval-valued symbolic data. Sklar (1959) introduced copulas as a vehicle for describing dependence between a joint distribution function and the corresponding marginal distributions in the context of classical data. Later, Deheuvels (1979) showed how to calculate empirical copulas for two-dimensional (classical) data. In Section 2 below, these ideas are extended to the evaluation of empirical copulas for two-dimensional interval-valued symbolic data. Then, in Section 3, these empirical copula results are used to find an estimate of Spearman's measure of association between two variables. A comparison with Pearson's product-moment correlation coefficient for interval-valued data is included.

2 Empirical Copulas for Interval-Valued Data

Let (Y, X) be a bivariate random variable. In the classical setting, suppose the data D are realizations (y_i, x_i), $i = 1, \ldots, n$. For symbolic data, let E be a dataset of m objects with descriptions $y(u)=[a(u), b(u)]$, $x(u)=[c(u), d(u])$, $u=1,\ldots,m$. It is assumed that values are uniformly distributed across the respective $y(u)$ and $x(u)$ intervals. For the sake of explanatory simplicity, it is also assumed that all individual descriptions in E satisfy a set of rules; adaptation to those cases where (a portion of the) data violate given rules can be made along the lines described in Bertrand and Goupil (2000) and Billard and Diday (2003).

From Sklar (1959), there exists a copula $C(x, y)$ such that

$$H(x, y) = C(F(x), G(y))$$

where $H(x, y)$ is the joint distribution function of (X, Y), and $F(x)$ and $G(y)$ are the marginal distribution functions of X and Y, respectively.

The empirical copula based on the data D, from Deheuvels (1979), is given by

$$C(\frac{i}{n}, \frac{j}{n}) = \frac{1}{n}[\#\text{pairs } (x, y) \text{ with } \ x < x_{(i)} \text{ and } y < y_{(j)}],$$

where $z_{(r)}$ is the rth order statistic, $r = 1, \ldots, n$.

For the symbolic dataset E, first calculate the midpoints

$$x_u = [c(u) + d(u)]/2, \qquad y_u = [a(u) + b(u)]/2.$$

Next, define x_i (and y_j) as the ith (jth) rank order of the x_u (y_u) statistics, $i, j = 1, \ldots, m$. Also, define the rectangles $R(x_i, y_j) = (s_x, x_i) \times (s_y, y_j)$, for $i, j = 1, \ldots, m$, where $s_x \leq \min_u(c(u))$ and $s_y \leq \min_u(a(u))$. Similarly, let $R(x_{m+1}, y_{m+1}) = (s_x, t_x) \times (s_y, t_y)$ where $t_x \geq \max_u(d(u))$ and $t_y \geq \max_u(b(u))$.

Then the empirical copula for the interval-valued data of E is given by

$$C'(x_i, y_j) = \frac{1}{m} \sum_{u \in E} \frac{\|Z(u) \cap R(x_i, y_j)\|}{\|Z(u)\|},$$

for $i, j = 1, \ldots, m+1$, where $Z(u)$ is the rectangle $X(u) \times Y(u)$ and $\|A\|$ is the area of the rectangle A.

To illustrate these ideas, we now calculate the empirical copula for the data of Table 1 where Y is a measure of hematocrit and X is a hemoglobin measure (these data are taken from Billard and Diday, 2002). The midpoint values (x_i, y_j) are shown in Table 2.

For example, suppose that we wish to calculate $C(x_1, y_3)$. Since

$$\begin{aligned} x_1 &= [\text{c}(11)+\text{d}(11)]/2 = 11.217, \\ y_3 &= [\text{a}(1)+\text{b}(1)]/2 \ \ = 36.453, \end{aligned}$$

then

$$C'(x_1, y_3) = \frac{1}{m}\left[0 + \cdots + 0 + \frac{(36.453 - 28.831)}{(41.980 - 28.831)}\frac{(11.217 - 9.922)}{(13.801 - 9.922)} + 0 + \frac{(36.453 - 27.713)}{(40.499 - 27.713)}\frac{(11.217 - 9.722)}{(12.712 - 9.722)} + 0 + \cdots + 0\right]$$

$$= 0.035457.$$

Table 1. Data: Hematocrit (Y), and Hemoglobin (X).

u	a b	c d	u	a b	c d
1	[33.296, 39.610]	[11.545, 12.806]	9	[28.831, 41.980]	[9.922, 13.801]
2	[36.694, 45.123]	[12.075, 14.177]	10	[44.481, 52.536]	[15.374, 16.755]
3	[36.699, 48.685]	[12.384, 16.169]	11	[27.713, 40.499]	[9.722, 12.712]
4	[36.386, 47.412]	[12.384, 15.298]	12	[34.405, 43.027]	[11.767, 13.936]
5	[39.190, 50.866]	[13.581, 16.242]	13	[30.919, 47.091]	[10.812, 15.142]
6	[39.701, 47.246]	[13.819, 15.203]	14	[39.351, 51.510]	[13.761, 16.562]
7	[41.560, 48.814]	[14.341, 15.554]	15	[41.710, 49.678]	[14.698, 15.769]
8	[38.404, 45.228]	[13.274, 14.601]	16	[35.674, 42.382]	[12.448, 13.519]

Table 2. Ranked Interval Midpoints (x, y).

i	1	2	3	4	5	6	7	8	9
u	11	9	1	12	13	16	2	4	8
x	11.2170	11.8615	12.1755	12.8515	12.9770	12.9835	13.1260	13 .8410	13.9375
i	10	11	12	13	14	15	16	17	
u	3	6	5	7	14	15	10		
x	14.2765	14.5110	14.9115	14.9475	15.1615	15.2335	16.0645	17.000	
j	1	2	3	4	5	6	7	8	9
u	11	9	1	12	13	16	2	8	4
y	34.1060	35.4055	36.4530	38.7160	39.0050	39.0280	40.9085	41.8160	41.8990
j	10	11	12	13	14	15	16	17	
u	3	6	5	7	14	15	10		
y	42.6920	43.4735	45.0280	45.1870	45.4305	45.6940	48.5085	53.000	

The complete set of $C'(x_i, y_j)$ values is displayed in Table 3. Furthermore, since $F(x)$ is the marginal distribution of X, it follows that the last column (for $j = 17$) corresponds to $F(x)$. Similarly, the last row (for $i = 17$) corresponds to the marginal $G(y)$. This determines the empirical copula for the symbolic data in Table 1.

Table 3. Empirical Copula $C'(x, y)$.

i/j	1	2	3	4	5	6	7	8	9
1	.025	.031	.035	.045	.047	.047	.054	.056	.056
2	.040	.052	.062	.084	.087	.087	.101	.104	.104
3	.048	.066	.081	.114	.119	.119	.138	.144	.144
4	.064	.094	.122	.192	.202	.202	.245	.262	.264
5	.065	.096	.125	.202	.212	.212	.262	.280	.281
6	.065	.096	.125	.202	.212	.213	.263	.281	.282
7	.067	.098	.129	.213	.224	.224	.280	.300	.302
8	.073	.109	.147	.258	.274	.275	.362	.398	.401
9	.073	.110	.150	.269	.286	.288	.393	.409	.412
10	.074	.111	.150	.269	.286	.288	.393	.438	.442
11	.075	.112	.151	.273	.291	.292	.405	.456	.460
12	.076	.113	.153	.279	.298	.299	.422	.662	.724
13	.076	.114	.153	.279	.298	.300	.423	.480	.486
14	.077	.114	.154	.282	.301	.303	.431	.491	.498
15	.077	.114	.154	.283	.302	.303	.433	.494	.500
16	.077	.114	.154	.285	.305	.307	.446	.510	.517
17	.077	.114	.154	.286	.305	.307	.446	.514	.521
i/j	10	11	12	13	14	15	16	17	
1	.056	.057	.057	.057	.057	.057	.058	.058	
2	.105	.106	.108	.108	.180	.108	.110	.110	
3	.147	.148	.151	.151	.151	.152	.153	.153	
4	.273	.279	.289	.290	.290	.291	.297	.297	
5	.293	.300	.311	.311	.312	.313	.320	.321	
6	.294	.301	.312	.313	.314	.315	.322	.322	
7	.312	.324	.336	.337	.339	.340	.348	.348	
8	.426	.443	.472	.474	.476	.478	.495	.497	
9	.440	.458	.491	.494	.496	.499	.518	.521	
10	.476	.501	.545	.550	.553	.557	.586	.593	
11	.499	.528	.583	.588	.593	.598	.637	.646	
12	.531	.569	.640	.647	.654	.662	.724	.741	
13	.534	.573	.645	.652	.660	.667	.733	.750	
14	.550	.594	.675	.683	.692	.702	.782	.804	
15	.554	.599	.684	.692	.702	.712	.796	.820	
16	.579	.633	.736	.747	.760	.774	.899	.952	
17	.584	.639	.747	.758	.772	.788	.928	1.00	

3 Dependence Measures

One common measure of dependence between two random variables X and Y is Spearman's rho ρ, which is defined as a function of the difference between the probability of concordance and the probability of discordance. Nelsen (1999) has shown that, for classical variables, this rho is related to the copula according to the formula

$$\rho = 12 \int\int [C(u,v) - uv]\, du\, dv.$$

Using this, Nelsen finds an estimate r of Spearman's rho based on Deheuvel's empirical coplua as

$$r = \frac{12}{n^2-1} \sum_{i=1}^{n} \sum_{j=1}^{n} \left[C(\frac{i}{n}, \frac{j}{n}) - \frac{i}{n}\frac{j}{n} \right].$$

Adapting Nelsen's estimator for classical variables to the present symbolic data case, we can estimate Spearman's rho for interval-valued data by

$$r' = \frac{12}{m^2-1} \left[\sum_{i=1}^{m+1} \sum_{j=1}^{m+1} C'(x_i, y_j) \right] - \left[\sum_{i=1}^{M+1} F(x_i) \right] \left[\sum_{j=1}^{m+1} G(y_j) \right].$$

For the present data, from the numbers for $C'(x_i, y_j)$ in Table 3, it can be shown that $r' = 0.8835$.

This estimated Spearman's rho can be compared with the correlation coefficient r_p based on Pearson's product-moment function, which is given in Billard and Diday (2003) as

$$r_p = S_{XY} / S_X S_Y$$

where, writing $a(u) = a$, $b(u) = b$, $c(u) = c$, $d(u) = d$, we have

$$S_{XY} = \frac{1}{4m} \sum_{u \in E} (a+b)(c+d) - \frac{1}{4m^2} \left[\sum_{u \in E} (a+b) \right] \left[\sum_{u \in E} (c+d) \right]$$

and

$$S_Y^2 = \frac{1}{3m} \sum_{u \in E} (a^2 + ab + b^2) - \frac{1}{4m^2} \left[\sum_{u \in E} (a+b) \right]^2,$$

with S_X^2 defined similarly. Then, using the dataset in Table 1, it follows that $r_p = 0.7013$.

In contrast, if we had tried a classical analysis with (x, y) values corresponding to the midpoints of the observed intervals (of Table 2, say), then Pearson's correlation coefficient for these data is $r_c = 0.9951$. That the symbolic r_p is less than the classical r_c is a reflection of the fact that the classical sample variance (in the divisor of the formula for the correlation coefficient) calculated at the respective interval midpoints is necessarily smaller than the symbolic sample variance since the symbolic variance across observations also incorporates the internal variance within each symbolic observation. The numerator is the same in both cases.

On the other hand, the empirical Spearman's rho for the symbolic data at $r' = 0.8835$ is larger than is the symbolic Pearson's $r_p = 0.7013$. This difference reflects the fact that the numerator in the calculation of Pearson's rho does not take into account any internal variation in the symbolic data point, whereas the empirical rho does. Accordingly, the empirical Spearman's rho as proposed here would be the preferred correlation coefficient, since it offers the more appropriate dependence measure for interval-valued symbolic data.

Acknowledgements

Partial support from an NSF-INRIA grant is gratefully acknowledged. Thanks are proferred to the University of Melbourne for providing facilities during execution of this work.

References

1. Bertrand, P., and Goupil, F. (2000). "Descriptive Statistics for Symbolic Data," in *Analysis of Symbolic Data: Exploratory Methods for Extracting Statistical Information from Complex Data*, eds. H.-H. Bock and E. Diday, Berlin:Springer-Verlag, pp. 103–124.
2. Billard, L., and Diday, E. (2003). "From the Statistics of Data to the Statistics of Knowledge:Symbolic Data Analysis," *Journal of the American Statistical Association*, **98**, 470–487.
3. Deheuvels, P. (1979). "La Fonction de Dependence Empirique et ses Proprietes: Un Test Non Parametrique d'Independence," *Académie Royale de Belgique Bulletin de la Classe des Sciences*, **65**, 274–292.
4. Nelsen, R. B. (1999). *An Introduction to Copulas.* Springer-Verlag, New York.

Clustering of Symbolic Objects Described by Multi-Valued and Modal Variables

André Hardy and Pascale Lallemand

University of Namur, Belgium
{andre.hardy,pascale.lallemand}@fundp.ac.be

Abstract: In this paper we investigate the problem of the determination of the number of clusters for symbolic objects described by multi-valued and modal variables. Three dissimilarity measures are selected in order to define distances on the set of symbolic objects. Methods for the determination of the number of clusters are applied to hierarchies of partitions produced by four hierarchical clustering methods, and to sets of partitions given by the symbolic clustering procedure SCLUST. Two real data sets are analysed.

1 Introduction

The aim of cluster analysis is to identify a structure within a data set. When hierarchical algorithms are used, a crucial problem is then to choose one solution in the nested sequence of partitions of the hierarchy. On the other hand, optimization methods for cluster analysis usually demand the a priori specification of the number of groups. So most clustering procedures require the user to fix the number of clusters, or to determine it in the final solution.

Symbolic data analysis (Bock and Diday, 2000) is concerned with the extension of classical data analysis and statistical methods to more complex data called symbolic data. In previous works we were interested in the determination of the number of clusters for symbolic objects described by interval variables (Hardy and Lallemand, 2002). In this paper we extend our research to multinominal and modal symbolic objects.

2 Multi-Valued and Modal Variables

Consider the classical situation with $E = \{x_1, ..., x_n\}$ a set of objects and a series of p variables $Y_1, ..., Y_p$. This paper is based on the following definitions (Bock and Diday, 2000).

(1) A variable Y is termed *set-valued* with the domain $\mathcal{Y}$, if for all $x_k \in E$,

$$\begin{aligned} Y : E &\rightarrow \mathcal{B} \\ x_k &\longmapsto Y(x_k) \end{aligned}$$

where $\mathcal{B} = \mathcal{P}(\mathcal{Y}) = \{U \neq \emptyset \mid U \subseteq \mathcal{Y}\}$.

(2) A set-valued variable is called *multi-valued* if its values $Y(x_k)$ are all finite subsets of the underlying domain $\mathcal{Y}$; so $|Y(x_k)| < \infty$, for all elements $x_k \in E$.

(3) A set-valued variable Y is called *categorical multi-valued* if it has a finite range $\mathcal{Y}$ of categories and *quantitative multi-valued* if the values $Y(x_k)$ are finite sets of real numbers.

A modal variable Y on a set $E = \{x_1, ..., x_n\}$ with domain $\mathcal{Y}$ is a mapping

$$Y(x_k) = (U(x_k), \pi_k) \quad \text{for all} \quad x_k \in E$$

where π_k is, for example, a frequency distribution on the domain $\mathcal{Y}$ of possible observation values and $U(x_k) \subseteq \mathcal{Y}$ is the support of π_k in the domain $\mathcal{Y}$.

3 Dissimilarity Measures for Symbolic Objects

Clustering algorithms and methods for the determination of the number of clusters usually require a dissimilarity matrix D which reflects the similarity structure of the n objects. In this section we present three distance measures on the set $E = \{x_1, ..., x_n\}$ in order to determine a $n \times n$ distance matrix D on E (Bock and Diday, 2000).

3.1 Multi-Valued Variables

The set $E = \{x_1, \ldots, x_n\}$ consists of n objects described by p multi-valued variables $Y_1, \ldots, Y_p$ with domains $\mathcal{Y}_1, \ldots, \mathcal{Y}_p$ respectively. Let m_j denote the number of categories taken by Y_j. The frequency value $q_{j,x_k}(c_s)$ associated with the category c_s $(s = 1, \ldots, m_j)$ of the variable Y_j is given by

$$q_{j,x_k}(c_s) = \begin{cases} |Y_j(x_k)|^{-1} & \text{if} \quad \mathrm{c_s \in Y_j(x_k)} \\ 0 & \text{otherwise.} \end{cases}$$

The symbolic representation of the object $x_k \in E$ is a vector in $(m_1 + \ldots + m_p)$-dimensional space, given by

$$x_k = ((q_{1,x_k}(c_1), \ldots, q_{1,x_k}(c_{m_1})), \ldots, (q_{p,x_k}(c_1), \ldots, q_{p,x_k}(c_{m_p}))).$$

So the original data matrix $\boldsymbol{X} = (Y_j(x_k)) \equiv (x_{kj})$ is transformed into a frequency matrix $\tilde{X}$ as shown below, where for all $x_k \in E$, and for all $j \in \{1, \ldots, p\}$, $\sum_{i=1}^{m_j} q_{j,x_k}(c_i) = 1$.

	Y_1			$\cdots$	Y_p		
	1	$\cdots$	m_1	$\cdots$	1	$\cdots$	m_p
x_1	$q_{1,x_1}(c_1)$	$\cdots$	$q_{1,x_1}(c_{m_1})$	$\cdots$	$q_{p,x_1}(c_1)$	$\cdots$	$q_{p,x_1}(c_{m_p})$
$\vdots$	$\vdots$		$\vdots$		$\vdots$		$\vdots$
x_k	$q_{1,x_k}(c_1)$	$\cdots$	$q_{1,x_k}(c_{m_1})$	$\cdots$	$q_{p,x_k}(c_1)$	$\cdots$	$q_{p,x_k}(c_{m_p})$
$\vdots$	$\vdots$		$\vdots$		$\vdots$		$\vdots$
x_n	$q_{1,x_n}(c_1)$	$\cdots$	$q_{1,x_n}(c_{m_1})$	$\cdots$	$q_{p,x_n}(c_1)$	$\cdots$	$q_{p,x_n}(c_{m_p})$

Let δ_j be a distance function defined on $\mathcal{B}_j$:

$$\begin{aligned} \delta_j : \ & \mathcal{B}_j \times \mathcal{B}_j \rightarrow R^+ \\ & (x_{kj}, x_{\ell j}) \longmapsto \delta_j(x_{kj}, x_{\ell j}). \end{aligned}$$

For each x_k, we denote by $x_{kj}^{(i)}$ the frequency value associated with the category c_i of Y_j. The L_1 and L_2 distances on $\mathcal{B}_j$ are respectively defined by:

$$\delta_j(x_{kj}, x_{\ell j}) = \sum_{i=1}^{|\mathcal{Y}_j|} |x_{kj}^{(i)} - x_{\ell j}^{(i)}| \text{ and } \delta_j(x_{kj}, x_{\ell j}) = \sum_{i=1}^{|\mathcal{Y}_j|} (x_{kj}^{(i)} - x_{\ell j}^{(i)})^2$$

and the de Carvalho distance by

$$\delta_j(x_{kj}, x_{\ell j}) = \sum_{i=1}^{|\mathcal{Y}_j|} (\gamma x_{kj}^{(i)} + \gamma' x_{\ell j}^{(i)})$$

where

$$\gamma = \begin{cases} 1 \text{ if } c_i \in Y_j(x_k) \text{ and } c_i \notin Y_j(x_\ell) \\ 0 \text{ otherwise} \end{cases}$$

$$\gamma\prime = \begin{cases} 1 \text{ if } c_i \notin Y_j(x_k) \text{ and } c_i \in Y_j(x_\ell) \\ 0 \text{ otherwise.} \end{cases}$$

We combine p dissimilarity indices $\delta_1, \ldots, \delta_p$ defined on the ranges $\mathcal{B}_j$ in to a global dissimilarity measure on E:

$$\begin{aligned} d : \ & E \times E \longrightarrow R^+ \\ & (x_k, x_\ell) \longmapsto d(x_k, x_\ell) = \left(\sum_{j=1}^{p} \delta_j^2(x_{kj}, x_{\ell j}) \right)^{1/2} \end{aligned}$$

where δ_j is one of the dissimilarity measures defined above.

3.2 Modal Variables

The case of modal variables is similar to the case of multi-valued variables. The frequencies $q_{j,x_k}(c_s)$ are simply replaced by the values of the distribution $\pi_{j,k}$ associated with the categories of $Y_j(x_k)$.

4 Clustering Procedures

The existence of dissimilarity matrices for multi-nominal and modal symbolic objects allows us to apply clustering algorithms to our set of symbolic objects in order to generate partitions. The first one is the symbolic clustering algorithm SCLUST (Verde et al., 2000). That clustering method is a generalization to symbolic objects of the well-known dynamic clouds clustering method (Celeux et al., 1989). It determines iteratively a series of partitions that improves at each step a mathematical criterion. We also consider four classical hierarchical clustering methods: the single link, complete link, centroid, and Ward algorithms.

5 Determination of the Number of Clusters

We select the five best stopping rules from the Milligan and Cooper (1985) study: the Caliński and Harabasz (1974) index (M_1), the Duda and Hart (1973) rule (M_2), the C-index (Hubert and Levin, 1985) (M_3), the Γ-index (Baker and Hubert, 1975) (M_4) and the Beale test (Beale, 1969) (M_5).

For the four hierarchical procedures, the indices associated with these rules are computed at each level of the hierarchies. Concerning SCLUST, we select the best partition into ℓ clusters, for each value of ℓ ($\ell = 1, \cdots, K$) where K is a reasonably large integer fixed by the user, and we compute the indices available for nonhierarchical classification (M_1, M_3 and M_4).

The analysis of theses indices should provide the "best" number of clusters. The Caliński and Harabasz method, the C-index and the Γ-index use various forms of sum of squares within and between clusters. The Duda and Hart rule and the Beale test are statistical hypothesis tests.

6 Examples

We describe result from applying these methods to two data sets. One data set concerns historical buckles, and the other concerns commercial fashion products.

6.1 Merovingian Buckles: VI-VIII Century A.C.

The set of symbolic data consists of 58 buckles described by six multi-valued symbolic variables. These variables and the corresponding categories are presented in Table 1. The complete data set is available at http://www-rocq.inria.fr/sodas/WP6/data/data.html.

The 58 buckles have been examined by archeologists. They identified two natural clusters. SCLUST and the four hierarchical clustering methods have been applied to that data set, with the three previously defined distances (L_1, L_2, and de Carvalho).

Variables	Categories
Fixation	iron nail; bronze bump; none
Damascening	bichromate; veneer; dominant inlaid; silver monochrome
Contours	undulations; repeating motifs; geometric frieze
Background	silver plate, hatching; geometric frame
Inlaying	filiform; hatching banner; dotted banner; wide ribbon
Plate	arabesque; large size; squared back; animal pictures; plait; circular

Table 1. Merovingian buckles: six categorical multi-valued variables.

Results Given by SCLUST

Table 2 presents the values of the indices given by the three stopping rules M_1, M_3, and M_4, as obtained with SCLUST and the de Carvalho dissimilarity measure.

k	M1	M3	M4
8	28.52599	0.03049	0.95382
7	30.37194	0.04221	0.95325
6	23.36924	0.05127	0.92168
5	31.03050	0.04869	0.93004
4	32.66536	0.05707	0.95822
3	41.24019	0.03788	0.96124
2	**51.13007**	**0.01201**	**0.99917**
1	-	-	-

Table 2. Number of clusters with SCLUST.

The first column indicates the number of clusters in each partition, and the other columns show the indices given by the three methods for the determination of the number of clusters applicable to nonhierarchical procedures.

The "optimal" number of clusters is the value of k corresponding to the maximum (respectively, the minimum) value of the indices for M_1 and M_4 (respectively, for M_3) (Milligan and Cooper, 1985). The three methods agree on two clusters in the set of Merovingian Buckles. Furthermore, these two clusters are the ones identified by the archeologists.

Results Given by Four Hierarchical Methods

The five best rules from the Milligan and Cooper (1985) study are applied at each level of the four hierarchies. The results for the complete link clustering method using the L_2 dissimilarity measure are presented in Table 3 below.

The Caliński and Harabasz method (M_1), the C-index (M_3) and the Γ-index (M_4) indicate that there are two clusters in the data set. For the Duda

Complete link	M1	M2	M3	M4	M5
7	33.83576	2.35439	0.00860	0.99117	0.00000
6	34.66279	2.28551	0.01338	0.98565	2.34051
5	28.87829	3.56668	0.03270	0.94615	**3.59244**
4	34.53483	1.48947	0.03986	0.93230	1.20779
3	29.45371	2.91271	0.02761	0.95592	1.88482
2	**51.47556**	1.53622	**0.00932**	**0.99010**	1.24133
1	-	**5.27061**	-	-	**3.20213**

Table 3. Number of clusters with the complete link method.

and Hart method (M_2) and the Beale test (M_5), standard scores have to be fixed. Adopting the recommended values (Milligan and Cooper, 1985), these methods detect two clusters for M_2, and either two or six clusters for M_5. The partition into six clusters given by M_5 is close to another classification of the Buckles into seven clusters given by the same archeologists.

Equivalent results are found with the complete link algorithm associated with the two other distances (L_1 and de Carvalho), and by the other clustering procedures (single link, centroid, and Ward) with the three distances.

6.2 Fashion Stores

The second data set describes the sales in a group of stores (items of clothing and accessories), belonging to six different countries. These sales concern the years 1999, 2000 and 2001. The 13 objects are the stores (Paris 6th, Lyon, Rome, Barcelona, Toulouse, Aix-Marseille, Madrid, Berlin, Milan, Brussels, Paris 15th, Paris 8th, London). Eight modal variables are recorded on each of the 13 objects, describing the items sold in these stores. For example, the variable "family product" has 13 categories (dress, sweater, T-shirt, etc.). The proportion of sales in each store is associated with all these categories. On the other hand, the variable "month" describes the proportion of sales for each month of the year.

We apply the five clustering methods (SCLUST, single link, complete link, centroid, Ward), with the three distances (L_1, L_2, de Carvalho). The resulting partitions are analysed by the previous methods for determining the number of clusters. The results are given in Table 4 (de Carvalho distance), Table 5 (L_1 distance) and Table 6 (L_2 distance).

The analysis of these tables and of the corresponding partitions leads to the following comments.

- The partition into two clusters seems to be interesting. In almost all the cases (except for SCLUST associated with the de Carvalho distance) the partition into two clusters is the same. In the first one we find the e-Fashion

	M1	M3	M4
SCLUST	2	4	1

	M1	M2	M3	M4	M5
Single link	2	2	2	2	2
Complete link	2	2	2	2	2
Centroid	2	2	2	2	2
Ward	2	2	2	2	2

Table 4. Number of clusters with the de Carvalho distance.

	M1	M3	M4
SCLUST	4	2	2

	M1	M2	M3	M4	M5
Single link	3	3	2	2	3
Complete link	4	3	2	2	3
Centroid	4	3	2	2	3
Ward	4	3	2	2	3

Table 5. Number of clusters with the L_1 distance.

	M1	M3	M4
SCLUST	2	2	2

	M1	M2	M3	M4	M5
Single link	2	2	2	2	2
Complete link	2	2	2	2	2
Centroid	2	2	2	2	2
Ward	2	2	2	2	2

Table 6. Number of clusters with the L_2 distance.

store of London, and all the other stores belong to the second cluster. If we look at the data, or if we examine the graphical representations (zoom-stars) associated with each of the symbolic variables, the e-Fashion store of London distinguishes itself from the other stores by two variables: the type of "sale promotion" and the number of "accessories" sold.

- When a classification into more than two clusters is taken into consideration, in all the cases a class appears with only two objects: the e-Fashion store of Madrid and the e-Fashion store of Rome. It can be mainly explained by the fact that these two stores sell mainly accessories, and that these sales are equally distributed during the year.

7 Conclusion

In this paper we were interested in the determination of the number of clusters for symbolic objects described by multi-valued and modal variables. The three distances used give similar results. Nevertheless, the de Carvalho distance seems to give better results in the multi-valued case.

Five clustering methods were used: a symbolic one (SCLUST) and four classical hierarchical methods. The classical methods produce results at least as good than the symbolic one.

Future research concerns the possibility of mixing the different types of symbolic variables in the same table.

References

1. Baker, F., and Hubert, L. (1975). "Measuring the Power of Hierarchical Cluster Analysis," *Journal of the American Statistical Association*, **70**, 31–38.
2. Beale, E. (1969). "Euclidean Cluster Analysis," *Bulletin of the International Statistical Institute*, **43**, 92–94.
3. Bock, H.-H., and Diday, E. (2000). *Analysis of Symbolic Data. Exploratory Methods for Extracting Statistical Information from Complex Data.* Springer-Verlag, Berlin.
4. Calinski, T., and Harabasz, J. (1974). "A Dendrite Method for Cluster Analysis," *Communications in Statistics*, **3**, 1–27.
5. Celeux, G., Diday, E., Govaert, G., Lechevallier, Y., and Ralan-Bondrainy, H. (1989). *Classification Automatique des Données.* Bordas.
6. Duda, R., and Hart, P. (1973). *Pattern Classification and Scene Analysis.* Wiley, New York.
7. Hubert, L., and Levin, J. (1976). "A General Statistical Framework for Assessing Categorical Clustering in Free Recall," *Psychological Bulletin*, **83**, 1072–1080.
8. Hardy, A., and Lallemand, P. (2002) "Determination of the Number of Clusters for Symbolic Objects Described by Interval Variables," in *Studies in Classification, Data Analysis and Knowledge Organisation*, eds. K. Jajuga, et al., Berlin:Springer, pp. 311–318.
9. Milligan, G., and Cooper, M. "An Examination of Procedures for Determining the Number of Cluster in a Data Set," *Psychometrika*, **50**, 159–179.
10. Verde, R., de Carvalho, F., and Lechevallier, Y. (2000). "A Dynamical Clustering Algorithm for Multinominal Data," *Data Analysis, Classification, and Related Methods*, eds. H. A. L. Kiers et al., Berlin:Springer, pp. 387–393.

A Hausdorff Distance Between Hyper-Rectangles for Clustering Interval Data

Marie Chavent

Université Bordeaux, France
chavent@math.u-bordeaux.fr

Abstract: The Hausdorff distance between two sets is used in this paper to compare hyper-rectangles. An explicit formula for the optimum class prototype is found in the particular case of the Hausdorff distance for the L_∞ norm. When used for dynamical clustering of interval data, this prototype will ensure that the clustering criterion decreases at each iteration.

1 Introduction and Notation

Symbolic Data Analysis (SDA) deals with data tables where each cell is not only a single value but also an interval of values, a set of categories, or a frequency distribution. SDA generalizes well-known methods of multivariate data analysis to this new type of data representations (Diday, 1988; Bock and Diday, 2000).

Throughout this paper, we consider the problem of clustering a set $\Omega = \{1, ..., i, ..., n\}$ of n objects into K disjoint clusters $\{C_1, ..., C_K\}$ by dynamical clustering (Diday and Simon, 1976). Iterative algorithms or dynamical clustering methods for symbolic data have already been proposed in Bock (2001) and Verde et al. (2000).

Here, we consider the particular case of objects i described on each variable j by an interval $x_i^j = [a_i^j, b_i^j]$ of $\mathbb{R}$. In other words, an object i is a hyper-rectangle in the Euclidean space $\mathbb{R}^p$ and is written as:

$$x_i = \prod_{j=1}^{p} \underbrace{[a_i^j, b_i^j]}_{x_i^j}.$$

In dynamical clustering, the prototype y of a cluster C is defined by optimizing an adequacy criterion f measuring the "dissimilarity" between the prototype and the cluster. In the particular case of interval data, this prototype is a hyper-rectangle (see Fig. 1).

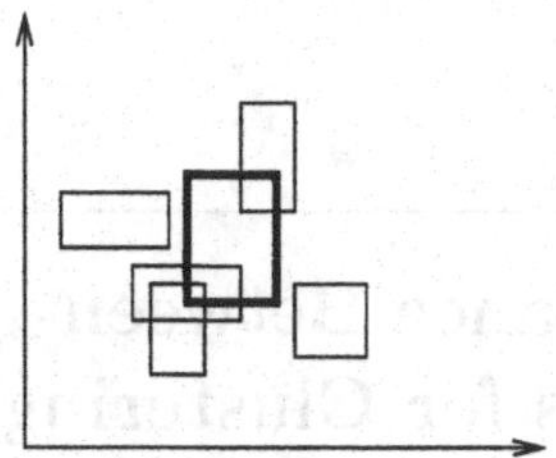

Fig. 1. A prototype y (thick line) of a set of rectangles (thin lines).

Here, the distance chosen to compare two p-dimensional hyper-rectangles is the Hausdorff distance d_H. This distance, defined to compare two sets of objects, depends on the distance chosen two compare two objects, here two points of $\mathbb{R}^p$. In the particular case where the Hausdorff distance is based on the L_∞ distance in $\mathbb{R}^p$, we are able to give an explicit formula for the prototype which minimizes:

$$f(y) = \max_{i \in C} d_H(x_i, y). \tag{1}$$

In the case of Hausdorff distances based on Euclidean or Manhattan distances between points, explicit formulas seem to be more difficult to find.

Chavent and Lechevallier (2002) give an explicit formula of the prototype $\hat{y}$ that minimizes the adequacy criterion

$$f(y) = \sum_{i \in C} d(x_i, y) \tag{2}$$

where d is not the Haudorff distance between two hyper-rectangles but the sum on each variable j of the one-dimensional Hausdorff distance d_H between two intervals.

In practice, the hyper-rectangle prototype defined in this article will probably be more sentitive to extreme values than the one defined in Chavent and Lechevallier (2002) but the distance used is a "real" Hausdorff distance on the $\mathbb{R}^p$-set.

2 The L_∞ Hausdorff Distance For Hyper-Rectangles

The Hausdorff distance (Nadler, 1978; Rote, 1991) is often used in image processing (Huttenlocher et al., 1993) to compare two sets A and B of objects. This distance depends on the distance d chosen to compare two objects u and v respectively in A and B.

We consider the L_∞ distance d_∞ between two points u and v of $\mathbb{R}^p$:

$$d_\infty(u, v) = \max_{j=1,\dots,p} |u_j - v_j| \tag{3}$$

and call "L_∞ Hausdorff distance" the Hausdorff distance associated to d_∞. Given that A and B are two hyper-rectangles in $\mathbb{R}^p$ denoted by

$$A = \prod_{j=1}^{p} A_j, \quad B = \prod_{j=1}^{p} B_j$$

where $A_j = [a_j, b_j]$ and $B_j = [\alpha_j, \beta_j]$ are intervals in $\mathbb{R}$, the L_∞ Hausdorff distance $d_{H,\infty}$ between A and B is defined by

$$d_{H,\infty}(A, B) = \max(h_\infty(A, B), h_\infty(B, A)) \tag{4}$$

where

$$h_\infty(A, B) = \sup_{u \in A} \inf_{v \in B} d_\infty(u, v). \tag{5}$$

In the one-dimensional case (i.e., $A_j = [a_j, b_j]$ and $B_j = [\alpha_j, \beta_j]$), we can drop the ∞ subscript:

$$h(A_j, B_j) = \sup_{u_j \in A_j} \inf_{v_j \in B_j} |u_j - v_j|, \tag{6}$$

and formula (4) simplifies to:

$$d_H(A_j, B_j) = \max\{|a_j - \alpha_j|, |b_j - \beta_j|\}. \tag{7}$$

This point will be used in the proof of properties 1 and 2, which are the basis for the explicit formulas for the optimum class prototype in Section 3.

Property 1. With the L_∞ distance, we have the following relation between asymmetric functions h in p dimensions and in one dimension:

$$h_\infty(A, B) = \max_{j=1,\ldots,p} h(A_j, B_j). \tag{8}$$

Proof.

$$\begin{aligned} h_\infty(A, B) &= \sup_{u \in A}\{\inf_{v \in B} \max_{j=1,\ldots,p} |u_j - v_j|\} \\ &= \sup_{u \in A}\{\max_{j=1,\ldots,p}\{\inf_{v_1 \in B_1} |u_1 - v_1|, \ldots, \inf_{v_p \in B_p} |u_p - v_p|\}\} \\ &= \max_{j=1,\ldots,p} \underbrace{\sup_{u_j \in A_j} \inf_{v_j \in B_j} |u_j - v_j|}_{h(A_j, B_j)}. \end{aligned}$$

Property 2. With the L_∞ distance, we have the following relation between the Haudorff distances d_H in p dimensions and in one dimension:

$$d_{H,\infty}(A, B) = \max_{j=1,\ldots,p} d_H(A_j, B_j). \tag{9}$$

Proof. From (8) we have:

$$h_\infty(A,B) = \max_{j=1,\dots,p} h(A_j,B_j)$$
$$h_\infty(B,A) = \max_{j=1,\dots,p} h(B_j,A_j).$$

Then

$$\begin{aligned} d_{H,\infty}(A,B) &= \max\{h_\infty(A,B), h_\infty(B,A)\} \\ &= \max_{j=1,\dots,p} \max\{h(A_j,B_j), h(B_j,A_j)\} \\ &= \max_{j=1,\dots,p} \underbrace{\max\{|a_j-\alpha_j|, |b_j-\beta_j|\}}_{d_H(A_j,B_j)}. \end{aligned}$$

3 The Optimum Class Prototype

We denote by y and $x_i \in C$ the hyper-rectangles which describe, respectively, the prototype and an object in cluster C:

$$y = \prod_{j=1}^{p} \underbrace{[\alpha^j, \beta^j]}_{y^j}$$

$$x_i = \prod_{j=1}^{p} \underbrace{[a_i^j, b_i^j]}_{x_i^j}.$$

We measure the "dissimilarity" between the prototype y and the cluster C by the mean of the function f defined in (1). In the particular case of the L_∞ Hausdorff distance (4),

$$f(y) = \max_{i\in C} d_{H,\infty}(x_i, y). \tag{10}$$

We define our prototype $\hat{y}$ as the hyper-rectangle which minimizes f. We see that:

$$f(y) = \max_{i\in C} \max_{j=1,\dots,p} d_H(x_i^j, y^j) \tag{11}$$
$$= \max_{j=1,\dots,p} \underbrace{\max_{i\in C} d_H(x_i^j, y^j)}_{\tilde{f}^j(y^j)}. \tag{12}$$

The equality (1) is due to property 2.

Now denote by $\hat{y}^j$ the minimizer of $\tilde{f}^j$ (see (2)) for $j=1,\dots,p$. Obviously, $\hat{y} = \prod_{j=1}^{p} \hat{y}^j$ is a minimizer of f, but for all indices j such that $\tilde{f}^j(\hat{y}^j) < f(\hat{y})$, all intervals $\tilde{y}^j$ such that $\tilde{f}^j(\tilde{y}^j) \leq f(\hat{y})$ also produce optimal solutions. Hence, the minimizer of f is not unique.

In the following, we shall use the minimizer $\hat{y} = \prod_{j=1}^{p} \hat{y}^j$, computable by the following explicit formulas (17) and (18).

We know from (2) and (7) that:

$$\tilde{f}^j(y^j) = \max_{i \in C} \max \{|a_i^j - \alpha^j|, |b_i^j - \beta^j|\}, \tag{13}$$

i.e.,

$$\tilde{f}^j(y^j) = \; max\, \{\max_{i \in C} |a_i^j - \alpha^j|, \max_{i \in C} |b_i^j - \beta^j|\}, \tag{14}$$

and so minimizing $\tilde{f}^j$ is equivalent to finding:

$$\min_{\alpha^j \in \mathbb{R}} \max_{i \in C} |a_i^j - \alpha^j| \tag{15}$$

and

$$\min_{\beta^j \in \mathbb{R}} \max_{i \in C} |b_i^j - \beta^j|. \tag{16}$$

The solutions $\hat{\alpha}^j$ and $\hat{\beta}^j$ are:

$$\hat{\alpha}^j = \frac{\max_{i \in C} a_i^j + \min_{i \in C} a_i^j}{2} \tag{17}$$

$$\hat{\beta}^j = \frac{\max_{i \in C} b_i^j - \min_{i \in C} b_i^j}{2}. \tag{18}$$

An example of the construction of this optimum prototype $\hat{y}$ is given in Figs.2 and 3.

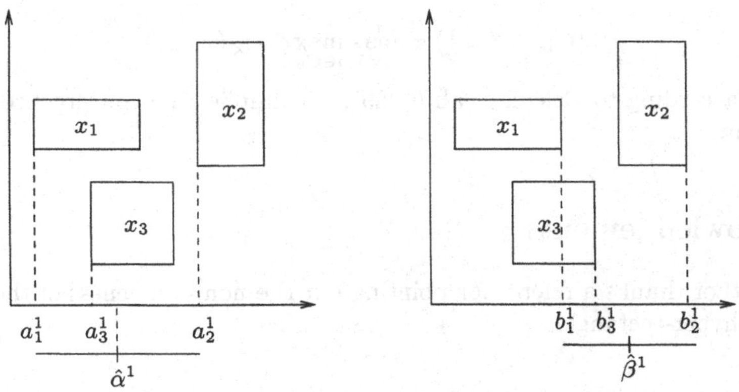

Fig. 2. Construction of a prototype $\hat{y}$ for $j = 1$; i.e., $\hat{y}^1 = [\hat{\alpha}^1, \hat{\beta}^1]$.

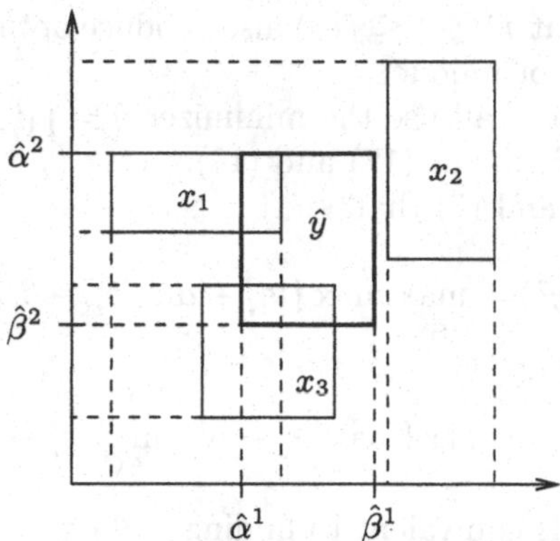

Fig. 3. Construction of a prototype $\hat{y}$.

4 Application to Dynamical Clustering

Dynamical clustering algorithm proceeds by iteratively determining the K class prototypes y_k and then reassigning all objects to the closest class prototype. The advantage of using the L_∞ Hausdorff distance and the adequacy criterion defined above is that we can get explicit and simple formulas for the prototypes.

As for the convergence of the algorithm, the prototypes which minimize the adequacy criterion ensure the decrease of any of the two clustering criteria (19) and (20), independently of the choice of the minimizer:

$$g(\{C_1, ..., C_K\}) = \sum_{k=1}^{K} \max_{i \in C_k} d_{H,\infty}(x_i, y_k) \tag{19}$$

$$g(\{C_1, ..., C_K\}) = \max_{k=1}^{K} \max_{i \in C_k} d_{H,\infty}(x_i, y_k). \tag{20}$$

Hence, according to Celeux et al. (1989), this implies the convergence of the algorithm.

Acknowledgements

The author thanks a referee for pointing out the non-uniqueness of the minimizing hyper-rectangle.

References

1. Bock, H.-H. (2001). "Clustering Algorithms and Kohonen Maps for Symbolic Data," in *ICNCB Proceedings*, Springer:Heidelberg, pp. 203–215.

2. Bock, H.-H., and Diday, E. (2000). *Analysis of Symbolic Data: Exploratory Methods for Extracting Statistical Information from Complex Data*, Studies in Classification, Data Analysis, and Knowledge Organisation, Springer-Verlag, Heidelberg.
3. Celeux, G., Diday, E., Govaert, G., Lechevallier, Y., and Ralambondrainy, H. (1989). *Classification Automatique des Données*. Dunod, Paris.
4. Chavent, M., and Lechevallier, Y. (2002). "Dynamical Clustering of Interval Data: Optimization of an Adequacy Criterion Based on Hausdorff Distance," in *Classification, Clustering, and Data Analysis*, eds. K. (Jajuga, A. Sokolowski, and H.-H. Bock, Berlin:Springer-Verlag, pp. 53–60.
5. Diday, E. (1988). "The Symbolic Approach in Clustering and Related Methods of Data Analysis: The Basic Choices," in *Classification and Related Methods of Data Analysis*, ed. H.-H. Bock, Amsterdam:North Holland, pp. 673–684
6. Diday, E., and Simon, J. C. (1976). "Clustering Analysis," in *Digital Pattern Classification*, ed. K. S. Fu, Berlin:Springer-Verlag, pp. 47–94.
7. Huttenlocher, D. P., Klanderman, G. A. and Rucklidge, W. J. (1993). "Comparing Images Using the Hausdorff Distance," *IEEE Transaction on Pattern Analysis and Machine Intelligence*, **15**, 850–863.
8. Nadler, S. B. Jr. (1978). *Hyperspaces of Sets*, Marcel Dekker, Inc., New York.
9. Rote, G. (1991). "Computing the Minimum Hausdorff Distance Between Two Point Sets on a Line Under Translation," *Information Processing Letters*, **38**, 123–127.
10. Verde, R., De Carvalho, F. A. T., and Lechevallier, Y. (2000). "A Dynamical Clustering Algorithm for Multinominal Data," in *Data Analysis, Classification and Related Methods*, eds. H. A. L. Kiers et al., Berlin:Springer-Verlag, pp. 387–394.

Kolmogorov-Smirnov for Decision Trees on Interval and Histogram Variables

Chérif Mballo[1,2] and Edwin Diday[2]

[1] Ecole Supérieure d'Informatique, Electronique et Automatique (ESIEA), France
mballo@esiea-ouest.fr
[2] Universite Paris Dauphine, France
diday@ceremade.dauphine.fr

Abstract: With advances in technology, data sets often contain a very large number of observations. Symbolic data analysis treats new units that are underlying concepts of the given data base or that are found by clustering. In this way, it is possible to reduce the size of the data to be treated by transforming the initial classical variables into variables called symbolic variables. In symbolic data analysis, we consider, among other types, interval and histogram variables. The algebraic structure of these variables leads us to adapt dissimilarity measures to be able to study them. The Kolmogorov-Smirnov criterion is used as a test selection metric for decision tree induction. Our contribution in this paper is to adapt this criterion of Kolmogorov-Smirnov to these types of variables. We present an example to illustrate this approach.

1 Introduction

In the last few years, the extension of the classical data analysis methods to new objects with more complex structure has been a prominent research topic (Bock and al., 2000). The aim of symbolic data analysis is to consider the data's particularities in the treatment methods without losing information.

Some authors (Perinel, 1996; Yapo, 2002) have been interested in building decision trees for symbolic variables. They treat explicitly probabilistic data (each unit is formally described by a probability distribution).

A variety of test selection metrics have been proposed, including gain and gain ratio (Quinlan, 1993), Gini's criterion (Breiman and al., 1984), and so on. We extend the metric proposed by Friedman (1977) based on Kolmogorov-Smirnov (KS) distance to the case of interval and histogram variables. The KS criterion (Utgoff and al., 1996) requires that individuals have to be ordered by their description (variable values). This criterion is used as a test selection metric (splitting criterion or attribute selection metric) to build a decision tree induction (Friedman, 1977). It is based on the cumulative distribution functions of the prior classes. Its advantage is that it gives the best split on each predictor in order that the two probability distributions associated to the two prior classes has the largest KS criterion value.

We have been interested in different possible orders of the variables (interval or histogram data). We consider a population of n objects (individuals). Each object is described by a symbolic data table with p variables: one response variable (the class variable) and the $p-1$ remaining variables are the predictors. In the beginning, the variable to explain is not partitioned. We transform this symbolic variable to explain, as in the example in Section 4, the class variable as discussed in Diday and al. (2003) with the Fisher algorithm (Fisher, 1958) to obtain the prior classes. The prior classes may be derived from supervised classification.

2 Ordering

This section describes issues that arise in ordering symbolic data that are interval-valued or histogram-valued.

2.1 Order of Interval Variables

A variable is called *interval type* if the value taken by each observation on this variable is a closed interval. We denote the set of closed intervals of real numbers by $\Im$. Thus, if $x \in \Im$, then $x = [l(x), r(x)]$ for some real numbers $l(x)$ ("l" as left bound), $r(x)$ ("r" as right bound) such that $l(x) \leq r(x)$. Taking two intervals $x = [l(x), r(x)]$ and $y = [l(y), r(y)]$, the by $x = y$ we mean, of course, that $l(x) = l(y)$ and $r(x) = r(y)$. To study an order relation on $\Im$, it is important to distinguish between two different situations: the case in which the intervals are disjoint or non-disjoint.

Some authors (Fishburn, 1985; Pirlot and al., 1997) have been interested in interval orders. The case of non-disjoint intervals has been broached by (Tsoukias and al., 2001) in the preference modelling area.

Disjoint Intervals

Let D be the subset of $\Im$ composed of all intervals such that

$$x_i \cap x_j = \emptyset \; \forall \, i \neq j.$$

By xRy, we mean that the interval x is *strictly before* the interval y. Mathematically, this relation R on D may be defined as follows:

$$xRy \Leftrightarrow r(x) < l(y).$$

This relation R is transitive and anti-reflexive, so it is a total order on D. It is clear that, graphically, when xRy, the interval x has a position which is "totally before" y. For example, ordering two intervals x and y for a time variable, x will be "totally before" y because x "finishes before" y 'starts".

Non-Disjoint Intervals

For overlapping intervals different situations may occur according to the position of the intervals.

-*Ordering Using Lower Bounds:* Two possibilities exist:

(i) lower bounds are distinct: the interval order is related to the position of the lower bounds;

(ii) lower bounds are equal: the interval order is related to the position of the upper bounds.

By xIy, we mean that the interval x is "almost before" the interval y. Mathematically, this relation I on $\Im$ may be defined as follows:

$$\begin{array}{l}\text{If } l(x) \neq l(y), \text{ then } xIy \Leftrightarrow l(x) < l(y);\\ \text{if } l(x) = l(y), \text{ then } xIy \Leftrightarrow r(x) < r(y).\end{array}$$

This relation I is transitive and anti-reflexive, so it is a total order on $\Im$.

The statement "almost before" is used just to point out that the intervals are non-disjoint and not every element in x is less than or equal to any element in y. For the interval x, we may say only that there is at least one element which is less than or equal to any element in y. Considering again the case of a time variable, x is "almost before" y if x "starts before" y but it does not matter which one "finishes" first; on the contrary, in the case in which x and y "start" at the same time, the interval which "finishes" first will be considered "almost before" the other one.

-*Ordering Using Upper Bounds:* Also in this case, two possibilities exist:

(i) upper bounds are distinct: the interval order is related to the position of the upper bounds;

(ii) upper bounds are equal: the interval order is related to the position of the lower bounds.

By sXy, we mean that the interval y is "almost after" the interval x. Mathematically, the following relation S on $\Im$ may be defined as follows:

$$\begin{array}{l}\text{If } r(x) \neq r(y), \text{ then } xSy \Leftrightarrow r(x) < r(y);\\ \text{if } r(x) = r(y), \text{ then } xSy \Leftrightarrow l(x) < l(y).\end{array}$$

The relation S is transitive and anti-reflexive, so it is a total order on $\Im$.

In analogy to the relation I introduced before, here the statement "almost after" is used to point out that the intervals are non-disjoint and not every element in y is greater than or equal to any element in x. In the interval y, there is at least one element which is greater than or equal to any element in x. In the case of a time variable, y is "almost after" x if y "ends after" x but it doesn't matter which one "starts" first; on the contrary, in the case in which y and x "end" at the same time, the interval which "starts after" will be considered "almost after" the other one.

Let us analyze the following four cases which refer to the possible different positions of the intervals to be ordered. The aim is to understand the difference between the two interval orders I and S in order to give to the reader the background to decide which order is the more suitable for treating his or her own data.

Case 1: $l(x) = l(y)$ and $r(y) < r(x)$
$l(x)$[——————] $r(x)$
$l(y)$[———] $r(y)$
yIx "y is *almost before* x"
ySx "*x is almost after y*"

Case 2: $l(x) < l(y)$ and $r(y) < r(x)$
$l(x)$[————]$r(x)$
$l(y)$[——] $r(y)$
xIy "*x* is *almost before y*"
ySx "*x is almost after y*"

Case 3: $l(x) < l(y)$ and $r(y) = r(x)$
$l(x)$[——————] $r(x)$
$l(y)$[————] $r(y)$
xIy "x is *almost before* y"
xSy "y is almost after x"

Case 4: $l(x) < l(y)$ and $r(x) < r(y)$
$l(x)$[————]$r(x)$
$l(y)$[————] $r(y)$
xIy "*x* is *almost before y*"
xSy "*y is almost after x*"

Considering two intervals x and y that are not strictly included one within another, as in Cases 1,3, and 4, if x is *almost before* y with respect to the relation I, then y is *almost after* x with respect to the relation S. In other words, I and S create the same relation of *precedence* between two intervals.

When the intervals are strictly included one within another as in Case 2, it turns out that x is *almost before* y with respect to the relation I, but x is also *almost after* y with respect to the relation S. This is the main difference between the two interval orders I and S. Taking into account this difference, the reader has to decide which one is more suitable for his own data.

An alternative, and the simplest, way to order intervals is to take into account the only position of the centers.

2.2 Order of Histogram Variables

A variable is called *histogram type* if the value taken by each observation for this variable is a histogram. We define a histogram by the weights associated with each category of a categorical variable. Several orderings of histogram variables are possible.

Ordering By the Average: The average of the weights is calculated for each individual. The order of the histograms is given by the natural order of the calculated values.

Ordering By the Median: The order of the histograms is established by the order of the respective medians calculated in the classical way.

Ordering By the Standard Deviation: The standard deviation is computed for each individual and the order of the histograms is established by the natural order of the calculated values.

It may happen that two histograms have the same average or median. In this instance, we proceed as follows: when two histograms have the same averages, we then compare their medians and when their medians are also equal, we then compare their standard deviations (this is a lexicographical order). Another alternative is also to order by the mode.

3 Decision Tree

To build a decision tree, we need a criterion in order to separate the population of one node, denoted C, into two subpopulations that are more homogeneous (two children nodes). We use the Kolmogorov-Smirnov criterion (KS).

Consider the case of two classes and suppose we need to find a single cut point x that partitions the values of an interval or a histogram variable into two blocks. One block (the left node) contains those values of X for which XRx (where R is one of the relations defined in Section 2) and the other block (the right node) contains the remaining values. When we have m classes, the principle consists of grouping these m classes into two classes ($2^{m-1} - 1$ possibilities) called superclasses. The KS criterion allows the separation of a population into two groups that are more homogeneous. It uses the two cumulative distribution functions resulting from grouping the m original classes into two superclasses. The method called *twoing* (Breiman and al., 1984) is used to generate, from the m classes, two superclasses C_1 and C_2 to which are associated the two cumulative distribution functions F_1 and F_2 of a symbolic random variable X. Because the calculation of KS distance involves only the cumulative distributions, we need only consider approximations. The empirical cumulative distribution function (approximate cumulative function) $\hat{F}_i$ (i=1,2) which estimates F_i is given by:

$$\hat{F}_i(x) = \frac{\#\{(XRx/X \in C) \cap C_i\}}{\#(C_i)} \tag{1}$$

where R is one of the relations defined in Section 2 and $\#A$ is the cardinality of set A. So the Kolmogorov-Smirnov criterion (or an optimal cut point x) is defined by :

$$KS(x) = \sup_x \left| \hat{F}_1(x) - \hat{F}_2(x) \right|, \tag{2}$$

This maximum value is the KS distance for this variable. It is a natural extension of this criterion KS, but the argument selected for the cutting is a closed interval or a histogram (according to the type of the selected predictor) and not a real number as in the classical case. Thus, we can use all the other steps (because these steps are common to all variable types) in order to build the decision tree. The principle consists of selecting, at each node, the most discriminating predictor (therefore the description of the corresponding individual) to maximize the KS criterion.

4 Partitioning a Symbolic Response Variable

When the response variable is not a class variable but a histogram or an interval type, how should we transform it into a class variable? To answer this question in an optimal way, we use the Fisher algorithm (Fisher, 1958). For example, in the case of two classes, the data are ordered and each of them is classified into one of the two classes $C_1 = \{i/i \leq w\}$ and $C_2 = \{i/i > w\}$. The partition C= (C_1, C_2) is the one which minimizes

$$W(C_1, C_2) = \sum_{l \in \{1,2\}} \sum_{i,j \in C_l} D(i, j) \tag{3}$$

where D is a numerical measure between intervals or histograms.

Table 1 uses data on developing and developed countries, as described in the following section. It contains the name of the individuals (first column), the initial values (second column), the order obtained by the lower bound (third column). Partitioning this variable into two classes, we obtain the fourth column. For the partitioning criterion used by the Fisher algorithm, we take the Hausdorff distance D between interval data defined as follows:

$$D([a, b]; [c, d]) = \max\left(|a - c|, |b - d|\right).$$

Table 1. Initial values, order, and class for life expectancy data.

Individuals	Life Exp.	Order	Class
DAMQ	[67.2;78.5]	SDAFR	2
SDAMQ	[64;76]	SDOCE	2
DEUR	[77.2;79.3]	DAFR	2
SDEUR	[66.1;78.2]	SDASI	2
DOCE	[68.4;78.7]	SDAMQ	2
SDOCE	[55.6;70.5]	DASI	1
DAFR	[56.7;70.7]	SDEUR	1
SDAFR	[40.6;52.3]	DAMQ	1
DASI	[65.1;80.5]	DOCE	2
SDASI	[62.3;71.9]	DEUR	1

The description of the Class 1 is [40.6;71.9] and the one for Class 2 is [64;80.5]. This partitioning enables us to transform a symbolic variable for explanation as a class variable; see Diday and al., (2003) for details. In this example, we chose just two classes. However, the method can be applied to k classes ($k < n$ where n is the number of the individuals).

5 Application

Table 2 shows data from countries in 2000, organized according to the composite indicators of development accepted by international organizations such as the World Bank, the International Monetary Fund and the United Nations. To obtain the data go to website

`www.ceremade.dauphine.fr/~touati/exemples.htm`

which is the URL for the free software SODAS (for Statistical Official Data Analysis Software).

Table 2. The initial database, obtained from SODAS.

Obs.	Population	PGR	NPR	Y
DAMQ	[15211;283230]	[0.9;1.8]	[0.857143;0.142857;0;0;0;0]	2
SDAMQ	[2576;25662]	[0.8;2.6]	[0.75;0.25;0;0;0;0]	2
DEUR	[4469;82017]	[0;0.5]	[0;0.833333;0.166667;0;0;0]	2
SDEUR	[1988;145491]	[-0.4;0.2]	[0.166667;0.833333;0;0;0;0]	2
DOCE	[814;19138]	[0.9;1.2]	[0;1;0;0;0;0]	2
SDOCE	[159;4809]	[0;2.7]	[0;1;0;0;0;0]	1
DAFR	[1161;67884]	[0.8;1.9]	[0.4;0.2;0.2;0.2;0;0]	1
SDAFR	[1757;35119]	[0.9;2.9]	[0.833333;0.166667;0;0;0;0]	1
DASI	[4913;1275130]	[0.3;2.9]	[0.2;0.4;0;0;0.2;0.2]	2
SDASI	[16189;1008940]	[1.4;2.6]	[0.4;0.2;0;0;0.4;0]	1

The first column of the table indicates the names of the individuals, which are groups of countries within continents. Countries are part of either of two economic entities: developed countries and developing countries. The initial data are from 50 countries on five continents. By crossing economic category with the continents this reduces to ten symbolic data points, one for each combination of economic category and continent.

The variable to explain is Y=*Life Expectancy*, partitioned as in Section 4. The remaining variables of this database are the predictors. There two predictors of the interval type; X_1 is Population and X_2 is Population Growth Rate (PGR). There is one predictor of histogram type; X_3 describes the nature of the political regime (NPR). This histogram variable has six categories: presidential, parliamentary, presidential-parliamentary, monarchy, constitutional, and popular. For the histogram data, the values in each category of an observed histogram are presented in brackets, in the order above.

In Table 2 we represent only the values of the categories. As these values are probabilistic, we notice that practically all the individuals have the same average and many of them also have the same medians. Therefore, we order the variable of histogram type by the standard deviation, as discussed in Section 2.2. We order the interval variables by lower bounds, as in Section

2.1, and thus obtain Table 3. In this table, we represent just the order of the individuals (increasing order) but this order is given by their description (we specify also the prior class of each individual for each predictor).

Table 3. Order and classes of the individuals by the predictor.

Pop.	Class	PGR	Class	NPR	Class
SDOCE	1	SDEUR	2	DAFR	1
DOCE	2	DEUR	2	DASI	2
DAFR	1	SDOCE	1	SDASI	1
SDAFR	1	DASI	2	SDAMQ	2
SDEUR	2	DAFR	1	DEUR	2
SDAMQ	2	SDAMQ	2	SDEUR	2
DEUR	2	DOCE	2	SDAFR	1
DASI	2	DAMQ	2	DAMQ	2
DAMQ	2	SDAFR	1	DOCE	2
SDASI	1	SDASI	1	SDOCE	1

It remains to calculate the KS criterion of each individual for each predictor (as indicated in Section 3) in order to deduce the most discriminanting predictor. This leads to Fig. 1.

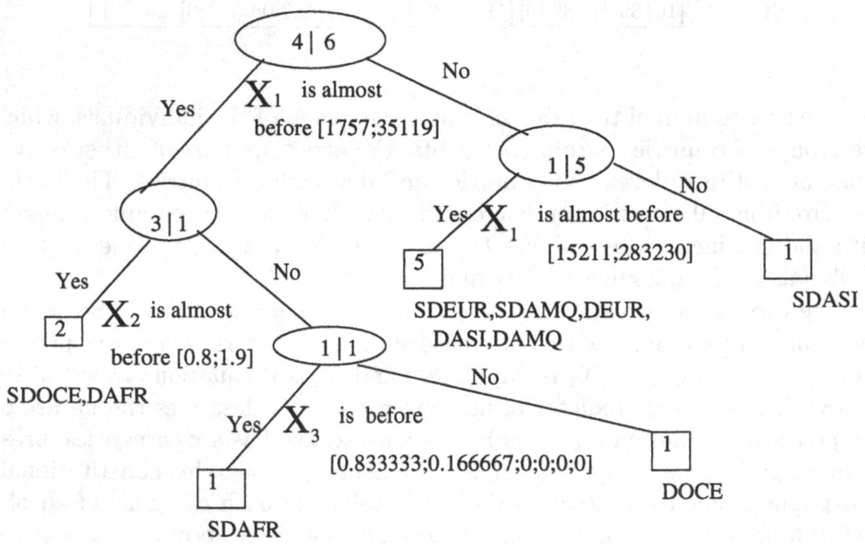

Fig. 1. Decision tree.

As we have a small file, a node is declared terminal (a leaf) when it is pure. In the case of a file having several individuals, one can declare, for example, a node as a terminal node when the size of one class is large with respect to the others (in this case, one can calculate the misclassification rate). Graphically, we represent an interior node by an ellipsis (containing at the left the size of the class 1 and at the right the one of the class 2) and a terminal node by a rectangle containing its size. We obtain five decision rules corresponding to the five terminal nodes. These decision rules permit the classification of new observations. For example, the decision rule for a new case w for the second terminal node is:

> If $X_1(w)$ is *almost before* $[1757; 35119]$ and $X_2(w)$ is *almost after* $[0.8; 1.9]$ and $X_3(w)$ is *before* $[0.833333; 0.166667; 0; 0; 0; 0]$, then the *Life Expectancy* of w is [40.6;71.9].

6 Conclusion and Perspectives

In this paper, we point out an extension of Kolmogorov-Smirnov criterion to the case where the variables are interval or histogram type. This criterion treats all the predictors together and it finds the most discriminating for each internal node. We propose in our future work to adapt the Kolmogorov-Smirnov criterion and the Fisher algorithm to other symbolic variables and to examine their complexity. The aim is to obtain a structured set of symbolic objects from the terminal nodes of the decision tree.

References

1. Bock, H. H., and Diday, E. (2000). *Analysis of Symbolic Data: Exploratory Methods for Extracting Statistical Information from Complex Data,* Springer, Berlin-Heidelberg.
2. Breiman, L., and Friedman, J. H., and Olshen, R., and Stone, C. J. (1984). *Classification and Regression Trees,* Belmont CA, Wadsworth.
3. Diday, E., and Gioia, F., and Mballo, C. (2003). "Codage Qualitatif d'une Variable Intervalle," *Journées de Statistique,* **35**, 415–418.
4. Fishburn, P. C. (1985). *Interval Orders and Interval Graphs: A Study of Partially Ordered Sets,* Wiley-Interscience, New York.
5. Fisher, W. D. (1958). "On Grouping for Maximum Homogeneity," *Journal of American Statistical Association,* **53**, 789–798.
6. Friedman, J. H. (1977). "A Recursive Partitioning Decision Rule for Nonparametric Classification," *IEEE Transactions on Computers,* **C-26**, 404–408.
7. Périnel, E. (1996). *Segmentation et Analyse des Données Symboliques : Application á des Données Probabilistes Imprécises.* Ph.D Thesis, Université Paris Dauphine, Paris.
8. Pirlot, M., Vincke, P. (1997). *Semi-orders: Properties, Representations, Applications,* Kluwer Academic Publishers, Dordrecht.
9. Quinlan, J. R. (1993). *C4.5: Programs for Machine Learning,* Morgan Kaufmann, San Mateo, CA.

10. Tsoukias, A., and The N. A. (2001). "Numerical Representation of PQI Interval Orders," *LAMSADE Université Paris Dauphine*, **184**, 1–27.
11. Utgoff, P. E., and Clouse, J. A. (1996). "A Kolmogorov-Smirnoff Metric for Decision Tree Induction," University of Massachusetts at Amherst Technical Report 96-3.
12. Yapo, J. P. A. (2002). *Méthodes de Segmentation sur un Tableau de Variables Aléatoires,* Ph.D Thesis, Université Paris Dauphine, Paris.

Dynamic Cluster Methods for Interval Data Based on Mahalanobis Distances

Renata M.C.R. de Souza[1], Francisco de A.T. de Carvalho[1], Camilo P. Tenório[1] and Yves Lechevallier[2]

[1] Cidade Universitaria, Brazil
fatc,rmcrs,cpt@cin.ufpe.br
[2] INRIA - Rocquencourt, France
Yves.Lechevallier@inria.fr

Abstract: Dynamic cluster methods for interval data are presented. Two methods are considered: the first method furnishes a partition of the input data and a corresponding prototype (a vector of intervals) for each class by optimizing an adequacy criterion which is based on Mahalanobis distances between vectors of intervals. The second is an adaptive version of the first method. Experimental results with artificial interval-valued data sets show the usefulness of these methods. In general, the adaptive method outperforms the non-adaptive one in terms of the quality of the clusters which are produced by the algorithms.

1 Introduction

Cluster analysis has been widely used in numerous fields including pattern recognition, data mining, and image processing. The goal in these problems is to group data into clusters such that objects within a cluster have high degree of similarity whereas objects belonging to different clusters have high degree of dissimilarity.

The dynamic cluster algorithm (Diday and Simon, 1976) is a partition clustering method whose aim is to obtain both a partition of the input data and the identification of a suitable representation or prototype (means, axes, probability laws, groups of elements, etc.) for each cluster by locally minimizing an adequacy criterion that measures the fit between the clusters and their representation. The k-means algorithm, in which the cluster centroid (the prototype in this case) is updated after all the objects have been considered for relocation, is a particular case of dynamic clustering with adequacy function equal to the squared error criterion (Jain, Murty, and Flynn, 1999).

In the adaptive version of the dynamic cluster method (Diday and Govaert, 1977), at each iteration there is a different measure for the comparison of each cluster with its own representation. The advantage of these adaptive distances is that the clustering algorithm is able to recognize clusters of different shapes and sizes.

Often, objects to be clustered are represented as a vector of quantitative features. However, the recording of interval-valued data has become a common practice in real world applications and nowadays this kind of data is widely used to describe objects. Symbolic Data Analysis (SDA) is a new area related to multivariate analysis and pattern recognition, and it has provided suitable data analysis methods for managing objects described as a vector of intervals (Bock and Diday, 2000).

Concerning partition clustering methods, SDA has provided suitable tools. Verde et al. (2001) introduced a dynamic cluster algorithm for interval data using context-dependent proximity functions. Chavent and Lechevallier (2002) proposed a dynamic cluster algorithm for interval data using an adequacy criterion based on Hausdorff distance. Souza and De Carvalho (2004) presented dynamic clustering algorithms for interval data based on adaptive and non-adaptive city-block distances.

The main contribution of this paper is to introduce two dynamic cluster methods for interval data. The first method furnishes a partition of the input data and a corresponding prototype (a vector of intervals) for each class by optimizing an adequacy criterion which is based on the Mahalanobis distances between vectors of intervals (section 2). The second is an adaptive version of the first method (section 3). In both methods, the prototype of each cluster is represented by a vector of intervals, where the bounds of each interval are, respectively, for a fixed variable, the average of the set of lower bounds, and the average of the set of upper bounds of the intervals of the objects belonging to the cluster for the same variable. In order to show the usefulness of these methods, several artificial interval data sets with different degrees of clustering difficulty were considered. The evaluation of the clustering results is based on an external validity index in the framework of a Monte Carlo experiment (section 4). Finally, in section 5 we describe our conclusions.

2 Clustering With Non-Adaptive Mahalanobis Distance

Let $E = \{s_1, \ldots, s_n\}$ be a set of n symbolic objects described by p interval variables. Each object s_i $(i = 1, \ldots, n)$ can be represented as a vector of intervals $\mathbf{x}_i = ([a_i^1, b_i^1], \ldots, [a_i^p, b_i^p])^T$. Let P be a partition of E into K clusters $C_1, \ldots, C_K$, where each cluster C_k $(k = 1, \ldots, K)$ has a prototype L_k that is also represented as a vector of intervals $\mathbf{y}_k = ([\alpha_k^1, \beta_k^1], \ldots, [\alpha_k^p, \beta_k^p])^T$.

According to the standard dynamic clustering algorithm, our method looks for both a partition $P = (C_1, \ldots, C_K)$ of a set of objects into K clusters and also the corresponding set of prototypes $L = (L_1, \ldots, L_K)$. This is done locally by minimizing an adequacy criterion that is usually defined in the following way:

$$W_1(P,L) = \sum_{k=1}^{K} \Delta_k^1(L_k) = \sum_{k=1}^{K} \sum_{i \in C_k} \delta(\mathbf{x}_i, \mathbf{y}_k) \tag{1}$$

where $\delta(\mathbf{x}_i, \mathbf{y}_k)$ is a distance measure between an object $s_i \in C_k$ and the class prototype L_k of C_k.

Let $\mathbf{x}_{iL} = (a_i^1, \ldots, a_i^p)^T$ and $\mathbf{x}_{iU} = (b_i^1, \ldots, b_i^p)^T$ be two vectors containing the lower and upper bounds, respectively, of the intervals describing $\mathbf{x}_i$. Consider also $\mathbf{y}_{kL} = (\alpha_k^1, \ldots, \alpha_k^p)^T$ and $\mathbf{y}_{kU} = (\beta_k^1, \ldots, \beta_k^p)^T$; these are two vectors containing the lower and upper bounds, respectively, of the intervals describing $\mathbf{y}_k$.

We define the distance between the two vectors of intervals $\mathbf{x}_i$ and $\mathbf{y}_k$ as

$$\delta(\mathbf{x}_i, \mathbf{y}_k) = d(\mathbf{x}_{iL}, \mathbf{y}_{kL}) + d(\mathbf{x}_{iU}, \mathbf{y}_{kU}) \tag{2}$$

where

$$d(\mathbf{x}_{iL}, \mathbf{y}_{kL}) = (\mathbf{x}_{iL} - \mathbf{y}_{kL})^T \mathbf{M}_L (\mathbf{x}_{iL} - \mathbf{y}_{kL}) \tag{3}$$

is the Mahalanobis distance between the two vectors $\mathbf{x}_{iL}$ and $\mathbf{y}_{kL}$ and

$$d(\mathbf{x}_{iU}, \mathbf{y}_{kU}) = (\mathbf{x}_{iU} - \mathbf{y}_{kU})^T \mathbf{M}_U (\mathbf{x}_{iU} - \mathbf{y}_{kU}) \tag{4}$$

is the Mahalanobis distance between the two vectors $\mathbf{x}_{iU}$ and $\mathbf{y}_{kU}$.

The matrices $\mathbf{M}_L$ and $\mathbf{M}_U$ are defined, respectively, as:

(i) $\mathbf{M}_L = (\det(\mathbf{Q}_{poolL}))^{1/p}\ \mathbf{Q}_{poolL}^{-1}$, where $\mathbf{Q}_{poolL}$ is the pooled covariance matrix with $\det(\mathbf{Q}_{poolL}) \neq 0$, i.e.,

$$\mathbf{Q}_{poolL} = \frac{(n_1 - 1)\mathbf{S}_{1L} + \ldots + (n_K - 1)\mathbf{S}_{KL}}{n_1 + \ldots + n_K - K}. \tag{5}$$

In eqn. (5), $\mathbf{S}_{kL}$ is the covariance matrix of the set of vectors $\{\mathbf{x}_{iL} : i \in C_k\}$ and n_k is the cardinality of C_k $(k = 1, \ldots, K)$.

(ii) $\mathbf{M}_U = (\det(\mathbf{Q}_{poolU}))^{1/p}\ \mathbf{Q}_{poolU}^{-1}$, where $\mathbf{Q}_{poolU}$ is the pooled covariance matrix with $\det(\mathbf{Q}_{poolU}) \neq 0$, i.e.,

$$\mathbf{Q}_{poolU} = \frac{(n_1 - 1)\mathbf{S}_{1U} + \ldots + (n_k - 1)\mathbf{S}_{KU}}{n_1 + \ldots + n_K - K}. \tag{6}$$

In eqn. (6), $\mathbf{S}_{kU}$ is the covariance matrix of the set of vectors $\{\mathbf{x}_{iU} : s_i \in C_k\}$ and n_k is again the cardinality of C_k $(k = 1, \ldots, K)$.

2.1 The Optimization Problem

In this method the optimization problem is stated as follows: Find the vector of intervals $\mathbf{y}_k = ([\alpha_k^1, \beta_k^1], \ldots, [\alpha_k^p, \beta_k^p])$ which locally minimizes the following adequacy criterion:

$$\Delta_k^1(L_k) = \sum_{i \in C_k} (\mathbf{x}_{iL} - \mathbf{y}_{kL})^T \mathbf{M}_L (\mathbf{x}_{iL} - \mathbf{y}_{kL}) + \sum_{i \in C_k} (\mathbf{x}_{iU} - \mathbf{y}_{kU})^T \mathbf{M}_U (\mathbf{x}_{iU} - \mathbf{y}_{kU}). \quad (7)$$

The problem now becomes that of finding the two vectors $\mathbf{y}_{kL}$ and $\mathbf{y}_{kU}$ which minimize the criterion $\Delta_1^k(L_k)$. According to Govaert (1975), the solution for $\mathbf{y}_{kL}$ and $\mathbf{y}_{kU}$ are obtained from the Huygens' theorem. The solutions are, respectively, the mean vectors of the sets $\{\mathbf{x}_{iL} : s_i \in C_k\}$ and $\{\mathbf{x}_{iU} : s_i \in C_k\}$.

Therefore, $\mathbf{y}_k$ is a vector of intervals whose bounds are, for each variable j, the average of the set of lower bounds and the average of the set of upper bounds, respectively, of the intervals of all of the objects that are members of the cluster C_k.

2.2 The Algorithm

The dynamic cluster algorithm with non-adaptive Mahalanobis distance has the following steps:

(1) *Initialization.* Randomly choose a partition $\{C_1 \ldots, C_K\}$ of E.
(2) *Representation step.*
For $k = 1$ to K compute $\mathbf{y}_k = ([\alpha_k^1, \beta_k^1], \ldots, [\alpha_k^p, \beta_k^p])$ where α_k^j is the average of $\{a_i^j : s_i \in C_k\}$ and β_k^j is the average of $\{b_i^j : s_i \in C_k\}$, $j = 1, \ldots, p$.
(3) *Allocation step.*
$test \leftarrow 0$

for $i = 1$ to n do
  define the cluster C_{k*} such that
    $k* = \text{argmin}_{k=1,\ldots,K} (\mathbf{x}_{iL} - \mathbf{y}_{kL})^T \mathbf{M}_L (\mathbf{x}_{iL} - \mathbf{y}_{kL}) + (\mathbf{x}_{iU} - \mathbf{y}_{kU})^T \mathbf{M}_U (\mathbf{x}_{iU} - \mathbf{y}_{kU})$
  if $i \in C_k$ and $k* \neq k$
    $test \leftarrow 1$
    $C_{k*} \leftarrow C_{k*} \cup \{s_i\}$
    $C_k \leftarrow C_k \setminus \{s_i\}$

(4) *Stopping criterion.*
If $test = 0$ then STOP, else go to Step 2.

3 Clustering With Adaptive Mahalanobis Distance

The dynamic clustering algorithm with adaptive distances (Diday and Govaert, 1977) also has a representation and an allocation step but there is a different distance associated with each cluster. The algorithm looks for a partition into K clusters, the corresponding K prototypes, and K different distances associated with the clusters. This is done by locally minimizing an adequacy criterion which is usually stated as:

$$W_2(P,L) = \sum_{k=1}^{K} \Delta_k^2(L_k, \delta_k) = \sum_{k=1}^{K} \sum_{i \in C_k} \delta_k(\mathbf{x}_i, \mathbf{y}_k) \tag{8}$$

where $\delta_k(\mathbf{x}_i, \mathbf{y}_k)$ is an adaptive dissimilarity measure between object $s_i \in C_k$ and the class prototype L_k for C_k.

To take account of the intra-class structure of the cluster C_k, we consider here an adaptive Mahalanobis distance between an object s_i and the prototype L_k, which is defined as:

$$\begin{aligned}\delta_k(\mathbf{x}_i, \mathbf{y}_k) = {} & (\mathbf{x}_{iL} - \mathbf{y}_{kL})^T \mathbf{M}_{kL} (\mathbf{x}_{iL} - \mathbf{y}_{kL}) + \\ & (\mathbf{x}_{iU} - \mathbf{y}_{kU})^T \mathbf{M}_{kU} (\mathbf{x}_{iU} - \mathbf{y}_{kU})\end{aligned} \tag{9}$$

where $\mathbf{M}_{kL}$ and $\mathbf{M}_{kU.}$ are matrices associated to the cluster C_k, both with determinants equal to 1.

3.1 The Optimization Problem

The optimization problem has two stages:

a) The class C_k and the matrices $\mathbf{M}_{kL}$ and $\mathbf{M}_{kU}$ $(k = 1, \ldots, K)$ are fixed. We look for the prototype L_k of the class C_k which locally minimizes

$$\begin{aligned}\Delta_k^2(L_k, \delta_k) = {} & \sum_{i \in C_k} (\mathbf{x}_{iL} - \mathbf{y}_{kL})^T \mathbf{M}_{kL} (\mathbf{x}_{iL} - \mathbf{y}_{kL}) + \\ & \sum_{i \in C_k} (\mathbf{x}_{iU} - \mathbf{y}_{kU})^T \mathbf{M}_{kU} (\mathbf{x}_{iU} - \mathbf{y}_{kU}).\end{aligned} \tag{10}$$

As we know from subsection 2.1, the solutions for α_{kL}^j and β_{kU}^j are, respectively, the average of $\{a_i^j : s_i \in C_k\}$, the lower bounds of the intervals $[a_i^j, b_i^j]$, $s_i \in C_k$, and the average of $\{b_i^j : s_i \in C_k\}$, the upper bounds of the intervals $[a_i^j, b_i^j]$, $s_i \in C_k$.

b) The class C_k and the prototypes L_k $(k = 1, \ldots, K)$ are fixed. We look for the distance δ_k of the class C_k which locally minimizes the criterion Δ_k^2 with $\det(\mathbf{M}_{kL}) = 1$ and $\det(\mathbf{M}_{kU}) = 1$. According to Diday and Govaert (1977), the solutions are: $\mathbf{M}_{kL} = (\det \mathbf{Q}_{kL})^{1/p}\, \mathbf{Q}_{kL}^{-1}$ where $\mathbf{Q}_{kL}$ is the covariance matrix of the lower bounds of the intervals belonging to the class C_k with $\det(\mathbf{Q}_{kL}) \neq 0$, and $\mathbf{M}_{kU} = (\det\, \mathbf{Q}_{kU})^{1/p}\, \mathbf{Q}_{kU}^{-1}$ where $\mathbf{Q}_{kU}$ is the covariance matrix of the upper bounds of the intervals belonging to the class C_k with $\det(\mathbf{Q}_{kU}) \neq 0$.

3.2 The Algorithm

The initialization, the allocation step, and the stopping criterion are nearly the same for the adaptive and non-adaptive dynamic clustering algorithms. The main difference between these algorithms occurs in the representation step when it computes for each class k, $(k = 1, \ldots, K)$ the matrices $\mathbf{M}_{kL} = (\det(\mathbf{Q}_{kL}))^{1/p}\, \mathbf{Q}_{kL}^{-1}$ and $\mathbf{M}_{kU} = (\det(\mathbf{Q}_{kU}))^{1/p}\, \mathbf{Q}_{kU}^{-1}$.

Remark. If a single number is considered as an interval with equal lower and upper bounds, the results furnished by these symbolic data methods are identical to those furnished by the standard numerical ones when traditional kinds of data (i.e., vector-valued observations) are used. Both the clusters and the corresponding prototypes are identical.

4 Experimental Results

To show the utility of these methods, experiments with two artificial interval data sets, having different degrees of clustering difficulty (clusters of different shapes and sizes, linearly non-separable clusters, etc), are considered. The experiments have three stages: generation of usual and interval data (stages 1 and 2), and evaluation of the clustering results in the framework of a Monte Carlo experiment.

4.1 Usual Data Sets

Initially, we consider two standard quantitative data sets in $\mathbb{R}^2$. Each data set has 450 points scattered among four clusters of unequal sizes and shapes: two clusters with elliptical shapes and sizes of 150 and two clusters with spherical shapes of sizes 50 and 100. The data points for each cluster in each data set were drawn according to a bivariate normal distribution with correlated components.

Data set 1, showing well-separated clusters, is generated according to the following parameters:

a) Class 1: $\mu_1 = 28$, $\mu_2 = 22$, $\sigma_1^2 = 100$, $\sigma_{12} = 21$, $\sigma_2^2 = 9$ and $\rho_{12} = 0.7$;
b) Class 2: $\mu_1 = 65$, $\mu_2 = 30$, $\sigma_1^2 = 9$, $\sigma_{12} = 28.8$, $\sigma_2^2 = 144$ and $\rho_{12} = 0.8$;
c) Class 3: $\mu_1 = 45$, $\mu_2 = 42$, $\sigma_1^2 = 9$, $\sigma_{12} = 6.3$, $\sigma_2^2 = 9$ and $\rho_{12} = 0.7$;
d) Class 4: $\mu_1 = 38$, $\mu_2 = -1$, $\sigma_1^2 = 25$, $\sigma_{12} = 20$, $\sigma_2^2 = 25$ and $\rho_{12} = 0.8$.

Data set 2, showing overlapping clusters, is generated according to the following parameters:

a) Class 1: $\mu_1 = 45$, $\mu_2 = 22$, $\sigma_1^2 = 100$, $\sigma_{12} = 21$, $\sigma_2^2 = 9$ and $\rho_{12} = 0.7$;
b) Class 2: $\mu_1 = 65$, $\mu_2 = 30$, $\sigma_1^2 = 9$, $\sigma_{12} = 28.8$, $\sigma_2^2 = 144$ and $\rho_{12} = 0.8$;
c) Class 3: $\mu_1 = 57$, $\mu_2 = 38$, $\sigma_1^2 = 9$, $\sigma_{12} = 6.3$, $\sigma_2^2 = 9$ and $\rho_{12} = 0.7$;
d) Class 4: $\mu_1 = 42$, $\mu_2 = 12$, $\sigma_1^2 = 25$, $\sigma_{12} = 20$, $\sigma_2^2 = 25$ and $\rho_\rho 12 = 0.8$.

4.2 Interval Data Sets

Each data point (z_1, z_2) of data sets 1 and 2 is the seed of a vector of intervals (i.e., a rectangle): $([z_1 - \gamma_1/2, z_1 + \gamma_1/2], [z_2 - \gamma_2/2, z_2 + \gamma_2/2])$. The parameters γ_1, γ_2 are uniformly selected from the same predefined interval. The intervals considered in this paper are: $[1, 8], [1, 16], [1, 24], [1, 32]$, and $[1, 40]$. Figure 1 shows interval data set 1 with well separated clusters and Fig. 2 shows interval data set 2 with overlapping clusters.

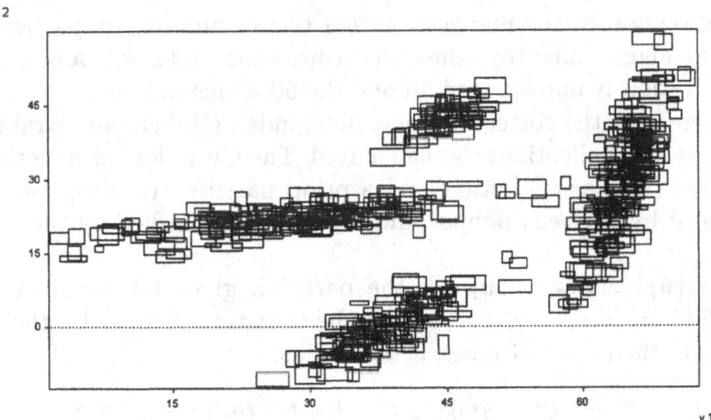

Fig. 1. Interval data set 1 showing well-separated classes.

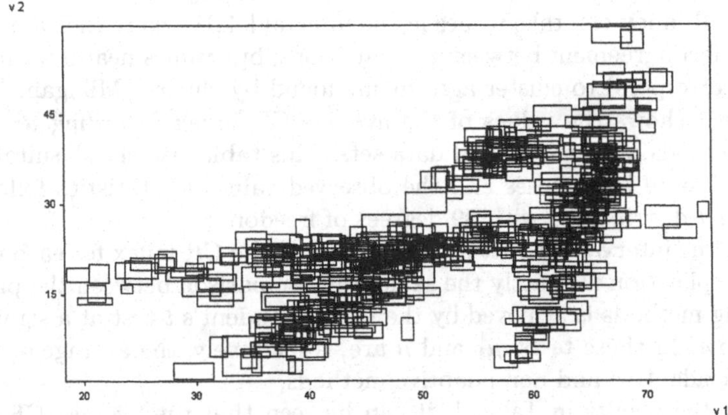

Fig. 2. Interval data set 2 showing overlapping classes.

4.3 The Monte Carlo Experiment

The evaluation of these clustering methods was performed in the framework of a Monte Carlo experiment: 100 replications are considered for each interval data set, as well as for each predefined interval. In each replication a clustering method was run (until convergence to a stationary value of the adequacy criterion W_1 or W_2) 50 times and the best result, according to criterion W_1 or W_2, is selected.

Remark. As in the standard (adaptive and non-adaptive) Mahalanobis distance methods for dynamic clustering, our methods sometimes have a problem with the inversion of the matrices. When this occurs, the implemented version of these algorithms stops the current iteration and starts a new one. The stopped iteration is not counted among the 50 which are run.

The average of the corrected Rand (CR) index (Hubert and Arabie, 1985) among these 100 replications was calculated. The CR index assesses the degree of agreement (similarity) between an a priori partition (in our case, the partition defined by the seed points) and a partition furnished by the clustering algorithm.

If $U = \{u_1, \ldots, u_r, \ldots, u_R\}$ is the partition given by the cluster analysis, and if $V = \{v_1, \ldots, v_c, \ldots, v_C\}$ is the partition defined by the *a priori* classification, then the CR index is defined as:

$$\mathrm{CR} = \frac{\sum_{i=1}^{R}\sum_{j=1}^{C}\binom{n_{ij}}{2} - \binom{n}{2}^{-1}\sum_{i=1}^{R}\binom{n_{i.}}{2}\sum_{j=1}^{C}\binom{n_{.j}}{2}}{\frac{1}{2}[\sum_{i=1}^{R}\binom{n_{i.}}{2} + \sum_{j=1}^{C}\binom{n_{.j}}{2}] - \binom{n}{2}^{-1}\sum_{i=1}^{R}\binom{n_{i.}}{2}\sum_{j=1}^{C}\binom{n_{.j}}{2}} \tag{11}$$

where n_{ij} represents the number of objects that are in clusters u_i and v_i; $n_{i.}$ indicates the number of objects in cluster u_i; $n_{.j}$ indicates the number of objects in cluster v_j; and n is the total number of objects.

The CR index can take values in the interval [-1,1], where the value 1 indicates perfect agreement between the partitions, but values near 0 (or negative values) correspond to cluster agreements found by chance (Milligan, 1996).

Table 1 shows the values of the average CR index according to the different methods and the interval data sets. This table also shows suitable null and alternative hypotheses and the observed values of statistics following a Student's t-distribution with 99 degrees of freedom.

Since the interval data set used to calculate the CR index for each method in each replication is exactly the same, the comparison between the proposed clustering methods is achieved by the paired Student's t-test at a significance level of 5%. In these tests, μ_1 and μ are, respectively, the average of the CR index for adaptive and non-adaptive methods.

From the results in Table 1, it can be seen that the average CR indices for the adaptive method are greater than those for the non-adaptive method in all situations. In addition, the statistical tests support the hypothesis that the average performance (measured by the CR index) of the adaptive method is superior to the non-adaptive method.

Table 1. Comparison between the clustering methods.

Range of values of γ_i $i = 1, 2$	Interval Data Set 1			Interval Data Set 2		
	Non-Adaptive Method	Adaptive Method	$H_0 : \mu_1 \leq \mu$ $H_a : \mu_1 > \mu$	Non-Adaptive Method	Adaptive Method	$H_0 : \mu_1 \leq \mu$ $H_a : \mu_1 > \mu$
$\gamma_i \in [1, 8]$	0.778	0.996	80.742	0.409	0.755	13.266
$\gamma_i \in [1, 16]$	0.784	0.986	82.182	0.358	0.688	22.609
$\gamma_i \in [1, 24]$	0.789	0.963	61.464	0.352	0.572	20.488
$\gamma_i \in [1, 32]$	0.802	0.937	39.181	0.349	0.435	18.204
$\gamma_i \in [1, 40]$	0.805	0.923	29.084	0.341	0.386	9.2851

5 Conclusions

In this paper, dynamic clustering methods for interval data are presented. Two methods are considered: the first method provides a partition of the input data and a corresponding prototype (a vector of intervals) for each class by optimizing an adequacy criterion which is based on Mahalanobis distances between vectors of intervals. The second is an adaptive version of the first method. In both methods the prototype of each class is represented by a vector of intervals, where the bounds of these intervals for a variable are, respectively, the average of the set of lower bounds and the average of the set of upper bounds of the intervals of the objects belonging to the class for the same variable. The convergence of these algorithms and the decrease of the partitioning criteria at each iteration is due to the optimization of the adequacy criteria at each representation step. The accuracy of the results furnished by these clustering methods was assessed by the using the corrected Rand index on results from simulated interval data sets with different degrees of clustering difficulty. In terms of the average CR index, the method that used adaptive distance clearly outperformed the method with non-adaptive distance.

Acknowledgments: The authors would like to thank CNPq (Brazilian Agency) for its financial support.

References

1. Bock, H. H., and Diday, E. (2000) *Analysis of Symbolic Data, Exploratory Methods for Extracting Statistical Information from Complex Data.* Springer, Heidelberg.
2. Chavent, M., and Lechevallier, Y. (2002). "Dynamical Clustering Algorithm of Interval Data: Optimization of an Adequacy Criterion Based on Hausdorff Distance," in *Classification, Clustering and Data Analysis*, eds. K. Jajuga and A. Sokolowsky, Heidelberg: Springer, pp. 53–59/

3. Diday, E., and Govaert, G. (1977). “Classification Automatique avec Distances Adaptatives,” *R.A.I.R.O. Informatique Computer Science*, **11** 329–349.
4. Diday, E., and Simon, J. J. (1976). “Cluster Analysis,” in *Digital Pattern Recognition*, ed K. S. Fu, pp. 47–94.
5. Govaert, G. (1975). *Classification Automatique et Distances Adaptatives*. Ph.D. dissertation, "hèse de 3ème cycle, Mathématique appliquée, Université Paris VI.
6. Hubert, L., and Arabie, P. (1985). “Comparing Partitions,” *Journal of Classification*, **2**, 193–218.
7. Jain, A. K., Murty, M. N., and Flynn, P. J. (1999). “Data Clustering: A Review,” *ACM Computing Surveys*, **31**, 264–323.
8. Milligan, G. W. (1996). “Clustering Validation: Results and Implications for Applied Analysis,” in *Clustering and Classification*, Singapore:Word Scientific, pp. 341–375.
9. Souza, R. M. C. R., and De Carvalho, F. A. T. (2004). “Clustering of Interval Data Based on City-Block Distances,” *Pattern Recognition Letters*, **25**, 353–365.
10. Verde, R., De Carvalho, F. A. T., and Lechevallier, Y. (2001). “A Dynamical Clustering Algorithm for Symbolic Data,” in *Tutorial on Symbolic Data Analysis*, GfKl Conference, Munich.

A Symbolic Model-Based Approach for Making Collaborative Group Recommendations

Sérgio R. de M. Queiroz and Francisco de A. T. de Carvalho

Universidade Federal de Pernambuco, Brazil
{srmq,fatc}@cin.ufpe.br

Abstract: In recent years, recommender systems have achieved great success. Popular sites give thousands of recommendations every day. However, despite the fact that many activities are carried out in groups, like going to the theater with friends, these systems are focused on recommending items for sole users. This brings out the need for systems capable of performing recommendations for groups of people, a domain that has received little attention in the literature. In this article we introduce a novel method of making collaborative recommendations for groups, based on models built using techniques from symbolic data analysis. Finally, we empirically evaluate the proposed method to see its behaviour for groups of different sizes and degrees of homogeneity, and compare the achieved results with a baseline methodology.

1 Introduction

You arrive at home and turn on your cable TV. There are 150 channels to choose from. How can you quickly find a program that will likely interest you? When one has to make a choice without full knowledge of the alternatives, a common approach is to rely on the recommendations of trusted individuals: a TV guide, a friend, a consulting agency. In the 1990s, computational *recommender systems* appeared to automatize the recommendation process. Nowadays, we have (mostly in the Web) various recommender systems. Popular sites, like *Amazon.com*, have recommendation areas where users can see which items would be of their interest.

One of the most successfully technologies used by these systems has been *collaborative filtering* (CF) (see e.g. Herlocker, 1999). The CF technique is based on the assumption that the best recommendations for an individual are those given by people with preferences similar to his/her preferences.

However, until now, these systems have focused only on making recommendations for individuals, despite the fact that many day-to-day activities are performed in groups (e.g. watching TV at home). This highlights the need of developing recommender systems for groups, that are able to capture the preferences of whole groups and make recommendations for them.

When recommending for groups, the utmost goal is that the recommendations should be the best possible for the group. Thus, two prime questions are raised: *What is the best suggestion for a group? How to reach this suggestion?*

The concept of making recommendations for groups has received little attention in the literature of recommender systems. A few works have developed recommender systems capable of recommending for groups (Hill et al., 1995, Lieberman et al., 1999, O'Connor et al. 2001), but none of them have delved into the difficulties involving the achievement of good recommendation for groups (i.e., the two fundamental questions previously cited).

Although little about this topic has been studied in the literature of recommender systems, how to achieve good group results from individual preferences is an important topic in many research areas, with different roots. Beginning in the XVIII century motivated by the problem of voting, to modern research areas like operational research, social choice, multicriteria decision making and social psychology, this topic has been treated by diverse research communities.

Developments in these research fields are important for a better understanding of the problem and the identification of the limitations of proposed solutions; as well as to the development of recommender systems that achieve similar results to the ones groups of people would achieve during a discussion.

A conclusion that can be drawn from these areas is that there is no "perfect" way to aggregate individual preferences in order to achieve a group result. Arrow's impossibility theorem (Arrow, 1963) showed that it is impossible for any procedure (termed a social function in social choice parlance) to achieve at the same time a set of simple desirable properties. Many empirical studies in social psychology have noted that the adequacy of a decision scheme (the mechanism used by a group of people to combine the individual preferences of its members into the group result) to the group decision process is very dependent to the group's intrinsic characteristics and the problem's nature (see e.g. Hinsz, 1999). Multi-criteria decision making strengthens the view that the achievement of an "ideal configuration" is not the most important feature when working with decisions (in fact, this ideal may not exist in most of the times) and highlights the importance of giving the users interactivity and permit the analysis of different possibilities.

However, the nonexistence of an ideal does not mean that we cannot compare different possibilities. Based on good properties that a preference aggregation scheme should have, we can define meaningful metrics to quantify the goodness of group recommendations. They will not be completely free of value judgments, but these will reflect desirable properties.

In this article we introduce a novel method of making recommendations for groups, based on the ideas of collaborative filtering and symbolic data analysis. Then we experimentally evaluate the proposed method to see its behaviour under groups of different sizes and degrees of homogeneity. For each group configuration the behaviour of the proposed method is compared with a baseline method. The metric used reflects good social characteristics for the group recommendations.

2 Recommending for Groups

The problem of recommendations for groups can be posed as follows: *how to suggest (new) items that will be liked by the group as a whole, given that we have a set of historical individual preferences from the members of this group as well as preferences from other individuals (who are not in the group).*

Thinking collaboratively, we want to know how to use the preferences (evaluations over items) of the individuals in the system to predict how one group of individuals (a subset of the community) will like the items available. Thence, we would be able to suggest items that will be valuable for this group.

To be used to recommend for groups, the CF methodology has to be adapted. We can think of two different ways to do this. The first is to use CF to recommend to the individual members of the group, and then combine the recommendations (we will call this approaches "aggregation-based methodologies"). The second is to modify the CF process so that it directly generates a recommendation for the group. This involves the modelling of the group as a single entity (we will call this approaches "model-based methodologies").

2.1 Symbolic Model-Based Approach

In this section we develop a model-based recommendation strategy for groups. During the recommendation process, it uses models for the items—which can be pre-computed—and does not require the computation of on-line user neighborhoods, not having this scalability problem present in many collaborative filtering algorithms (for individuals). To create the models and compare them tecniques from symbolic data analysis (Bock and Diday, 2000) are used.

The intuition behind our approach is that for each item we can identify the group of people who like it and the group of people that do not like it. We assume that the group for which we will make a recommendation will appreciate an item if the group has similar preferences to the group of people who like the item and is dissimilar to the group of people who do not like it.

To implement this, first the group of users for whom the recommendations will be computed is represented by a prototype that contains the histogram of rates for each item evaluated by the group. The target items (items that can be recommended) are also represented in a similar way, but now we create two prototypes for each target item: a positive prototype, that contains the histogram of rates for (other) items evaluated by individuals who liked the target item; and a negative prototype that is analogous to the positive one, but the individuals chosen are those who did not like the target item. Next we compute the similarity between the group prototype and the two prototypes of each target item. The final similarity between a target item and a group is given by a simple linear combination of the similarities between the group prototype and both item prototypes using the formula: $sim_f = \frac{sim_{pos}+1-sim_{neg}}{2}$, where sim_f is the final similarity value, sim_{pos} is the similarity between the group prototype and the positive item prototype and sim_{neg} analogously for the negative one. Finally, we order the target items by decreasing order of similarity values. If we want to recommend k items to the users, we can take the first k items of this ordering. Figure 1 depicts the recommendation process. Its two main aspects, the creation of prototypes and the similarity computation will be described in the following subsections.

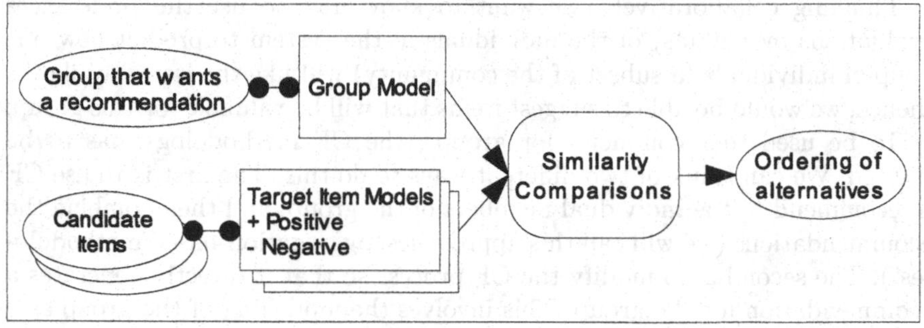

Fig. 1. The recommendation process

Prototype Generation

A fundamental step of this method is the prototype generation. The the group and the target items are represented by the histograms of rates for items. Different weights can be attributed to each histogram that make up the prototypes. In other words, each prototype is described by a set of p symbolic variables Y_j. Each item corresponds to a categorical modal variable Y_j that may also have an associated weight. The modalities of Y_j are the different grades that can be given to items. In our case, we have six modalities.

Group Prototype

In the group prototype we have the grade histograms for every item that has been evaluated by at least one member of the group. The grade histogram is built by computing the frequency of each modality in the ratings of the group members for the item being considered. The used data has a discrete set of 6 grades: $\{0.0, 0.2, 0.4, 0.6, 0.8, 1.0\}$, where 0.0 is the worst and 1.0 is the best grade. For example, if an item i_1 was evaluated by 2 users in a group of 3 individuals and they gave the ratings 0.4 and 0.6 for the item, the row in the symbolic data table corresponding to the item would be: $\{i_1, \{0.0, 0.0, 0.5, 0.5, 0.0, 0.0\}, 0.667\}$, assuming the weight as the fraction of the group that has evaluated the item.

Item Prototypes

To build a prototype for a target item, the first step is to decide which users will be selected to have their evaluations in the prototype. This users have the role of characterizing the profile of those who like the target item, for the positive profile; and of characterizing the profile of those who do not like the target item, for the negative profile. Therefrom, for the positive prototype only the users that evaluated the target item highly are chosen. Users that have given grades 0.8 or 1.0 were chosen as the "positive representatives" for the group. For the negative prototype the users that have given 0.0 or 0.2 for the target item were chosen. One parameter for the building of the models is how many users will be chosen for each target item. We have chosen 300 users for each prototype, after experimenting with 30, 50, 100, 200 and 300 users.

Similarity Calculation

To compute the similarity between the prototype of a group and the prototype of a target item, we only consider the items that are in both prototypes. As similarity measure we tried Bacelar-Nicolau's weighted affinity coefficient (presented in Bock and Diday 2000) and two measures based on the Euclidean distance and the Pearson correlation, respectively. At the end we used the affinity coefficient, as it achieved slightly better results. The similarity between two prototypes k and k' based on the affinity coefficient is given by:

$$\text{protsim}(k,k') = \sum_{j=1}^{p} w_j \times \sum_{l=1}^{m_j} \sqrt{n_{kjl} \times n_{k'jl}} \quad (1)$$

where:

- p is the number of items present in both prototypes;
- w_j is the weight attributed to item j;
- m_j is the number of modalities (six, for the six different rates);
- n_{kjl} and $n_{k'jl}$ are the relative frequencies obtained by rate l in the prototypes k and k' for the item j, respectively.

3 Experimental Evaluation

To run our experiments, we used the Eachmovie dataset. Eachmovie was a recommender service that run as part of a research project at the Compaq Systems Research Center. During that period, 72,916 users gave 2,811,983 evaluations to 1,628 different movies. Users' evaluations were registered using a 6-level numerical scale (0.0, 0.2, 0.4, 0.6, 0.8, 1.0). The dataset can be obtained from Compaq Computer Corporation (available at the URL: `http://www.research.compaq.com/SRC/eachmovie/`). The Eachmovie dataset has been used in various experiments involving recommender systems.

We restricted our experiments to users that have evaluated at least 150 movies (2,551 users). This was adopted to allow an intersection (of evaluated movies) of reasonable size between each pair of users, so that more credit can be given to the comparisons related to the homogeneity degree of a group.

3.1 Data Preparation: The Creation of Groups

To conduct the experiments, it was necessary the existence of groups of users with varying sizes and homogeneity degrees. The EachMovie dataset is only about individuals, therefore it was needed to build the groups first.

Four group sizes were defined: 3, 6, 12 and 24 individuals. We believe that this range of sizes includes the majority of scenarios where recommendation for groups can be used. For the degree of homogeneity factor, 3 levels were used: high, medium and low homogeneity. The groups don't need to be a partition of the set of users, i.e. the same user can be in more than one different group. The next subsections describe the methodology used to build the groups.

Obtaining a Dissimilarity Matrix

The first step in the group definition was to build a dissimilarity matrix for the users. That is, a matrix m of size $n \times n$ (n is the number of users) where each m_{ij} contains the dissimilarity value between users i and j. To obtain this matrix, the dissimilarity of each user against all the others was calculated.

The dissimilarities between users will be subsequently used to construct the groups with the three desired homogeneity degrees. To obtain the dissimilarity between two users i and j, we calculated the Pearson correlation coefficient ρ_{ij} between them (which is in the interval $[-1, 1]$) and transformed this value into a dissimilarity using the formula: $\text{dissim}(i, j) = 1 - (\rho_{ij} + 1)/2$. The Pearson correlation coefficient is the most common measure of similarity between users used in collaborative filtering algorithms (see e.g. Herlocker et al., 1999). To compute ρ_{ij} between two users we consider only the items x that both users have graded and use the formula: $\rho_{ij} = \frac{\sum_x (i_x - \bar{i})(j_x - \bar{j})}{\sqrt{\sum_x (i_x - \bar{i})^2}\sqrt{\sum_x (j_x - \bar{j})^2}}$, where i_x is the grade that user i has given for item x and $\bar{i}$ is the average grade (over the items x) for user i (analogously for user j).

For our experiments, the movies were randomly separated in three sets: a profile set with 50% of the movies, a training set with 25% and a test set with 25% of the movies. Only the user's evaluations which refer to elements of the first set were used to obtain the dissimilarity matrix. The evaluations that refer to movies of the other sets were not used at this stage. The rationale behind this procedure is that the movies from the test set will be the ones used to evaluate the behavior of the model (Section 3.2). That is, it will be assumed that the members of the group did not know them previously. The movies from the training set were used to adjust the model parameters.

Group Formation

High homogeneity groups. We wanted to obtain 100 groups with high homogeneity degree for each of the desired sizes. To this end, we first randomly generated 100 groups of 200 users each. Then the hierarchical clustering algorithm divisive analysis (diana) was run for each of these 100 groups. To extract a high homogeneity group of size n from each tree, we took the the "lowest" branch with at least n elements. If the number of elements of this branch was larger than n we tested all combinations of size n and selected the one with lowest total dissimilarity (sum of all dissimilarities between the n users). For groups of size 24, the number of combinations was too big. In this case we used a heuristic method, selecting the n users which have the lowest sum of dissimilarities in the branch (sum of dissimilarities between the user in consideration and all others in the branch).

Low homogeneity groups. To select a group of size n with low homogeneity from one of the groups with 200 users, we first calculated for each user its sum of dissimilarities (between this user and all the other 199). The n elements selected were the ones with the n largest sum of dissimilarities.

Medium homogeneity groups. To select a group of size n with medium homogeneity degree, n elements were randomly selected from the total population of users. To avoid surprises due to randomness, after a group was generated, a test to compare a single mean (the one of the extracted group) to a specified value (the mean of the population) was done (using $\alpha = 0.05$).

3.2 Experimental Methodology

For each of the 1200 generated groups (4 sizes $\times$ 3 homogeneities $\times$ 100 repetitions) recommendations for itens from the test set were generated. We also generated recommendations using a baseline model, inspired by a "null model" used in group experiments in social psychology (e.g. Hinsz, 1999).

The null model takes the opinion of one randomly chosen group member as the group decision. Taking this to the domain of recommender systems, we randomly selected one group member and make recommendations for this individual (using traditional neighbourhood-based collaborative filtering). These recommendations are taken as the group recommendations.

To evaluate the behaviour of the strategies with the various sizes and degrees of homogeneity of the groups, a metric is needed. As we have a set of rankings as the input and a ranking as the output, a ranking correlation method was considered a good candidate. We used the Kendall's rank correlation coefficient (τ). For each generated recommendation, we calculated τ between the final ranking generated for the group and the users' individual rankings (obtained from the users' grades available in the test set). Then we calculated the average τ, for the recommendation. The $\bar{\tau}$ has a good social characteristic. One ranking with largest $\bar{\tau}$ is a Kemeny optimal aggregation (it is not necessarily unique). Kemeny optimal aggregations are the only ones that fulfill at the same time the principles of neutrality and consistency of the social choice literature and the extended Condorcet criterion (Dwork et al., 2001), which is: If a majority of the individuals prefer alternative a to b, then a should have a higher ranking than b in the aggregation. Kemeny optimal aggregations are NP-hard to obtain when the number of rankings to aggregate is ≥ 4 (Dwork et al., 2001). Therefore, it is not possible to implement an optimal strategy in regard of the $\bar{\tau}$, making it a good reference for comparison.

The goal of the experiment was to evaluate how $\bar{\tau}$ is affected by the variation on the size and homogeneity of the groups, as well as by the strategy used (symbolic approach *versus* null model). To verify the influence of each factor, we did a three-way (as we have 3 factors) analysis of variance (ANOVA). After the verification of significant relevance, a comparison of means for the levels of each factor was done. To this end we used Tukey Honest Significant Differences test at the 95% confidence level.

4 Results and Discussion

Figure 2 shows the observed $\bar{\tau}$'s for the symbolic and the null approaches.

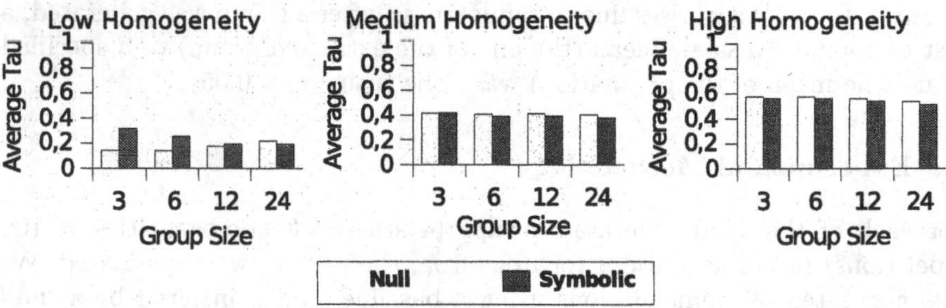

Fig. 2. Observed $\bar{\tau}$'s by homogeneity degree for the symbolic approach and the null model.

The symbolic approach was significantly better than the null model in heterogeneous groups of 3 and 6 people (achieving a $\bar{\tau}$ 2.19 and 1.76 times better than the null model, respectively). The results were statistically equivalent for groups of 12 people, and the null model had a better result for groups of 24 people (the null model was 1.19 times better in this case). It is not clear if the symbolic model is inadequate for larger heterogeneous group, or if this result is due to the biases present in the data used. Due to the process of group formation, larger heterogeneous groups (even in the same homogeneity degree) are more homogeneous than smaller groups, as it is much more difficult to find a large group strongly heterogeneous than it is to find a smaller one. Experiments using synthetic data where the homogeneity degree was more carefully controlled would be more useful to do this comparisons.

Under medium and high homogeneity levels, the null model shows that for more homogeneous groups it is a good alternative. It was statistically equivalent to the symbolic model for groups of 3 people and better for the others. The difference, however, was not very large. This suggests that the symbolic strategy should be improved to better accommodate this cases.

Making comparisons for the factor homogeneity, in all cases the averages of the levels differed significantly. Besides, we had: high average > medium avg. > low avg., i.e. the compatibility degree between the group recommendation and the individual preferences was proportional to the group's homogeneity degree. These facts were to be expected if the strategies were coherent.

For the group size, in many cases the differences between its levels were not significative, indicating that the size of a group is less important than its homogeneity degree for the performance of recommendations.

Acknowledgments: The authors would like to thank CNPq and CAPES (Brazilian Agencies) for their financial support.

References

1. Arrow, K. J. (1963). *Social Choice and Individual Values.* Wiley, New York.
2. Bock, H.-H. and Diday, E. (2000). *Analysis of Symbolic Data: Exploratory Methods for Extracting Statistical Information from Complex Data.* Springer, Berlin Heidelberg.
3. Dwork, C., Kumar, R., Moni, N., and Sivakumar, D. (2001). "Rank Aggregation Methods for the Web," in *Proceedings of the WWW10 Conference*, Hong Kong:World Wide Web Conference Committee, pp. 613–622.
4. Herlocker, J. L., Konstan, J. A., Borchers, A., and Riedl, J. (1999). "An Algorithm Framework for Performing Collaborative Filtering," in *Proceedings of the 22nd ACM SIGIR Conference*, Berkeley:ACM, pp. 230–237.
5. Hill, W., Stead, L., Rosenstein, M., and Furnas, G. (1995). "Recommending and Evaluating Choices in a Virtual Community of Use," in *Proceedings of the ACM CHI'95 Conference*, Denver:ACM, pp. 194–201.
6. Hinsz, V. B. (1999). "Group Decision Making with Responses of a Quantitative Nature: The Theory of Social Schemes for Quantities," *Organizational Behavior and Human Decision Processes*, **80**, 28–49.
7. Lieberman, H., Van Dyke, N. W., Vivacqua, A.S. (1999). "Let's Browse: A Collaborative Web Browsing Agent," in *Proceedings of the IUI-99,* Los Angeles:IUI, pp. 65–68.
8. O'Connor, M., Cosley, D., and Konstan, J. A. and Riedl, J. (2001). "PolyLens: A Recommender System for Groups of Users," in *Proceedings of the 7th ECSCW conference*, Bonn:ECSCW, pp. 199–218.

Probabilistic Allocation of Aggregated Statistical Units in Classification Trees for Symbolic Class Description

Mohamed Mehdi Limam[1], Edwin Diday[1], and Suzanne Winsberg[2]

[1] Université Paris IX Dauphine, France
{limam,diday}@ceremade.dauphine.fr
[2] Institut de Recherche et Coordination Acoustique/Musique, France
winsberg@ircam.fr

Abstract: Consider a class of statistical units, in which each unit may be an aggregate of individual statistical units. Each unit is decribed by an interval of values for each variable. Our aim is to develop a partition of this class of aggregated statistical units in which each part of the partition is described by a conjunction of characteristic properties. We use a stepwise top-down binary tree method and we introduce a probabilistic approach to assign units to the nodes of the tree. At each step we select the best variable and its best split to optimize simultaneously a discrimination criterion given by a prior partition and a homogeneity criterion. Finally, we present an example of real data.

1 Introduction

One of the aims of many classification methods is to split a population of n statistical individuals to obtain a partition into L classes, where $n > L$. Although in most cases the partition is designed either to optimize an intra-class homogeneity criterion as in classical clustering, or an inter-class discrimination criterion, as in classical decision or regression trees, both Vrac et al. (2002) and Limam et al. (2002) have developed methods which consider both criteria simultaneously. When the aim is class description, they found that by combining the two criteria they achieve an almost optimal discrimination, while retaining homogeneity, thus leading to improved class description. Their work differs from previous work not only because it combines supervised and unsupervised learning, itself an innovation, but because it can deal with data that are histograms or intervals, which arise in situations with aggregated statistical units.

These data are inherently richer, possessing potentially more information than the classical numerical data previously considered in classical algorithms such as CART and ID3. We encounter the former type of data when dealing with the more complex, aggregated statistical units found when analyzing huge data sets. For example, it may be useful to deal with aggregated units such as countries rather than with the individual inhabitants of the country. Notice that here the statistical unit is the country not the individual citizen. Then the resulting data set, after the aggregation, will more than likely contain symbolic data rather than classical data values. By symbolic data we mean that rather than having a specific single value for an observed variable, an observed value for an aggregated statistical unit may be multivalued. For example, in the case under consideration, the observed value may be an interval of values. For a detailed description of symbolic data analysis see Bock and Diday (2001).

In this paper we further develop the analysis of interval-valued variables, using a probabilistic approach to assign units to classes. In our case the aggregated statistical unit is described by an interval of values for each variable. So, instead of the usual practice of allocating the unit to a single or unique class or node of the partition, as is done in Limam et al. (2002) and elsewhere, we determine the probability that the unit belongs to each class of the partition. Périnel (1999) has used this probabilistic approach in supervised learning.

We shall now review the main features of the method using an illustrative example. Let the class to describe, C, be young people between the ages of 15 and 25, described by variables such as student grades and hours of participation in sports activities. The discriminatory categorical variable or prior partition could be smokers and nonsmokers of all age groups. We want to obtain a description of C which induces a partition of C consisting of homogenous classes of young people each of which is well discriminated with respect to smokers and non smokers. Of course, due to Huygens' theorem, we obtain classes of young people, each of which will be homogeneous with respect to the variables describing them while being well-discriminated from each other with respect to these same variables. Here, in addition they will be discriminated from each other with respect to the prior partition, i.e., smokers and non smokers. Thus we calculate the homogeneity criterion for the class we want to describe, but the discrimination criterion is based on the prior partition of the population. At each step in growing the binary tree, any given unit is not assigned to just one of the two descendent nodes but has a probability of being assigned to each of them. For example if 22 is the cutting value, the interval [18, 25] is not assigned with certainty to either the right node or the left node of this value.

Our approach is based on divisive top-down methods, which successively divide the population into two classes until a suitable stopping rule prevents further divisions. We use a monothetic approach such that each split is carried out using only one variable, as it provides a clearer interpretation of the clusters obtained. Divisive methods of this type are often referred to as tree-structured classifiers with acronyms such as CART and ID3 (see Breiman et al. (1984) and Quinlan (1986)).

Naturally, classical data are a special case of the interval-valued type of data considered here. Others have developed divisive algorithms for data types encountered when dealing with symbolic data, considering either a homogeneity criterion or a discrimination criterion based on an a priori partition, but not both simultaneously. Chavent (1997) has proposed a method for unsupervised learning, while Périnel (1999) and Gettler (1999) have proposed ones for supervised learning. Our method is an extension of that proposed by Limam et al. (2003).

To describe our method, this paper defines a cutting or split for interval type variables, and it defines a cutting value for this type of data. We describe in detail our new probabilistic allocation rule. Finally, we outline the approach used to combine the two criteria of homogeneity and discrimination.

2 The Underlying Population and the Data

Consider a population $\Omega = \{1, ..., n\}$ with n units. The Ω is partitioned into J known disjoint classes $G_1, ..., G_J$ and into M other disjoint classes $C_1, ..., C_M$, also known, which could be the same or different from the partition $G_1, ..., G_J$. Each unit $k \in \Omega$ of the population is described by three categories of variables:

- G : the a priori partition variable, which is a nominal variable defined on Ω with J categories $\{1, ..., J\}$;
- y_C : the class that describe the data; this is a nominal variable defined on Ω with M categories $\{1, ..., M\}$;
- $y_1, ..., y_p$: p explanatory variables.

Here $G(k)$ is the index of the class of the unit $k \in \Omega$ and G is a mapping defined on Ω with domain $\{1, ..., J\}$ which generates the a priori partition into J classes that discriminate the sample.

Also, $y_C(k)$ is the index of the class of the unit $k \in \Omega$ and y_C is a mapping defined on Ω with domain $\{1, ..., M\}$ which generates the second partition into M classes $C_1, ..., C_M$. One of the above classes will be chosen to be described. We denote this class to be described as C.

To each unit k and to each explanatory variable y_j is associated a symbolic description (with *imprecision* or *variation*). The description denoted by $[y_j(k)]$ that is associated with a quantitative y_j to a unit $k \in \Omega$ is an interval $y_j(k) \subset Y_j$ where Y_j is the set of possible values for y_j. Naturally, the case of an single-valued quantitative variable is a special case of this type of variable.

3 The Method

Four inputs are required for this method: 1) the data, consisting of n statistical units, each described by K symbolic or classical variables; 2) the prior partition of either some defined part of the population or the entire population;

3) the class C that the user aims to describe, which consists of n statistical units coming from the population of $n + n_0$ statistical units; 4) a coefficient, α, which gives more or less importance to the discriminatory power of the prior partition or to the homogeneity of the description of the given class C.

The method uses a monothetic hierarchical descending approach that works by dividing a node into two nodes, which we call sons. At each step l (l nodes correspond to a partition into l classes), one of the nodes (or leaves) of the tree is cut into two nodes in order to optimize a quality criterion Q for the constructed partition into $l + 1$ classes. The division of a node N sends a proportion of units to the left node N_1 and the other proportion to the right node N_2. This division is done by a "cutting" (y, c), where y is called the cutting variable and c the cutting point.

The algorithm always generates two kinds of output. The first is a graphical representation, in which the class to be described, C, is represented by a binary tree. The final leaves are the clusters constituting the class and each branch represents a cutting (y, c). The second is a description: each final leaf is described by the conjunction of the cutting points from the top of the tree to this final leaf. The class C is then described by a disjunction of these conjunctions. If the user wishes to choose an optimal value of α using the data-driven method described in Vrac et al. (2002), a graphical representation enabling this choice is also generated as output.

Let $H(N)$ and $h(N_1; N_2)$ be, respectively, the homogeneity criterion of a node N and of a couple of nodes $(N_1; N_2)$. Then we define $\Delta H(N) = H(N) - h(N_1; N_2)$. Similarly we define $\Delta D(N) = D(N) - d(N_1; N_2)$ for the discrimination criterion. The quality Q of a node N (respectively q of a couple of nodes $(N_1; N_2)$) is the weighted sum of the two criteria, namely $Q(N) = \alpha H(N) + \beta D(N)$ (respectively $q(N_1; N_2) = \alpha h(N_1; N_2) + \beta d(N_1; N_2)$) where $\alpha + \beta = 1$. So the quality variation induced by the splitting of N into $(N_1; N_2)$ is $\Delta Q(N) = Q(N) - q(N_1; N_2)$. We maximize $\Delta Q(N)$. Note that since we are optimizing two criteria the criteria must be normalized. The user can modulate the values of α and β so as to weight the importance that is given to each criterion.

To determine the cutting $(y; c)$ and the node to split, we must first, for each node N, select the cutting variable and its cutting point to minimize $q(N_1; N_2)$. Then, we select and split the node N which maximizes the difference between the quality before the cutting and the quality after the cutting, $\max \Delta Q(N)$.

Recall that we are working with interval variables. So we must define what constitutes a cutting for this type of data and what constitutes a cutting point. Among the many possibilities for choosing a cutting point, we recommend using the mean of the interval in defining a cutting point c for an interval variable. First we order the means of the intervals for all units; the cutting point is then defined as the mean of two successive interval means.

To illustrate this, suppose we have n statistical units in class N (take $n = 3$), and consider variable y_j (say size). Let A have value $[5, 7]$, B have value

$[1, 3]$, and D have value $[9, 11]$. So we first order the units in increasing order of the means of the intervals. We obtain $B(2) < A(6) < D(10)$. We can determine $n - 1 = 2$ cutting points by taking the mean of two consecutive values (two consecutive means of intervals). Here, one cutting point is $(2 + 6)/2 = 4$ and the other cutting point is $(6 + 10)/2 = 8$. Therefore we can also determine $n-1$ partitions into two classes (here Partition 1 is $\{N_1 = \{B\}; N_2 = \{A; D\}\}$ and Partition 2 is $\{N_1 = \{B; A\}; N_2 = \{D\}\}$, and so we have $n - 1$ quality criterion values $q(N_1, N_2)$.

We denote by p_{kq} the probability that the description $y_j(k)$ of unit k assigns the property $[y_j \leq c]$ associated with the question q (cf. Périnel, 1999). We assume that the membership in the left node N_1 depends on the property $[y_j \leq c]$ while the membership in the right node depends on the property $[y_j > c]$. That is:

- p_{kq}= probability that k is assigned to the left node, using $y_j(k)$
- $1 - p_{kq}$= probability that k is assigned to the right node, using $y_j(k)$.

We calculate these probabilities p_{kq} for a quantitative variable y_j with $y_j(k) = [y_j^{\min}(k), y_j^{\max}(k)]$ and $q = [y_j \leq c]$ as follows:

$$p_{kq} = \begin{cases} c - y_j^{\min}(k)/y_j^{\max}(k) - y_j^{\min}(k) & \text{if } c \in [y_j^{\min}(k), y_j^{\max}(k)] \\ 0 & \text{if } c < y_j^{\min}(k) \\ 1 & \text{if } c > y_j^{\max}(k). \end{cases}$$

First, we compute the probability that an object k belongs to the son nodes N_1 or N_2 of the node N:

$$p_k(N_1) = p_k(N) \times p_{kq}$$
$$p_k(N_2) = p_k(N) \times (1 - p_{kq}).$$

where p_{kq} is calculated above and $p_k(N)$ is the membership probability of an object k for node N. At the first step of the algorithm, we have, of course, $p_k(N) = 1$, $k = 1, ..., n$, because all the individuals belong "completely" to the root node; in the following steps, the probabilities p_{kq} are computed on each cutting (y_j, c). The sizes of the nodes N_1 and N_2 are denoted by $n_{N_1}$and n_{N_2}, respectively, and are calculated on the basis of the formulae:

$$n_{N_1} = \sum_{k=1}^{n} p_k(N_1)$$
$$n_{N_2} = \sum_{k=1}^{n} p_k(N_2).$$

The probability of having the class G_i from the a priori partition inside the nodes N_1 and N_2 is denoted, respectively, by $P_{N_1}(G_i)$ and $P_{N_2}(G_i)$. These are calculated on the basis of the formulae:

$$P_{N_1}(G_i) = \sum_{k \in C \cap G_i} p_k(N_1)/n_{N_1}$$
$$P_{N_2}(G_i) = \sum_{k \in C \cap G_i} p_k(N_2)/n_{N_2}$$

where C is the class to describe and has n units.

The probabilities calculated above are used to calculate the homogeneity and the discrimination criteria. We shall now define the homogeneity criterion for interval type data.

The clustering or homogeneity criterion we use is an inertia criterion. This criterion is used in Chavent (1997). The inertia of a node t which could be N_1 or N_2 is

$$H(t) = \sum_{w_i \in t} \sum_{w_j \in t} \frac{p_i p_j}{2\mu} \Delta(w_i, w_j),$$

where p_i = the weight of the individual w_i. In our case $p_i = p_k(t)$, $\mu = \sum_{w_i \in N} p_i$ is the weight of class t, Δ is a distance between individuals defined as $\Delta(w_i, w_j) = \sum_{k=1}^{K} \delta^2(w_i, w_j)$ with K the number of variables, for

$$\delta^2(w_i, w_j) = m_k^{-2} \left| \frac{y_k^{\min}(w_i) + y_k^{\max}(w_i)}{2} - \frac{y_k^{\min}(w_j) + y_k^{\max}(w_j)}{2} \right|^2,$$

where $[y_k^{\min}(w_i), y_k^{\max}(w_i)]$ is the interval value of the variable y_k for the unit w_i and $m_k = \left|\max_{w_i} y_k^{\max} - \min_{w_i} y_k^{\min}\right|$ which represents the maximum area of the variable y_k. We remark that δ^2 falls in the interval [0, 1]. Moreover, the homogeneity criterion must be normalized to fall in the interval [0, 1].

Let us turn to the discrimination criterion. The discrimination criterion we choose is an impurity criterion, Gini's index, which we denote as D. This criterion was introduced by Breiman et al. (1984) and measures the impurity of a node t (which could be N_1 or N_2) with respect to the prior partition $(G_1, G_2, ..., G_J)$ as:

$$D(t) = \sum_{l \neq i} p_l p_i = 1 - \left(\sum_{i=1}^{J} p_i^2\right)$$

with $p_i = P_t(G_i)$. We require that $D(N)$ be normalized to fall in the interval [0, 1].

To assign each object k with vector description $(Y_1, ..., Y_p)$ to one class G_i of the prior partition, the following rule is applied :

$$G(k) = G_i \iff p_k(G_i) > p_k(Gj) \quad j = 1, ..., J,\ i \neq j.$$

The membership probability $p_k(G_i)$ is calculated as the weighted average (over all terminal nodes) of the conditional probability $P_t(G_i)$, with weights $p_k(t)$:

$$p_k(G_i) = \sum_{t=1}^{T} P_t(G_i) \times p_k(G_i).$$

In other words, it consists of summing the probabilities that an individual belongs to the class G_i over all terminal nodes t, with these probabilities being weighted by the probability that this individual reaches the corresponding terminal node.

The set of individuals is assigned to t on the basis of the majority rule. The membership in t is

$$\text{node}(t) = \{k : p_k(t) > p_k(s) \, \forall s \neq t\}.$$

Therefore we can calculate the size of the class G_i inside a terminal node t as $n_t(G_i) = \{k : k \in \text{node}(k) \text{ and } k \in G_i\}$.

4 Example

Our example deals with real symbolic data. The class to describe contains 18 soccer teams in the French league from a population Ω of 50 teams in Europe. The aim is to explain the factors which discriminate the ten best teams of one championship (G_1) from the worst teams (G_2) which are the other teams in the same championship. But we also wish to have good descriptors of the resulting homogeneous clusters.

Because we have aggregated data for the players on each team, we are not dealing with classical data that has a single value for each variable for each statistical unit. Here, each variable for each team is an interval. There are $K = 2$ interval variables: age and weight of each player of each team. These interval variables describe the variation for all the players of each team.

In the analysis we stop the division at four terminal nodes. We obtain a disjunction of descriptions. Each description corresponds to a final leaf. An example of such a description is: [the weight of the players is between 73.50 and 79.5] and [the age of the players is between 26 and 29]. In terms of a "symbolic object," this description is denoted by

$$a(w) = [\text{ weight}(w) \in [73.50, 79.50]] \wedge [\text{ age}(w) \in [26, 29]]], \; w \in \Omega.$$

Of course, we can also describe it by using all the explanatory variables.

For each terminal node t of the tree T associated with class G_s we can calculate the corresponding misclassification rate $R(s|t) = \sum_{r=1}^{L} P(r/t)$ where $r \neq s$ and $P(r|t) = \frac{n_t(G_r)}{n_t}$ is the proportion of the individuals at the node t allocated to the class G_s but belonging to the class G_r with $n_t(G_r)$ and n_t defined in the previous section. The misclassification MR of the tree T is $MR(A) = \sum_{t \in T} \frac{n_i}{n} R(s/t)$, where $r \neq s$. For each terminal node of the tree T we can calculate the corresponding inertia, $H(t)$, and we can calculate the total inertia by summing over all the terminal nodes. So,

$$H(t) = \sum_{w_i \in t} \sum_{w_j \in t} \frac{p_i p_j}{2\mu} \Delta(w_i, w_j) \quad \text{for } p_i = 1/n_t.$$

The total inertia of T is $I(A) = \sum_{t \in T} H(t)$.

When we use only a homogeneity criterion, i.e., we fix $\alpha = 1$ ($\beta = 0$), each description gathers homogenous groups of teams. The total inertia of the terminal nodes is minimized and equal to 0.84. However, the misclassification rate is high, equal to 33%. When we use only a discrimination criterion, i.e., we fix $\alpha = 0$, ($\beta = 1$) with an initial partition such that P1 = the best teams and P2 = the worst teams, we have a misclassification rate of 27%. However the inertia is equal to 0.90, which is larger than before.

When we vary alpha to optimize both the inertia and the misclassification rate simultaneously, we find that: the inertia varies when we increase α; the misclassification rate increases when we increase α. If we choose a data-driven value of $\alpha = 0.6$ (cf. Vrac et al., 2002), the resulting inertia is 0.89 and the misclassification rate is 30%. So we have a good misclassification rate and a better class description than that which we obtain when considering only a discrimination criterion; and we have a better misclasification rate than that which we obtain when considering only a homogeneity criterion.

5 Conclusion

In this paper we present a new approach to obtaining a description of a class. The class to describe can be a class from a prior partition, the whole population, or any class from the population. Our approach is based on a divisive top-down tree method, restricted to recursive binary partitions, until a suitable stopping rule prevents further divisions. This method is applicable to interval type data.

We have two main ideas. The first is that we combine a homogeneity criterion and a discrimination criterion to describe a class explaining an a priori partition. The user may weight these criteria depending on their relative importance to reaching the goal of the analysis. The second idea is that because we are treating symbolic variables with multivalued observed values, we use a probabilistic approach to assign units to nodes.

References

1. Bock, H., and Diday, E. (2001). "Symbolic Data Analysis and the SODAS Project: Purpose, History, and Perspective," *Analysis of Symbolic Data*, **1**, 1–23.
2. Breiman, L., Friedman, J. H., Olshen,R. A., and Stone, C. J. (1984). *Classification and Regression Trees*, Wadsworth, Belmont, California.
3. Chavent, M. (1997). *Analyse de Données Symboliques, Une Méthode Divisive de Classification*. Ph.D. dissertation, Université Paris IX Dauphine, Paris.
4. Gettler-Summa, M. (1999). *MGS in SODAS : Marking and Generalization by Symbolic Objects in the Symbolic Official Data Analysis Software*. Cahiers du CEREMADE, Paris, France.
5. Limam, M., Diday, E., and Winsberg, S. (2003). "Symbolic Class Description with Interval Data," *Journal of Symbolic Data Analysis*, **1**, to appear.

6. Limam, M., Vrac, M., Diday, E., and Winsberg,S. (2002). "A Top Down Binary Tree Method for Symbolic Class Descriptions," Proceedings of the Ninth International Conference on Information Processing and Management of Uncertainty (IPMU), *Université de Savoie*, 877–882.
7. Périnel, E. (1999). "Construire un Arbre de Discrimination Binaire à Partir de Données Imprécises," Revue de Statistique Appliquée, **47**, 5–30.
8. Quinlan, J. R. (1986). "Induction of Decision Trees," *Machine Learning*, **1**, 81–106.
9. Vrac, M., Limam, M., Diday, E., and Winsberg, S. (2002). "Symbolic Class Description," in *Classification, Clustering, and Data Analysis*, eds. K. Jajuga and A. Sokolowski, Heidelberg:Springer, pp. 329–337.

Building Small Scale Models of Multi-Entity Databases By Clustering

Georges Hébrail[1] and Yves Lechevallier[2]

[1] ENST Paris, France
hebrail@enst.fr
[2] INRIA - Rocquencourt, France
Yves.Lechevallier@inria.fr

Abstract: A framework is proposed to build small scale models of very large databases describing several entities and their relationships. In the first part, it is shown that the use of sampling is not a good solution when several entities are stored in a database. In the second part, a model is proposed which is based on clustering all entities of the database and storing aggregates on the clusters and on the relationships between the clusters. The last part of the paper discusses the different problems which are raised by this approach. Some solutions are proposed: in particular, the link with symbolic data analysis is established.

1 Introduction and Motivation

Every day, more and more data are generated by computers in all fields of activity. Operational databases create and update detailed data for management purposes. Data from operational databases are transferred into data warehouses when they need to be used for decision-aid purposes. In some cases, data are summarized (usually by aggregation processes) when loaded into the data warehouse, but in many cases detailed data are kept. This leads to very large amounts of data in data warehouses, especially due to the fact that historical data are kept. On the other hand, many analyzes operated on data warehouses do not need such detailed data: data cubes (i.e., n-way arrays) are often used at a very aggregated level, and some data mining or data analysis methods only use aggregated data.

The goal of this paper is to discuss methods for reducing the volume of data in data warehouses, preserving the possibility to perform needed analyses. An important issue in databases and data warehouses is that they describe several entities (populations) which are linked together by relationships. This paper tackles this fundamental aspect of databases and proposes solutions to deal with it.

The paper is organized as follows. Section 2 is devoted to the presentation of related work, both in the fields of databases and statistics. Section 3 describes how several entities and their relationships are stored in databases and data warehouses. In Section 4, it is shown that the use of sampling is not appropriate for several reasons. Section 5 presents the model we propose for building small scale models (SSM) of multi-entity databases: the model is based on a clustering of all entities and a storage of information on the clusters instead of the detailed entities. Section 6 discusses the main outcome problems to this approach: (1) the choice of the clustering method, (2) the use of the SSM, (3) the updatability of the SSM. Section 7 finally establishes a link between this work and the approach of symbolic data analysis proposed by (Diday 1988).

2 Related Work

This work is related both to the database and statistical data analysis fields.

For many years, work has been done in the field of databases to improve response time for long queries in large databases, or to provide quickly approximate answers to long queries. Summaries of data are built and updated to do so. Two main approaches have been developed: the construction of histograms (see for instance Gibbons et al. (1997), Chaudhuri (1998), Poosala and Ganti 1999), and the use of sampling techniques (see for instance Gibbons and Matias (1998), Chaudhuri et al. 2001). In these approaches summaries are built at a table level and do not take into account that tables in relational databases may store either entities or relationships between entities. Consequently, the management of summaries on several entities linked together is not truly supported.

Still in the area of databases, work has been done on the use of data compression techniques to improve response time, by storing compressed data on disk instead of original data (cf. Ng and Ravishankar 1995; Westmann et al. 2000). In this situation compressed data have no interpretation and cannot be used unless decompressing them. Our work differs from this work in the sense that our compression technique has a semantic basis.

At the edge between databases and statistics, much work has been done in the field of scientific and statistical databases. In this field, the concept of summary tables (storing aggregated data) has been introduced for many years and some models and query languages have been proposed and developed (see for instance Shoshani, 1982; Ozsoyoglu and Ozsoyoglu, 1985). More recently, the concept of multidimensional databases (sometimes referred as OLAP systems) has been introduced which enables the user to query interactively summary tables (see for instance Chaudhuri and Dayal, 1997).

In the field of statistics, our work is related to clustering methods and to sampling methods. These two domains have been studied extensively for many years (see for instance Duda et al., 2001, and Cochran, 1997). Our work and discussion benefits from known results from these domains.

More recently, a new direction has been explored at the edge of statistical data analysis and artificial intelligence. The concept of symbolic objects has been introduced to describe objects which are not individuals but have the ability to represent characteristics of groups of individuals. For a complete presentation of this approach, see Bock and Diday (2000). Section 7 shows that our model can benefit from the concept of symbolic objects.

Finally, in Hou (1999), it is shown that most data mining tasks can be achieved using only some summary tables. This work differs from ours in the sense that the summary tables store clusters of individuals which are not based on a clustering process. Also, this approach does not support multi-entity information.

3 Storing Several Entities in the Same Database

Relational databases are used in business information systems to store data needed for the management of the company; e.g., data about orders, bills, suppliers, customers, and so forth. Such business databases store data corresponding to several populations (so-called in the statistical community) known as several entities in the database community. The information systems community has developed models for describing the contents of such databases. A very famous model, proposed by Chen (1976) describes the contents of a database as a set of entities and relationships between entities. More recent models, such as UML (see Booch et al., 1999), are more complete, taking into account the object oriented approach. In this paper, we will refer to a simplified entity-relationship (ER) model proposed by Chen, to clarify the presentation.

Within the ER model, the contents of a database are described by sets of entities (for instance cars, customers, or products, as in the example of Fig. 1), and relationships between entities. Relationships are represented in Fig. 1 by ellipses linked to the corresponding sets of entities. Both entities and relationships can be described by attributes (for instance NAME, ADDRESS for CUSTOMER, and QUANTITY for the relationship linking CUSTOMER, PRODUCT and SUPPLIER). Relationships may link together two or more entities. Relationships are also described by some cardinality information: in the example of Fig. 1, a car is owned by exactly one customer and a customer may have from 0 to several cars, and a customer may be involved in from 0 to several relationships with a couple of products and suppliers. Table 1 describes the attributes of the entities of Fig. 1. Note that attributes identifying entities (called keys) are prefixed by ID.

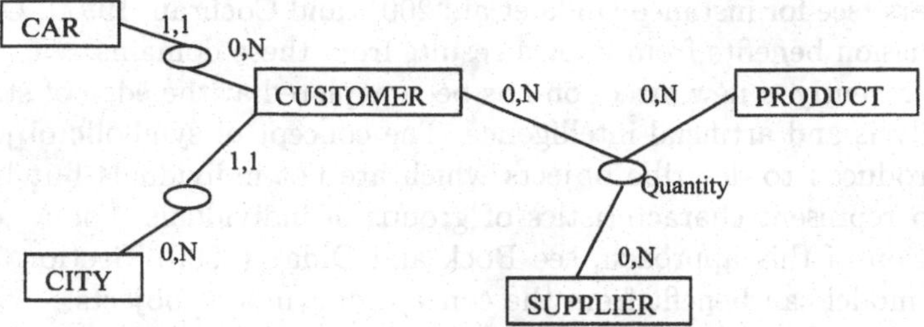

Fig. 1. Example of an ER diagram describing the contents of a database.

Table 1. Attributes of entities (SPC stands for Socio-Professional Category).

SETS OF ENTITIES	ATTRIBUTES
CUSTOMER	IDCUST, NAME, ADDRESS, AGE, SALARY, SPC
CITY	IDCITY, NAME, RURAL/URBAN, #POPULATION, #BUSLINES
CAR	IDCAR, NAME, BRAND, PRICE, SPEED, WEIGHT
SUPPLIER	IDSUPP, NAME, ACTIVITY, TURNOVER, EMPLOYEES
PRODUCT	IDPROD, NAME, CATEGORY, SUBCATEGORY, PRICE, WEIGHT

Each line in Fig. 2 corresponds to a table in the relational database. Underlined attributes are primary keys.

CUSTOMER (IDCUST, NAME, ADDRESS, AGE, SALARY, SPC, IDCITY)
IDCITY refers to CITY
CITY (IDCITY, NAME, RURAL/URBAN, POPULATION, #BUSLINES)
CAR (IDCAR, NAME, BRAND, PRICE, WEIGHT, IDCUST)
IDCUST refers to CUSTOMER
SUPPLIER (IDSUPP, NAME, ACTIVITY, TURNOVER, #EMPLOYEES)
PRODUCT (IDPROD, NAME, CATEGORY, SUBCATEGORY, PRICE, WEIGHT)
ORDER (IDCUST, IDPROD, IDSUPP, QUANTITY)
IDCUST refers to CUSTOMER
IDPROD refers to PRODUCT
IDSUPP refers to SUPPLIER

Fig. 2. Relational database schemata of the ER diagram of Figure 1.

4 Aggregation Versus Sampling

Considering the example described above, we address now the following problem:

Assuming that the size of the database is very large (for instance millions of customers, cars, products, orders, and thousands of cities), build a small scale model (SSM) of the database, so that further analyzes may be performed on the SSM (computation of cross tables, principal component analysis, clustering, construction of decision trees, and so forth).

For a statistician, a natural way to achieve this goal is to sample the database. Many methods have been developed to do so (see Cochran, 1977); characteristics of a whole population (for instance the average salary of customers) can be approximated by only considering a sample of it. But several problems appear when applying sampling theory to solve our problem. They are discussed below.

4.1 Representativeness of the Sample

Inference from a sample requires that the sample be large enough and representative. This can be achieved by using simple random or stratified random sampling. Randomization ensures that the inference is correct. Stratified sampling is used when some subsets of the population are too small to be sufficiently represented in the sample, or when data collection makes it necessary. In this case, calibration is performed to correct bias. But stratified sampling needs the definition of a goal for the analysis: this constraint is not compatible with our problem since we wish to build a small scale model of the database which can be used for any further analysis. In particular, individuals corresponding to a "niche" (small sub-population) may be either absent from the sample or insufficiently represented to consider inference on them.

4.2 Update of the Sample

The contents of databases and data warehouses are subject to changes over time. So there is a need for updating the SSM of the database when the initial database changes. Updating a sample is a difficult problem, especially if we want to keep the sample representative and to limit its size.

4.3 Sampling Several Entities and Their Relationships

The most important difficulty we meet in using sampling as a solution to our problem refers to the management of a SSM describing several sets of entities and their relationships. Since sampling theory applies to one population of individuals, one can sample separately all sets of entities stored in the database. But doing this, there is no chance that relationships between entities are sampled correctly: cars in the car sample do not correspond in general to owners belonging to the customer sample. One can imagine procedures to complement the samples so that the relationships between objects in the sample are complete. But, depending on the cardinalities of the relationships, these procedures may lead one to keep the whole database as the sample.

Though efficient algorithms exist to sample relational databases (Olken, 1993), we consider that this approach is not practical to build SSMs of databases.

5 Small Scale Models of Multi-Entity Databases

We propose to build the small scale model (SSM) of a database as follows:

- Each set of entities (in our example: CAR, CUSTOMER, CITY, etc.) is partitioned into a large number of classes (typically 10,000 to 100,000) using a clustering algorithm.
- Classes of entities are stored in the SSM, being described by the size of the class and by aggregated information associated with entity attributes.
- Relationships between entities are aggregated at the entity class level. They are described by the size of every non-empty combination of classes, and by aggregated information associated with relationship attributes.

Recalling the example, the structure of the SSM, expressed as a relational database, is shown in Fig. 3.

SSM_CUSTOMER (C_CUST, D_AGE, D_SALARY, D_SPC, COUNT)
SSM_CITY (C_CITY, D_RURAL/URBAN, D_POPULATION, D_#BUSLINES, COUNT)
SSM_CAR (C_CAR, D_BRAND, D_PRICE, D_WEIGHT, COUNT)
SSM_SUPPLIER (C_SUPP, D_ACTIVITY, D_TURNOVER, D_#EMPLOYEES, COUNT)
SSM_PRODUCT (C_PROD, D_CATEGORY, D_SUBCATEGORY,
D_PRICE, D_WEIGHT, COUNT)
SSM_CUST_CITY (C_CUST, C_CITY, COUNT)
C_CUST refers to CUSTOMER
C_CITY refers to CITY
SSM_CAR_CUST (C_CAR, C_CUST, COUNT)
C_CAR refers to CAR
C_CUST refers to CUSTOMER
SSM_ORDER (C_CUST, C_PROD, C_SUPP, D_QUANTITY, COUNT)
C_CUST refers to CUSTOMER
C_PROD refers to PRODUCT
C_SUPP refers to SUPPLIER

Fig. 3. Relational database schemata of the SSM.

The interpretation of this relational schemata is the following:

- Each class of entities is identified by a value appearing in a column prefixed by C_. For instance C_CUST identifies classes of customers.
- Classes of entities are described by aggregated descriptions of entity attributes (prefixed by D_). The simplest way to build such aggregated descriptions is to compute the sum of values for numerical attributes, and frequency distributions for others. More accurate descriptions can be considered, such as histograms. Columns prefixed by D_ correspond to complex data types in an object-relational database. Note that attributes such as NAME have been removed from the class description since different entities have different names. Note also that all tables describing classes of entities include a COUNT attribute featuring the number of entities in each class. Fig. 4 shows an example of the contents of the CAR SSM.

- Relationships between entities are described by the number of associations of all non-empty combination of classes of entities involved in the relationship. For instance, the tuple ("cluster_car_121," "cluster_cust_342," 26) in table SSM_CAR_CUST means that there are 26 instances of cars of cluster 121 linked to customers of cluster 342 in the detailed database. When relationships also show attributes (like QUANTITY in the ORDER relationship), these attributes are aggregated just as entity attributes are.

C_CAR	D_BRAND	D_PRICE	D_WEIGHT	COUNT
cluster_car_1	RENAULT : 2 CITROEN : 87	1098705	93628	89
cluster_car_2	PEUGEOT : 12 CITROEN : 1	293046	15899	13
...	...	...	...	...

Fig. 4. Sample contents of SSM_CAR.

6 Follow-Up Problems

There are many problems raised by this approach. This section lays out some of these issues.

6.1 Choice of the clustering method

The clustering method must meet the following main requirements: (1) ability to process a very large number of entities (up to several millions), (2) ability to produce a large number of clusters (from 10,000 to 100,000), (3) ability to handle attributes (variables) of heterogeneous type.

Requirements (1) and (2) lead naturally to iterative methods like k-means (cf. Duda et al., 2001) or Self Organizing Maps (SOM) (Kohonen, 1995).

As for requirement (3), we first need to eliminate attributes like NAME or ADDRESS, which show a different value for almost all entities. A simple criterion to do so is to eliminate attributes showing more than a threshold of distinct values, for instance 100. Another solution is to use possibly existing taxonomies on these attribute values, available as metadata. A simple solution to handle variables of heterogeneous type is to do the following: (1) transform all categorical variables into a complete disjunctive representation, (2) use a weight on each variable related to its variance.

6.2 Using the Small Scale Model of a Database

We give here some examples to show typical queries which can be addressed to a SSM.

Computation of Statistics on Entities

First, SSM tables corresponding to entities can be queried as a whole. For instance the following queries can be answered exactly: Average salary of customers; Total population in all cities; Total number of bus lines in all cities; Total number of cars.

Selections may be applied to SSM tables corresponding to entities, possibly leading to exact answers to queries (Total number of Renault cars, Number of rural cities) or to approximate answers, for instance: Average salary for customers having SPC = "Farmer." To answer the latter query, all customer classes with a minimum of 1 customer with SPC = "Farmer" are selected (the frequency distribution kept for SPC is used to do this). Selected classes may either contain only farmers or customers with some other SPCs. An interval of values can then be computed for the average salary over selected classes. Since the clustering has been done with a large number of classes, there is a good chance that most selected classes contain only or mainly farmers.

Computation of Statistics Using Entities and Relationships

SSM tables corresponding to relationships can be used to answer queries involving relationships between entities, for instance: Average salary of farmer customers owning a Renault car. This query can be answered by following the steps below:

- Selection in SSM_CUSTOMER of customer classes with frequency of SPC = "Farmer" not equal to zero.
- Selection in SSM_CAR of car classes with frequency of BRAND = "Renault" not equal to zero.
- Selection in SSM_CAR_CUST of all couples (car class, customer class) where the car class or the customer class have been previously selected. This procedure eliminates some customer classes selected before.
- Computation of an interval of values for the requested average salary.

Performing Data Mining on Entities

For entities showing only numerical attributes, methods like Principal Component Analysis (PCA) can be applied to the SSM representation, considering that all entities belonging to the same class have the same value for the numerical variable. Intra-class inertia is lost, but this loss is minimized by the clustering process. The same approach can be followed to perform clustering on the SSM. Most methods of data analysis can analyze individuals associated with a weight. For entities showing categorical variables, Section 7 shows that symbolic data analysis can be applied.

6.3 Updating the Small Scale Model of the Database

The update of the SSM is straightforward. When the detailed database changes, the SSM can be updated incrementally in the following way:

- For every created/modified/suppressed entity, its class is computed using a function derived from the clustering process. The SSM table associated with the entity is updated: numerical descriptions are updated by a simple addition/substraction, and frequency distribution of categorical attributes are updated by modifying the corresponding frequency value(s).
- SSM tables associated with the relationships in which the updated entity is involved are also updated (both the COUNT column and possible relationship aggregated attributes).

After many updates, the clustering of entities may become inaccurate; the intra-class inertia may be increasing so that approximate answers to queries addressed to the SSM may be not precise enough. In this case, it may be necessary to rebuild the SSM, by applying again the clustering of some entities.

7 Link with Symbolic Data Analysis

Symbolic data analysis (Bock and Diday, 2000) aims at analyzing objects that describe groups of individuals instead of single individuals. Standard methods of data analysis have been extended to analyze such symbolic objects. Software (called SODAS) is available to run these extended methods. The link between our study and symbolic data analysis can be established at three levels:

- Assertions (which are particular symbolic objects) can be used to describe SSMs of entities, but not SSMs of relationships. As a matter of fact, assertions can describe intervals of values, histograms, and probability distributions.
- The methods available in the SODAS software can be applied to SSMs of entities.
- The introduction of the SSM structure gives new perspectives for symbolic data analysis: more complex structures such as hords, synthesis, or composite objects can be used to manage relationships between symbolic objects.

8 Conclusion and Further Work

We have presented a new model for building small scale models (SSMs) of large databases. Both entities and relationships between entities stored in the database are summarized. This is achieved by clustering entities of the database, and storing aggregates about clusters of entities and relationships between clusters of entities. Much further work can be considered on SSMs, mainly:

- The study of relevant clustering methods to build SSMs, including the stability of clusters against database updates,
- The definition of a language to query SSMs (inspired from those described in Ozsoyoglu and Ozsoyoglu, 2000) and the evaluation of the precision of answers obtained by querying SSMs instead of the whole database,
- The study of the use of symbolic object structures to deal with relationships between assertions.

References

1. Bock, H.-H., and Diday, E. (eds.) (2000). *Analysis of Symbolic Data. Exploratory Methods for Extracting Statistical Information from Complex Data*, Data Analysis and Knowledge Organization, Springer Verlag, Heidelberg.
2. Booch, G., Rumbaugh, J., and Jacobson, I. (1999). *Unified Modeling Language User Guide*, Object Technology Series, Addison-Wesley, New York.
3. Chaudhuri, S. (1998). "An Overview of Query Optimization in Relational Systems," in *Proceedings of the Seventeenth ACM SIGACT-SIGMOD-SIGART Symposium on Principles of Database Systems*, pp. 34-43.
4. Chaudhuri, S., Das, G., and Narasayya, V. (2001). "A Robust, Optimization-Based Approach for Approximate Answering of Aggregate Queries," *Proceedings of ACM SIGMOD 2001.*
5. Chaudhuri, S., and Dayal, U., (1997). "An Overview of Data Warehousing and OLAP Technologies," *ACM SIGMOD Record.*
6. Chen, P. P., (1976). "The Entity-Relationship Model: Towards a Unified View of Data," in *ACM TODS*, Vol. 1, No. 1.
7. Cochran, W. G., (1977). *Sampling Techniques*, 3rd edition, John Wiley & Sons, New York.
8. Diday, E. (1988). "The Symbolic Approach in Clustering and Related Methods of Data Analysis: The Basic Choice," in *Classification and Related Methods of Data Analysis*, H.-H. Bock, ed., Amsterdam:North Holland, pp. 673-684.
9. Duda, R. O., Hart, P. E., and Stork, D. G. (2001). "Chapter 10 : Unsupervised Learning and Clustering," in *Pattern Classification*, Wiley Interscience, New York.
10. Gibbons, P. B., and Matias, Y. (1998). "New Sampling-Based Summary Statistics for Improving Approximate Query Answers," in *Proceedings of ACM SIGMOD 1998.*
11. Gibbons, P. B, Matias, Y., and Poosala, V. (1997). "Fast Incremental Maintenance of Approximate Histograms," *Proceedings of the 23rd International Conference on Very Large Data Bases.*
12. Hou, W. (1999). "A Framework for Statistical Data Mining with Summary Tables,"in *Proceeding of 11th International Conference on Scientific and Statistical Database Management*, Columbus, Ohio.
13. Kohonen T. (1995). *Self-Organizing Maps*, Springer, Berlin.
14. Ng, W. K., Ravishankar, C. V. (1995). "Relational Database Compression Using Augmented Vector Quantization," in *Proceedings of the 11th Conference on Data Engineering*, Taiwan.
15. Olken, F. (1993). *Random Sampling from Databases*, Ph.D. Dissertation, University of California at Berkeley, USA.

16. Ozsoyoglu, G., and Ozsoyoglu, Z. M. (1985). "Statistical Database Query Languages," *IEEE Transactions on Software Engineering*, **12**, 1071–1081.
17. Poosala, V., and Ganti, V. (1999). "Fast Approximate Answers to Aggregate Queries on a Data Cube," in *11th International Conferemce on Scientific and Statistical Database Management*, Cleveland.
18. Shoshani, A. (1982). "Statistical Databases, Characteristics, Problems and Some Solutions," in *Proceedings of the 1982 Conference on Very Large Data Bases, VLDB.*
19. Westmann, T., Kossmann, D., Helmer, S., and Moerkotte, G. (2000). "The Implementation and Performance of Compressed Databases," *SIGMOD Record*, **29**, 55–67.

Part V

Taxonomy and Medicine

Phylogenetic Closure Operations and Homoplasy-Free Evolution

Tobias Dezulian[1] and Mike Steel[2]

[1] University of Tübingen, Germany
dezulian@informatik.uni-tuebingen.de
[2] University of Canterbury, New Zealand
M.Steel@math.canterbury.ac.nz

Abstract: Phylogenetic closure operations on partial splits and quartet trees turn out to be both mathematically interesting and computationally useful. Although these operations were defined two decades ago, until recently little had been established concerning their properties. Here we present some further new results and links between these closure operations, and show how they can be applied in phylogeny reconstruction and enumeration. Using the operations we study how effectively one may be able to reconstruct phylogenies from evolved multi-state characters that take values in a large state space (such as may arise with certain genomic data).

1 Phylogenetic Closure Operations

Meacham (1983), building on the earlier work of Estabrook and McMorris (1977) and others, described two formal rules for deriving new phylogenetic relationships from pairs of compatible characters. These rules are particularly simple and appealing, and we describe them in the following subsections. There are interesting mathematical relationships between these rules, and we develop and those and indicate new results that support their use in modern phylogenetic modeling.

1.1 Rules for Partial Splits

In this paper a *partial X-split* refers to a partition of some subset of X into two disjoint nonempty subsets, say A and B, and we denote this by writing $A|B$ (= $B|A$). Also we say that a phylogenetic X–tree $\mathcal{T}$ *displays* a partial X–split $A|B$ if there exists at least one edge of $\mathcal{T}$ whose deletion from $\mathcal{T}$ separates the leaves labeled by the species in A from the species in B. This concept is illustrated in Fig. 1.

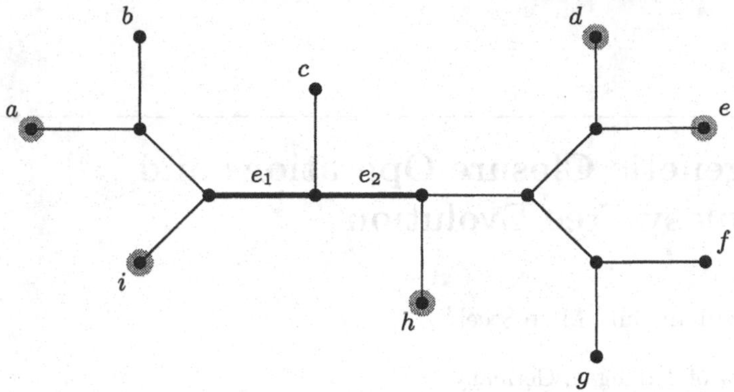

Fig. 1. The phylogenetic X–tree shown above displays the partial X–split $\{a,i\}|\{d,e,h\}$. Deleting edge e_1 or e_2 separates $\{a,i\}$ from $\{d,e,h\}$.

Given a collection Σ of partial X–splits and a partial X–split $A|B$, we write $\Sigma \vdash A|B$ if every phylogenetic X–tree that displays each partial X–split in Σ also displays $A|B$. Let $A_1|B_1$ and $A_2|B_2$ be two partial X-splits. Meacham's two rules can be stated as follows.

(M1): If $A_1 \cap A_2 \neq \emptyset$ and $B_1 \cap B_2 \neq \emptyset$ then

$$\{A_1|B_1, A_2|B_2\} \vdash A_1 \cap A_2|B_1 \cup B_2, A_1 \cup A_2|B_1 \cap B_2.$$

(M2): If $A_1 \cap A_2 \neq \emptyset$ and $B_1 \cap B_2 \neq \emptyset$ and $A_1 \cap B_2 \neq \emptyset$ then

$$\{A_1|B_1, A_2|B_2\} \vdash A_2|B_1 \cup B_2, A_1 \cup A_2|B_1.$$

The underlying theorem (Meacham, 1983) that justifies these two rules is the following:

ANY PHYLOGENETIC X–TREE THAT DISPLAYS THE PARTIAL X–SPLITS ON THE LEFT OF **(M1)** OR **(M2)** ALSO DISPLAYS THE CORRESPONDING PARTIAL X–SPLITS ON THE RIGHT.

1.2 Rules for Quartet Trees

At around the same time as Meacham's paper, researchers in stemmatology in Holland, building on the earlier pioneering work of Colonius and Schulze (1981), described rules for combining quartet trees. In particular, Marcel Dekker in his MSc thesis (1986) investigated two 'dyadic' rules, which take as their input two quartet trees and produce one or more output quartet trees.

Standard terminology refers to a fully-resolved phylogenetic tree on four leaves as a *quartet tree* and we write it as $ab|cd$ if the interior edge separates the pair of leaves a, b from the pair of leaves c, d. Also we say that a phylogenetic X–tree $\mathcal{T}$ *displays* the quartet tree $ab|cd$ if there is at least one interior edge of

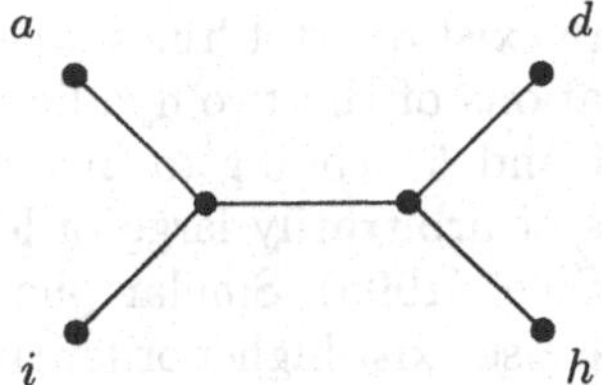

Fig. 2. A quartet tree $ai|dh$ that is displayed by the tree in Fig.1.

$\mathcal{T}$ that separates the pair a, b from the pair c, d. These concepts are illustrated in Fig.1 and Fig.2. For any phylogenetic X–tree $\mathcal{T}$ we let $\mathcal{Q}(\mathcal{T})$ denote the set of all quartet trees that are displayed by $\mathcal{T}$.

Returning now to quartet rules, for a set $\mathcal{Q}$ of quartet trees we write $\mathcal{Q} \vdash ab|cd$ precisely if every phylogenetic tree that displays $\mathcal{Q}$ also displays $ab|cd$. We call the statement $\mathcal{Q} \vdash ab|cd$ a *quartet rule*, and it is *dyadic* if $|\mathcal{Q}| = 2$. There are precisely two dyadic quartet rules:

(Q1): $\{ab|cd, ab|ce\} \vdash ab|de$ and

(Q2): $\{ab|cd, ac|de\} \vdash ab|ce, ab|de, bc|de$.

The underlying (and easily proved) theorem that justifies these two rules is the following:

ANY PHYLOGENETIC X–TREE THAT DISPLAYS THE QUARTET TREES ON THE LEFT OF **(Q1)** OR **(Q2)** ALSO DISPLAYS THE CORRESPONDING QUARTET TREE(S) ON THE RIGHT.

Thus for a set $\mathcal{Q}$ of quartet trees we may form the *dyadic closure* of $\mathcal{Q}$ subject to either or both rules. More precisely, for $\theta \subseteq \{1, 2\}$, let qcl_θ denote the minimal set of quartet trees that contains $\mathcal{Q}$ and is closed under rule **(Qi)** for each $i \in \theta$. In practice $\mathrm{qcl}_\theta(\mathcal{Q})$ can be obtained from $\mathcal{Q}$ by constructing a sequence

$$\mathcal{Q} = \mathcal{Q}_1 \subseteq \mathcal{Q}_2 \subseteq \cdots$$

where $\mathcal{Q}_{i+1}$ consists of $\mathcal{Q}_i$ together with all additional quartets that can be obtained from a pair of quartets in $\mathcal{Q}_i$ by applying the rule(s) allowed by θ. Then $\mathrm{qcl}_\theta(\mathcal{Q})$ is just $\mathcal{Q}_i$ for the first index i for which $\mathcal{Q}_{i+1} = \mathcal{Q}_i$. Note that the sequence $\mathcal{Q}_i$ is uniquely determined by $\mathcal{Q}$ and $\mathrm{qcl}_\theta(\mathcal{Q})$ is the minimal subset of quartet trees containing $\mathcal{Q}$ that is closed under the rule(s) in θ.

The construction of $\mathrm{qcl}_\theta(\mathcal{Q})$ is useful for the following reasons. First, if $\mathcal{Q}$ is incompatible, we may discover this by finding a pair of contradictory quartets (of the form $ab|cd, ac|bd$ in $\mathrm{qcl}_\theta(\mathcal{Q})$). Second, we may find that $\mathrm{qcl}_\theta(\mathcal{Q})$ consists of all the quartets of a tree, from which we can thereby not only verify that $\mathcal{Q}$ is compatible, but easily construct a tree that displays $\mathcal{Q}$. This is precisely what Dekker found for some of his trees describing the copying history of manuscripts.

Dekker showed that there exist quartet 'rules' of order 3 that could not be reduced to repeated applications of the two dyadic rules. Dekker also found irreducible rules of order 4 and 5, leading to his conjecture that there exist irreducible quartet rules of arbitrarily large order, a result subsequently established in Bryant and Steel (1995). Similar phenomena occur with split closure rules, for which there also exist higher order rules for combining partial X–splits, and indeed a third order rule was described by Meacham (1983).

Since dyadic quartet rules are provably incomplete, why then should we bother with them? Two reasons seem compelling. First, in an area where most interesting questions are NP-complete (cf. Ng, Steel,and Wormald, 2000; Steel, 1992), computing dyadic quartet closure can, reassuringly, be carried out in polynomial-time. Second, there are now several sufficient conditions known where quartet closure will yield all the quartets of a tree. We shall describe one of these now, after recalling some terminology.

Definitions: We say that a set $\mathcal{Q}$ of quartet trees *defines a phylogenetic X–tree $\mathcal{T}$* precisely if $\mathcal{T}$ is the only phylogenetic X–tree that displays each quartet tree in $\mathcal{Q}$. In this case it is easily shown that $\mathcal{T}$ must be fully resolved, and $|\mathcal{Q}| - (|X| - 3) \geq 0$; if in addition we have $|\mathcal{Q}| - (|X| - 3) = 0$ then we say that $\mathcal{Q}$ is *excess-free*. □

Theorem 1. *Suppose $\mathcal{Q}$ is a set of quartet trees and $\mathcal{Q}$ contains an excess-free subset that defines a phylogenetic tree $\mathcal{T}$. Then* $\mathrm{qcl}_2(\mathcal{Q}) = \mathcal{Q}(\mathcal{T})$.

The only known proof of this result, in Böcker et al. (2000), is an easy consequence of the 'patchwork' theory in Böcker (1999) and Böcker, Dress and Steel (1999). This in turn is based on one of the most mysterious and apparently difficult results in phylogenetics, which concerns the proof an innocuous-looking yet powerful theorem: *Any set $\mathcal{Q}$ of two or more quartet trees that is excess-free and defines a phylogenetic tree is the disjoint union of two non-empty, excess-free subsets.*

In Section 2 we shall provide another sufficient condition under which dyadic quartet closure, in this case using rule (**Q1**), will yield all the quartets of any fully resolved tree.

1.3 The (Almost) Happy Marriage

The reader may now be wondering what, if any, connection exists between the rules that Meacham described and those of Dekker. It turns out there is a very close (but not exact) correspondence between these operations, and to explain this we introduce some further notation.

Definitions: We say that a partial split $A'|B'$ *refines* another partial split $A|B$ precisely if $A \subseteq A'$ and $B \subseteq B'$ (or $A \subseteq B'$ and $B \subseteq A'$) and we denote this by writing $A|B \preceq A'|B'$. Note that $\preceq$ is a partial order on the set $\Sigma(X)$ of all partial X–splits, and if $A|B \preceq A'|B'$ but $A|B \neq A'|B'$, then as is usual we shall write $A|B \prec A'|B'$. Given a set Σ of partial X–splits, we define the *reduction* of Σ to be the set $\rho(\Sigma)$ of partial X–splits defined by:

$$\rho(\Sigma) = \{A|B \in \Sigma : \text{ there is no } A'|B' \in \Sigma \text{ for which } A|B \prec A'|B'\}.$$

□

We should note that a set of partial X–splits Σ conveys no more phylogenetic information than does its reduction. This is due to the following, easily established result: The set of phylogenetic X–trees that displays each split in Σ is identical to the set of phylogenetic X–trees that displays each split in $\rho(\Sigma)$. Therefore it will be convenient for us to reduce whenever we feasible to ensure that the sets of partial X–splits do not become excessively large.

Definitions: For a set Σ of partial X–splits and $\theta \subseteq \{1, 2\}$ let

$$W_\theta(\Sigma) := \{\Sigma' \subseteq \Sigma(X) : \Sigma \subseteq \Sigma' \text{ and } \Sigma' \text{ is closed under } (\mathbf{Mi}) \text{ for all } i \in \theta\}.$$

Notice that $W_\theta(\Sigma) \neq \emptyset$ since $\Sigma(X) \in W_\theta(\Sigma)$, and if $\Sigma_1, \Sigma_2 \in W_\theta(\Sigma)$ then $\Sigma_1 \cap \Sigma_2 \in W_\theta(\Sigma)$. Thus the set $\cap W_\theta(\Sigma)$ $(= \cap\{\Sigma : \Sigma \in W_\theta(\Sigma)\}$ is well-defined, and it is the (unique) minimal set of partial X–splits that contains Σ and which is also closed under Meacham's rules (**Mi**) for all $i \in \theta$. Finally, let

$$\mathrm{spcl}_\theta(\Sigma) := \rho(\cap W_\theta(\Sigma)).$$

Thus $\mathrm{spcl}_\theta(\Sigma)$ is the reduction of the set $\cap W_\theta(\Sigma)$. □

We can construct $\mathrm{spcl}_\theta(\Sigma)$ by repeatedly applying the rules allowed by θ to construct a sequence $\Sigma = \Sigma_1 \subseteq \Sigma_2 \subseteq \cdots$ until the sequence stabilizes. At this point (as well as at any point along the sequence that we wish) we can then apply reduction. This construction was suggested by Meacham (1983) and our aim here is to establish some of its useful features.

Example 1. Let

$$\Sigma = \{\{a, b\}|\{c, d\}, \{a, b\}|\{c, e\}, \{a, c\}|\{d, e\}, \{b, c\}|\{d, e\}\}.$$

Then $\mathrm{spcl}_1(\Sigma) = \{\{a, b\}|\{c, d, e\}, \{a, b, c\}|\{d, e\}\}$. □

Example 2. Let

$$\Sigma = \{\{b, f\}|\{e, g\}, \{a, f\}|\{d, g\}, \{a, e\}|\{c, d\}, \{a, e\}|\{b, c\}, \{a, d\}|\{c, g\}\}.$$

Then $\mathrm{spcl}_2(\Sigma) = \{\{c, g\}|\{a, b, d, e, f\}, \{b, f\}|\{a, c, d, e, g\}, \{a, e\}|\{b, c, d, f, g\}, \{a, b, e, f\}|\{c, d, g\}\}$. □

Notice that rule (**M2**) has the property that the derived partial splits refine the two input partial splits. Consequently

$$|\mathrm{spcl}_2(\Sigma)| \leq |\Sigma|.$$

Rule (**M1**) does not have this property. Note also that $\mathrm{spcl}_{1,2}(\Sigma)$ is not necessarily equal to $\mathrm{spcl}_1(\mathrm{spcl}_2(\Sigma))$ or to $\mathrm{spcl}_2(\mathrm{spcl}_1(\Sigma))$.

For a set Σ of partial X–splits, let $\mathcal{Q}(\Sigma)$ denote the set of *induced* quartet trees, defined by

$$\mathcal{Q}(\Sigma) := \{aa'|bb' : a, a' \in A, b, b' \in B, A|B \in \Sigma\}.$$

A phylogenetic X–tree displays the partial X–splits in Σ if and only if $\mathcal{T}$ displays the quartet trees in $\mathcal{Q}(\Sigma)$. Note that $\mathcal{Q}(\Sigma) = \mathcal{Q}(\rho(\Sigma))$ and so

$$\mathcal{Q}(\mathrm{spcl}_\theta(\Sigma)) = \mathcal{Q}(\cap W_\theta(\Sigma)). \tag{1}$$

Given a set Σ of quartet splits we may construct the quartet closure (under rules in θ) of $\mathcal{Q}(\Sigma)$, or we may construct the induced quartets of the split closure (under rules in θ) of Σ. By either route we derive a collection of quartet trees from a collection of partial X–splits. A fundamental questions is: When are the resulting sets of quartet trees identical? In other words, when does the following diagram commute?

$$\begin{array}{ccc} \Sigma & \xrightarrow{\mathcal{Q}} & \mathcal{Q}(\Sigma) \\ {\scriptstyle \mathrm{spcl}_\theta}\downarrow & & \downarrow{\scriptstyle \mathrm{qcl}_\theta} \\ \mathrm{spcl}_\theta(\Sigma) & \xrightarrow{\mathcal{Q}} & (*) \end{array}$$

The answer to this question is given in the following result.

Theorem 2. *Let Σ be a collection of partial X–splits. Then*

$$\mathrm{qcl}_\theta(\mathcal{Q}(\Sigma)) = \mathcal{Q}(\mathrm{spcl}_\theta(\Sigma))$$

for $\theta = \{1\}$ and $\theta = \{1,2\}$. For $\theta = \{2\}$ we have

$$\mathrm{qcl}_\theta(\mathcal{Q}(\Sigma)) \subseteq \mathcal{Q}(\mathrm{spcl}_\theta(\Sigma))$$

and containment can be strict.

Theorem 2 ensures that $\mathcal{Q}(\mathrm{spcl}_1(\Sigma))$ and $\mathcal{Q}(\mathrm{spcl}_{1,2}(\Sigma))$ can both be computed in polynomial time, which is not obvious since $\mathrm{spcl}_1(\Sigma)$ and $\mathrm{spcl}_{1,2}(\Sigma)$ could presumably be very large.

Proof of Theorem 2: First note that

$$\mathrm{qcl}_2(\mathcal{Q}(\Sigma)) \subseteq \mathcal{Q}(\mathrm{spcl}_2(\Sigma)) \tag{2}$$

by Semple and Steel (2001). And Example 2 shows that containment can be strict, for in this example $ab|cd \in \mathcal{Q}(\mathrm{spcl}_2(\Sigma)) - \mathrm{qcl}_2(\mathcal{Q}(\Sigma))$. Note that containment can be strict even when, as in Example 2, we have $\mathcal{Q}(\mathrm{spcl}_2(\Sigma)) = \mathcal{Q}(\mathcal{T})$ for a tree $\mathcal{T}$ defined by Σ.

Next we show that

$$\mathcal{Q}(\text{spcl}_1(\Sigma)) = \text{qcl}_1(\mathcal{Q}(\Sigma)). \tag{3}$$

To do so, we first show that

$$\mathcal{Q}(\text{spcl}_1(\Sigma)) \subseteq \text{qcl}_1(\mathcal{Q}(\Sigma)). \tag{4}$$

Consider the sequence $\Sigma = \Sigma_0, \Sigma_1, \Sigma_2, \ldots, \Sigma_N = \text{spcl}_1(\Sigma)$, where each Σ_{i+1} is obtained from Σ_i by using **(M1)**whenever applicable on any pair of splits in Σ_i.

We prove by induction on i that $\mathcal{Q}(\Sigma_i) \subseteq \text{qcl}_1(\mathcal{Q}(\Sigma))$, which suffices to establish (4). For $i = 0$, we have $\mathcal{Q}(\Sigma_0) = \mathcal{Q}(\Sigma) \subseteq \text{qcl}_1(\mathcal{Q}(\Sigma))$. Now suppose that the induction hypothesis holds for i where $0 \leq i < N$. For the induction step let $q \in \mathcal{Q}(\Sigma_{i+1})$. If $q \in \mathcal{Q}(\Sigma_i)$, then $q \in \text{qcl}_1(\mathcal{Q}(\Sigma))$ as claimed. Thus we may suppose that $q \in \mathcal{Q}(\Sigma_{i+1}) - \mathcal{Q}(\Sigma_i)$. In this case, referring to **(M1)** we may suppose, without loss of generality, that q is induced by the split $A_1 \cup A_2 | B_1 \cap B_2$. In this case we may further suppose (since we assume $q \notin \mathcal{Q}(\Sigma_i)$) that $q = a_1a_2|b_1b_2$, where $a_1 \in A_1 - A_2$, $a_2 \in A_2 - A_1$, and $b_1, b_2 \in B_1 \cap B_2$. Furthermore, there exists an element $a \in A_1 \cap A_2$ for spcl_1 to be applicable and yield q, and thus $a_1a|b_1b_2 \in \mathcal{Q}(\Sigma_i)$ and $a_2a|b_1b_2 \in \mathcal{Q}(\Sigma_i)$. The induction hypothesis yields that $a_1a|b_1b_2 \in \text{qcl}_1(\mathcal{Q}(\Sigma))$ and $a_2a|b_1b_2 \in \text{qcl}_1(\mathcal{Q}(\Sigma))$. Application of **(Q1)** to the latter two quartets yields $q = a_1a_2|b_1b_2 \in \text{qcl}_1(\mathcal{Q}(\Sigma))$, which establishes the induction step and thereby the proof of (4).

We now establish the reverse inclusion, namely:

$$\text{qcl}_1(\mathcal{Q}(\Sigma)) \subseteq \mathcal{Q}(\text{spcl}_1(\Sigma)). \tag{5}$$

Consider the sequence of quartet sets $\mathcal{Q}(\Sigma) = \mathcal{Q}_0, \mathcal{Q}_1, \mathcal{Q}_2, \ldots, \mathcal{Q}_N = \text{qcl}_1(\mathcal{Q}(\Sigma))$, where each $\mathcal{Q}_{i+1}$ is obtained from $\mathcal{Q}_i$ by using **(Q1)** whenever applicable on any pair of quartets in $\mathcal{Q}_i$.

We prove by induction on i that $\mathcal{Q}_i \subseteq \mathcal{Q}(\text{spcl}_1(\Sigma))$, thus establishing the theorem. For $i = 0$, we have $\mathcal{Q}_0 = \mathcal{Q}(\Sigma) \subseteq \mathcal{Q}(\text{spcl}_1(\Sigma))$. Now suppose that the induction hypothesis holds for some i where $0 \leq i < N$. Let $q \in \mathcal{Q}_{i+1}$. If $q \in \mathcal{Q}_i$ then $q \in \mathcal{Q}(\text{spcl}_1(\Sigma))$ as claimed, so we may assume that $q \in \mathcal{Q}_{i+1} - \mathcal{Q}_i$. In this case, without loss of generality, $q = ab|cd$ and there is some x and two quartet trees $q_1 = ab|cx$, $q_2 = ab|dx \in \mathcal{Q}_i$, so that one application of **(Q1)** yields q. By the induction hypothesis $q_1, q_2 \in \mathcal{Q}(\text{spcl}_1(\Sigma))$. Let $\sigma_1 = \{a, b, a'_1, a'_2, \cdots, a'_j\}|\{c, x, b'_1, b'_2, \cdots, b'_l\} \in \text{spcl}_1(\Sigma)$ be a split from which q_1 is derived, and let $\sigma_2 = \{a, b, a''_1, a''_2, \cdots, a''_m\}|\{d, x, b''_1, b''_2, \cdots, b''_n\} \in \text{spcl}_1(\Sigma)$ be a split from which q_2 is derived. Note that $\sigma_1 \neq \sigma_2$ due to $q \in \mathcal{Q}_{i+1} - \mathcal{Q}_i$. Application of **(M1)** to σ_1 and σ_2 yields $\sigma_3 \in \text{spcl}_1(\Sigma)$ where

$$\begin{aligned}\sigma_3 = \{a, b\} \cup (\{a'_1, a'_2, \cdots, a'_j\} \cap \{a''_1, a''_2, \cdots, a''_m\})\\ |\{c, d, x, b'_1, b'_2, \cdots, b'_l, b''_1, b''_2, \cdots, b''_n\}.\end{aligned}$$

Since $q \in \mathcal{Q}(\{\sigma_3\}) \subseteq \mathcal{Q}(\text{spcl}_1(\Sigma))$, this establishes (5). And combining (4) and (5) establishes (3).

We now show that

$$\mathcal{Q}(\mathrm{spcl}_{1,2}(\Sigma)) = \mathrm{qcl}_{1,2}(\mathcal{Q}(\Sigma)). \tag{6}$$

To do so we first establish that

$$\mathrm{qcl}_{1,2}(\mathcal{Q}(\Sigma)) \subseteq \mathcal{Q}(\mathrm{spcl}_{1,2}(\Sigma)). \tag{7}$$

Construct a sequence of quartet sets $\mathcal{Q}(\Sigma) = \mathcal{Q}_0, \mathcal{Q}_1, \ldots, Q_N = \mathrm{qcl}_{1,2}(\mathcal{Q}(\Sigma))$ where $\mathcal{Q}_{i+1} = \mathrm{qcl}_{p(i)}(\mathcal{Q}_i)$, and where

$$p(i) = \begin{cases} 1 & \text{if } i \text{ is odd;} \\ 2 & \text{if } i \text{ is even;} \end{cases}$$

We use induction to show that for each i we have $\mathrm{qcl}_{p(i)}(\mathcal{Q}_i) \subseteq \mathcal{Q}(\mathrm{spcl}_{1,2}(\Sigma))$. The case $i = 0$ is clear, and the inductive step for i odd follows the argument used to establish (5), while the inductive step for i even follows the argument used in Semple and Steel (2001) to establish (2).

It remains to establish the reverse inclusion, namely:

$$\mathcal{Q}(\mathrm{spcl}_{1,2}(\Sigma)) \subseteq \mathrm{qcl}_{1,2}(\mathcal{Q}(\Sigma)). \tag{8}$$

Consider the sequence $\Sigma = \Sigma_0, \Sigma_1, \Sigma_2, \ldots, \Sigma_N = \mathrm{spcl}_{1,2}(\Sigma)$, where each Σ_{i+1} is obtained from Σ_i by using **(M1) and (M2)**whenever applicable on any pair of splits in Σ_i.

We use induction on i to show that $\mathcal{Q}(\Sigma_i) \subseteq \mathrm{qcl}_{1,2}(\mathcal{Q}(\Sigma))$ holds for any i between 0 and N, thus establishing the claim. For $i = 0$, $\Sigma_0 = \Sigma$, and so $\mathcal{Q}(\Sigma_i) \subseteq \mathrm{qcl}_{1,2}(\mathcal{Q}(\Sigma))$. Now suppose that the induction hypothesis holds for i where $0 \leq i < N$. For the induction step let $q \in \mathcal{Q}(\Sigma_{i+1})$. If $q \in \mathcal{Q}(\Sigma_i)$ then $q \in \mathrm{qcl}_{1,2}(\mathcal{Q}(\Sigma))$, as claimed, so we may suppose that $q \in \mathcal{Q}(\Sigma_{i+1}) - \mathcal{Q}(\Sigma_i)$.

Now q can only have been derived by either using **(M1)**, in which case we refer to the argument used to establish (4) to show that $q \in \mathrm{qcl}_1(\mathcal{Q}(\Sigma)) \subseteq \mathrm{qcl}_{1,2}(\mathcal{Q}(\Sigma))$, or by using **(M2)**, which we consider now. For $\mathrm{spcl}_{1,2}$ to be applicable on Σ_i and yield q, there exist two splits $\sigma_1 = A_1|B_1$ and $\sigma_2 = A_2|B_2$ with $\sigma_1, \sigma_2 \in \Sigma_i$ and elements x, y, z with $x \in A_1 \cap A_2, y \in A_2 \cap B_1, z \in B_1 \cap B_2$. Furthermore, without loss of generality, $q = a_1a_2|b_1b_2$, where $a_1 \in A_1 - A_2$ and $b_1, b_2 \in B_2$. Note that x, y, z are distinct, since otherwise σ_1 or σ_2 would contain an identical element on both sides of the split. Also note that $x \neq a_1$.

The following cases arise:

(I) $a_2 \in A_2$.

(a) $z \notin \{b_1, b_2\}$.

Consider the quartets $q_1 = a_1x|zy, q_2 = yx|zb_1, q_3 = yx|zb_2$ obtained from σ_1 and σ_2, and also the quartet $q_7 = a_2x|b_1b_2$. By the induction hypothesis, $\{q_1, q_2, q_3, q_7\} \subseteq \mathrm{qcl}_{1,2}(\mathcal{Q}(\Sigma))$. Application of **(Q2)** on $\{q_1, q_3\}$ and $\{q_1, q_2\}$ produces $q_4 = a_1x|zb_2$ and $q_5 = a_1x|zb_1$, respectively, and one application of **(Q1)** on $\{q_4, q_5\}$ yields $q_6 = a_1x|b_1b_2$. Finally, an application of **(Q1)** on $\{q_6, q_7\}$ yields $q = a_1a_2|b_1b_2 \in \mathrm{qcl}_{1,2}(\mathcal{Q}(\Sigma))$.

(b) $z = b_1$.

Proceed as in argument (a), to define and obtain q_1, q_3, q_4 and q_7. Since $q_4 = a_1x|b_1b_2$, application of (**Q2**) on $\{q_4, q_7\}$ yields $q = a_1a_2|b_1b_2 \in \mathrm{qcl}_{1,2}(\mathcal{Q}(\Sigma))$.

(c) $z = b_2$.

Proceed symmetrically to argument (b).

(II)$a_2 \in A_1 - A_2$.

Proceed as in argument (I), and similarly define and obtain $q_1, \ldots, q_6 \in \mathrm{qcl}_{1,2}(\mathcal{Q}(\Sigma))$ with $q_6 = a_1x|b_1b_2$. In contrast to argument (I), obtain $q_7 = a_2x|b_1b_2$ by the same line of argument used to obtain q_6, taking advantage of the symmetry of a_1 and a_2. As in (I), one application of (**Q1**) on $\{q_6, q_7\}$ yields $q = a_1a_2|b_1b_2 \in \mathrm{qcl}_{1,2}(\mathcal{Q}(\Sigma))$.

Combining (7) and (8) establishes (6) and thereby the theorem. □

1.4 The Extended Family: Characters and Trees

The operations described above, on partial X–splits and on quartet trees, are not confined to these seemingly specialized inputs. Indeed they apply easily to more familiar phylogenetic objects—namely characters and trees. We pause to describe this connection here as it will be useful in Section 4.

Given a sequence $\mathcal{C} = (\chi_1, \ldots, \chi_k)$ of partitions of X, which we shall refer to as (qualitative, unordered) *characters*, one can associate with $\mathcal{C}$ a set $\Sigma(\mathcal{C})$ of partial X–splits and a set $\mathcal{Q}(\mathcal{C})$ of quartet trees, defined as follows:

$$\Sigma(\mathcal{C}) = \{A|B : A, B \in \chi_i, \text{ for some } i \in \{1, \ldots k\}\}$$
$$\mathcal{Q}(\mathcal{C}) = \mathcal{Q}(\Sigma(\mathcal{C})).$$

Similarly, given a collection $\mathcal{P}$ of phylogenetic X–trees on overlapping leaf sets we may associate a set $\Sigma(\mathcal{P})$ of partial X–splits and a set $\mathcal{Q}(\mathcal{P})$ of quartet trees, defined as follows:

$$\Sigma(\mathcal{P}) = \cup_{\mathcal{T} \in \mathcal{P}} \Sigma(\mathcal{T}), \text{ and } \mathcal{Q}(\mathcal{P}) = \cup_{\mathcal{T} \in \mathcal{P}} \mathcal{Q}(\mathcal{T}).$$

The following result (Steel, 1992) shows that the phylogenetic compatibility of characters (or of trees with overlapping leaf sets) can be completely transformed into questions involving either partial X–splits or quartet trees.

Proposition 1. *Let $\mathcal{T}$ be a phylogenetic X-tree, $\mathcal{C}$ a collection of characters on X, and $\mathcal{P}$ a collection of phylogenetic trees whose leaf sets are subsets of X. The following are equivalent:*

- *$\mathcal{T}$ displays the characters in $\mathcal{C}$ (respectively the trees in $\mathcal{P}$).*
- *$\mathcal{T}$ displays the partial X-splits in $\Sigma(\mathcal{C})$ (respectively the partial X-splits in $\Sigma(\mathcal{P})$).*
- *$\mathcal{T}$ displays the quartet trees in $\mathcal{Q}(\mathcal{C})$ (respectively the quartet trees in $\mathcal{Q}(\mathcal{P})$).*

2 Meacham's First Rule Yields All Quartets from a Generous Cover

In this section we show that a sufficiently 'rich' subset of quartets from a fully resolved phylogenetic tree $\mathcal{T}$ suffices for the reconstruction of $\mathcal{T}$ by the quartet rule (**Q1**). We begin by introducing some terminology.

For any two vertices x, y of an X-tree $\mathcal{T}$, let *path set* $p(x,y) := \{x = v_1, v_2, .., v_i = y\}$ denote the set of all vertices traversed by the path from x to y in $\mathcal{T}$ and let *length* $l(x,y) := |p(x,y)| - 1$ denote the number of edges traversed by this path. The path between two inner vertices u, v of a phylogenetic tree $\mathcal{T}$, is said to be *distinguished* by a resolved quartet tree $ab|cd$ precisely if $p(a,b) \cap p(u,v) = \{u\}$ and $p(c,d) \cap p(u,v) = \{v\}$. A collection $\mathcal{Q}$ of quartet trees is a *generous cover* of $\mathcal{T}$ if $\mathcal{Q} \subseteq \mathcal{Q}(\mathcal{T})$ and if, for all pairs of interior vertices u, v of $\mathcal{T}$, there exists a quartet tree $ab|cd \in \mathcal{Q}$ that distinguishes the path uv.

In Mossel and Steel (2003) it was shown that if $\mathcal{Q}$ is a generous cover of $\mathcal{T}$ then $\mathcal{T}$ is the only tree that displays $\mathcal{T}$ and, furthermore, $\mathcal{T}$ can be reconstructed from $\mathcal{Q}$ by a polynomial-time algorithm. The aim of this section is to show a further result, namely that if $\mathcal{Q}$ is a generous cover of $\mathcal{T}$ then $\mathrm{qcl}_1(\mathcal{Q}) = \mathcal{Q}(\mathcal{T})$. First, however, we establish a definition and two lemmas.

Definition: An unordered pair $\{x, y\}$ of distinct leaves of a tree are said to form a *cherry* precisely if x and y are adjacent to a common vertex.

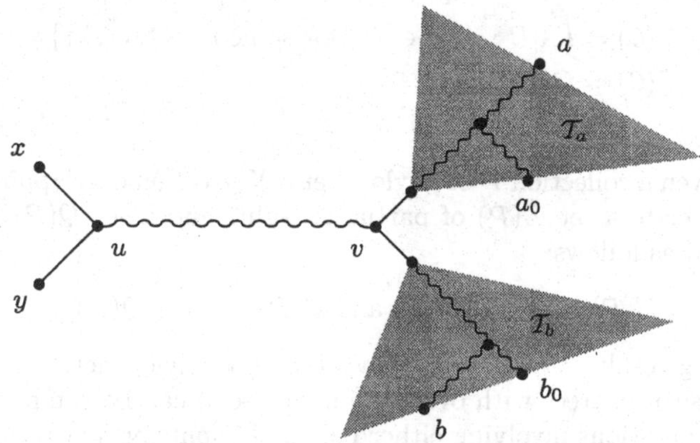

Fig. 3. Quartet $xy|a_0b_0$ distinguishes path uv.

Lemma 1. *Let $\mathcal{Q} \subseteq \mathcal{Q}(\mathcal{T})$ be a generous cover for a binary phylogenetic X-tree $\mathcal{T}$ and $\{x, y\}$ be a cherry of $\mathcal{T}$. Then $xy|ab \in \mathrm{qcl}_1(\mathcal{Q})$ for all $a, b \in X - \{x, y\}$.*

Proof. For any $a, b \in X - \{x, y\}$, consider the path uv uniquely distinguished by the quartet tree $xy|ab$ with vertex u adjacent to $\{x, y\}$ as in Figure 3.

Let the *distinguished path length* $dpl_{xy}(a,b) := l(u,v)$ for this path uv and let $dpl_{xyMAX} := max(\{dpl_{xy}(a,b) : a,b \in X - \{x,y\}\})$. Consider the three subtrees of $\mathcal{T}$ that would be derived by deleting vertex v. Let $\mathcal{T}_a$ be the subtree of $\mathcal{T}$ pendant to v containing a. Similarly, let $\mathcal{T}_b$ be the subtree of $\mathcal{T}$ pendant to v containing b.

We show that $ab|xy \in \mathrm{qcl}_1(\mathcal{Q})$ by applying induction on $\Delta(a,b) := dpl_{xyMAX} - dpl_{xy}(a,b)$. For $\Delta(a,b) = 0$, $\{a,b\}$ forms a cherry and due to the generous cover property of $\mathcal{Q}$: $xy|ab \in \mathcal{Q} \subseteq \mathrm{qcl}_1(\mathcal{Q})$. Suppose now that the result holds whenever $\Delta(a',b') = k$. Then, for $\Delta(a,b) = k+1$, since $\mathcal{Q}$ is a generous cover $\exists\ a_0 \in \mathcal{T}_A, b_0 \in \mathcal{T}_B : xy|a_0b_0 \in \mathcal{Q}$. We consider the following cases:

(i) $a = a_0, b = b_0$.
In this case $xy|ab \in \mathcal{Q} \subseteq \mathrm{qcl}_1(\mathcal{Q})$ as claimed.

(ii) $a = a_0, b \neq b_0$.
Since $\Delta(b,b_0) \leq k$, the induction hypothesis implies that $xy|bb_0 \in \mathrm{qcl}_1(\mathcal{Q})$. Furthermore $xy|a_0b_0 = xy|ab_0 \in \mathrm{qcl}_1(\mathcal{Q})$ and thus $xy|ab \in \mathrm{qcl}_1(\{xy|bb_0, xy|ab_0\}) \subseteq \mathrm{qcl}_1(\mathcal{Q})$.

(iii) $a \neq a_0, b = b_0$.
Symmetric argument to case (ii).

(iv) $a \neq a_0, b \neq b_0$.
As $\Delta(b,b_0) \leq k$, the induction hypothesis implies $xy|bb_0 \in \mathrm{qcl}_1(\mathcal{Q})$. Similarly, $xy|aa_0 \in \mathrm{qcl}_1(\mathcal{Q})$. So $xy|a_0b \in \mathrm{qcl}_1(\{xy|bb_0, xy|a_0b_0\})$ and thus $xy|ab \in \mathrm{qcl}_1(\{xy|aa_0, xy|a_0b\}) \subseteq \mathrm{qcl}_1(\mathcal{Q})$.

Thus, in all possible cases $xy|ab \in \mathrm{qcl}_1(\mathcal{Q})$, which completes the proof of Lemma 1.

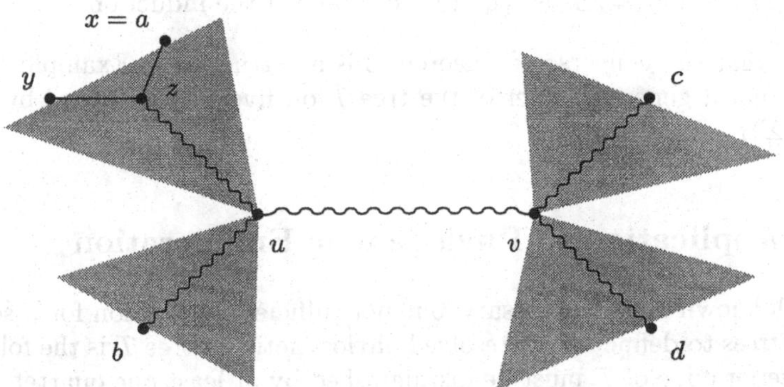

Fig. 4. Transition from $\mathcal{T}$ to $\mathcal{T}' = \mathcal{T}|X - \{x\}$ deletes x and suppresses z.

Lemma 2. *Let $\mathcal{Q} \subseteq \mathcal{Q}(\mathcal{T})$ be a generous cover for a binary phylogenetic tree $\mathcal{T}$ and let $\{x, y\}$ be a cherry of $\mathcal{T}$. Then* $\mathrm{qcl}_1(\mathcal{Q})$ *is a generous cover for $\mathcal{T}' = \mathcal{T}|X - \{x\}$.*

Proof. Let u, v be any interior vertices of $\mathcal{T}'$. Since $\mathcal{Q}$ is a generous cover, there exists a quartet $ab|cd \in \mathcal{Q}$ that *distinguishes* the path uv (cf. Fig. 4). Now, either $x \notin \{a, b, c, d\}$, in which case we are done, or, without loss of generality, $x = a$. Note that then $y \notin \{b, c, d\}$. And since $xb|cd \in \mathcal{Q} \subseteq \mathrm{qcl}_1(\mathcal{Q})$ and, by Lemma 1, $xy|cd \in \mathrm{qcl}_1(\mathcal{Q})$, the quartet tree $yb|cd \in \mathrm{qcl}_1(\{xb|cd, xy|cd\}) \subseteq \mathrm{qcl}_1(\mathcal{Q})$ distinguishes uv independently of x, thus establishing Lemma 2.

Theorem 3. *Let $\mathcal{T}$ be a binary phylogenetic tree and suppose that quartet set $\mathcal{Q} \subseteq \mathcal{Q}(\mathcal{T})$ is a generous cover. Then* $\mathrm{qcl}_1(\mathcal{Q}) = \mathcal{Q}(\mathcal{T})$.

Proof. We use induction on $|X|$. For $|X| = 4$, $\mathrm{qcl}_1(\mathcal{Q}) = \mathcal{Q}(\mathcal{T})$ as needed. For $|X| = k + 1$ choose any cherry $\{x, y\}$ of $\mathcal{T}$. By Lemma 2, $\mathrm{qcl}_1(\mathcal{Q})$ contains a subset $\mathcal{Q}_x$ that is a generous cover of $\mathcal{T}|X - \{x\}$. By the induction hypothesis therefore $\mathcal{Q}(\mathcal{T}|X - \{x\}) = \mathrm{qcl}_1(\mathcal{Q}_x)$. Similarly, $\mathrm{qcl}_1(\mathcal{Q})$ contains a subset $\mathcal{Q}_y$ that is a generous cover of $\mathcal{T}|X - \{y\}$ and so $\mathcal{Q}(\mathcal{T}|X - \{y\}) = \mathrm{qcl}_1(\mathcal{Q}_y)$. Finally, Lemma 1 yields that $\mathcal{Q}_{xy} := \{xy|ab : a, b \in X - \{x, y\}\} \subseteq \mathrm{qcl}_1(\mathcal{Q})$.

Now,

$$\begin{aligned}
\mathcal{Q}(\mathcal{T}) &= \mathcal{Q}(\mathcal{T}|X - \{x\}) \cup \mathcal{Q}(\mathcal{T}|X - \{y\}) \cup \mathcal{Q}_{xy} \\
&\subseteq \mathrm{qcl}_1(\mathcal{Q}_x) \cup \mathrm{qcl}_1(\mathcal{Q}_y) \cup \mathrm{qcl}_1(\mathcal{Q}) \\
&\subseteq \mathrm{qcl}_1(\mathcal{Q}) \cup \mathrm{qcl}_1(\mathcal{Q}) \cup \mathrm{qcl}_1(\mathcal{Q}) \\
&= \mathrm{qcl}_1(\mathcal{Q}) \\
&\subseteq \mathcal{Q}(\mathcal{T}),
\end{aligned}$$

hence $\mathcal{Q}(\mathcal{T}) = \mathrm{qcl}_1(\mathcal{Q})$ as is required to establish the induction step.

Note that the converse of Theorem 3 is not true, as in Example 1 where $\mathcal{Q}(\Sigma)$ is not a generous cover of the tree $\mathcal{T}$ on five leaves defined by Σ, yet $\mathrm{qcl}_1(\mathcal{Q}(\Sigma)) = \mathcal{Q}(\mathcal{T})$.

3 An Application to Phylogenetic Enumeration

It is well known that a necessary, but not sufficient, condition for a set $\mathcal{Q}$ of quartet trees to define a fully resolved phylogenetic X–tree $\mathcal{T}$ is the following: each interior edge of $\mathcal{T}$ must be distinguished by at least one quartet. Consequently we must have $|\mathcal{Q}| \geq n - 3$, where $n = |X|$. Consider the case where we have a set $\mathcal{Q}$ of size $n - 3$. A natural question is how many fully resolved phylogenetic trees have the property that each of their interior edges is distinguished by $\mathcal{Q}$. When $n \leq 5$ this number can be at most 1, but when $n = 6$ this number can be 2 (an example is provided by the set $\mathcal{Q} = \{12|35, 34|26, 56|14\}$).

In the following result we use one of the dyadic quartet closure rules to establish an upper bound on this number in general. First we state a lemma (cf. Steel, 1992, or Theorem 6.8.8 of Semple and Steel, 2003) that is central to the proof.

Lemma 3. *Suppose $\mathcal{Q}$ is a collection of quartet trees that distinguishes every interior edge of some fully-resolved phylogenetic X-tree $\mathcal{T}$. If, in addition, there is some element $y \in X$ that is a leaf in each quartet tree in $\mathcal{Q}$, then $\mathcal{Q}$ defines $\mathcal{T}$.*

Theorem 4. *Suppose $\mathcal{Q}$ is a set of quartet trees of size $n-3$ where n is the size of the set X of leaf labels of $\mathcal{Q}$. Let $\mathrm{d}(\mathcal{Q})$ denote the set of fully-resolved phylogenetic X-trees for which each interior edge is distinguished by exactly one quartet tree in $\mathcal{Q}$. Then*

$$\log_2 |\mathrm{d}(\mathcal{Q})| \leq n-3-\lceil \frac{4(n-3)}{n} \rceil.$$

Proof. For each element $x \in X$ let $n(x)$ denote the number of quartet trees in $\mathcal{Q}$ that have leaf x. Consider the set of pairs (q, x) where $q \in \mathcal{Q}$ and x is a leaf of q. Counting this set in the two obvious ways, we obtain $\sum_{x \in X} n(x) = 4|\mathcal{Q}| = 4(n-3)$, and so the average value of $n(x)$ over all choices $x \in X$ is exactly $4(n-3)/n$. Consequently there exists an element $y \in X$ that lies in at least $r := \lceil 4(n-3)/n \rceil$ quartet trees from $\mathcal{Q}$. Now, for the set $\mathcal{Q}'$ consisting of the $n-3-r$ quartet trees in $\mathcal{Q}$ that do not contain leaf y, let us replace each quartet $q = ab|cd$ by either $S_1(q) := \{ab|cy, ab|dy\}$ or $S_2 := \{ay|cd, by|cd\}$. For each map $\pi : \mathcal{Q}' \to \{1,2\}$ consider the collection

$$\mathcal{Q}[\pi] := (\mathcal{Q} - \mathcal{Q}') \cup (\cup_{q \in \mathcal{Q}'} S_{\pi(q)}(q)).$$

We claim that there exists a bijection

$$\beta : \mathrm{d}(\mathcal{Q}) \to \{\pi : \mathcal{Q}' \to \{1,2\} : \mathcal{Q}[\pi] \text{ is compatible }\}.$$

This bijection associates to each phylogenetic X-tree $\mathcal{T}$ in $\mathrm{d}(\mathcal{Q})$ the map $\pi : \mathcal{Q}' \to \{1,2\}$. Consider a quartet tree $ab|cd \in \mathcal{Q}'$. Since $ab|cd$ distinguishes some interior edge, say $e = \{u, v\}$, of $\mathcal{T}$, then leaf y is connected to precisely one of a, b, c, d in the forest obtained from $\mathcal{T}$ by deleting u and v. If y is connected to c or d in this forest then set $\pi(ab|cd) = 1$, otherwise set $\pi(ab|cd) = 2$. Note that $\mathcal{Q}[\pi]$ is compatible, since each quartet tree in $\mathcal{Q}(\pi)$ is displayed by $\mathcal{T}$, thus the function β that we have just described is well defined. To see that β is one-to-one, suppose that $\beta(\mathcal{T}) = \beta(\mathcal{T}') = \pi$. Then $\mathcal{T}$ and $\mathcal{T}'$ both display all the quartet trees in $\mathcal{Q}(\pi)$. Furthermore, each quartet tree in $\mathcal{Q}[\pi]$ contains leaf y, and $\mathcal{Q}[\pi]$ distinguishes every interior edge of $\mathcal{T}$. Thus, by Lemma 3, $\mathcal{T}' = \mathcal{T}$ and so β is one-to-one, as claimed. Finally, β is onto, since if $\pi : \mathcal{Q}' \to \{1,2\}$ has the property that $\mathcal{Q}[\pi]$ is compatible, then if $\mathcal{T}$ is a tree that displays $\mathcal{Q}(\pi)$ then $\mathcal{T}$ displays each quartet tree in $\mathcal{Q}$; this follows by applying (**Q1**)—any tree that displays $S_1(q)$ (or $S_2(q)$) also displays q.

The existence of the bijection β immediately implies that

$$\log_2 |\mathrm{d}(\mathcal{Q})| \leq \log_2 |\{\pi : \mathcal{Q}' \rightarrow \{1,2\}\}| = |\mathcal{Q}'| = n - 3 - r$$

which establishes the theorem.

4 Tree Construction In Homoplasy-Free Evolution

Markov models are now standard for modeling the evolution of aligned genetic sequence data. These models are routinely used as the basis for phylogenetic tree construction using techniques such as maximum likelihood (cf. Swofford et al., 1996). In these models the state space (the set of possible values each character can take) is typically samll; for DNA sequence data it is 4, but occasionally 2 for purine-pyrimidine data, or 20 for amino acid sequences. For such models the subsets of the vertices of a phylogenetic tree $\mathcal{T}$ that are assigned to particular states do not generally form connected subtrees of $\mathcal{T}$ (in biological terminology this is because of 'homoplasy,' which is the evolution of the same state more than once in the tree).

4.1 The Random Cluster Model

Recently, there is increasing interest in genomic characters such as gene order where the underlying state space may be very large (cf. Gallut and Barriel, 2002; Moret et al., 2001; Moret et al., 2002; and Rokas and Holland, 2000). For example, the order of k genes in a signed circular genome can take any of $2^k(k-1)!$ values. In these models whenever there is a change of state (e.g., a reshuffling of genes by a random inversion of a consecutive subsequence of genes), it is likely that the resulting state (gene arrangement) is a unique evolutionary event, arising for the first time in the evolution of the genes under study. Indeed Markov models for genome rearrangement such as the (generalized) Nadeau-Taylor model (cf. Moret et al., 2002; Nadeau and Taylor, 1984) confer a high probability that any given character generated is homoplasy-free on the underlying tree, provided the number of genes is sufficiently large relative to $|X|$ (Semple and Steel, 2002). In this setting the random cluster model is the appropriate (limiting case) model, and may be viewed as the phylogenetic analogue of what is known in population genetics as the 'infinite alleles model' of Kimura and Crow (1964).

We now consider the following random process on a phylogenetic tree $\mathcal{T}$. For each edge e let us independently either cut this edge with probability $p(e)$ or leave it intact. The resulting disconnected graph (forest) G partitions the vertex set $V(\mathcal{T})$ of $\mathcal{T}$ into non-empty sets according to the equivalence relation that $u \sim v$ if u and v are in the same component of G. This model thus generates random partitions of $V(\mathcal{T})$, and thereby of X by connectivity. In this way we can generate a character on X, as illustrated in Fig. 5, or more generally, a sequence $\mathcal{C}$ of independently-generated characters. Following Mossel and Steel (2003), we call resulting probability distribution on partitions of X the *random cluster model* with parameters $(\mathcal{T}, p)$ where p is the map $e \mapsto p(e)$.

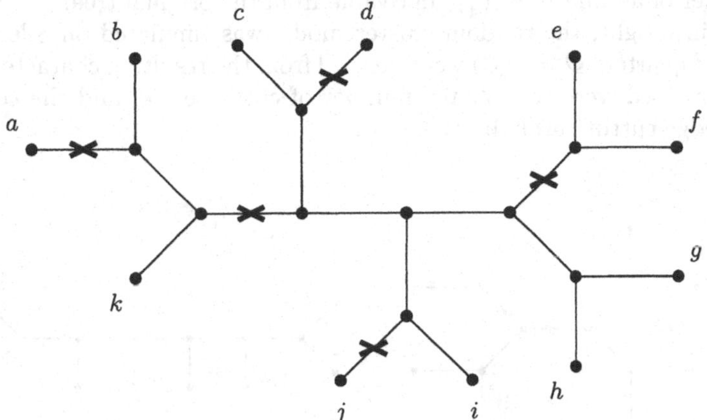

Fig. 5. Cutting the marked edges yields the character $\{a|bk|cghi|d|ef|j\}$.

Mossel and Steel (2003) show that the number of characters required to correctly reconstruct a fully resolved tree with n leaves grows at the rate $\log(n)$ provided the range of p is constrained to lie between any two fixed values that are less than 0.5. Here we use simulations to investigate how much phylogenetic information can be accessed using the various dyadic closure rules, when characters evolve according to this model.

4.2 Quantitative Closure Gains

For a compatible set $\mathcal{Q}$ of quartet trees, let

$$\mathrm{cl}(\mathcal{Q}) = \bigcap_{\mathcal{T} \in \mathrm{co}(\mathcal{Q})} \mathcal{Q}(\mathcal{T})$$

where $\mathrm{co}(\mathcal{Q})$ is the set of phylogenetic trees that display each of the trees in $\mathcal{Q}$. Thus $\mathrm{cl}(\mathcal{Q})$ consists of precisely those quartet trees that are displayed by every phylogenetic tree that displays $\mathcal{Q}$, and so $\mathrm{qcl}_1(\mathcal{Q}), \mathrm{qcl}_2(\mathcal{Q}), \mathrm{qcl}_{1,2}(\mathcal{Q})$ are all subsets of $\mathrm{cl}(\mathcal{Q})$.

This set $\mathrm{cl}(\mathcal{Q})$ is called the *closure* of $\mathcal{Q}$ and it has the property that $|\mathrm{cl}(\mathcal{Q})| = \binom{n}{4}$ precisely when $\mathcal{Q}$ defines $\mathcal{T}$. No polynomial-time algorithm is known for computing the closure of a set of quartets, whereas the dyadic closure can clearly be computed in polynomial time.

This situation poses interesting questions in the random cluster model that have practical consequences. For a sequence $\mathcal{C}$ of characters generated independently under the random cluster model, consider the induced set $\mathcal{Q} = \mathcal{Q}(\mathcal{C})$ of quartet trees (as described in Section 1.4). How large are $\mathcal{Q} = \mathcal{Q}(\mathcal{C}), \mathrm{qcl}_1(\mathcal{Q}), \mathrm{qcl}_2(\mathcal{Q}), \mathrm{qcl}_{1,2}(\mathcal{Q})$ on average in relation to $\mathrm{cl}(\mathcal{Q})$; i.e., how many 'forced' quartet relationships can be derived using only quartet rules of order two? And, similarly, how does the size of these sets compare to the number of all quartets ($\binom{n}{4}$) derivable from the original tree?

To gain insight, the random cluster model was simulated on 8-leaf trees and sets of quartets $\mathcal{Q} = \mathcal{Q}(\mathcal{C})$ were derived from the resulting characters. The parameters used were tree shape, number of characters k, and the common value of edge-cutting probability ($p(e)$).

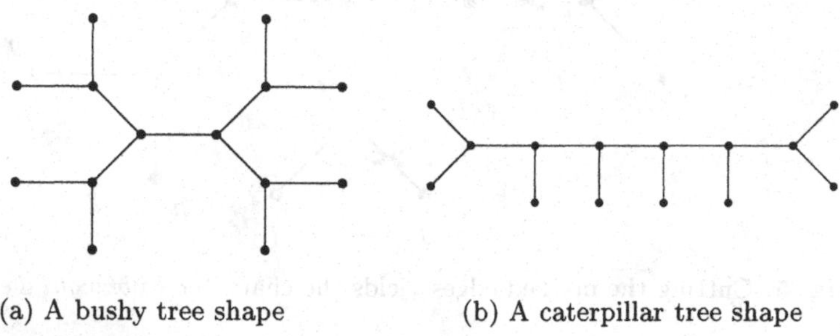

(a) A bushy tree shape (b) A caterpillar tree shape

Fig. 6. Two extreme tree shapes on eight leaves used for random cluster model simulation: (a) shows a bushy tree shape, with minimal length for the longest inner path; (b) shows a caterpillar tree shape, with maximal length of the longest inner path.

We first simulated the model on trees having the bushy tree shape in Fig. 6(a). We ran averaged the results of 500 runs of the random cluster model for each set of parameter values. Each run gave a set of k characters $\mathcal{C}$ and the quartet sets $\mathcal{Q} = \mathcal{Q}(\mathcal{C})$, $\mathrm{qcl}_1(\mathcal{Q})$, $\mathrm{qcl}_2(\mathcal{Q})$, $\mathcal{Q}(\mathrm{spcl}_2(\mathcal{Q}))$, $\mathrm{qcl}_{1,2}(\mathcal{Q})$ and $\mathrm{cl}(\mathcal{Q})$, where $\mathrm{spcl}_2(\mathcal{Q}) = \mathrm{spcl}_2(\Sigma(\mathcal{Q}))$ with $\Sigma(\mathcal{Q}) = \{\{a,b\}|\{c,d\} : ab|cd \in \mathcal{Q}\}$ in line with Proposition 1. >From these quartet sets we computed the following values:

$$\frac{|\mathcal{Q}|}{|\mathrm{cl}(\mathcal{Q})|}, \frac{|\mathrm{qcl}_1(\mathcal{Q})|}{|\mathrm{cl}(\mathcal{Q})|}, \frac{|\mathrm{qcl}_2(\mathcal{Q})|}{|\mathrm{cl}(\mathcal{Q})|}, \frac{|\mathcal{Q}(\mathrm{spcl}_2(\mathcal{Q}))|}{|\mathrm{cl}(\mathcal{Q})|}, \frac{|\mathrm{qcl}_{1,2}(\mathcal{Q})|}{|\mathrm{cl}(\mathcal{Q})|}.$$

These values for the bushy tree shape on eight leaves, using 16 (respectively 32) characters, are shown graphically for varying $p(e)$ in the range $\{0, \ldots, .95\}$ (in steps of .01) in Fig. 7(a) (respectively Fig. 7(b)).

Furthermore, the number of quartets in each of the sets $\mathcal{Q}$, $\mathrm{qcl}_1(\mathcal{Q})$, $\mathrm{qcl}_2(\mathcal{Q})$, $\mathcal{Q}(\mathrm{spcl}_2(\mathcal{Q}))$, $\mathrm{qcl}_{1,2}(\mathcal{Q})$ and $\mathrm{cl}(\mathcal{Q})$ was put in relation to the total number of quartets obtainable from the original tree, yielding the values:

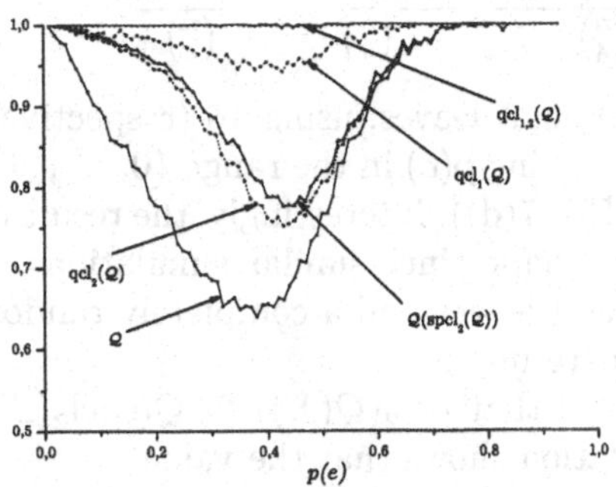

(a) The case $k = 16$. We plot the ratio of the size of the labeled quartet sets to the size of the closure.

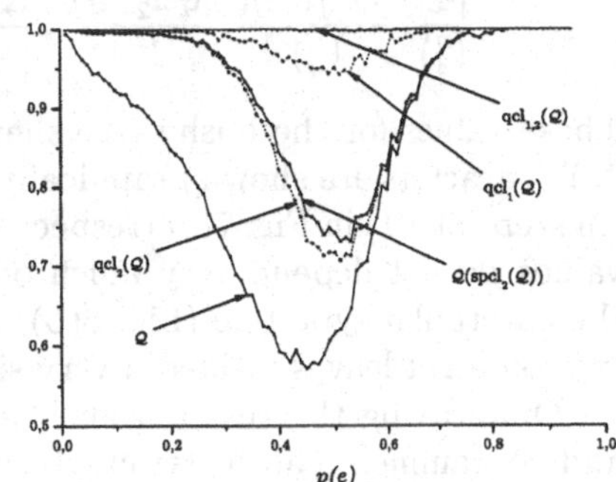

(b) The case $k = 32$. We plot the ratio of the size of the labeled quartet sets to the size of the closure.

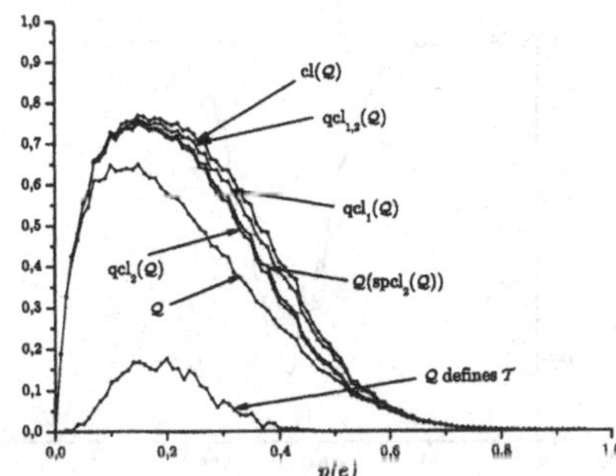

(c) The case $k = 16$. We plot the ratio of the size of the labeled quartet sets to the size of all quartets of the original tree. The average fraction of cases in which $\mathcal{Q}$ defines a tree is depicted and labeled "$\mathcal{Q}$ defines $\mathcal{T}$".

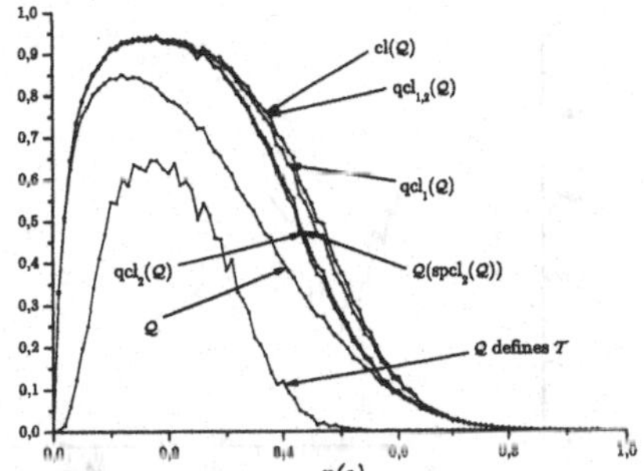

(d) The case $k = 32$. We plot the ratio of the size of the labeled quartet sets to the size of all quartets of the original tree. The average fraction of cases in which $\mathcal{Q}$ defines a tree is depicted and labeled "$\mathcal{Q}$ defines $\mathcal{T}$".

Fig. 7. Above Figures show the result of a random cluster model simulation on a bushy tree on 8 leaves yielding 16 (respectively 32) characters.

$$\frac{|\mathcal{Q}|}{\binom{n}{4}}, \frac{|\mathrm{qcl}_1(\mathcal{Q})|}{\binom{n}{4}}, \frac{|\mathrm{qcl}_2(\mathcal{Q})|}{\binom{n}{4}}, \frac{|\mathcal{Q}(\mathrm{spcl}_2(\mathcal{Q}))|}{\binom{n}{4}}, \frac{|\mathrm{qcl}_{1,2}(\mathcal{Q})|}{\binom{n}{4}}, \frac{|\mathrm{cl}(\mathcal{Q})|}{\binom{n}{4}}.$$

These values for the bushy tree shape on eight leaves, using 16 (respectively 32) characters are shown graphically for varying $p(e)$ in the range $\{0, \ldots, .95\}$ (in steps of .01) in Fig. 7(c) (respectively Fig. 7(d)). Interestingly, the resulting values do not depend very much on tree shape since similar simulations on the caterpillar type tree (Fig. 6(b)) on eight leaves and a completely random tree on eight leaves yielded a very similar result.

Quantifying the result from Theorem 2 that $\mathrm{qcl}_2(\mathcal{Q}(\Sigma)) \subseteq \mathcal{Q}(\mathrm{spcl}_2(\Sigma))$ and containment can be strict, the simulation shows that the value

$$\tau = |\mathrm{qcl}_2(\mathcal{Q})| / |\mathcal{Q}(\mathrm{spcl}_2(\mathcal{Q}))|$$

is larger than .95 on average in this setting. Its curve against $p(e)$ has a distinctive V-shape as shown in Fig. 8.

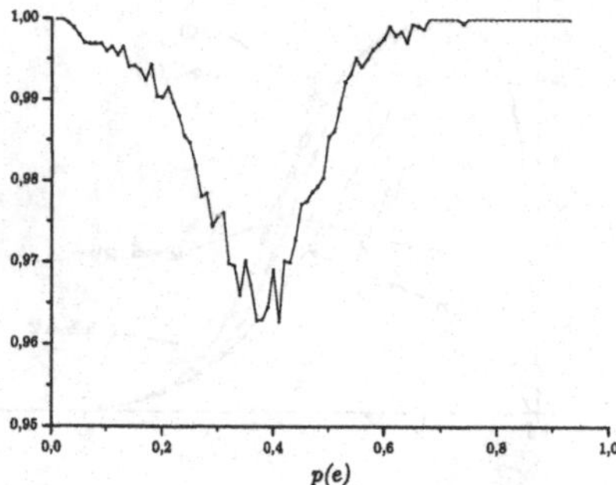

(a) The ratio τ for the case $k = 16$.

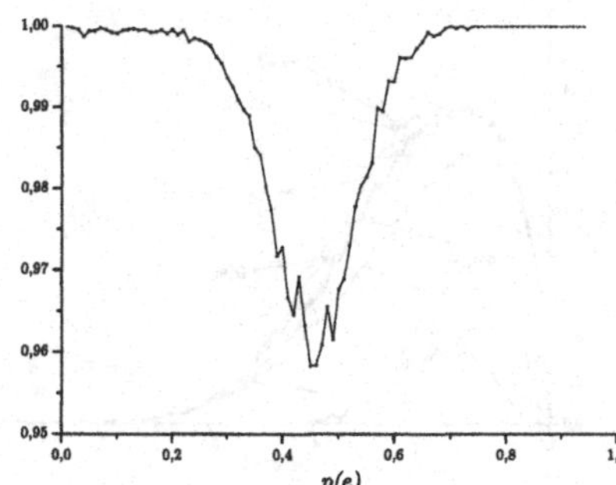

(b) The ratio τ for the case $k = 32$.

Fig. 8. The ratio τ is graphed against $p(e)$ in a random cluster model simulation with parameters: bushy tree shape, 8 leaves, quartets derived from k characters, 500 runs.

Note that in this simulation, the values $|\mathrm{qcl}_{1,2}(\mathcal{Q})|/\binom{n}{4}$ and $|\mathrm{cl}(\mathcal{Q})|/\binom{n}{4}$ are so close that they are indistinguishable in Fig. 7(c) and Fig. 7(d). This indicates that $|\mathrm{qcl}_{1,2}(\mathcal{Q})|/|\mathrm{cl}(\mathcal{Q})|$ is very close to 1 as is visible in Fig. 7(a) and Fig. 7(b), and thus the vast majority of quartets is already gained by $\mathrm{qcl}_{1,2}(\mathcal{Q})$. To explore this phenomenon further, we recorded the values of $|\mathrm{qcl}_{1,2}(\mathcal{Q})|/|\mathrm{cl}(\mathcal{Q})|$ separately, depending on whether $\mathcal{Q}$ defines a tree or not. These values are depicted in Fig. 9(a) (respectively Fig. 9(b)) for 16 (respectively 32) characters along with the average number of cases in which $\mathcal{Q}$ defines a tree. We found that in the majority of cases where Q did not define a tree, $\mathrm{qcl}_{1,2}(\mathcal{Q}) = \mathrm{cl}(\mathcal{Q})$, but occasionally $\mathrm{qcl}_{1,2}(\mathcal{Q}) \neq \mathrm{cl}(\mathcal{Q})$, as expected by the comments in Section 1.2. However, an observation that was made consistently in all conducted simulations is that whenever $\mathcal{Q}$ defines a tree, $\mathrm{qcl}_{1,2}(\mathcal{Q})$ yields all the quartets of this tree; i.e., $\mathrm{qcl}_{1,2}(\mathcal{Q}) = \mathrm{cl}(\mathcal{Q})$. But in general this equality need not hold for a set $\mathcal{Q}$ that defines a tree (Steel, 1992). A further observation is that the average size of the quartet sets $\mathcal{Q}$ that define a tree decreases with $p(e)$ (results not shown).

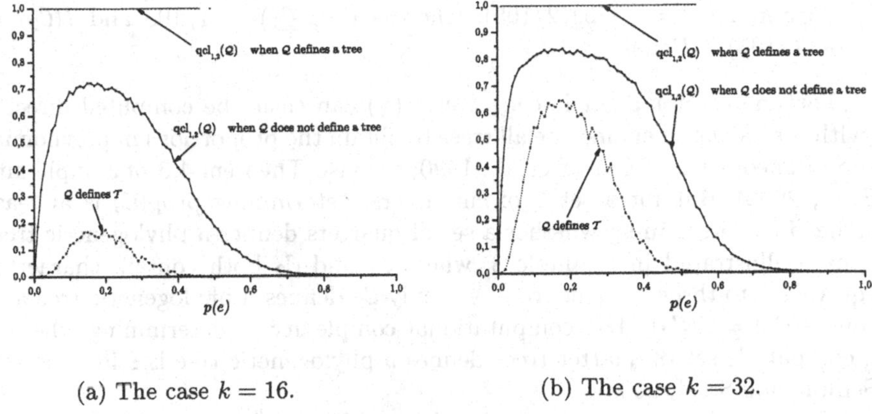

(a) The case $k = 16$. (b) The case $k = 32$.

Fig. 9. This plots the ratio of the size of the labeled quartet sets to the size of all quartets of the original tree. Furthermore, the average fraction of cases where $\mathcal{Q}$ defines a tree is depicted and labeled "$\mathcal{Q}$ defines $\mathcal{T}$".

4.3 Phylogenetic Information Content

Finally, we investigate a measure for the information content of characters described by Semple and Steel (2002). For a single character χ, a natural measure for the phylogenetic information content I of χ is the following:

$$I(\chi) = -\log(\mathrm{prop}(\chi))$$

where $\mathrm{prop}(\chi)$ is the proportion of fully-resolved phylogenetic X-trees for which χ is homoplasy-free. At the two extremes, when χ partitions X into singleton sets, or when χ has just one set (namely X), we have $I(\chi) = 0$, since then every tree is homoplasy-free under χ. Similarly, for a compatible set of characters $\mathcal{C} = \{\chi_1, \ldots, \chi_k\}$, we can define

$$I(\mathcal{C}) = -\log(\mathrm{prop}(\mathcal{C}))$$

where $\mathrm{prop}(\mathcal{C})$ is the proportion of fully-resolved phylogenetic X-trees $\mathcal{T}$ on which each $\chi \in \mathcal{C}$ is homoplasy-free.

Example 3. Assume

$$\chi_1 = \{\{1,2\},\{4,5\},\{3\},\{6\}\}$$
$$\chi_2 = \{\{3,4\},\{1,6\},\{2\},\{5\}\}$$
$$\chi_3 = \{\{5,6\},\{2,3\},\{1\},\{4\}\}$$
$$\chi_4 = \{\{5,6\},\{1,3\},\{2\},\{4\}\}$$

with $\mathcal{C}_1 = \{\chi_1, \chi_2, \chi_3\}$ and $\mathcal{C}_2 = \{\chi_1, \chi_2, \chi_4\}$. Then $\text{prop}(\chi_i) = 35/105$ and $I(\chi_i) = -\log(35/105)$ for all $i \in \{1,2,3,4\}$. On the other hand, $\text{prop}(\mathcal{C}_1) = 2/105$ and $I(\mathcal{C}_1) = -\log(2/105)$, whereas $\text{prop}(\mathcal{C}_2) = 1/105$ and $I(\mathcal{C}_2) = -\log(1/105) \neq I(\mathcal{C}_1)$.

Fortunately, for a single character, $I(\chi)$ can easily be computed directly (without having to enumerate all trees to obtain the proportion) in polynomial time (Theorem 2 of Carter et al., 1990; see also Theorem 4.3 of Semple and Steel, 2002). But for a set $\mathcal{C}$ of characters, determining $\text{prop}(\mathcal{C})$ is at least as hard as determining whether a set of quartets defines a phylogenetic tree. This is illustrated in Example 3, where $\mathcal{C}_1$ and $\mathcal{C}_2$ both contain characters equivalent to three quartet trees, yet only $\mathcal{C}_2$ defines a phylogenetic tree and thus $I(\mathcal{C}_1) \neq I(\mathcal{C}_2)$. The computational complexity of determining whether a compatible set of quartet trees defines a phylogenetic tree is still open (cf. Semple and Steel, 2003).

For $\mathcal{C} = \{\chi_1, \dots, \chi_k\}$, consider $I_{approx}(\mathcal{C}) = \sum_{1 \le i \le k} I(\chi_i)$, which can easily be computed in polynomial time. For a fully resolved phylogenetic X–tree $\mathcal{T}$, selected uniformly at random from the set of all such trees, if the events (for $i = 1, \dots k$) defined by $E_i := \{\mathcal{T} \text{ displays } \chi_i\}$ were independent (in the statistical sense), then $I(\mathcal{C}) = I_{approx}(\mathcal{C})$. In general, however, $I(\mathcal{C}) \neq I_{approx}(\mathcal{C})$ and it is of interest to compare $I(\mathcal{C})$ with $I_{approx}(\mathcal{C})$ when $\mathcal{C}$ is generated under the random cluster model.

Figures 10(a) and 10(b) depict the values of $I(\mathcal{C})$ and $I_{approx}(\mathcal{C})$ in same random cluster model setting described in the previous section and shown in Fig. 7 for 16 (respectively 32) characters. The results suggest that $I_{approx}(\mathcal{C})$ tends to overestimate $I(\mathcal{C})$ (i.e, the events E_i are positively correlated), and that $I_{approx}(\mathcal{C})$ is only close to $I(\mathcal{C})$ when $p(e)$ is close to either 0 or 1.

5 Acknowledgments

We thank the New Zealand Institute for Mathematics and its Applications (NZIMA) for support under the *Phylogenetic Genomics* programme. We also thank two referees for some helpful comments on an earlier version of this manuscript.

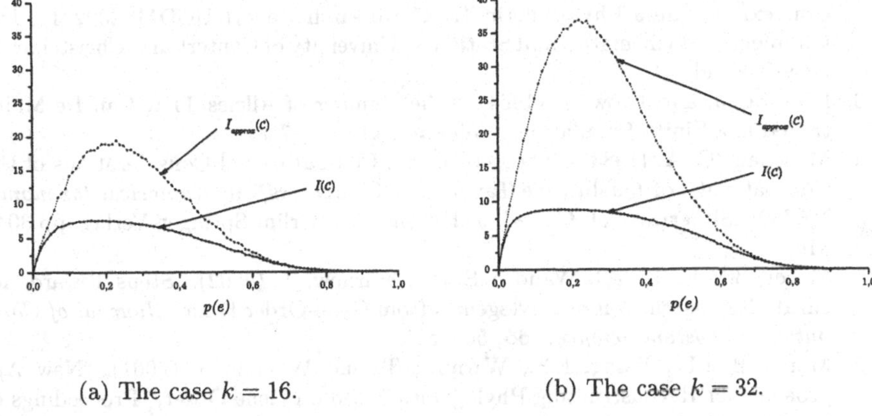

(a) The case $k = 16$. (b) The case $k = 32$.

Fig. 10. Figures (a) and (b) depict the values of $I(\mathcal{C})$ and $I_{approx}(\mathcal{C})$ as discussed in Section 4.3.

References

1. Aho, A. V., Sagiv, Y., Szymanski, T. G., and Ullman, J. D. (1981). "Inferring a Tree from Lowest Common Ancestors with an Application to the Optimization of Relational Expressions," *SIAM Journal on Computing*, **10**, 405–421.
2. Bandelt, H.-J., and Dress, A.W.M. (1986). "Reconstructing the Shape of a Tree from Observed Dissimilarity Data," *Advances in Applied Mathematics*, **7**, 309–343.
3. Bryant, D. and Steel, M. (1995). "Extension Operations on Sets of Leaf-Labelled Trees," *Advances in Applied Mathematics*, **16**, 425–453.
4. Böcker, S. (1999). *From Subtrees to Supertrees*. Unpublished PhD thesis. Fakultät für Mathematik, Universität Bielefeld, Bielefeld.
5. Böcker, S., Dress, A. W. M., and Steel, M. (1999). "Patching Up X-Trees," *Annals of Combinatorics*, **3**, 1–12.
6. Böcker, S., Bryant, D., Dress, A. W. M., and Steel, M. A. (2000). "Algorithmic Aspects of Tree Amalgamation," *Journal of Algorithms*, **37**, 522–537.
7. Carter, M., Hendy, M. D., Penny, D., Székely, L. A., and Wormald, N. C. (1990). "On the Distribution of Lengths of Evolutionary Trees," *SIAM Journal on Discrete Mathematics*, **3**, 38–47.
8. Colonius, H. and Schulze, H. H. (1981). "Tree Structures for Proximity Data," *British Journal of Mathematical and Statistical Psychology*, **34**, 167–180.
9. Dekker, M. C. H. (1986). *Reconstruction Methods for Derivation Trees*. Unpublished Masters thesis. Vrije Universiteit, Amsterdam, Netherlands.
10. Estabrook, G. F. and McMorris, F. R. (1977). "When Are Two Qualitative Taxonomic Characters Compatible?" *Journal of Mathematical Biology*, **4**, 195–200.
11. Gallut, C. and Barriel, V. (2002). "Cladistic Coding of Genomic Maps," *Cladistics*, **18**, 526–536.

12. Huber, K.T., Moulton, V. and Steel, M. (2002). "Four Characters Suffice to Convexly Define a Phylogenetic Tree," Research Report UCDMS2002/12, Department of Mathematics and Statistics, University of Canterbury, Christchurch, New Zealand.
13. Kimura, M. and Crow, J. (1964). "The Number of Alleles That Can Be Maintained in a Finite Population," *Genetics*, **49**, 725–738.
14. Meacham, C. A. (1983). "Theoretical and Computational Considerations of the Compatibility of Qualitative Taxonomic Characters," in *Numerical taxonomy*, NATO ASI Series, Vol. G1, ed. J. Felsenstein, Berlin: Springer-Verlag, pp.304–314.
15. Moret, B.M.E. Tang,J. Wand, L.S. and Warnow, T. (2002). "Steps Toward Accurate Reconstruction of Phylogenies from Gene-Order Data," *Journal of Computer and System Sciences*, **65**, 508–525.
16. Moret, B.M.E., Wang, L.S., Warnow, T. and Wyman, S. (2001). "New Approaches for Reconstructing Phylogenies Based on Gene Order," Proceedings of the 9th International Conference on Intelligent Systems for Molecular Biology ISMB-2001, *Bioinformatics*, **17**, S165–S173.
17. Nadeau, J.J. and Taylor, B.A. (1984). "Lengths of Chromosome Segments Conserved Since Divergence of Man and Mouse," *Proceedings of the National Academy of Sciences USA*, **81**, 814–818.
18. Ng, M. P., Steel, M., and Wormald, N. C. (2000). "The Difficulty of Constructing a Leaf-Labelled Tree Including or Avoiding a Given Subtree," *Discrete Applied Mathematics*, **98**, 227–235.
19. Rokas, A., Holland P.W.H. (2000). "Rare Genomic Changes as a Tool for Phylogenetics," *Trends in Ecology and Evolution*, **15**, 454-459.
20. Semple, C. and Steel, M. (2001). "Tree Reconstruction Via a Closure Operation on Partial Splits," in *Proceedings of Journées Ouvertes: Biologie, Informatique et Mathématique*, Lecture Notes in Computer Science, eds. O. Gascuel and M.-F. Sagot, Berlin: Springer-Verlag, pp.126–134.
21. Semple, C. and Steel, M. (2002). "Tree Reconstruction from Multi-State Characters," *Advances in Applied Mathematics*, **28**, 169–184.
22. Semple, C. and Steel, M. (2003). *Phylogenetics*, Oxford, U.K.: Oxford University Press.
23. Steel, M. (1992). "The Complexity of Reconstructing Trees from Qualitative Characters and Subtrees," *Journal of Classification*, **9**, 91–116.
24. Swofford, D.L., Olsen, G.J., Waddell, P.J., and Hillis, D.M. (1996). "Phylogenetic Inference," in *Molecular Systematics* (2nd edn.), eds. D. M. Hillis, C. Moritz, B. K. Marble, Sunderland U.S.A.: Sinauer, pp. 407–514.
25. Mossel, E. and Steel, M. (2003). "A Phase Transition for a Random Cluster Model on Phylogenetic Trees," *Mathematical Biosciences* (in press).

Consensus of Classification Systems, with Adams' Results Revisited

Florent Domenach[1] and Bruno Leclerc[2]

[1] Tsukuba University, Japan
domenach@sk.tsukuba.ac.jp
[2] L'Ecole des Hautes Etudes en Sciences Sociales, France
leclerc@ehess.fr

Abstract: The problem of aggregating a profile of closure systems into a consensus closure system has interesting applications in classification. We first present an overview of the results obtained by a lattice approach. Then, we develop a more refined approach based on overhangings and implications that appears to be a generalization of Adams' consensus tree algorithm. Adams' uniqueness result is explained and generalized.

1 Introduction

Let S be a finite set. In this paper, we consider the problem of aggregating a profile (k-tuple) $\mathcal{F}^* = (\mathcal{F}_1, \mathcal{F}_2, \dots, \mathcal{F}_k)$ of closure systems on S (families of subsets including S and preserving intersection) into a consensus closure system $\mathcal{F} = c(\mathcal{F}^*)$.

One main purpose for research on such a consensus is the classification of a set S described by variables of different types. In this situation, a similar approach was independently considered by Régnier (1965) and Mirkin (1974,1975). Each variable v induces a partition on S by the equivalence relation R_v defined by $sR_vs' \iff v(s) = v(s')$. So a set of k variables leads to a k-tuple profile $\pi^* = (\pi_1, \dots, \pi_k)$ of k partitions. The idea is to aggregate the elements of π^* into a unique partition π that summarizes π^* in some useful sense.

Régnier, then Mirkin (1974), proposed, as an output of clustering, a partition called the *median* of π^* which minimizes the quantity $\Sigma_{1 \leq i \leq k}\, \delta(\pi, \pi_i)$, where δ is the *symmetric difference metric* on equivalences. This often results in difficult linear integer programming problems, with an extensive literature that includes algorithms (see the survey in Barthélemy and Leclerc, 1995).

Mirkin (1975) also considered an axiomatic approach, with axioms (desirable properties) of the kind stated by Arrow (1951) in his celebrated work on social choice. Mirkin concluded that only the partition obtained as the intersection of the classes of some elements of the profile could satisfy those axioms. Generalizations of Mirkin's result were obtained in Leclerc (1984), especially for ultrametrics, and in Monjardet (1990a) for lattice structures (cf. Day and McMorris, 2003).

The same approach, but replacing partitions by closure systems, presents several advantages. First, structural information (order, tree structure) provided by the input variables is totally or partly retained (while partitions just take equality into account). As the example of Galois lattices (and their generalizations; see for instance Domenach and Leclerc (2002)) shows, closure systems are a basic tool in symbolic data analysis and also in logic, relational data bases, and, more generally, the mathematics of social sciences.

Another reason for research on this kind of consensus is that several consensus problems already studied in the literature are particular cases of the consensus of closure systems. The basic example is provided by hierarchies, where many works have followed those of Adams (1972) and Margush and McMorris (1981)—see the surveys by Leclerc (1998) and Bryant (2003). Also, several other common classification models are closure systems, possibly after adding the empty and full sets.

Closure systems and some of their uses are presented in Section 2.1. Some equivalent structures are recalled in Section 2.2, one of which results from a recent extension of work in Adams (1986). Section 2.3 discusses lattice structures. Section 3 presents the main results provided by the application to closure systems of general results on the consensus problem in lattices. These results are interesting, but also somewhat disappointing, because they only use the presence or absence of classes in the families of the profile. A more refined approach appears necessary, and so we begin to develop in Section 4 a generalization of the Adams algorithm (Adams, 1972) and characterization (Adams, 1986) for trees.

2 A Consensus Problem on Systems of Classes

A classification on a finite given set S will be just a set $\mathcal{F} \subseteq \mathcal{P}(S)$ of classes (subsets) of S. A class $C \in \mathcal{F}$ is interpreted as a cluster, and its elements are supposed to share common features, or to be similar in some sense, or both.

2.1 Classification and Closure Systems

The following simple conditions are natural in the context of classes:

(C1) $S \in \mathcal{F}$ (the entire universe is a class)
(C2) $C, C' \in \mathcal{F} \Rightarrow C \cap C' \in \mathcal{F}$ (the class of all elements belonging to C and to C' is a class).

With these two properties, $\mathcal{F}$ is a *closure system* (or a *Moore family*) on S.

Although we interpret all closure systems (which we shall abbreviate as CSs) as classifications, we call *classification systems* those satisfying the further condition (C3):

(C3) for any $s \in S$, $\{s\} \in \mathcal{F}$ (particularization of single elements).

Note that (C2) frequently (and always with (C3)) implies that the empty set is a class; this is an unusual convention, but it will prove useful.

In many contexts, the difference between CSs and classification systems is not very significant, since adding singletons (and possibly the empty set) changes any CS into a classification system. In fact, Condition (C2) is quite restrictive and it is not satisfied by all the types of families of subsets used in classification.

If we consider the data side of a classification process, we observe that several types of closure systems are naturally associated to descriptions of objects by variables of various types. Consider a variable v with values in a codomain D ($v(s) \in D$ for all $s \in S$). If, for instance, D is linearly ordered (an ordinal or numerical variable), then its observed values naturally induce a closure system on S, precisely the collection of subsets $\{\{s \in S : v(s) \leq \alpha\} : \alpha \in D\}$. A similar scheme appears for other types of variables, as summarized in Table 1 below.

Variable Type	**Structure of D**	**Subsets of S**	**Closure Space Type**
Numerical, ordinal	Linear order	$\{s \in S : v(s) \leq \alpha\}$, $\alpha \in D$	Nested
Nominal	Finite set $D = \{v_1, \ldots, v_k\}$	$\{s \subset S : v(s) = v_i\}$	Tree of subsets
Taxonomic	Rooted tree	$\{s \in S : v(s) \leq \alpha\}$, $\alpha \in D$	Tree of subsets
Multicriterion evaluation	Product of linear orders	$\{s \in S : v(s) \leq \alpha\}$, $\alpha \in D$	Distributive

Table 1. Closure systems induced by description variables.

To explain the first row in Table 1, recall that the case of a linearly ordered set D leads to a *nested* CS $\mathcal{F}$; i.e., $\mathcal{F}$ is totally ordered by set inclusion—for all $C, C' \in \mathcal{F}$, $C \cap C' \in \{C, C'\}$. For the second and third rows, a CS is a *tree of subsets* if, for all $C, C' \in \mathcal{F}$, $C \cap C' \in \{\emptyset, C, C'\}$. A nominal variable induces a partition $\pi = \{S_1, \ldots, S_k\}$ of S, and the closure system $\pi \cup \{S, \emptyset\}$ is a tree of subsets. Note that nested CSs are particular trees of subsets, and that the empty set belongs to any tree of subsets which is not nested. In the foruth row, multicriterion evaluation occurs, for instance, in the optimal choice domain: the set $\mathcal{F}$ of the classes induced on S as indicated satisfies (C1), (C2) and the property: $C, C' \in \mathcal{F} \Rightarrow C \cup C' \in \mathcal{F}$. Such a CS is said to be *distributive*. Of course, this list is not exhaustive.

In these examples, when the primary set of classes $\mathcal{A}$ was not directly a CS, it was in fact completed into $\Phi(\mathcal{A}) = \{S\} \cup \{\cap\mathcal{B} : \mathcal{B} \subseteq \mathcal{A}\}$, the smallest (for inclusion) closure system that includes $\mathcal{A}$.

The output of a classification process is also frequently a closure system and, moreover, a classification system as defined above. For instance, a tree of subsets $\mathcal{H}$ satisfying (C3) will be said to be a *hierarchical system*. Then $\mathcal{H} - \emptyset$ is a hierarchy, in the usual sense. Pyramids (or quasi-hierarchies) and weak hierarchies, in their preserving-intersection version, provide other examples (with the empty set added). Recall finally that the Galois lattice (Barbut and Monjardet, 1970) and concept analysis (Ganter and Wille, 1999) have a double closure system as the output.

2.2 Equivalent Structures

In this section, three notions are defined which, together with CSs, turn out to be equivalent. A *closure operator* is a mapping onto the power set $\mathcal{P}(S)$ of S, satisfying properties of *isotony* (for all $A, B \subseteq S$, $A \subseteq B$ implies $\varphi(A) \subseteq \varphi(B)$), *extensivity* (for all $A \subseteq S$, $A \subseteq \varphi(A)$) and *idempotence* (for all $A \subseteq S$, $\varphi(A) = \varphi(\varphi(A))$). Then, the image $\mathcal{F}_\varphi = \varphi(\mathcal{P}(S))$ of $\mathcal{P}(S)$ by φ is exactly the set of all the fixed points of φ, which are called the elements of $\mathcal{P}(S)$ *closed* by φ, and $\mathcal{F}_\varphi$ is a closure system on S. Conversely, a closure operator $\varphi_\mathcal{F}$ on $\mathcal{P}(S)$, given by $\varphi_\mathcal{F}(A) = \bigcap\{F \in \mathcal{F} : A \subseteq F\}$, is associated to any closure system $\mathcal{F}$ on S.

A *full implicational system* (FIS), denoted by I, $\rightarrow_I$, or simply $\rightarrow$, is a binary relation on $\mathcal{P}(S)$ satisfying the following conditions:

(I1) $B \subseteq A$ implies $A \rightarrow B$;
(I2) for any $A, B, C \in S$, $A \rightarrow B$ and $B \rightarrow C$ imply $A \rightarrow C$;
(I3) for any $A, B, C, D \in S$, $A \rightarrow B$ and $C \rightarrow D$ imply $A \cup C \rightarrow B \cup D$.

An *overhanging relation* (OR) on S, denoted by $\Subset$, is also a binary relation on $\mathcal{P}(S)$ satisfying:

(O1) $A \Subset B$ implies $A \subset B$;
(O2) $A \subset B \subset C$ implies $A \Subset C \iff [A \Subset B$ or $B \Subset C]$;
(O3) $A \Subset A \cup B$ implies $A \cap B \Subset B$.

The sets of, respectively, closure systems, closure operators, full implicational systems, and overhanging relations on S are denoted, respectively, as $\mathcal{M}$, $\mathcal{C}$, $\mathcal{I}$ and $\mathcal{O}$. In fact, these sets are in a one-to-one correspondence with each other. The equivalence between closure systems and closure operators has been recalled above. Concerning a closure operator φ and its associated FIS $\rightarrow$ and OR $\Subset$, the first of the equivalences below is due to Armstrong (1974) and the second is given in Domenach and Leclerc (2003):

$$A \rightarrow B \iff B \subseteq \varphi(A)$$
$$A \Subset B \iff A \subset B \text{ and } \varphi(A) \subset \varphi(B)$$

In terms of classification, $A \to B$ (A implies B) means that any cluster including A includes also B, while $A \Subset B$ (B overhangs A) means that A is included in B and A does not imply B (there is at least one class including A, but not B).

There is a significant literature on implications, due to their importance in domains such as logic, lattice theory, relational databases, knowledge representation, and lattice data analysis (see the survey paper Caspard and Monjardet, 2003). Overhanging relations derive from Adams (1986), who called them 'nestings' and found characterizations in the case of hierarchical systems. Their recent generalization to all closure systems (Domenach and Leclerc, 2003) make them a further tool for the study of closure systems. We have introduced the term 'overhanging relation' because the original one, nesting, may be confused with nested families (of subsets), which in some mathematical contexts corresponds to a family totally ordered by inclusion. Although FISs and ORs are strongly related (every result about one of them is in fact also a result on the other), it can be useful to consider overhangings rather than implications; e.g., the work in Adams provides an example of this.

2.3 Lattices

The results of this section may be found in Caspard and Monjardet (2003) and, for overhangings, in Domenach and Leclerc (2003). First, each of the sets $\mathcal{M}$, $\mathcal{C}$, $\mathcal{I}$ and $\mathcal{O}$ is naturally ordered as follows:

- $\mathcal{M}$ is ordered by inclusion: for $\mathcal{F}, \mathcal{F}' \in \mathcal{M}$, $\mathcal{F} \subseteq \mathcal{F}'$ means that any class of $\mathcal{F}$ is also a class of $\mathcal{F}'$;
- $\mathcal{I}$ and $\mathcal{O}$ are ordered by inclusion too: given $I, I' \in \mathcal{I}$, $I \subseteq I'$ means that, for all $A, B \subseteq S$, $A \to_I B$ implies $A \to_{I'} B$. Similarly, given $\Subset, \Subset' \in \mathcal{O}$, $\Subset \subseteq \Subset'$ means that, for all $A, B \subseteq S$, $A \Subset B$ implies $A \Subset' B$.
- $\mathcal{C}$ is ordered by the pointwise order: given $\varphi, \varphi' \in \mathcal{C}$, $\varphi \leq \varphi'$ means that $\varphi(A) \subseteq \varphi'(A)$ for any $A \subseteq S$.

Moreover, with the same notations as above, all these sets are isomorphic or dually isomorphic:

$$\mathcal{F} \subseteq \mathcal{F}' \iff \varphi' \leq \varphi \iff I' \subseteq I \iff \Subset \subseteq \Subset'$$

where φ, I, and $\Subset$ (respectively, φ', I' and $\Subset'$) are the closure operator, full implicational system, and overhanging relation associated to $\mathcal{F}$ (respectively, to $\mathcal{F}'$).

The sets $\mathcal{M}$ and $\mathcal{I}$ preserve set intersection, while $\mathcal{O}$ preserves set union. It is not difficult to see that the maximum elements of, respectively, $\mathcal{M}$, $\mathcal{I}$, and $\mathcal{O}$ are $\mathcal{P}(S)$, $(\mathcal{P}(S))^2 = \{(A, B) : A, B \subseteq S\}$, and the set $\{(A, B) : A, B \subseteq S, A \subset B\}$, while their minimum elements are, respectively, $\{S\}$, $\{(A, B) : A, B \subseteq S, B \subseteq A\}$, and the empty relation on $\mathcal{P}(S)$.

From these results, $\mathcal{M}$ and $\mathcal{I}$ are closure systems on $\mathcal{P}(S)$ and $(\mathcal{P}(S))^2$, respectively. The operator Φ defined in Section 2.1 is the closure operator associated with $\mathcal{M}$. It is well-known that, with the inclusion order, any closure system $\mathcal{F}$ on S is a lattice $(\mathcal{F}, \vee, \cap)$ with the meet $F \cap F'$ and the join $F \vee F' = \varphi(F \cup F')$ for all $F, F' \in \mathcal{F}$. If $F \subseteq F'$, F' *covers* F (denoted as $F \prec F'$) if $F \subseteq G \subseteq F'$ implies $G = F$ or $G = F'$.

An element J of $\mathcal{F}$ is join irreducible if $\mathcal{G} \subseteq \mathcal{F}$ and $J = \bigvee \mathcal{G}$ imply $J \in \mathcal{G}$; an equivalent property is that J covers exactly one element, denoted as J^-, of $\mathcal{F}$. The set of all the join irreducibles is denoted by $\mathcal{J}$; we set $\mathcal{J}(F) = \{J \in \mathcal{J} : J \subseteq F\}$ for any $F \in \mathcal{F}$, with $F = \bigvee \mathcal{J}(F)$ for all $F \in \mathcal{F}$. If $F = \bigvee \mathcal{J}'$, with $\mathcal{J}' \subseteq \mathcal{J}(F)$, $\mathcal{J}'$ is called a *representation* of F. A join irreducible is an *atom* if it covers the minimum element of $\mathcal{F}$, and the lattice $\mathcal{F}$ is *atomistic* if all its join irreducibles are atoms. The lattice $\mathcal{F}$ is *lower semimodular* if, for every $F, F' \in \mathcal{F}$, $F \prec F \vee F'$ and $F' \prec F \vee F'$ imply $F \cap F' \prec F$ and $F \cap F' \prec F'$. The lattice $\mathcal{F}$ is *ranked* if it admits a numerical *rank function* r such that $F \prec F'$ implies $r(F') = r(F) + 1$. Lower semimodular lattices are ranked.

The lattice $\mathcal{F}$ is a *convex geometry* if it satisfies one of the following equivalent conditions (among many other characterizations, see Monjardet, 1990a):

(CG1) Every element F of $\mathcal{F}$ admits a unique minimal representation;
(CG2) $\mathcal{F}$ is ranked with rank function $r(F) = |\mathcal{J}(F)|$;
(CG3) $\mathcal{F}$ is lower semimodular with a rank function as in (CG2.

Since it is a closure system on $\mathcal{P}(S)$, the ordered set $\mathcal{M}$ is itself a lattice. This lattice is an atomistic convex geometry (its atoms are the closure systems $\{S, F\}, F \subset S$, with exactly one non-trivial class). Now, if $\mathcal{J}$ is the set of all the atoms of $\mathcal{M}$, we have $\mathcal{J}(\mathcal{F}) = \{\{S, A\} : A \subset S, A \in \mathcal{F}\}$ and $|\mathcal{J}(\mathcal{F})| = |\mathcal{F}| - 1$.

3 Lattice Consensus Applied to Closure Systems

In this section we consider the main consequences of the lattice structure of $\mathcal{M}$ for the consensus problem on closure systems, that is aggregation of a profile $\mathcal{F}^* = (\mathcal{F}_1, \mathcal{F}_2, \ldots, \mathcal{F}_k)$ of CSs into a CS $\mathcal{F} = c(\mathcal{F}^*)$. General results on the consensus problem in lattices may be found in, among others, Monjardet (1990b), Barthélemy and Janowitz (1991) and Leclerc (1994). Their consequences were investigated for classification trees (Barthélemy, et al., 1986), partitions (Barthélemy, et al., 1995), and orders (Leclerc 2003). The last reference contains useful results for the consensus in $\mathcal{M}$ because the semilattice of the orders defined on a given set has common features with convex geometries.

3.1 An Axiomatic Result

We now review the main results on closure systems (together with choice functions) obtained by Raderanirina (2001). Consider a consensus function

$c : \mathcal{M}^k \rightarrow \mathcal{M}$, and set $K = \{1, \ldots, k\}$. The function c is $\mathcal{J}$*-neutral monotonic* if, for all $A, B \subset S$, $\mathcal{F}^*$, $\mathcal{F}'^* \in \mathcal{M}^k$,

$$\{i \in K : A \in \mathcal{F}_i\} \subseteq \{i \in K : B \in \mathcal{F}'_i\} \text{ implies } [A \in c(\mathcal{F}^*) \Rightarrow B \in c(\mathcal{F}'^*)].$$

The function c is *Paretian* if for every $\mathcal{F}^* \in \mathcal{M}^k$, $\bigcap_{1 \leq i \leq k} \mathcal{F}_i \subseteq c(\mathcal{F}^*)$. These properties seem very natural: neutral monotonicity means that, if a subset of K has the power to impose the presence of a class A in some consensus $c(\mathcal{F}^*)$, then a greater subset has also this power, even for another class B in another profile. Pareto (unanimity) means that a class present in all the items of $\mathcal{F}^*$ must be in $c(\mathcal{F}^*)$.

A *federation* on K is a family $\mathcal{K}$ of subsets of K satisfying the monotonicity property: $[L \in \mathcal{K}, L' \supseteq L] \Rightarrow [L' \in \mathcal{K}]$. A federation consensus function $c_{\mathcal{K}}$ on $\mathcal{M}$ is then associated with $\mathcal{K}$ by $c_{\mathcal{K}}(\mathcal{F}^*) = \bigvee_{L \in \mathcal{K}} (\bigcap_{i \in L} \mathcal{F}_i)$. Especially, if $\mathcal{K} = \{L \subseteq K : L \supseteq L_0\}$ for a fixed subset L_0 of K, then $c_{\mathcal{K}}(\mathcal{F}^*) = \bigcap_{i \in L_0} \mathcal{F}_i$ is an *oligarchic* consensus function. So, an oligarchic consensus function retains those classes that are present in all systems corresponding to a fixed set of indices.

Another class of federation consensus functions includes the *quota rules*, where $\mathcal{K} = \{L \subseteq K : |L| \geq q\}$, for a fixed number q, with $0 \leq q \leq k$. Such a quota rule is equivalently defined as :

$$c_q(\mathcal{F}^*) = \Phi(\mathcal{A}_q)$$

where $\mathcal{A}_q = \{A \subset S : |\{i \in K : A \in \mathcal{F}_i\}| \geq q\}$, the set of non-trivial classes appearing in at least q elements of the profile, and Φ is the operator defined in Section 2.1 above. Especially, for $q = k/2$, $c_q(\mathcal{F}^*) = m(\mathcal{F}^*)$ is the so-called (weak) *majority rule* and, for $q = k$, it is the *unanimity rule* $u(\mathcal{F}^*)$, which is also the particular oligarchic consensus function with $L_0 = K$.

Starting from the axiomatic results in Monjardet (1990) and the studies on the lattice $\mathcal{M}$ in Caspard and Monjardet (2003), Raderanirina obtained several axiomatic characterizations of federation consensus functions on sets of closure systems and choice functions. Here we just recall the most general one:

Theorem 1 (Raderanirina, 1990). *A federation consensus function c on $\mathcal{M}$ is $\mathcal{J}$-neutral monotonic and Paretian if and only if it is oligarchic.*

3.2 Bounds on Medians

For a metric approach to the consensus in $\mathcal{M}$, we first have to define metrics. For that, we just follow Barthélemy et al. (1981) and Leclerc (1994). A real function v on $\mathcal{M}$ such that $\mathcal{F} \subseteq \mathcal{F}'$ implies $v(\mathcal{F}) < v(\mathcal{F}')$ is a *lower valuation* if it satisfies one of the following two equivalent properties:

(LV1) For all $s, t \in L$ such that $s \vee t$ exists, $v(s) + v(t) \leq v(s \vee t) + v(s \wedge t)$;

(LV2) The real function d_v defined on $\mathcal{M}^2$ by the following formula is a metric on $\mathcal{M}$: $d_v(\mathcal{F}, \mathcal{F}') = v(\mathcal{F}) + v(\mathcal{F}') - 2v(\mathcal{F} \cap \mathcal{F}')$.

A characteristic property of lower semimodular semilattices is that their rank functions are lower valuations. Using property (CG2), the *rank metric* is obtained by taking $v(\mathcal{F}) = |\mathcal{F}|$ and, so, $d_v(\mathcal{F}, \mathcal{F}') = \delta(\mathcal{F}, \mathcal{F}') = |\mathcal{F} \Delta \mathcal{F}'|$, where Δ is the symmetric difference on subsets. The equality between the rank and the symmetric difference metric is characteristic of convex geometries or close structures (Leclerc, 2003).

Consider the consensus procedure which consists of searching for the *medians* of the profile $\mathcal{F}^*$ for the metric δ, that is, the elements $\mathcal{M}$ of $\boldsymbol{\mathcal{M}}$ such that the *remoteness* $\rho(\mathcal{M}, \mathcal{F}^*) = \Sigma_{1 \leq i \leq k}\, \delta(\mathcal{M}, \mathcal{F}_i)$ is a minimum (see Barthélemy and Monjardet, 1981)). Note that the solution may not be unique.

Set $\mathcal{J}_m = \{\{S, A\} : A \in \mathcal{A}_{k/2}\}$ (the set of majority atoms). From results in Leclerc (1994, 2003), every median $\mathcal{M}$ of $\mathcal{F}^*$ is the join of some subset of $\mathcal{J}_m$. In other words, $\mathcal{M} = \Phi(\mathcal{B})$, for some $\mathcal{B} \subseteq \mathcal{A}_{k/2}$. It follows that:

Theorem 2. *For any profile $\mathcal{F}^*$ and for any median $\mathcal{M}$ of $\mathcal{F}^*$, the inclusion $\mathcal{M} \subseteq m(\mathcal{F}^*)$ holds.*

4 Overhangings and Generalized Adams' Results

The consensus systems of Section 3 retain classes that are present in enough (oligarchies, majorities) or all (unanimity) families of the profile. In the case of hierarchies, it was observed that considering only classes is a serious limitation that may prevent us from recognizing actual common features. This criticism remains valid for general closure systems. For an example, the set $\{b, c\}$ appears in the two classification systems $\mathcal{F}_1$ and $\mathcal{F}_2$ of Figure 1, but never as an entire class. So, the link between b and c exist in both families, but disappears in the output of any consensus method uniquely based on classes.

Moreover, consensus systems based on classes may frequently be trivial. For instance, if there does not exist any majority non-trivial class in a profile of closure systems, then the majority rule (and unique median) closure system is reduced to $\{S\}$. It is almost the same for the 2-profile of Figure 1, where majority (or unanimity) on classes just provides trivial classes: the empty and full sets and the singletons. This drawback may be thought of as a consequence of the loss of information observed just above.

The implication (or overhanging) relations are defined on all the subsets on S, i.e., without limitation on the potential classes. They may be a good tool for a finer approach of consensus. Indeed, from the results in Adams (1986) and Domenach and Leclerc (2003), it appears that in the hierarchical case, the Adams method is based on overhangings. Here we begin a similar study for general closure systems.

4.1 A Uniqueness Theorem on the Fitting of Overhangings

The elements assembled in Section 2 allows us to state a very general uniqueness result. Let Ξ be a binary relation on $\mathcal{P}(S)$, with only the assumption that

$(A,B) \in \Xi$ implies $A \subset B$. Consider the following two properties for a closure system $\mathcal{F}$, with associated closure operator φ and overhanging relation $\Subset$:

(AΞ1) $\Xi \subseteq \Subset$;

(AΞ2) for all $F, G \in \mathcal{F}$, $F \subset G$ implies $(F,G) \in \Xi$.

Let $\mathcal{F}'$ an alternative closure system, with closure operator φ' and overhanging relation $\Subset'$.

Theorem 3. *If both $\mathcal{F}$ and $\mathcal{F}'$ satisfy Conditions (AΞ1) and (AΞ2), then $\mathcal{F} = \mathcal{F}'$.*

Proof. Observe first that the maximum set S is in $\mathcal{F}$ and $\mathcal{F}'$. If $\mathcal{F} \neq \mathcal{F}'$, then the symmetric difference $\mathcal{F}\Delta\mathcal{F}'$ is not empty. Let F be a maximal element of $\mathcal{F}\Delta\mathcal{F}'$. It may be assumed without lost of generality that F belongs to $\mathcal{F}$. Since F is not equal to S, it is covered by at least one element G of $\mathcal{F}$, with $G \in \mathcal{F}'$. By (AΞ2), $(F,G) \in \Xi$ and, by (AΞ1), $F \Subset' G$. Set $F' = \varphi'(F)$. We have $F \subset F'$, since $F \notin \mathcal{F}'$ and $F' \Subset' G$, as $F' = \varphi'(F) = \varphi'(F') \subset \varphi'(G) = G$. But, according to the hypotheses, $F \subset F'$ implies $F' \in \mathcal{F}$, with $F \subset F' \subset G$, a contradiction with the hypothesis that G covers F in $\mathcal{F}$. □

This result generalizes the Adams uniqueness result, where $\mathcal{F}_1, \mathcal{F}_2, \ldots, \mathcal{F}_k$ are hierarchical closure systems and $\Xi = \bigcap_{1 \leq i \leq k} \Subset_i$. It is even stronger, since it proves that no other closure system, even a non-hierarchical onhe, can share properties (AΞ1) and (AΞ2) with the Adams consensus tree.

The following question then arises: for a given binary relation Ξ on $\mathcal{P}(S)$, does there exist an overhanging relation $\Subset$ satisfying conditions (AΞ1) and (AΞ2)? According to the Theorem 3, a solution, when it exists, is unique. Adams provides such a solution in the particular case that he considers (see also Semple and Steel, 2000 for supertrees).

Such a question is of major interest in consensus problems, where a profile $(\mathcal{F}_1, \mathcal{F}_2, \ldots, \mathcal{F}_k)$ of closure systems on S, with their associated overhanging relations, respectively $\Subset_1, \Subset_2, \ldots, \Subset_k$, is considered. In that context, Ξ may be any convenient combination of $\Subset_1, \Subset_2, \ldots, \Subset_k$, for instance $\Xi = \bigcup_{L \subseteq K, 2|L| > k} \bigcap_{i \in L} \Subset_i$ corresponds to a majority rule on overhangings.

It is worth noticing that, due to the properties of $\mathcal{O}$, there always exists a maximum overhanging relation $\Subset_0$ such that $\Subset \subseteq \Xi$. For instance, if $\Xi = \bigcap_{1 \leq i \leq k} \Subset_i$, then $\Subset_0 = \bigwedge_{1 \leq i \leq k} \Subset_i$ is the meet of the $\Subset_i$'s in the lattice $\mathcal{O}$. According to the isomorphism results of Section 2.3, it just corresponds to the unanimity rule on closure systems, as already considered.

4.2 A Generalization of Adams' Algorithm

In this section, we present a tentative algorithm generalizing Adams' method to closure systems.

With the notations of the previous sections, we first construct a family $\mathcal{G}$ of subsets of S in the following way: we initialize it with the ground set S.

Then, for each element F of $\mathcal{G}$ not already marked and maximal, we consider for every $i, 1 \leq i \leq k$, the elements in $\mathcal{F}_i$ covered by $\varphi_i(F)$. We then take all the non-empty intersections of these elements, one per CS of the profile, which will belong to the family $\mathcal{G}$. This algorithm is presented in Table 2. If $\mathcal{G}$ is a closure system, then the consensus family $\mathcal{F}$ is equal to $\mathcal{G}$. Otherwise, $\mathcal{F} = \Phi(\mathcal{G})$.

Algorithm :
Initialization :
$p := 0$;
$\mathcal{G} := \{S\}$;
For all $F \in \mathcal{G}$ unmarked, F maximal :
For all $x \in F$:
$\mathcal{G} := \mathcal{G} \cup \{F_1 \cap \ldots \cap F_k, F_i \prec_{\mathcal{F}_i} \varphi_i(F), x \in F_i\}$;
Mark F;

Table 2. Consensus algorithm.

Example 1. Consider the closure systems $\mathcal{F}_1$ and $\mathcal{F}_2$ of Figure 1 on $S = \{a, b, c, d, e\}$. They are not hierarchical, but of the "2-3 hierarchy" type, a particular class of pyramids defined in Bertrand (2002). Observe that these two CSs have no common classes, but an obvious common structure. The algorithm presented in Table 2 extracts this common structure. It directly computes the closure system of Figure 2.

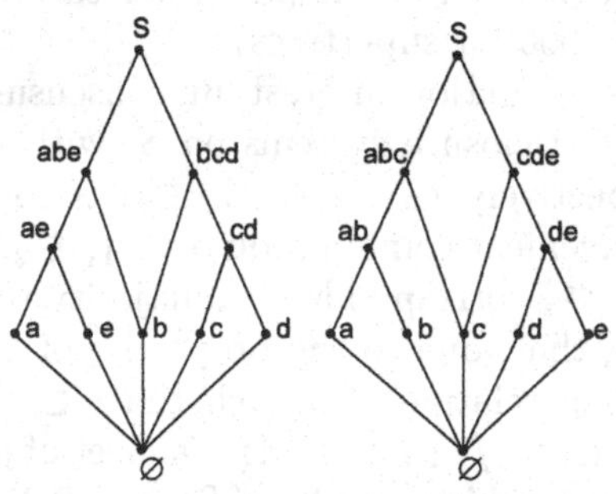

Fig. 1. Two closure systems $\mathcal{F}_1$ and $\mathcal{F}_2$.

At this time, the study of the properties satisfied by the output leads to many questions. For instance, is $\mathcal{G}$ always a closure system or, otherwise, for what kind of other systems is that property true (as for hierarchical systems)? When does the overhanging relation of $\mathcal{F}$ satisfy (AΞ1) and (AΞ2)?

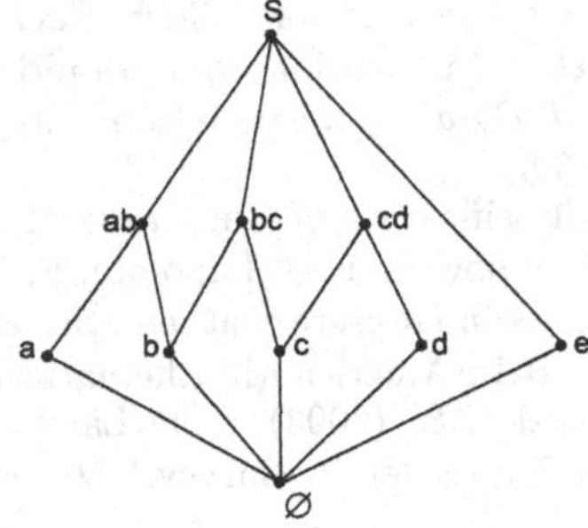

Fig. 2. The consensus closure system of $\mathcal{F}_1$ and $\mathcal{F}_2$.

5 Conclusion

The last section outlines further work on the consensus of closure systems. One problem is to recognize binary relations Ξ on $\mathcal{P}(S)$ for which an overhanging relation $\Subset$ satisfying (AΞ1) and (AΞ2) exists. For instance, starting from $\Xi = \bigcup_{L \subseteq K, 2|L|>k} \bigcap_{i \in L} \Subset_i$ allows one to use the fact that a CS appears several times in a profile, which is impossible with intersection rules. Another problem concerns finding efficient algorithms for overhanging relations.

References

1. Adams III, E.N. (1972). "Consensus Techniques and the Comparison of Taxonomic Trees," *Systematic Zoology*, **21**, 390–397.
2. Adams III, E.N. (1986). "N-Trees as Nestings: Complexity, Similarity and Consensus," *Journal of Classification*, **3**, 299–317.
3. Armstrong, W.W. (1974). "Dependency Structures of Data Base Relationships," *Information Processing*, **74**, 580–583.
4. Arrow, K.J. (1951). *Social Choice and Individual Values.* Wiley, New York.
5. Barbut, M., and Monjardet, B. (1970). *Ordre et Classification, Algèbre et Combinatoire.* Hachette, Paris .
6. Barthélemy, J.-P., and Janowitz, M.F. (1991). "A Formal Theory of Consensus," *SIAM Journal of Discrete Mathematics*, **4**, 305–322.
7. Barthélemy, J.-P., and Leclerc, B. (1995). "The Median Procedure for Partitions," in *Partitioning Data Sets*, eds. I.J. Cox, P. Hansen, and B. Julesz, DIMACS Series in Discrete Mathematics and Theoretical Computer Science, **19**. Providence, RI: American Mathematical Society, pp. 3–34.
8. Barthélemy, J.-P., Leclerc, B., and Monjardet, B. (1986). "On the Use of Ordered Sets in Problems of Comparison and Consensus of Classifications," *Journal of Classification*, **3**, 187–224.
9. Barthélemy, J.-P., and Monjardet, B. (1981). "The Median Procedure in Cluster Analysis and Social Choice Theory," *Mathematical Social Sciences*, **1**, 235–238.

10. Bertrand, P. (2002). "Set Systems for Which Each Set Properly Intersects at Most One Other Set - Application to Pyramidal Clustering," in *Classification, Clustering, and Data Analysis*, eds. K. Jajuga and A. Sokolowski, Berlin:Springer, pp. 38–39.
11. Bryant, D. (2003). "A Classification of Consensus Methods for Phylogenetics," in *Bioconsensus*, eds. M. Janowitz, F.-J. Lapointe, F. McMorris, B. Mirkin, and F. Roberts, DIMACS Series in Discrete Mathematics and Theoretical Computer Science, **61**, Providence, R.I.: American Mathematical Society, pp. 163–184.
12. Caspard, N., and Monjardet, B. (2003). "The Lattices of Moore Families and Closure Operators on a Finite Set: A Survey," *Discrete Applied Mathematics*, **127**, 241–269.
13. Domenach, F., and Leclerc, B. (2002). "On the Roles of Galois Connections in Classification," in *Explanatory Data Analysis in Empirical Research*, eds. M. Schwaiger and O. Opitz, Berlin:Springer, pp. 31–40.
14. Domenach, F., and Leclerc, B. (2003). "Closure Systems, Implicational Systems, Overhanging Relations and the case of Hierarchical Classification," *Mathematical Social Sciences*, to appear.
15. Day, W.H.E., and McMorris, F.R. (2003). *Axiomatic Consensus Theory in Group Choice and Biomathematics*, SIAM, Philadelphia.
16. Ganter, B., and Wille, R. (1999). *Formal Concept Analysis*. Springer, Berlin.
17. Leclerc, B. (1984). "Efficient and Binary Consensus Functions on Transitively Valued Relations," *Mathematical Social Sciences*, **8**, 45–61.
18. Leclerc, B. (1994). "Medians for Weight Metrics in the Covering Graphs of Semilattices," *Discrete Applied Mathematics*, **49**, 281–297.
19. Leclerc, B. (1998). "Consensus of Classifications: The Case of Trees," in *Advances in Data Science and Classification, Studies in Classification, Data Analysis and Knowledge Organization*, eds. A. Rizzi, M. Vichi, and H.-H. Bock, Berlin:Springer-Verlag, pp. 81–90.
20. Leclerc, B. (2003). "The Median Procedure in the Semilattice of Orders," *Discrete Applied Mathematics*, **127**, 285–302.
21. Margush, T., and McMorris, F.R. (1981). "Consensus n-Trees," *Bulletin of Mathematical Biology*, **43**, 239–244.
22. Mirkin, B. (1974). "The Problems of Approxmation in Spaces of Relations and Qualitative Data Analysis," *Automatika y Telemecanika*, English translation *Information and Remote Control*, **35**, 1424–1431.
23. Mirkin, B. (1975). "On the Problem of Reconciling Partitions,"in *Quantitative Sociology, International Perspectives on Mathematical and Statistical Modelling*, New York:Academic Press, pp. 441-449.
24. Monjardet, B. (1990). "Arrowian Characterization of Latticial Federation Consensus Functions," *Mathematical Social Sciences*, **20**, 51–71.
25. Monjardet, B. (1990). "Comments on R.P. Dilworth's 'Lattices with Unique Irreducible Decompositions'," in *The Dilworth Theorems: Selected Works of Robert P. Dilworth,* eds. K. Bogart, R. Freese, and J. Kung, Boston, MA:Birkhauser, pp. 192–201.
26. Raderanirina, V. (2001). *Treillis et Agrégation de Familles de Moore et de Fonctions de Choix*, Ph.D. Thesis, University Paris 1 Panthéon-Sorbonne, Paris.
27. Régnier, S. (1965). "Sur Quelques Aspects Mathématiques des Problèmes de Classification Automatique," *ICC Bulletin*, **4**, 175-191.
28. Semple, C., and Steel, M.A. (2000). "A Supertree Method for Rooted Trees," *Discrete Applied Mathematics*, **105**, 147–158.

Symbolic Linear Regression with Taxonomies

F. Afonso[1,2], L. Billard[2], and E. Diday[1]

[1] Ceremade/Université Paris 9 Dauphine, France
{afonso,diday}@ceremade.dauphine.fr
[2] Lamsade/Université Paris 9 Dauphine, France
[3] University of Georgia, U.S.A.
lynne@stat.uga.edu

Abstract: This work deals with the extension of classical linear regression to symbolic data and constitutes a continuation of previous papers from Billard and Diday on linear regression with interval and histogram-valued data. In this paper, we present a method for regression with taxonomic variables. Taxonomic variables are variables organized in a tree with several levels of generality. For example, the towns are aggregated up to their regions, the regions are aggregated up to their country.

1 Introduction

In practice data sets often contain a very large number of observations. Rather than any one individual in a database, we may be interested in the patterns of specific groups (concepts in symbolic data language). Alternatively, because of the sheer size of the data sets, aggregation of the individual data in some form, has to occur to make the data of a manageable size in order to carry out an appropriate analysis. The key point is that after this aggregation, each data "point" is now no longer a single point in p-dimensional space as in classical data sets, but rather each observation consists of lists, intervals, histograms or other manifestations of symbolic data (Billard et al., 2003). The purpose of the present work is to propose ways to adapt classical ideas in regression analysis to enable regression analysis on symbolic data. Billard and Diday introduced regression for interval-valued symbolic data in (Billard et al., 2000) and histogram-valued symbolic data in (Billard et al., 2002). The present work considers how to implement regression analysis in the presence of taxonomy variables.The method is described and tested on a data set simulated from real statistics. Finally,we will present an example of symbolic linear regression in order to study concepts.

2 Some Preliminaries

In linear regression, we want to explain a dependent variable Y with a linear equation of explanatory variables:

$$X_i, i = 1, ..., k : Y = b_0 + b_1X_1 + ... + b_kX_k + e = bX + e$$

where e is the residual error vector. In order to find the best vector b, we minimize this residual error. We obtain: $b^* = (X'X)^{-1}X'Y$. In the following sections, we will highlight the matrices X and Y to be regressed.

2.1 The SODAS Software

The different methods have been implemented in the SODAS software for the European project of symbolic analysis ASSO (Bock et al., 2000). The Symbolic REGression module SREG provides methods and tests for multiple linear regression with the symbolic data intervals, quantitative and qualitative histograms, taxonomies and mother-daughters variables.

2.2 Taxonomic Variables

Taxonomic variables are variables with several levels of generality. They are useful, e.g., to classify fauna and flora, geographical zones, etc. For example, Table 1 presents the three levels of a taxonomy variable relating to geographical zones ('zone' say).

Table 1. Taxonomy zone.

Level 1	2	3
town1	region1	country1
town2	region1	country1
town3	region2	country1
town4	region2	country1
town5	region3	country2
town6	region3	country2
town7	region4	country2
town8	region4	country2

3 Regression for Taxonomic Variables

In general suppose there are t taxonomy variables, with the jth such variable having t_j levels, $j = 1, \ldots, t$. To illustrate the methodology, suppose there are two taxonomy variables 'color' and 'zone'. Suppose the taxonomy variable 'color' divides into light and dark tones (at level $v = 2$, X_2=tone, say) with these in turn dividing into white and yellow, and brown and black, respectively (at level $v = 1$, $X_1 =$ shade, say.) Here, $t_1 = 2$. Suppose that 'zone' consists of two possible countries each of which has two possible regions with the regions in turn comprising two towns (as in Table 1). There are three levels, at level $v = 1, Z_1 \equiv$ town, at level $v = 2, Z_2 \equiv$ region, and at level $v = 3, Z_3 \equiv$ country, with $t_2 = 3$.

Then, assume the data are as in Table 2 where 'color' and 'zone' are the explanatory variables and Y is the quantitative dependent variable. The problem is that we deal with values at different levels of generality. Indeed, for the individuals 5, 10, 17 we know the tone of the color but not the shade. For the individuals 5, 6, 8 and 19, we know the country or the region but not the town.

Table 2. Data matrix with taxonomies.

Individual	Color	Zone	Y	Individual	Color	Zone	Y
1	yellow	town1	3500	11	brown	town7	1500
2	black	town2	2300	12	yellow	town6	2200
3	white	town3	3600	13	black	town3	2000
4	black	town3	2100	14	white	town2	3800
5	light	region1	4000	15	white	town5	3000
6	yellow	country1	3500	16	brown	town5	2000
7	black	town5	1700	17	light	town4	2900
8	brown	region3	2600	18	yellow	town 1	3500
9	yellow	town7	2100	19	brown	country1	2400
10	light	town8	3200	20	brown	town7	1500

Remark 1. We will regress the ordered and non-ordered qualitative variables after having replaced the initial matrix by a binary matrix where each variable is a category of the initial variables taking the values 0 *or* 1. Consequently, we will have to remove one category by variable in order to obtain a reversible matrix.

3.1 Method of Regression

In this method, one regression at each level is performed. Each regression uses only those observations which provide relevant data value at that level.

Thus in the example of Table 2, at the first level, we do not use the observations 5, 6, 8, 10, 17 and 19; at the second level specific colors are identified by the tones and towns by their region and only the observations 6 and 19 are not used; and at the third level all the observations are used but the taxonomic values are those at the top of the trees, tone for the color variable and country for the zone variable. The first ten observations are displayed in Table 3a, 3b, 3c, respectively. For example, after the transformation of the data matrix into a binary matrix and the suppression of the categories dark and region4, we will obtain, at level 2, the regression equation

$$Y = \hat{\alpha} + \hat{\beta}\text{light} + \hat{\partial}_1\text{region1} + \hat{\partial}_2\text{region2} + \hat{\partial}_3\text{region3}$$

i.e.,

$$Y = 1566.25 + 1017.5(\text{light}) + 1039.75(\text{region1}) + 575(\text{region2}) \\ +326.75(\text{region3}). \quad (1)$$

where *light*, *region*1 and *region*3 take the values 0 or 1, as appropriate.

An advantage of this method is that there is no modification of the actual data set. Each decomposed level has its own regression equation. However, as the number of taxonomic variables increases, then the method becomes less efficient as more observations would perforce be removed at least at the lowest levels to be replaced by its higher level values.

Table 3a, 3b, 3c. Matrices for the regressions at the levels 1, 2 and 3.

First level

i	Color	Zone	Y
1	yellow	town1	3500
2	black	town2	2300
3	white	town3	3600
4	black	town3	2100
7	black	town5	1700
9	yellow	town7	2100

Second level

i	Color	Zone	Y
1	light	region1	3500
2	dark	region1	2300
3	light	region2	3600
4	dark	region2	2100
5	light	region1	4000
7	dark	region3	1700
8	dark	region3	2600
9	light	region4	2100
10	light	region4	3800

Third level

i	Color	Zone	Y
1	light	country1	3500
2	dark	country1	2300
3	light	country1	3600
4	dark	country1	2100
5	light	country1	4000
6	light	country1	3500
7	dark	country2	1700
8	dark	country2	2600
9	light	country2	2100
10	light	country2	3800

3.2 Prediction of Missing Values in the Taxonomies

Suppose further we want to predict shade at level 1, viz., the X_1 missing value for observation $i = 10$. Thus, by setting color as the dependent variable, we can determine the appropriate regression equation for each level. We give the codes white = 1, yellow = 2, brown = 3 and black =1 to X_1 and light = 1, dark = 2 to X_2. At level 1, we obtain the equation

$$X_1 = 6.075 - 0.002Y + 2.9(\text{town1}) + 2.5(\text{town2}) + 2.1(\text{town3}) + 1.1(\text{town5}) \\ +0.34(\text{town6}).$$

Hence, for observation $i = 10$, we obtain $\hat{X}_1 = 2.2$. This value is not sufficient to tell us whether the shade is yellow or brown. In this case we know the tone value at the next higher level is light; so we would take the shade to be yellow. If the tone were unknown, we would execute the regression at the second level producing

$$X_2 = 2.863 - 0.0007Y + 0.74(\text{region1}) + 0.5(\text{region2}) + 0.355(\text{region3})$$

with $\hat{X}_2 = 0.61$ for observation $i = 10$. This suggests that the tone is light and hence the shade is likely to be yellow (rather than brown). In this manner, predictions at higher levels of generality can be used to tighten predictions made at lower levels in the taxonomy tree.

Note that we have to delete one of the possible values (here black for color, and town7 for zone) in order to be able to invert the "$(X'X)$" matrix.

3.3 Example

Now, we test the method with a data set simulated from real statistics.

Test 1: All the Explanatory Variables are Taxonomies

The data set to be used consists of 10000 individuals with dependent variable Y as income. The predictor variables are two taxonomic variables, work characteristics X and zone Z. The work variable has two levels, $t_1 = 2$. Thus, at the second level representing the type of work X_2, individuals either work Full time $X_2 = 1$, Part time $X_2 = 2$ or Do not work $X_2 = 3$. At the first level the variable X_1 is weeks worked and X_1 takes four possible values where each of $X_2 = 1$ and $X_2 = 2$ has three branches corresponding to Number of weeks worked with values 50 weeks or more ($X_1 = 1$), 27 to 49 weeks ($X_1 = 2$) and 26 weeks or less ($X_1 = 3$). The fourth $v = 1$ level value is $X_1 = 4$ which is the only branch of the $X_2 = 3$ possibility.

The zone variable Z has four levels, $t_2 = 4$. At the top of the tree, Z_4 represents the variable Division with $Z_4 = 1, 2, 3, 4$ being the NorthEast, MidWest, South, and West, respectively. Each division has branches at the third level ($v = 3$) corresponding to the variable Region Z_3 with two regions in each division except for the South which has three regions. Each region has two branches at the second, $v = 2$, level corresponding to $Z_2 = 1, 2$, if the observation is from a metro, or nonmetro area, respectively. Finally, at level $v = 1$, Z_1 takes values 1(2) if the metro area is a central city with fewer (more) than one million inhabitants, respectively, $Z_1 = 3(4)$ if the metro area is a noncentral city with fewer (more) than 1 million inhabitants, and $Z_1 = 5$ if it is a nonmetro area.

Test 2: Non-Taxonomic Variables

In addition to the taxonomy variables X and Z described in the Test 1, the dataset also contains values for nontaxonomy quantitative variables, viz., W_1 (age), W_2 (glucose), W_3 (cholesterol), W_4 (hemoglobin), W_5 (hematocrit), W_6 (red blood count) W_7 (white blood count) and nontaxonomy qualitative variables W_8 (race $= 1, 2$ for white, black), W_9 (age group, $W_9 = 1, \ldots, 7$ for age groups 15-24 year olds, 25-34, 35-44, 45-54, 55-64, 65-74, and over 74 years old) and W_{10} (diabetes with $W_{10} = 0, 1, 2$ for No diabetes, Mild diabetes and Yes, respectively). Let $\boldsymbol{V} \equiv (X, Z, W_1, \ldots, W_{10})$; and let V_j take possible values (modules in the taxonomy tree) $m_{j1}, \ldots, m_{jn_j}$.

Let us consider the role played by the taxonomy variables at the respective levels. Table 4 provides the relevant calculations of the weights when there are not missing values

$$w_j = \sum_{i=1}^{n_j} |\text{coeff}(V_j, m_{ji})| \tag{2}$$

for the jth variable $j = 1, \ldots, 12$ and for the regressions fitted at each level. These weights provide a measure of the importance of the respective variables to the overall regression model. Thus, for level 1, we see that the two taxonomy variables Work and Zone together contribute a weight of 139644 or 75.7% of the total, while the ten nontaxonomy variables together contribute a weight of 332312 or 18.0%, along with the regression constant of 11690 contributing 6.3%. However, as the regression moves to higher levels in the taxonomy tree, the taxonomy variables become increasingly less important. Thus, at the top of the tree at level $v = 4$, the taxonomy variables account for only 6.1% (down from 75.7%) of the coefficient weights, while the nontaxonomy variables now account for 62.9% of the regression weights. This is partly explained by the fact there are fewer modalities (tree branches) as the levels increase. In this example, we have 45 branches at level Z_1 but only four at Z_4.

Table 4. Weight of the taxonomy variables at the respective levels.

	level 1		level 2	level 3	level 4
Variable	w_j	%	%	%	%
Constant	11690	6.3%	7.1	21.4	31.0
Z	134971	73.1%	63.5	23.8	2.7
X	4673	2.5%	1.5	2.9	3.4
Total of the taxonomies	139644	75.7%	65.1	26.7	6.1
Total of the other variables(W_j)	33232	18.0%	27.8	51.9	62.9
Total	184566	100%	100	100	100

Conclusions from the Tests

Since typically a dataset will contain some observations with missing values on (some) lower branches, what seems to be interesting is what happens in these situations. To study this, three different sets of missing data are generated by random selection. Thus, in the first case all the data is used (see Table 5 column removed data=1), in the second case only a few values are missing (12% of the first level of the taxonomy, 6% of the level 2 and 3% of the level 3, column removed data=2) whereas in the third case there is a large percentage of lower level values missing (40%, 20%, 10% at the levels 1, 2, 3 respectively, column removed data=3). In order to capture the impact of the missing values on the measure, we use a correlation performance measure $R_p = (1-p)R^2$, where p is the proportion of the values missing at each level, and R^2 is the usual correlation coefficient. We can see the R_p values of Test 1 and Test 2 in Table 5.

Table 5. R_p values for the tests 1 and 2.

		Test 1			Test 2		
	levels:	(1,2,3,4)	(1,2,3,4)	(1,2,3,4)	(1,2,3,4)	(1,2,3,4)	(1,2,3,4)
Removed data %:		(0,0,0,0)	(12,6,3,0)	(40,20,10,0)	(0,0,0,0)	(12,6,3,0)	(40,20,10,0)
Level	R^2 or R_p:	Value of R^2 or R_p			Value of R^2 or R_p		
1	R^2	0.33	0.33	0.34	0.86	0.87	0.89
1	R_p	0.33	0.26	0.12	0.86	0.66	0.31
2	R_p	0.16	0.16	0.15	0.72	0.71	0.66
3	R_p	0.05	0.05	0.05	0.59	0.59	0.59
4	R_p	0.03			0.56		

If we look at the R_p values, we can note that level 1 seems to be clearly the best level when there are only few missing values (Column removed data=1, test 1: $R_p = 0.33$). However, in the presence of a lot of missing values at the first level, the R_p values suggest that we should look at the second level (removed data=3, test2, level 1: $R_p = 0.31$, level 2: $R_p = 0.66$). Level 3 and 4 are not good levels. Indeed, for the test 1 with no missing values $R_p = 0.05(0.03)$ at level 3(4). Moreover, we can see that in the presence of nontaxonomy variables the decrease of the R_p values is more important. This is due to the fact that like the taxonomy variables, the classical (or other symbolic) variables are penalized by the removal of individuals.

4 Applications of Symbolic Regression

While the results so far have dealt with individuals $i = 1, \ldots, n$ ($n = 10,000$ in the example), wherein each variable takes a single (classical) value, the method developed apply equally to symbolic data. In this case, we wish to study concepts. For example, we may be interested in the regression relation between variables for the concept defined by an age × race (or age × race × gender, or age × region, or etc) descriptor. Here, the particular choices of concepts will depend on the fundamental questions or interest, and as such there can be many such choices. In other situations, the data can describe predefined concepts. For example, we have a data set where each individual is a football team player but we do not wish to study the players but the teams. To illustrate, assume we are interested in concepts defined by an agegroup × work descriptor where agegroup is the qualitative variable and work the taxonomy variable defined in Section 3.3. Therefore, we will study $7 \times 7 = 49$ concepts. Hence, we may be interested in the relation between cholesterol as the quantitative dependent variable with the variables hematocrit(quantitative), hemogroup (categories are 10 intervals of hemoglobin [10,11], [11.1,11.4], ..., [13.9,14.2], [14.3,15.2]) and work(see Table 6a). After the creation of the concepts, the quantitative variables hematocrit and cholesterol become interval-valued variables (with the DB2SO module of Sodas). Moreover, the hemogroup variable becomes a quantitative histogram-valued variable because the categories are intervals. Finally, as the variable work is a part of the concepts definition, work remains a taxonomy variable (see Table 6b).We present the results (Fisher test F and determination coefficient R^2) of the simple symbolic linear regressions and the multiple linear regression with all the explanatory variables in Table 7. We can conclude that hematocrit and hemogroup seem to be quite good predictors ($F > f(0.95)$ and $R_{\text{hematocrit}} = 0.42$ and $R_{\text{hemogroup}} = 0.40$) whereas the taxonomy variable work is refused by the F-test.

Table 6a. Initial classical data matrix.

i	concepts	chol	agegroup	X_2	X_1	X=work	hemat	hemogroup
1	3 × 11	151	3	1	1	11	33	[12.3, 12.6]
2	3 × 11	154	3	1	1	11	37	[12.7, 13]
3	3 × 11	158	3	1	1	11	36	[12.3, 12.6]
4	5 × 21	173	5	2	1	21	42	[13.1, 13.4]
5	5 × 21	179	5	2	1	21	40	[13.5, 13.8]
...								

Table 6b. Concepts built from Table 6a.

concepts	cholesterol	work	hematocrit	hemogroup
3 × 11	[151, 158]	11	[33, 37]	2/3[12.3, 12.6], 1/3[12.7, 13]
5 × 21	[173, 179]	21	[40, 42]	$\frac{1}{2}$[13.1, 13.4], $\frac{1}{2}$[13.5, 13.8]

Table 7. Fisher Tests and Determination Coefficients of the Symbolic Regressions. Dependent Variable=cholesterol.

Explanatory variables	Fisher test F	Quantile $f(0.95)$	R^2
hematocrit	34.5	4.17	0.42
hemogroup	32.3	4.17	0.40
work (level 1)	0.05	2.42	0.007
multiple regression	17.1	3.31	0.43

5 Conclusions

This work has first developed methodology to fit regression models to data which internally contain taxonomies. Other methods of regression with taxonomic variables have been discussed and tested in (Afonso et al., 2004) and (Afonso et al., 2003). This symbolic linear regression is useful when we wish to study concepts instead of individuals. Moreover, what seems to be interesting is to extend this work to other symbolic variables. Also, this symbolic method can be directly extended to other regressions as the Bayesian regression. Indeed, we will use the same matrices. Consequently, a future work with regard to non-linear regression can be interesting too. Finally, the need to develop mathematical rigor to these new linear regression methods remains an open problem.

Acknowledgement

Partial support from an NSF-INRIA grant is gratefully acknowledged.

References

1. Afonso, F., Billard, L., and Diday, E.(2004). "Régression Linéaire Symbolique avec Variables Taxonomiques," in *Actes des IVèmes Journées d'Extraction et Gestion des Connaissance, EGC Clermont-Ferrand 2004*, eds. Hébrail and al., RNTI-E-2, Vol. 1, pp. 205–210.
2. Afonso, F., Billard, L., and Diday, E. (2003). "Extension des Méthodes de Régression Linéaire aux cas des Variables Symboliques Taxonomiques et Hiérarchiques," *Actes des XXXVèmes journées de Statistique, SFDS Lyon 2003*, Vol. 1, pp. 89–92.
3. Billard, L., and Diday, E. (2003). "From the Statistics of Data to the Statistics of Knowledge: Symbolic Data Analysis," *Journal of the American Statistical Association*, **98**, 470–487
4. Billard, L., and Diday, E.(2002). "Symbolic Regression Analysis," in *Classification, Clustering and Data Analysis*, eds. H.-H. Bock et al., Berlin:Springer-Verlag, pp. 281–288.
5. Billard, L., and Diday, E. (2000). "Regression Analysis for Interval-Valued Data," in *Data Analysis, Classification and Related Methods*, eds. H. Kiers et al., Berlin:Springer-Verlag, pp. 369–374.
6. Bock, H.-H., and Diday E.(2000). *Analysis Data Sets: Exploratory Methods for Extracting Statistical Information from Complex Data*, Springer-Verlag, Berlin.

Determining Horizontal Gene Transfers in Species Classification: Unique Scenario

Vladimir Makarenkov, Alix Boc and Abdoulaye Baniré Diallo

Université du Québec à Montréal, Canada
makarenkov.vladimir@uqam.ca, boc.alix@courrier.uqam.ca,
banire@math.uqam.ca

Abtract: The problem of species classification, taking into account the mechanisms of reticulate evolution such as horizontal gene transfer (HGT), species hybridization,or gene duplication, is very delicate. In this paper, we describe a new algorithm for determining a unique scenario of HGT events in a given additive tree (i.e., a phylogenetic tree) representing the evolution of a group of species. The algorithm first establishes differences between topologies of species and gene-additive trees. Then it uses a least-squares optimization procedure to test for the possibility of horizontal gene transfers between any pair of edges of the species in the tree, considering all previously added HGTs in order to determine the next one. We show how the proposed algorithm can be used to represent possible ways in which the rubisco *rbcL* gene has spread in a species classification that includes plastids, cyanobacteria, and proteobacteria.

1 Introduction

Species classification has been often modeled using an additive tree in which each species can only be linked to its closest ancestor and interspecies relationships are not allowed. However, such important evolutionary mechanisms as gene convergence, gene duplication, gene loss, and horizontal gene transfer (i.e. lateral gene transfer) can be appropriately represented only by using a network model (see Olsen and Woese, 1998, or Doolittle, 1999). This paper addresses the problem of detection of horizontal gene transfer events. Several attempts to use network-based evolutionary models to represent horizontal gene transfers can be found in the scientific literature (cf. Page, 1994, or Page and Charleston, 1998). Recently we proposed a new method (Boc and Makarenkov, 2003) for detecting HGT events based on a mathematically sound model using a least-squares mapping of a gene tree into a species tree. The latter method proceeds by obtaining a classification of probable HGTs that may have occurred in course of the evolution; the biologists should then be able to select appropriate HGTs from the classification established.

In this article, we propose a new approach that allows one to establish a unique scenario of horizontal gene transfers. This approach exploits topological discrepancies existing in the species and gene-additive trees. To reconcile topological differences between the species and gene trees, we recompute the edge lengths of the species tree with respect to the gene data. Then, each pair of edges of the species tree will be evaluated for the possibility of a horizontal gene transfer, and the best one of those, according to the least-squares criterion, will be added to the species tree. All further HGT edges will be added to the species tree in the same way, leading to the construction of an HGT network. A number of computational rules that are plausible from the biological point of view are incorporated in our model. In the application section, we discuss a unique scenario for the lateral gene transfers of the *rbcl* gene in a bacteria classification considered in Delwiche and Palmer (1996).

2 Description of the New Method

The new algorithm allows one to determine the best possible least-squares fit for horizontal gene transfer events in a group of organisms under consideration. It proceeds first by mapping gene data into a species tree followed by consecutive addition of new HGT edges with directions. The algorithm is comprised of the two main steps described below:

Step 1. Let T be an additive species tree whose leaves are labeled according to the set X of n taxa and let T_1 be a gene tree whose leaves are labeled according to the same set X of n taxa. Then T and T_1 can be inferred from sequence or distance data using an appropriate tree-fitting algorithm. Without loss of generality, we assume that T and T_1 are binary trees, whose internal nodes are all of degree 3 and whose number of edges is $2n$-3. The species tree should be explicitly rooted; the position of the root is important in our model. If the topologies of T and T_1 are identical, we conclude that the evolution of the given gene followed that of the species, and no horizontal gene transfers between edges of the species tree should be indicated. However, if the two additive trees are topologically different, it may be the result of horizontal gene transfers. In the latter case, the gene tree T_1 can be mapped into the species tree T by least-squares fitting of the edge lengths of T to the pairwise distances in T_1 (see Barthélemy and Guénoche (1991) or Makarenkov and Leclerc (1999) for more details on this technique).

Step 2. The goal of this step is to establish a classification of all possible HGT connections between pairs of edges in T. In our model, the HGT edges providing the greatest contribution to decreasing the least-squares statistic will correspond to the most probable cases of horizontal gene transfer. Thus, the first HGT in this list will be added to the species tree T, transforming it into a phylogenetic network. Once the first HGT edge is added to T, all its edges, including the new HGT edge, will be reestimated to fit the best the inter-leaf distances in the gene tree T_1. To add this first HGT edge to the network under construction, the algorithm considers $(2n\text{-}3)(2n\text{-}4)$ possibilities, which is the maximum number of different directed inter-edge connections in a binary phylogenetic tree with n leaves. Then, the best second, third, and so forth, HGT edges are added to T in the same way. The addition of any new HGT edge starting from the second one is done by taking into account all previously added HGTs. The algorithm stops when a prespecified number of HGT edges have been added to T. The resulting phylogenetic network represents a possible evolutionary scenario, and it is the best scenario, in terms of the least-squares criterion, among all the horizontal gene transfers considered.

3 Computing the Least-Squares Coefficient

The addition of a new edge may create an extra path between any pair of nodes in a phylogenetic network. Figure 1 illustrates the only possible case when the minimum path-length distance between taxa (i.e. species) i and j is allowed to pass across the new HGT edge (a,b) directed from b to a. From the biological point of view it would be plausible to allow the horizontal gene transfer between b and a to affect the evolutionary distance between the pair of taxa i and j, where the position of i in T is fixed, if and only if j is located in the shaded area in Fig. 1.

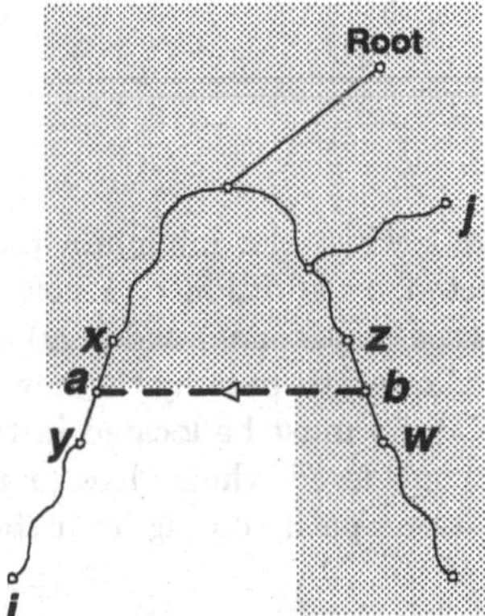

Fig. 1. The minimum path-length distance between the taxa i and j can be affected by addition of a new edge (a,b) representing horizontal gene transfer between edges (z,w) and (x,y) in the species tree if the leaf j is located in the shaded area of the picture. The path between the taxa i and j can pass by the new edge (a,b).

In all other cases than the one shown in Fig. 1, the path between the taxa i and j should not be permitted to pass by the new edge (a,b) representing the gene transfer from b to a. These cases are illustrated in Fig. 2(a) to 2(d).

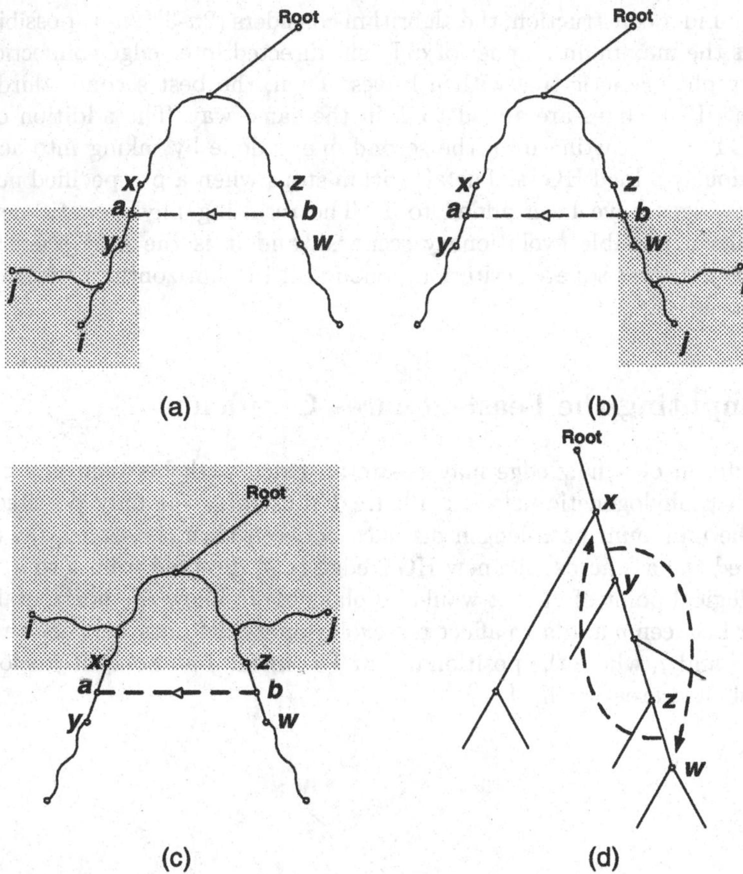

Fig. 2. (a-c) Three situations when the minimum path-length distance between the taxa i and j is not affected by addition of a new edge (a,b) representing the horizontal gene transfer between edges (z,w) and (x,y) of the species tree. The path between taxa i and j is not allowed to pass by the new edge (a,b). In Figures 2(a), 2(b), and 2(c), both leaves i and j must be located in the shaded area. Figure 2(d) shows that no HGT can be considered when edges (x,y) and (z,w) are located on the same lineage (i.e. on the same path coming from the root).

To compute the value of the least-squares coefficient Q for a given HGT edge (a,b) the following four-part strategy was adopted. First, we define the set of all pairs of taxa such that the path between them can be allowed to pass by a new HGT edge (a,b). Second, for this set we determine all pairs of taxa such that the minimum path-length distance between them may decrease after addition of (a,b). Third, we look for an optimal value l of the length of (a,b), while keeping fixed the lengths of all other tree edges. And finally, fourth, all edge lengths are reassessed one at a time.

Let us define the set A(a,b) of all pairs of taxa ij such that the distances between them may change if an HGT edge(a,b) is added to the tree T. Then A(a,b) is the set of all pairs of taxa i,j such that they are located in T as shown in Fig. 1 and:

$$\min\{d(i,a)+d(j,b);\ d(j,a)+d(i,b)\} < d(i,j), \qquad (1)$$

where $d(i,j)$ is the minimum path-length distance between taxa i and j in T. The vertices a and b are located in the middle of the edges (x,y) and (z,w), respectively.

The following function can be defined:

$$\mathrm{dist}(i,j) = d(i,j) - \min\{d(i,a)+d(j,b);\ d(j,a)+d(i,b)\}, \qquad (2)$$

so that A(a,b) is a set of all leaf pairs i,j with $\mathrm{dist}(i,j) > 0$. Then the least-squares objective function to be minimized, with l used as an unknown variable, can be formulated as follows:

$$Q(ab,l) = \sum_{\mathrm{dist}(i,j)>l} (\min\{d(i,a)+d(j,b);\ d(j,a)+d(i,b)\} + l - \delta(i,j))^2 + \sum_{\mathrm{dist}(i,j)\le l} (d(i,j)-\delta(i,j))^2 \rightarrow \min \qquad (3)$$

where $\delta(i,j)$ is the minimum path-length distance between the taxa i and j in the gene tree T_1. The function $Q(ab,l)$ measures the gain in fit when a new HGT edge (a,b) with length l is added to the species tree T.

When the optimal value of a new edge (a,b) is determined, this computation can be followed by an overall polishing procedure for all edge lengths in T. To reassess the length of any edge of T, one can use equations (1), (2), and (3) assuming that the lengths of all the other edges are fixed. These computations are repeated for all pairs of edges in the species tree T. When all pairs of edges in T are tested, only the HGT corresponding to the smallest value of Q is retained for addition to T. This algorithm requires $\mathcal{O}(kn^4)$ operations to provide one with a unique HGT scenario including k transfer edges.

4 HGT of the *rbcL* Gene: Unique Scenario

The new algorithm described in previous sections was applied to analyze the plastids, cyanobacteria, and proteobacteria data considered in Delwiche and Palmer (1996). These authors found that the gene classification based on the *rbcL* gene contains a number of conflicts compared to the species classification (built for 48 species) based on 16S ribosomal RNA and other evidence. To carry out the analysis we reduced the number of species to 15, as shown by the trees in Figs. 3(a) and 3(b). Each species shown in Fig. 3 represents a group of bacteria or plastids from the original phylogeny provided by Delwiche and Palmer (1996, Fig.2). We decided to conduct our study with three α-proteobacteria, three β-proteobacteria, three γ-proteobacteria, two cyonobacteria, one green plastid, one red and brown plastid and two single plastid species *Gonyaulax* and *Cyanophora*.

The new algorithm used as input the species and gene additive trees in Fig. 3 (a) and 3(b) and provided a unique scenario of horizontal gene transfers of the *rbcL* gene. The topological conflicts between the trees in Fig. 3 can be explained either by lateral gene transfers that may have taken place between the species indicated or by ancient gene duplication followed by gene loss—these two hypotheses are not mutually exclusive (see Delwiche and Palmer (1996) for more detail). In this paper, the lateral gene transfer hypothesis was examined to explain the conflicts between the species and gene classifications.

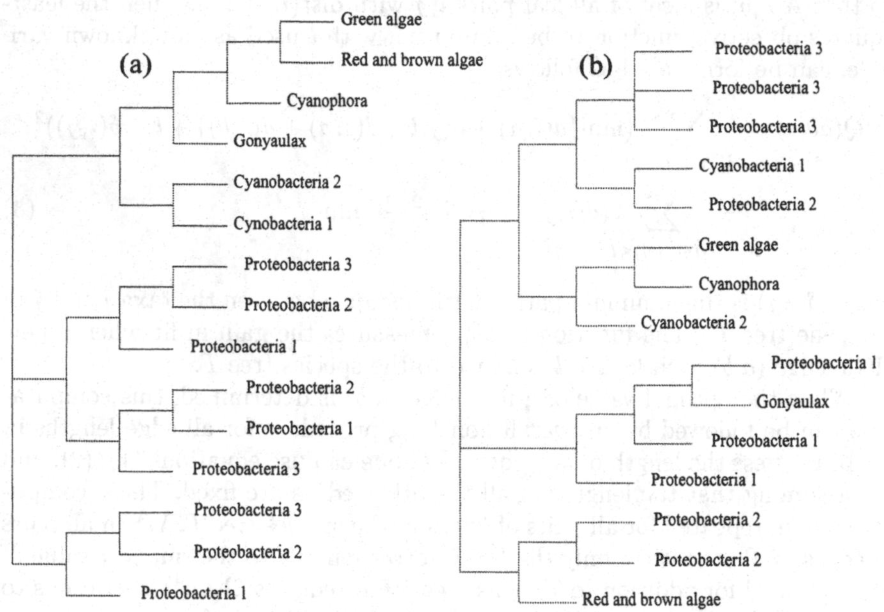

Fig. 3. (a) Species tree for 15 taxa representing different groups of bacteria and plastids from Delwiche and Palmer (1996, Fig. 2). Each taxon represents a group of organisms reported in Boc and Makarenkov (2003). The species tree is built on the base of 16S rRNA sequences and other evidence. (b) *rbcL* gene tree for 15 taxa representing different groups of bacteria and plastids constructed by contracting nodes of the 48-taxa phylogeny from Delwiche and Palmer (1996, Fig. 2).

The solution network depicting the species tree with 10 horizontal gene transfers is shown in Fig. 4. The numbers at the HGT edges correspond to their position in the scenario of transfers. Thus the transfer between α-proteobacteria1 and *Gonyaulax* was found in the first iteration of the algorithm, then the transfer between *Gonyaulax* and β-proteobacteria1, followed by that from *Gonyaulax* to γ-proteobacteria1, and so forth. Delwiche and Palmer (1996, Fig. 4) indicated these as the most probable four HGT events of the rubisco genes including those between cyanobacteria and γ-proteobacteria, γ-proteobacteria and α-proteobacteria, γ-proteobacteria and β-proteobacteria, and finally, between α-proteobacteria and plastids. The three last transfers can be found in our unique scenario in Fig. 4, whereas the first one, between cyanobacteria and γ-proteobacteria, goes in the opposite direction. It is worth noting that the obtained solution is also different from that found in Boc and Makarenkov (2003).

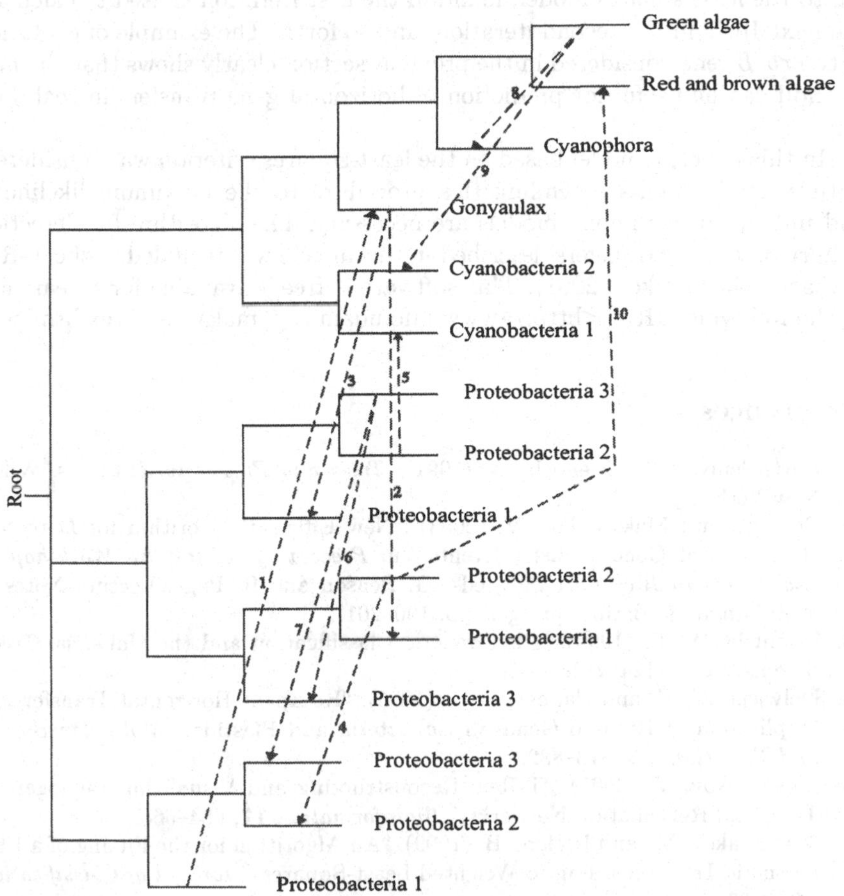

Fig. 4. Species tree from Fig. 3a with 10 dashed, arrow-headed edges representing horizontal gene transfers of the *rbcL* gene. Numbers on the HGT edges indicate their order of appearance.

5 Conclusion

The algorithm described in this article allows one to establish a unique scenario of horizontal gene transfer events that may have occurred in course of the evolution. The algorithm exploits the discrepancy between the species and gene additive trees built for the same set of observed species by mapping the gene data into the species tree and then by estimating the possibility of a horizontal gene transfer between each pair of edges in the species tree.

A number of plausible biological rules not treated in Boc and Makarenkov (2003) are incorporated in the reconstruction process. The best HGT, according to the least-squares model, found in the first iteration is used to calculate the next HGT in the second iteration, and so forth. The example of evolution of the *rbcL* gene considered in the previous section clearly shows that the new method can be useful for prediction of horizontal gene transfers in real data sets.

In this paper, a model based on the least-squares criterion was considered. Future developments extending this procedure to the maximum likelihood and maximum parsimony models are necessary. The algorithm for detection of horizontal gene transfers described in this article was included in the T-Rex package (Makarenkov, 2001). This software is freely available for researchers at the following URL: <http://www.info.uqam.ca/~makarenv/trex.html>.

References

1. Barthélemy, J-P., Guénoche A. (1991). *Trees and Proximity Relations.* Wiley, New York.
2. Boc, A., and Makarenkov, V. (2003). "New Efficient Algorithm for Detection of Horizontal Gene Transfer Events," in *Proceedings of the 3rd Workshop on Algorithms in Bioinformatics,* eds. G. Benson and R. Page, Lecture Notes in Bioinformatics, Berlin:Springer, pp. 190–201.
3. Doolittle, W. F. (1999). "Phylogenetic Classification and the Universal Tree," *Science*, **284**, 2124–2128.
4. Delwiche, C. F. and Palmer, J. D. (1996). "Rampant Horizontal Transfer and Duplication of Rubisco Genes in Eubacteria and Plastids," *Molecular Biology and Evolution*, **13**, 873–882.
5. Makarenkov, V. (2001). "T-Rex: Reconstructing and Visualizing Phylogenetic Trees and Reticulation Networks," *Bioinformatics*, **17**, 664–668.
6. Makarenkov, V., and Leclerc, B. (1999). "An Algorithm for the Fitting of a Phylogenetic Tree According to Weighted Least-Squares," *Journal of Classification*, **16**, 3–26.
7. Olsen, G., and Woese, C. (1998). "Archael Genomics Overview," *Cell*, **89**, 991–994.
8. Page, R. (1994). "Maps Between Trees and Cladistic Analysis of Historical Associations Among Genes, Organism and Areas," *Systematic Biology*, **43**, 58–77.
9. Page, R., and Charleston, M. A. (1998). "From Gene to Organismal Phylogeny: Reconciled Trees," *Bioinformatics*, **14**, 819–820.

Active and Passive Learning to Explore a Complex Metabolism Data Set

Susan J. Simmons[1], Xiaodong Lin[2], Chris Beecher[3], and Young Truong[4] and S. Stanley Young[5]

[1] University of North Carolina at Wilmington, USA
simmonssj@uncw.edu
[2] Statistical and Applied Mathematical Sciences Institute, USA
linxd@samsi.info
[3] Metabolon, USA
cbeecher@metabolon.com
[4] University of North Carolina, USA
truong@bios.unc.edu
[5] National Institute of Statistical Sciences, USA
young@niss.org

Abstract: Metabolomics is the new 'omics' science that concerns biochemistry. A metabolomic dataset includes quantitative measurements of all small molecules, known as metabolites, in a biological sample. These datasets are rich in information regarding dynamic metabolic (or biochemical) networks that are unattainable using classical methods and have great potential, conjointly with other omic data, in understanding the functionality of genes. Herein, we explore a complex metabolomic dataset with the goal of using the metabolic information to correctly classify individuals into different classes. Unfortunately, these datasets incur many statistical challenges: the number of samples is less than the number of metabolites; there is missing data and non-normal data; and there are high correlations among the metabolites. Thus, we investigate the use of robust singular value decomposition, rSVD, and recursive partitioning to understand this metabolomic data set. The dataset consists of 63 samples, in which we know the status of the individuals (disease or normal and for the diseased individuals, if they are on drug or not). Clustering using only the metabolite data is only modestly successful. Using distances generated from multiple tree recursive partitioning is more successful.

1 Introduction

Complex data sets are becoming available in the post-genomic era; there is an increasing interest in the analysis of genetic information (genomics), and their transcription (transcriptomics) and subsequent translation into protein (proteomics). The recently emerging science of metabolomics completes the primary omics ladder of DNA, RNA, proteins and metabolites. As such, it provides a prototypic means of understanding of cellular function. Metabolomics is the biochemical profiling of all small molecules, biochemicals or metabolites, in an organism. Even though the dynamic nature of metabolites makes them difficult to measure, recent advances in technology allows robust quantification of the concentrations of hundreds of metabolites from a biological sample (Stitt and Fernie, 2003). This new omics science offers insight into the dynamic interactions in metabolic pathways and an unambiguous representation of cellular physiology (Beecher, 2002). Furthermore, patterns of metabolites can be used to identify biomarkers of specific disease, understand pathological development, and propose targets for drug intervention.

Data obtained through a metabolomic experiment posses a number of challenges to statistical modeling. The number of metabolites measured (=p), usually in the hundreds is much larger than the number of biological samples (=n): n « p. Additionally, there may be severe distributional difficulties such as non-normal distributions, outliers (unusual data values), missing values, and high correlations among metabolites. Common objectives are finding "patterns" in the data, in particular, clustering of the biological samples (rows) into groups with similar metabolic expression profiles; and clustering the metabolic concentrations (columns) into groups where the level of metabolic expression is similar in the samples.

Due to the challenges of modeling this dataset, many clustering techniques may produce erroneous results. For example, most clustering techniques are influenced by outliers and can not accommodate missing values. Further disadvantages of hierarchical clustering techniques are that the dendrograms produce orderings of rows (biological samples) that are not unique (Liu et al., 2003). Thus, we investigate two methods that have appealing features and overcome these challenges. The first method is rSVD that was proposed by Liu et al (2003). This technique is by-product of 'ordination', which involves finding suitable permutations of the rows and columns that lead to a steady progression of data values going down the rows and across the columns. The clusters are determined by placing vertical and possibly horizontal lines in the dataset that divide it into homogeneous blocks. The second method we examine that is useful in overcoming these statistical challenges is recursive partitioning, RP, which provides a powerful classification algorithm resulting in a tree diagram. The tree diagram identifies the metabolites that are useful in partitioning the sample into smaller, more homogeneous groups. RP uses information on the classification of the objects whereas rSVD uses only the information on the metabolites.

We explore these two techniques on a metabolomic dataset. The dataset contains 63 biological samples in which there are four different groups. There are two primary groups, diseased and healthy individuals. We will attempt to find other groups within the data set. Note, the data contains blanks where the metabolic concentrations were below detection limits. The goal of this study is to use rSVD and recursive partitioning in an exploratory manner to identify metabolites that cluster samples into consistent groups based on their biological function.

2 Robust Singular Value Decomposition

The robust clustering technique described by Liu et al. (2003) is used to cluster the metabolomic data by biological samples and metabolic concentrations. The method involves a systematic approach of ordering the rows and columns so the underlying homogeneous clusters may be found. The technique involves approximating the dataset, which we will denote as X, with a bilinear form. The array X is viewed as an n by p array with n representing the number of biological samples (rows) and p representing the metabolic concentrations (columns). Thus, the approximate bilinear form is

$$x_{ij} = r_i c_j + e_{ij}, \tag{1}$$

where r_i is a parameter corresponding to the ith biological sample, c_j corresponds to the jth concentration, and e_{ij} is a 'residual'. Estimating the array with this bilinear form allows the dataset to be permuted by ordering the r_i values of the rows and the c_j values of the columns, which results in an array with high and low values in the corners and medium values in the middle, leading to an informative display (Liu et al., 2003).

Subsequently, grouping values of r_i that are similar will result in clusters of biological samples, and grouping similar values of c_j will give clusters of metabolites. If the residuals are small so that the $r_i c_j$ captures all the important structure of the data matrix, then the ordination and ensuing clustering using the r or c values is essentially unique.

The method proposed by Liu et al. (2003) focuses on an algorithm proposed by Gabriel-Zamir (1979) that uses an alternating least squares approach to reconcile the problem of missing values. This algorithm begins with an initial estimate of the column factors c_j which are used to provide a matching scaling for the rows. Viewing

$$x_{ij} = r_i c_j + e_{ij} \tag{2}$$

as a regression of the ith row of X on the column factors identifies r_i as the coefficient of a no-intercept regression. The regression is fit row by row using all non-empty cells, which results in an estimate of the row factors r_i. The algorithm proceeds by switching the roles of the rows and columns so that bilinear form is now regarded as a regression of the jth column of X on the row factors. The regression is fit column by column using all non-empty cells in exactly the same way to calculate fresh estimates of the column factors c_j.

This approach uses all the observed data, and does not require imputation of missing data.

The alternating least squares algorithm is effective in solving the missing information problem; however, it does not address the issue of sensitivity to outliers. Using a robust regression method instead of ordinary least squares (OLS) in the alternating regressions can solve this problem. Various forms of outlier-resistant regression methods are possible, such as L1 (Hawkins et al., 2001), weighted L1 (Croux et al., (2003), least trimmed squares (Ukkelberg and Borgen, 1993), or an M-estimation method. In this analysis, we choose to use the L1 method proposed by Hawkins et al. (2001).

Thus, the resulting alternating robust fitting, ARF, algorithm handles missing information smoothly, without requiring a separate 'fill-in' step, and it is impervious to a minority of outlier cells. Outliers will, of course, create a problem for the ARF, as with almost any conceivable method, if they constitute the majority of the elements of any row or column.

Finding k clusters based on biological samples may be found by sorting the rows by their r_i values and finding 'breakpoints' $b(0) = 0 < b(1) < b(2) < b(k-1) < b(k) = n$ and allocating to cluster h those metabolites which, in the reordering, have index $b(h-1) < i <= b(h)$. The breakpoints need to be chosen so that the biological samples within each cluster have r_i values as similar as possible. This can be made operational by the criterion that the pooled sum of squared deviations of the r_i broken down into the k clusters should be a minimum (Liu et al., 2003). Exact algorithms for finding breakpoints to attain this minimum are given by Venter and Steel (1996), and by Hawkins et al. (2001). Similarly, applying the optimal segmentation algorithm to the column factors c_j clusters the metabolites into any specified number of clusters such that the metabolites within clusters have c_j values as similar as possible.

Figure (1) illustrates the log transform of the raw data. Rows correspond to biological samples and the columns correspond to metabolites. In order to create the following illustration, many outliers need to be truncated. We will proceed with the rSVD analysis by permuting the rows and columns of this matrix and we will display the smoothed result by plotting the outer product of the first eigenvectors.

Figure (2) illustrates the outer product of the sorted first eigenvector pairs. Notice the shaded cluster around the lower left corner of the figure; this is the strong response outlier group, including the four samples X44, X20, X43 and X48, Group 4. The other disease groups, however, are not as clear even using the second and third eigenvector pairs. To further identify the biological clusters of the samples, we investigate recursive partitioning.

3 Recursive Partitioning, Results and Discussion

Recursive partitioning is an algorithm that searches through all of the variables and identifies the single variable produces the best 'split' among groups

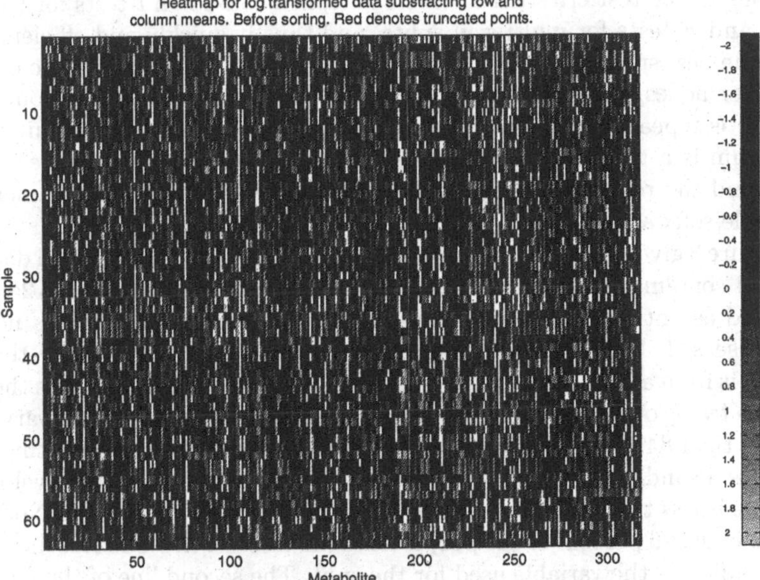

Fig. 1. Heat map of the assay values for 63 samples and 317 metabolites.

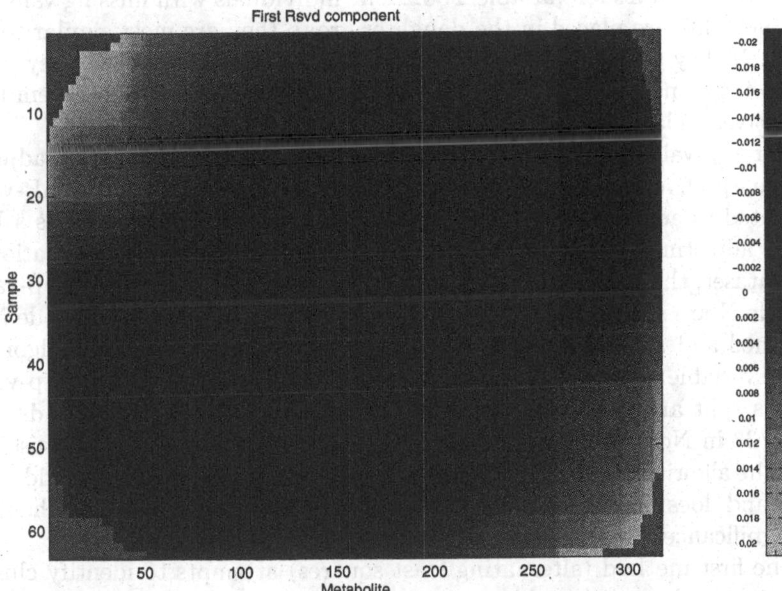

Fig. 2. Heatmap constructed from the outer product of the first row and the first column eigenvectors.

(samples). The test criterion for the best split is based on t-tests for two-way splits and F-tests for multi-way splits, and thus it quickly and efficiently decides the best split. When a split occurs, the group is broken into two or more daughter nodes, which are more homogeneous than the starting group. This process is repeated until no significant splits are possible. The result of this algorithm is a tree diagram that identifies the variables used to create each split, and the resulting groups or daughter nodes. We use the commercially available software FIRMPlus^{TM} to perform the RP analysis.

Figure 3 gives one tree from a multiple-tree analysis of the medical data set. Node N contains 61 observations (duplicate observations, X26 and X26b were removed as outliers for this analysis). The samples are classified as normal, 0, or diseased, 1, so the average for Node N (u=) is the probability that the sample is from a diseased person. The first step of the algorithm splits the data set into two groups depending on variable Y302. If the level of this variable is greater than 84.1, the sample is placed into Node $N2$. Notice that this Node contains 18 individuals and all of them have the disease. If the level of the variable is less than or equal to 84.1, then the sample is placed into Node $N1$. In this node, 26 percent of the people have the disease. In Node N1, the header Y302 indicates the variable used for the split. The second line of the header is $x \leq 84.1$ or "?", which indicates that this node constitutes biological samples with values less than or equal to 84.1 for variable Y302 and any samples with missing values for variable Y302. The individuals with missing values for variable Y302 are placed in the daughter group they are most similar to, $N1$ or $N2$. If they were statistically distinct from those groups, then they would be put into a new group. This treatment of missing values allows them to be predictive in classifying the samples.

Three p-values are used to judge the validity of a split; the unadjusted p-value (p=), computed without regard to multiple testing; the aP-value, computed to adjust for the segmentation; and the bP-value, which is a Bonferroni adjustment reflecting the number of predictors under consideration. In this dataset, there are 317 continuous predictors. We see that all the p-values in Node N are suitably small. As Node $N2$ is pure, it is not split. Node N1 is examined and after looking at all predictors and split points, the algorithm selects variable Y15 as the split variable and a split point of 73.1. The p-values for this split are suitably small. 9/10 individuals in Node $N11$ are diseased and 2/33 in Node $N12$ are diseased. Of the 61 samples, three are misclassified. The algorithm examines both Nodes $N11$ and $N12$ looking for additional splits and does not find any more significant splits ($bP < 0.05$ was chosen as the significance level).

The first method (alternating least squares) attempts to identify clusters of sample without using their class labels; the second method (RP) is very different as it uses the disease indicator (0=control, 1=disease). In Figure 2, the last 8 samples shown in the lower left corner of the heat map are (from bottom up): $X43$, $X48$, $X44$, $X20$, $X23$, $X4$, $X31$ and $X26$. The first four of these constitute a clinically recognized sub-set of the disease population. The

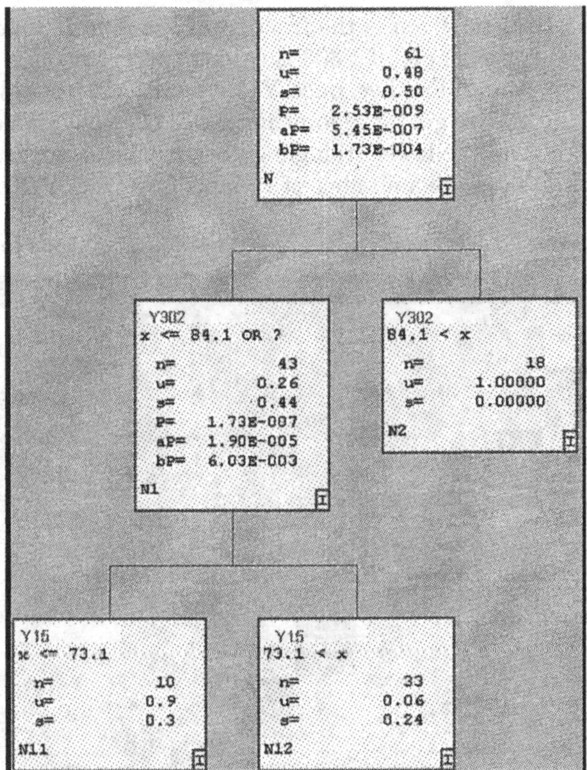

Fig. 3. A single recursive partitioning tree from a 100-tree analysis.

next three are arguably within this class but were not clinically recognized. Case $X26$ was ultimately considered an outlier.

The corresponding first 20 variables from left to right are: Y303, Y313, Y316, Y237, Y197, Y262, Y314, Y297, Y309, Y301, Y213, Y308, Y193, Y310, Y274, Y312, Y196, Y162, Y295, and Y307. Biochemical experts recognized some of these as significant markers for the disease population; RP found previously recognized variables and found new important variables.

For data sets with a relatively small number of observations, it is advantageous to build many trees. FIRMPlus builds multiple trees by randomizing the split variable used at each split point over a specified number of statistically significant variables. We use the default of 10. We build 100 trees. From the forest of trees there are a number of things that can be learned about the predictor variables and the samples. Variables that are used often over the forest of trees are important. Variables that are seldom or never used together in a tree are likely to be correlated. Variables that are used in the same tree are likely to be synergistic. Figure 4 gives the frequency that a variable is used in the forest of trees along the diagonal. We see that the variable Y15 is used often (the statistic given is the fraction of the data in a tree controlled by the variable). For example, if Y303 is used, then Y15 is often used, i.e. the variables are synergistic. Further, once Y15 is used, Y215 is never used. The upper part of the matrix gives the joint incidence of two variables being used together in a tree and the lower triangle gives the joint incidence in standard deviation units. We can see a number of variable pairs, e.g. Y18 and Y6, Y215 and Y307.

	Y15	Y302	Y215	Y18	Y6	Y39	Y300	Y224	Y307	26	Y294	Y22	Y114
Y15	0.26	0.049	0	0	0	0	0.078	0.079	0	0.036	0	0	0
Y302	0.1	0.16	0.042	0	0	0	0	0	0	0	0.015	0	0
Y215	-1.4	1.2	0.11	0	0	0	0	0	[illegible]	0	0	0	0
Y18	-1.2	-1.0	-0.8	0.097	[illegible]	0	0	0	0	0.0054	0	0	0
Y6	-1.4	-1.2	-1.0	5.5	0.13	0	0	0	0	0	0	0	0
Y39	-1.1	-1.0	-0.8	-0.7	-0.8	0.082	0	0	0	0	0.023	[illegible]	0
Y300	2.3	-1.1	-0.9	-0.6	-0.9	-0.7	0.11	0	0	0	0	0	0
Y224	2.5	-1.1	-0.8	-0.8	-0.9	-0.7	-0.8	0.1	0	0	0	0	0
Y307	-1.3	-1.1	4.1	-0.8	-0.9	-0.7	-0.8	-0.8	0.11	0	0	0	0
Y26	0.6	-1.0	-0.8	-0.3	-0.9	-0.7	-0.8	-0.8	-0.8	0.094	0	0	0
Y294	-1.3	-0.2	-0.8	-0.8	-0.9	1.3	-0.8	-0.8	-0.8	-0.8	0.1	0	0
Y22	-1.2	-1.0	-0.8	-0.7	-0.8	[illegible]	-0.8	-0.7	-0.8	-0.7	-0.7	0.09	0
Y114	-1.1	-0.9	-0.7	-0.7	-0.8	-0.6	-0.7	-0.7	-0.7	-0.7	-0.7	-0.7	0.08

Fig. 4. Joint incidence of variables used in 100 TP trees.

Next we can judge the similarity between two samples by using a RP tree-based distance. Distance is computed as the proportion of the total sample of the smallest node where two observations occur together. If they only occur together in the parent node the proportion, distance, is 1.00. If they always occur together in a small terminal node, then the proportion, distance, is small. If they are immediately sent to different daughter nodes on the first split, then they are dissimilar. If they always occur together in a terminal node, then they are similar. Figure 5 gives a heat map of the similarity of samples.

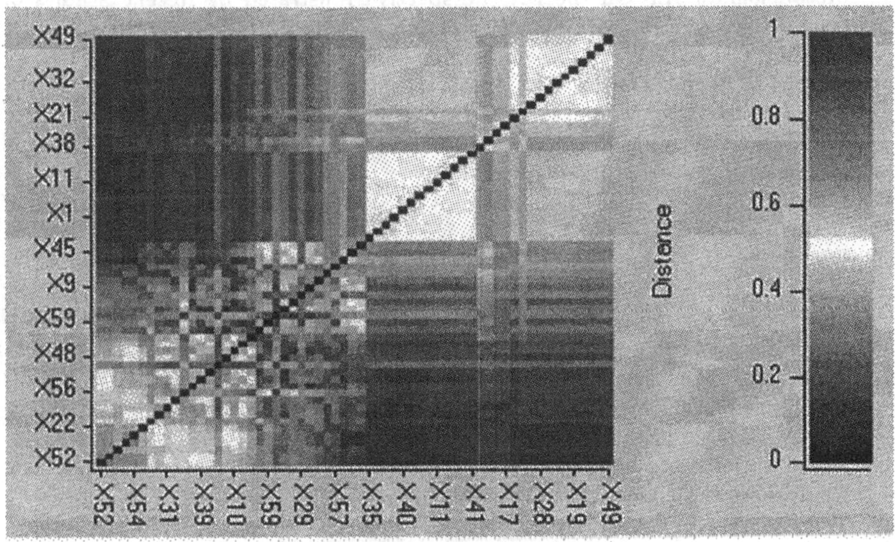

Fig. 5. RP-based distance matrix of the 61 samples.

Each sample is perfectly similar to itself so we have shaded dots through the diagonal. We also see interesting patterns of three or four groups. The upper right hand group is of normal individuals. The group in the center of Figure 5 is of diseased, drug-treated individuals. The lower left hand group is of diseased, non-drug-treated individuals. The small shaded group in the lower left hand of Figure 5 is of individuals that appear to have a somewhat different manifestation of the disease. There is an ongoing effort to better identify the nature of these individuals.

Acknowledgements

The authors gratefully acknowledge Dr.s Bruce Kristal, Steve Rozen, Rima Kaddurah-Daouk, Wayne MAtson, Misha Bogdanov, Flint Beal and Dr. Merit E Cudkowicz and Dr. Robert Brown at Massachusetts General Hospital for their contribution to the organization of the original data set.

References

1. Stitt, M. and Fernie, A. R. (2003). "From Measurements of Metabolites to Metabolomics: An 'On the Fly' Perspective Illustrated by Recent Studies of Carbon-Nitrogen Interactions", *Current Opinion in Biotechnology*, **14**, 136–144.
2. Beecher, C. (2002). "Metabolomics: The Newest of the 'omics' Sciences", *Innovations of Pharmaceutical Technology*, 57–64.
3. Liu, L., Hawkins, D. M., Ghosh, S., Young, S. S. (2003). "Robust Singular Value Decomposition Analysis of Microarray Data," *Proceedings of the National Academy of Sciences*, **23**, 13167–13172.
4. Weckwerth, W. (2003). "Metabolomics in Systems Biology," *Annual Review of Plant Biology*, **54**, 669–689.
5. Gabriel, K. R., Zamir , S. (1979). "Lower Rank Approximation of Matrices by Least Squares with any Choice of Weights," *Technometrics*, **21**, 489–498.
6. Hawkins, D. M., Liu, L., Young, S. S. (2001). "Robust Singular Value Decomposition," Technical Report, NISS 122, *www.niss.org/downloadabletechreports.html.*
7. Croux, C., Filzmoser, P., Pison, G. and Rousseeuw, P.J. (2003). "Fitting Multiplicative Models by Robust Alternating Regressions," *Statistics and Computing*,**13**, 23–26.
8. Ukkelberg, A and Borgen, O. (1993). "Outlier Detection by Robust Alternating Regression," *Analytica Chemica Acta*, **277**, 489–494.
9. Venter, J. H., and Steel, S. J. (1996). "Finding Multiple Abrupt Change Points," *Computational Statistics and Data Analysis*, **22**, 481–504.
10. Hawkins, D. M. (2001). "Fitting Multiple Change-Points to Data," *Computational Statistics and Data Analysis*, **37**, 323–341.
11. FIRMPlus^{TM}: Golden Helix Inc., Bozeman, MT (www.goldenhelix.com).

Mathematical and Statistical Modeling of Acute Inflammation

Gilles Clermont[1], Carson C. Chow[1], Gregory M. Constantine[1], Yoram Vodovotz[1], and John Bartels[2]

[1] University of Pittsburgh, U.S.A.
clermontg@ccm.upmc.edu, ccchow@pitt.edu, gmc@euler.math.pitt.edu, vodovotzy@upmc.edu

[2] Immunetrics Inc., Pittsburgh, U.S.A.

Abstract: A mathematical model involving a system of ordinary differential equations has been developed with the goal of assisting the design of therapies directed against the inflammatory consequences of infection and trauma. Though the aim is to build a model of greater complexity, which would eventually overcome some existing limitations (such as a reduced subset of inflammatory interactions, the use of mass action kinetics, and calibration to circulating but not local levels of cytokines), the model can at this time simulate certain disease scenarios qualitatively as well as predicting the time course of cytokine levels in distinct paradigms of inflammation in mice. A parameter search algorithm is developed that aids in the identification of different regimes of behaviour of the model and helps with its calibration to data. Extending this mathematical model, with validation in humans, may lead to the in silico development of novel therapeutic approaches and real-time diagnostics.

1 Introduction

Acute systemic inflammation is triggered by stresses on a living organism such as infection or trauma. This response involves a cascade of events mediated by a network of cells and molecules. The process localizes and identifies an insult, strives to eliminate offending agents, and initiates a repair process. If the system functions properly, inflammation eventually abates and the body returns to equilibrium. However, the inflammatory response can also compromise healthy tissue, further exacerbating inflammation(Nathan (2002), Jarrar et al. (1999)). The systemic inflammation that results from severe infection (sepsis) or trauma can lead to a shock state and organ dysfunction, possibly culminating in death (Jarrar et al. (1999), Marshall (2001), Hotchkiss and Karl (2003).). Shock is a major healthcare problem that afflicts victims of both trauma and sepsis. In 1999, a quarter of a million deaths were associated with sepsis in the US alone.(Carrico (1994), Angus et al. (2001))

Much has been learned regarding the cellular and molecular mechanisms of the acute inflammatory response. However, except for recombinant human activated protein C (Bernard et al. (2001)), this knowledge has not led to effective therapies for inflammation-induced shock. Many attempted anti-inflammatory strategies have failed to improve outcome in large, randomized clinical trials, despite showing promise in animal and early phase human studies (Bone (1996)). One reason for this failure is that inflammation-induced shock is a complex process. Hence, the full consequences of modulating single pathways or mediators are difficult to predict from the knowledge of those pathways or mediators in isolation.

It has been suggested that mathematical modeling might provide an effective tool to grapple with the complexity of the inflammatory response to infection and trauma (Nathan (2002), Buchman et al. (2001), Neugebauer et al. (2001)). Modeling is increasingly being used to address clinically relevant biological complexity, in some cases leading to novel predictions (Kitano (2002)). We embarked on an iterative process of model generation, verification and calibration in animal models, and subsequent hypothesis generation. The model, described by a system of differential equations, aims to explain the reaction of the immune system in three different scenarios, by engaging processes that take place at the molecular level. In the next section we describe the biological basis of the model in greater detail. Section 3 describes a global search strategy of the parameter space that aids in predicting regime behaviour of the model as well as optimizing the fit of the model to observed data. The regime classification and prediction is based on a multinomial logistic model described in Section 4. An application to in silico simulation using the model is then described.

2 Building a Mathematical Model of Acute Inflammation

In the model, neutrophils and macrophages are activated directly by bacterial endotoxin (lipopolysaccharide [LPS]) or indirectly by various stimuli elicited systemically upon trauma and hemorrhage. Although not included explicitly in our model, early events such as mast cell degranulation and complement activation (Nathan (2002)) are incorporated implicitly in the dynamics of our endotoxin and cytokine variables. These stimuli, including endotoxin, enter the systemic circulation quickly and activate circulating monocytes and neutrophils (Parker and Watkins (2001)). Activated neutrophils also reach compromised tissue by migrating along a chemoattractant gradient (Bellingan (1999)). Once activated, macrophages and neutrophils produce and secrete effectors that activate these same cells and also other cells, such as endothelial cells. Pro-inflammatory cytokines–tumor necrosis factor (TNF), interleukin

(IL)-6, and IL-12 in our mathematical model–promote immune cell activation and pro-inflammatory cytokine production (Freeman and Natanson (2000)). The concurrent production of anti-inflammatory cytokines counterbalances the actions of pro-inflammatory cytokines. In an ideal situation, these anti-inflammatory agents serve to restore homeostasis. However, when overproduced, they may lead to prolonged immunosupression and failure to appropriately respond to repeated challenges (Volk et al. (2000)). Following prolonged hemorrhage, severe trauma, and/or persistent infection, the biological components of inflammation become more specific and focused, giving way to the adaptive immune response (Medzhitov and Janeway (2000)). Additional interactions, e.g. production of NO from the endothelial nitric oxide synthase (eNOS), add granularity to our model (Bone (1996), Pinsky (2001)). The model is explicitely provided in the Appendix, and was constructed from known interactions among components as documented in the existing literature. In deriving the mathematical model, we balanced biological realism with simplicity. Our goal is to find a fixed set of parameters that would qualitatively reproduce many known scenarios of inflammation found in the literature, correctly describe our data, and be able to make novel predictions to be tested experimentally.

The model was trained on data sets for three separate scenarios (surgical trauma; surgical trauma/hemorrhage; and 3 and 6 mg/kg doses of endotoxin [Fig. 1]) and then used to predict data from subsequent scenarios in mice (12 mg/kg endotoxin, combined surgery, hemorrhage and endotoxin). The paradigm of endotoxin administration reproduces several clnical and laboratory features of severe infections. We used a single set of equations and parameters in those equations, changing only the starting conditions, to account for all three inflammatory scenarios. More recently, the model was also verified and partially calibrated in humans treated with endotoxin.

The model and parameters were specified in two stages. In the preliminary stage, the model was constructed so it could reproduce qualitatively several different scenarios that exist in the literature. In this stage, direct values of parameters such as cytokine half-lives were used when available. The resulting qualitatively correct model was then calibrated to experimental data in mice (described in greater detail below) using three different inflammatory paradigms: surgical trauma, surgical trauma followed by hemorrhage, and endotoxemia. In the later stage, the model was matched to our experimental data by adjusting the parameters using our knowledge of the biological mechanisms together with the dynamics of the model, to attain desired time course shapes. An algorithm described in the sections to follow was used to obtain optimal sets of parameters for qualitatively correct behavior of the model as well as optimal fit to the data.

Specifically, we sought to determine whether the mathematical model could reproduce qualitatively published data showing divergent outcomes in endotoxemia and hemorrhagic shock. We approximated survival as tissue dysfunc-

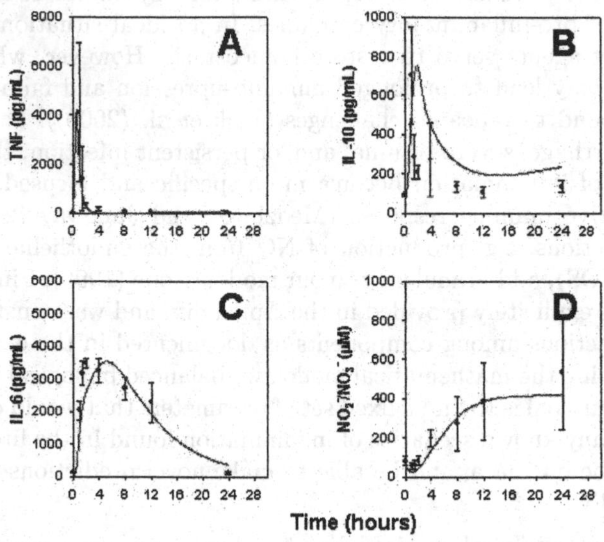

Fig. 1. Simulation and calibration of the cytokine response to endotoxin in mice. Mice received 6 mg/kg LPS i.p. At various time points following this injection, the mice were euthanized and sera obtained. Black symbols represent mean SD for 3-8 separate animals. Curved lines indicate prediction of mathematical model.

tion that returns to baseline, while considering persistently elevated tissue dysfunction as a proxy for death. Such desparate time evolutions represent two drastically different regimes, though more refined behavioral distinctions are usually made.

3 A Parameter Optimization Algorithm Based on Optimal Codes

The algorithm was developed out of the need to survey a high dimensional space in which varying one or two parameters at a time, while keeping the others fixed, is simply not practical. It has at its core a (binary) code with efficient covering properties of the high dimensional parameter space. For simplicity we worked with Hamming codes, but other codes with optimal covering properties may be used. The setting is that of a finite dimensional vector space V of dimension n over F_2, the binary field, endowed with the usual inner product with values in F_2. We specify the code as the orthogonal complement of the space generated by the row vectors of a parity check matrix H of full row rank. The code is, therefore,

$$C = \{x : Hx = 0\}.$$

Let the dimension of C be k. Of equal interest are the cosets of the code. A coset C_y is specified as follows:

$$C_y = \{x : Hx = y\},$$

where y is the "syndrome" vector defining the coset in question. Since C has dimension k, the vector y is a column vector of dimension $n-k$. The set $\{C_y\}$ represents the set of 2^{n-k} cosets of C, as y runs over the set of all binary vectors of dimension $n-k$. The reader is refered to MacWilliams and Sloane (1978) for material on coding theory. We write out some of the details for the Hamming code in 7 dimensions, assuming that we have seven parameters, defined by the parity check matrix

$$H = \begin{pmatrix} 1\,0\,1\,0\,1\,0\,1 \\ 0\,1\,1\,0\,0\,1\,1 \\ 0\,0\,0\,1\,1\,1\,1 \end{pmatrix}.$$

This matrix H yields a code of dimension 4, consisting of 16 binary vectors.

We shall make use of a binary code C in the following way. The response function f of n (usually real) parameters $x_1, \ldots, x_n$ is to be investigated over a product space $B = \prod_{i=1}^{n} [a_i, b_i]$, with $a_i \leq x_i \leq b_i$; $1 \leq i \leq n$. For illustrative purposes we assume that the usually vector-valued response function is a scalar function. This function is in practice obtained by integrating the ODE system numerically. To describe how the algorithm works we assume that we want to numerically find the minimum of f over B. Take a vector $x = (x_1, \ldots, x_n) \in B$. Code x as a binary vector by placing a 0 in coordinate position i if $x_i \in [a_i, \frac{a_i+b_i}{2}]$ and a 1 otherwise; write $\bar{x}$ for the coded x.

By a deliberate or a random process, select a point $x_{i0} \in [a_i, (a_i + b_i)/2] = B_{i0}$ and a point $x_{i1} \in ((a_i + b_i)/2, b_i] = B_{i1}$; $1 \leq i \leq n$. A point $(x_{1j_1}, \ldots, x_{nj_n})$, with j_m being either 0 or 1, belongs to the "cell" $\prod_{i=1}^{n} B_{ij_i}$. Consider now the set of coded points of B,

$$\{(\bar{x}_{1j}, \ldots, \bar{x}_{nj}) : j = 0, 1\}.$$

This process defines 2^n binary vectors which we now view as the elements of an $n-$dimensional vector space V over the field with two elements F_2. Indeed, with the points x_{ij} fixed, the correspondence

$$(x_{1j_1}, \ldots, x_{nj_n}) \leftrightarrow (\bar{x}_{1j_1}, \ldots, \bar{x}_{nj_n}),$$

with $j_m = 0$ or 1, is a bijection by way of which we shall identify the selected points of B, which we denote by $V(B)$, with elements of V. In particular, any subset S of points of V identifies through this bijection a corresponding set of points in B, which we write as $S(B)$. This is the case with the set of vectors in a linear code C of V as well. If C is a linear code of dimension k, the subset $C(B)$ consists of 2^k points in B. By abuse of language, we may on occasion refer to $C(B)$ as the points of the code C.

If the objective is to minimize function f over B, the algorithm first identifies the cells B_{ij} associated with the code C. Within each cell B_{ij} the algorithm replicates itself, that is, it treats cell B_{ij} as a new space B. It selects points in B_{ij} in accordance to (a code equivalent to) C. [Two codes are called equivalent if one is obtained from the other upon a permutation of coordinates.] We evaluate the function f at all points selected in B_{ij}, for all cells B_{ij}. This allows us to identify a subset L of cells that yield the smallest values of f. If the minimum obtained so far is satisfactory, we stop. Else we iterate the procedure within each of the cells in L. This allows evaluation of the function f on a finer local mesh (at a deeper level of iteration). The nested level may be repeated any number of times. We stop when the minimum reached on f is sufficiently low. The list L keeps tabs of the adresses of the cells of interest at the various levels of iteration. All this happens only for cells associated with the code C. We can thus select from list L a point x_C (found in some cell of code C) such that $f(x_C)$ is the smallest value of f found so far. Produce the list of differences $L = \{(f(x) - f(x_C))/||x - x_C|| : x \in C(B)\}$ and select $x_0 \in C(B)$ such that $(f(x_0) - f(x_C))/||x_0 - x_C||$ is maximal. [In general x in the list L actually runs over the set of cosets selected so far.] Along the line $x_C - t(x_0 - x_C)$ find a smallest positive value t_0 of t such that $x_C - t_0(x_0 - x_C)$ is in a cell of $V(B)$ not examined thus far. The coded version of $x_C - t_0(x_0 - x_C) = y$ defines a vector in V not previously considered, and hence identifies a new coset $C_y = y + C$ of C.

The coset C_y thus identified has the same optimal covering properties of V as does C. The process followed for code C is now repeated for the coset C_y. After examining $m \leq n - k$ cosets of C, call them $\{C_{y_1}, \ldots, C_{y_m}\}$ (let $y_1 = 0$, so $C_{y_1} = C$), we obtain m points $P = \{x_{C_{y_i}} : 1 \leq i \leq m\}$ from the corresponding m lists. The point in P at which f attains a minimum is the point the algorithm gives as solution to the optimization problem. The algorithm thus combines local gradient properties with global reach throughout the region B by way of the cosets of the code C.

4 Classifying Parameter Sets Yielding Different Regimes

Though minimizing an objective function occurs any time one fits a model to data, our focus is to predict the correct regime for a given vector of parameters. The first step is to identify originally a set of regimes that the system of ODE's could produce; see also Neugebauer (2001). While several potential regimes may be suspected to exist a priori, not all possible regimes will usually be known. However, each time we evaluate the model at a parameter set (i.e., numerically integrate it) we either classify the resulting function in one of the known regimes or decide to create a new regime. We can thus eventually expand the set of regimes as the computer simulation progresses. Comparison of regimes involves defining a measure that compares two regimes and computes a distance between them. We decided to use a measure that matches only "qualitatively defining features" of the functions in questions, such as notable peaks, tail behaviour, or other qualitatively relevant traits. We shall then say that two functions are in the same regime if they have qualitatively similar features; else they represent different regimes.

We now describe how we can use the algorithm in the previous section in conjunction with a multinomial logistic distribution to classify any point in the parameter space. The outcomes of the logistic distribution are the r distinct regimes. We now start the algorithm. At each parameter point selected, by integrating the ODE system, we obtain the response function. We compute distances to each of the r regimes and classify that parameter point in one of them. The code ensures that the parameter space is optimally covered each time we select a new coset of parameter points. After a sufficiently large number of iterations we may notice points in the parameter space where bifurcations seem to occur. In the neighborhood of such points (should they prove of investigative interest) we can locally replicate the search just described.

To classify an arbitrary parameter point θ we use the multinomial logistic as follows: think of the points in the parameter space that we evaluated and classified as *data* for the logistic model. Using maximum likelihood estimation, in the usual way, estimate from this data the coefficients in the logistic function. Use the logistic model thus created to predict that θ yields a response in regime i with probability p_i (with the p_i summing to 1). The probabilities p_i are estimated from the predictive equations generated by the logistic model. We now classify θ in the class corresponding to regime j, where j is defined by $p_j = \max_{1 \leq i \leq r} p$.

We have carried out simulated population studies/clinical trials involving therapeutics, e.g. Anti-tumor necrosis factor (TNF), an agent that decreased acute inflammation by binding to TNF, a major early stimulant of the inflammatory response. We constructed a simulated clinical trial of anti- TNF treatment in a population of 1000 individuals with Gram-negative infection. We initially created the trial population by varying the following characteristics across individuals: initial pathogen load, pathogen virulence, timing of the intervention (antibiotics and anti-TNF administered upon "admission" of the virtual patient), which occurred earlier in those cases having a higher pathogen load, and genetic variability (cytokine gene polymorphisms). Accordingly, we varied across individuals the ability of macrophages and neutrophils to produce TNF, anti- inflammatories, and nitric oxide, a small molecule that has several effects as can be seen from model equations. In this simulation, we found that anti-TNF was effective at all three doses, with a slight additional gain at the two higher doses (data not shown), but only in cases of severe infection (high pathogen load). Individuals presented late with modest pathogen load see only marginal, if any, improvement. The intervention is detrimental in individuals with low pathogen loads treated early. It would be difficult to identify these individuals a priori in the setting of a clinical trial, while a simulation can provide some identifying characteristics. A multinomial logistic model, using four qualitative outcomes, was used to classify the cases in a validation cohort not used to develop the regression model.

If a strategy to treat only patients predicted to be helped by treatment were adopted, 28 patients would be harmed by treatment. However, harm would be prevented in 175 patients. Treatment would not have changed outcome in 24 patients as opposed to 553 patients if all patients are treated. Thus, the 28 patients harmed by adopting a treatment strategy based on the statistical model's recommendation is nevertheless lower than the 181 harmed by indiscriminate administration. Furthermore, since only 250 patients are ultimately treated, this strategy also results in substantial cost savings. In summary, the combination of a mechanistic model and a multinomial regression model permitted to optimize the selection of patients who should receive therapy with anti-TNF, on the basis of a one time measurement of a subset of independent variables.

5 Appendix: ODEs for the Model

The following ordinary differential equations describe the mathematical model.

$$
\begin{aligned}
PE' &= -k_{pe} \cdot PE \\
MR' &= -(k_{m0} + k_{mpe} \cdot f2(PE, x_{mpe}) + k_{md} \cdot f2(D, x_{md}) + k_{mb} \cdot fb(B)) \\
&\quad \cdot k_{mtrauma} \cdot tr(t, k_{tr}) + f2(TNF, x_{mtnf})/x_{mtnf}^2 \\
&\quad + k_{m6} \cdot f2(IL6, x_{m6})/x_{m6}^2) \cdot fs2(CA, x_{mca}) \cdot fs2(IL10, x_{m10}) \cdot MR \\
&\quad + k_{mm} \cdot (TNF - CA)) - k_{mr} \cdot (MR - Sm) \\
MA' &= (k_{m0} + k_{mpe} \cdot f2(PE, x_{mpe}) + k_{md} \cdot f2(D, x_{md}) + k_{mb} \cdot fb(B)) \\
&\quad \cdot (k_{mtrauma} \cdot tr(t, k_{tr}) + f2(TNF, x_{mtnf})/x_{mtnf}^2 \\
&\quad + k_{m6} \cdot f2(IL6, x_{m6})/x_{m6}^2) \cdot fs2(CA, x_{mca}) \cdot fs2(IL10, x_{m10}) \cdot MR \\
&\quad - k_{ma} \cdot MA - k_{mape} \cdot f(PE, x_{mape}) \cdot MA \\
&\quad - k_{mano} \cdot f2(iNOS, x_{maNO}) \cdot MA \\
NR' &= -(k_{npe} \cdot f(PE, x_{npe}) + k_{ntf} \cdot f(TNF, x_{ntf}) + k_{n6} \cdot f(IL6, x_{n6}) \\
&\quad + k_{nb} \cdot fb(B) + k_{nd} \cdot f(D, x_{nd}) + k_{ntrauma} \cdot tr(t, k_{tr})) \cdot NR \\
&\quad + k_{nr}(Sn - NR)
\end{aligned}
$$

$$
\begin{aligned}
NA' &= (k_{npe} \cdot f(PE, x_{npe}) + k_{ntf} \cdot f(TNF, x_{ntf}) + k_{n6} \cdot f(IL6, x_{n6}) \\
&\quad + k_{nb} \cdot fb(B) + k_{nd} \cdot f(D, x_{nd}) + k_{ntrauma} \cdot tr(t, k_{tr})) \cdot NR \\
&\quad - k_{nn0} \cdot fs2(iNOS, x_{nn0}) \cdot NA - k_n \cdot fs(TNF, x_{ntnfs}) \cdot NA \\
iNOS' &= (k_{inosn} \cdot NA + k_{inosm} \cdot MA + k_{inosec}) \cdot fs2(CA, x_{inosca}) \\
&\quad \cdot fs2(IL10, x_{inos10}) \cdot fs2(TNF, x_{inostnf}) \cdot f(PE, x_{inospe}) \\
&\quad + k_{inos6} \cdot fs2(IL6, x_{inos6})) \cdot fs2(iNOS, x_{inosno}) - k_{inos} \cdot iNOS \\
eNOS' &= k_{enos} \cdot (k_{enosec} \cdot fs(TNF, x_{enostnf}) \cdot fs(PE, x_{enospe}) \\
&\quad \cdot fs4(tr(t, k_{tr}), x_{enostr}) \cdot (1 + f(CA, x_{enosca})) - eNOS) \\
NO3in' &= k_{no23in} \cdot (iNOS - NO3in) \\
NO3' &= k_{no23} \cdot (eNOS - NO23in - NO3) \\
TNF' &= (k_{tnfmr} \cdot MR \cdot PE + k_{tnfn} \cdot NA + k_{tnfm} \cdot MA) \\
&\quad \cdot (1 + k_{tnfno} \cdot f(iNOS, x_{tnfno}) + k_{tnftnf} \cdot f(TNF, x_{tnftnf})) \\
&\quad \cdot fs4(CA, x_{tnfca}) \cdot fs2(IL10, x_{tnf10}) \cdot fs2(IL6, x_{tnf6}) \\
&\quad - k_{tnf} \cdot TNF \\
IL6' &= (k_{6mrpe} \cdot MR \cdot PE + k_{6m} \cdot MA) \\
&\quad \cdot (1 + k_{6tnf} \cdot f2(TNF, x_{6tnf})/x_{6tnf}^2 + k_{66} \cdot f2(IL6, x_{66})/x_{66}^2 \\
&\quad + k_{6NO} \cdot f2(iNOS, x_{6no})/x_{6no}^2) \cdot fs2(CA, x_{6ca}) \cdot fs2(IL10, x_{610}) \\
&\quad + k_6 \cdot fs2(D, x_{6d}) \cdot (S6 - IL6) \\
IL10' &= (k_{10n} \cdot NA + k_{10m} \cdot MA) \\
&\quad \cdot (k_{10mr} + k_{10tnf} \cdot f4(TNF, x_{10tnf})/x_{10tnf}^4 + k_{10ca} \cdot CA \\
&\quad + k_{106} \cdot IL6 + k_{10no} \cdot iNOS) \cdot fs2(IL12, x_{1012}) \\
&\quad + k_{10} \cdot (S10 - IL10) \\
CA' &= (k_{can} \cdot NA + k_{cam} \cdot MA) \cdot (1 + k_{catnf} \cdot f(TNF, x_{catnf}) \\
&\quad + k_{ca6} \cdot f(IL6, x_{ca6}) + k_{cano} \cdot f(iNOS, x_{cano})) \cdot fs2(CA, x_{caca}) \\
&\quad - k_{ca} \cdot CA \\
IL12' &= k_{12m} \cdot MA \cdot (1 + k_{12tnf} \cdot f(TNF, x_{12tnf}) + k_{126} \cdot f(IL6, x_{126})) \\
&\quad \cdot fs2(IL10, x_{1210}) - k_{12} \cdot IL12 \\
B' &= k_b \cdot ((1 - k_{bh} \cdot square(t_{bon}, t_{boff}))/ \\
&\quad (1 + k_{bno} \cdot (iNOS + eNOS - x_{bno})) - B) \\
D' &= (k_{db} \cdot fb(B) + k_{dtnf} \cdot TNF + k_{d6} \cdot IL6 + k_{dd} \cdot f2(D, x_{dd})) \\
&\quad \cdot (1 - k_{dno} \cdot f(iNOS + eNOS - x_{dno})) - k_d \cdot D + k_{dtr} \cdot tr(t, k_{tr})
\end{aligned}
$$

The equations represent the dynamics of circulating or systemic levels of immune cells, cytokines, and molecules. In addition, there are three systemic variables representing blood pressure, tissue dysfunction, and tissue trauma. The latter is expressed as an exponential decay from an initial insult. For numerical ease, the variables of the equations are defined in abstract units of concentration. The actual units are restored with a simple scaling factor when comparing to experimental data. The time unit is fixed at hours. Exact mathematical descriptions of the equations and the parameters that enter appear in some of our more detailed writings on this subject.

Acknowledgements

This work was funded under NIH grant GM67240.

References

1. Angus, D.C., Linde-Zwirble, W.T., Lidicker, J., et al. (2001). "Epidemiology of Severe Sepsis in the United States: Analysis of Incidence, Outcome, and Associated Costs of Care," *Critical Care Medicine*, **29**, 1303–1310.
2. Bellingan, G. (1999). "Inflammatory Cell Activation in Sepsis", *British Medical Bulletin*, **55**, 12–29.
3. Bernard, G.R., Vincent, J.L., Laterre, P.F., et al. (2001). "Efficacy and Safety of Recombinant Human Cctivated Protein C for Severe Sepsis," *New England Journal of Medicine*, **344**, 699–709.
4. Bone, R.C. (1996). "Why Sepsis Trials Fail," *Journal of the American Medical Association*, **276**, 565–566.
5. Bone, R.C. (1996). "Immunologic Dissonance: A Continuing Evolution in Our Understanding of the Systemic Inflammatory Response Syndrome (SIRS) and the Multiple Organ Dysfunction Syndrome (MODS)," *Annals of Internal Medicine*, **125**, 680–687.
6. Buchman, T.G., Cobb, J.P., Lapedes, A.S., et al. (2001). "Complex Systems Analysis: A Tool for Shock Research," *Shock*, **16**, 248–251.
7. Carrico, C.J. (1994). "1993 Presidential Address, American Association for the Surgery of Trauma: It's Time to Drain the Swamp," *Journal of Trauma*, **37**, 532–537.
8. Chow, C. C. et al. (2003). "Quantitative Dynamics of the Acute Inflammatory Response in Shock States," submitted to *Critical Care Medicine*.
9. Freeman, B.D., Natanson, C. (2000). "Anti-Inflammatory Therapies in Sepsis and Septic Shock," *Expert Opin. Investig. Drugs*, **9**, 1651–1663.
10. Hill, A.V. (1998). "The Immunogenetics of Human Infectious Diseases", [Review] [128 refs]. *Annu. Rev. Immunol.*, **16**, 593–617.
11. Hotchkiss, R.S., Karl, I.E. (2003). "The Pathophysiology and Treatment of Sepsis," *New England Journal of Medicine*, **348**, 138–150.
12. Jarrar, D., Chaudry, I.H., Wang P. (1999). "Organ Dysfunction Following Hemorrhage and Sepsis: Mechanisms and Therapeutic Approaches (Review)", *International Journal of Molecular Medicine*, **4**, 575–583.
13. Kitano, H. (2002). "Systems Biology: A Brief Overview," *Science*, **295**, 1662–1664.
14. MacWilliams, F.J., and Sloane, N.J.A. (1978). *The Theory of Error Correcting Codes*, North Holland, Amsterdam.
15. Majetschak, M., Flohe, S., Obertacke, U., et al. (1999). "Relation of a TNF Gene Polymorphism to Severe Sepsis in Trauma Patients," *Annals of Surgery*, **230**, 207–214.

16. Marshall, J.C. (2001). "Inflammation, Coagulopathy, and the Pathogenesis of Multiple Organ Dysfunction Syndrome," *Critical Care Medicine*, **29**, S99–106.
17. Marshall, R.P., Webb, S., Hill, M.R., et al. (2002). "Genetic Polymorphisms Associated with Susceptibility and Outcome in ARDS", *Chest*, **121**, 68S–69S.
18. Medzhitov, R., Janeway, C.J. (2000). "Innate Immunity," *New England Journal of Medicine*, **343**, 338–344.
19. Mira, J.P., Cariou, A., Grall, F., et al. (1999). "Association of TNF2, a TNF-a Promoter Polymorphism, with Septic Shock Susceptibility and Mortality. A Multicenter Study," *Journal of the American Medical Association*, **282**, 561–568.
20. Nathan, C. (2002). "Points of Control in Inflammation," *Nature*, **420**, 846–852.
21. Neugebauer, E.A., Willy, C., Sauerland, S. (2001). "Complexity and Non-Linearity in Shock Research: Reductionism or Synthesis?" *Shock*, **16**, 252–258.
22. Parker, S.J., Watkins, P.E. (2001). "Experimental Models of Gram-Negative Sepsis", *British Journal of Surgery*, **88**, 22–30.
23. Pinsky, M.R. (2001). "Sepsis: A Pro- and Anti-Inflammatory Disequilibrium Syndrome," *Contrib. Nephrol.*, 354–366.
24. Seydel, R. (1994). *Practical Bifurcation and Stability Analysis: From Equilibrium to Chaos*, 2nd edition, Springer Verlag, New York.
25. Schroder, J., Kahlke, V., Book, M., et al. (2000). "Gender Differences in Sepsis: Genetically Determined?" *Shock*, **14**, 307-310.
26. Schluter, B., Raufhake, C., Erren, M., et al. (2002). "Effect of the Interleukin-6 Promoter Polymorphism (-174 G/C) on the Incidence and Outcome of Sepsis", *Critical Care Medicine*, **30**, 32–37.
27. Stuber, F. (2001). "Effects of Genomic Polymorphisms on the Course of Sepsis: Is There a Concept for Gene Therapy?", *J. Am. Soc. Nephrol.*, **12** Suppl. 17, S60–S64.
28. Volk, H.D., Reinke, P., Docke, W.D. (2000). "Clinical Aspects: From Systemic Inflammation to 'Immunoparalysis'," *Chem. Immunol.*, **74**, 162–177.
29. Walley, K.R., Holmes, C.L., Sandford, A.J., et al. (2002). "Differential Association of the TNF? - 308 G/A Polymorphism in Critically Ill Patients With and Without Septic Shock," *American Journal of Respiratory Critical Care Medicine*, **165** (Suppl):A519.

Combining Functional MRI Data on Multiple Subjects

Mark G. Vangel

Athinoula A. Martionos Center for Biomedical Imaging, U.S.A.
vangel@nmr.mgh.harvard.edu

Abstract: Worsley et al. (2002) propose a practical approach to multiple-subject functional MRI data analyses which uses the EM algorithm to estimate the between-subject variance component at each voxel. The main result of this article is a demonstration that the much more efficient Newton-Raphson algorithm can be reliably used for these calculations. This result follows from an extension of a simple algorithm proposed by Mandel and Paule (1970) for the one-way unbalanced ANOVA model, two variants of which have been shown to be equivalent to modified ML and REML, in which the "modification" is that the within-subject variances as treated as known.

1 Introduction

Magnetic resonance imaging (MRI) is a versatile technique which uses differences in magnetic susceptibility to visualize internal anatomy, often in extraordinary detail. Functional magnetic resonance imaging (fMRI) is a related technique which makes essential use of the fact that the magnetic susceptibility of hemoglobin differs depending on whether the molecule is oxygenated (*oxy*hemoglobin) or not (*deoxy*hemoglobin). In contrast to ordinary (structural) MRI, fMRI datasets are 4-dimensional (3D+time), with a typical spatial resolution of $3mm^3$, and a temporal resolution of about 2 seconds. The *BOLD* (Blood Oxygen Level Dependent) response which is the output measure of fMRI of the brain appears to be related to average synaptic activity (without regard to whether the activity is excitatory or inhibitory)(e.g., Tagamets and Horwitz (2002), and references given there), and so one can use this technique to explore the activity of a living, working brain. The ubiquity of MRI scanners combined with the (usually) non-invasive nature of the technique has led to a vast amount of research during the last decade. In particular, it is probably no exaggeration to say that the influence of fMRI on experimental psychology has been revolutionary.

In addition to the data itself, an fMRI experiment usually includes an *experimental paradigm*, which describes the nature, time of onset and duration of various stimuli. Datasets tend to be quite large: a typical brain scan has 32 slices, each of 64 × 64 voxels, with the entire brain imaged every 2 seconds, for a total of several hundred time values per voxel. Two or more such scans are often available for each subject, and a typical study of modest size will consist of 10-15 subjects. Statistical challenges are everywhere, from preprocessing the data through clustering and classification of voxels in summary statistical maps. In the present article, however, we will focus on the fitting of linear models to individual voxels, and specifically to an approach for combining analyses in order to obtain consensus inferences from multiple subjects.

2 Voxel-Level Linear Models

The approach usually taken in fMRI data analysis is to fit a linear model to each voxel in a single data file (i.e., a single scan on a single subject), in which coefficients of the model reflect the stimuli of interest in the paradigm, as well as nuisance drift. Following Worsley et al. (2002), we express this linear model for the ith voxel as

$$\begin{aligned} Y_i &= \underbrace{x_{i1}\beta_1 + \cdots + x_{ik}\beta_k}_{\text{fMRI Response}} \\ &\quad + \underbrace{x_{i,k+1}\beta_{k+1} \cdots + x_{i,m}\beta_m}_{\text{drift}} + \epsilon_i \\ &= x_i'\beta + \epsilon_i, \end{aligned} \tag{1}$$

where $x_i' = [x_{i1}, \ldots, x_{im}]'$ and $\beta = [\beta_1, \ldots, \beta_m]'$, and ϵ is Gaussian error, for which one can assume independence, or perhaps an autoregressive correlation structure.

One way to generalize this approach to multiple subjects, multiple sessions within a subject, or subject-level covariates (e.g., age, gender) is to introduce these as additional factors, and thus extend (1) to a mixed model. After transforming each scanned brain onto a common anatomical space, the data from corresponding voxels can be gathered from the various subjects and sessions and combined in voxelwise analyses. A simple calculation, though, shows that computational difficulties can arise because of the volume of data involved; a typical experiment can consist of 32×64×64 voxels, each containing a time series of length 200, for each of 15 subjects scanned twice leading to 32 × 64 × 64 × 200 × 15 × 2 words, or approximately 3.1 gigabytes of data.

Worsley et al. (2002) address these computational concerns by performing analyses hierarchically, with successive computations in the hierarchy employing only the sufficient statistics from the level below. Specifically, for an experiment consisting of a single session for $j = 1, \ldots, n$ subjects, let C_j and

S_j denote estimated voxel-level coefficient contrasts and standard errors, respectively, perhaps reflecting the difference in BOLD activation between an experimental condition of interest and a baseline fixation. Let γ denote a vector of subject-level coefficients. (In the simplest case where there are no subject-level covariates, γ will be a scalar multiplying a column of n ones.) For each voxel, we consider the model

$$C_j = z_j'\gamma + \eta_j, \tag{2}$$

where z_j is a vector of known covariates, and η_j is normally distributed with mean zero and variance $\sigma^2 + S_j^2$, independently for $j = 1, \ldots, n$.

Treating the within-subject standard errors S_j as known, Worsley et al. (2002) show how σ^2 can be estimated using the EM algorithm. By employing a simple computational trick, these authors report that reasonable estimates can be obtained in approximately 10 iterations. It is the purpose of this article to demonstrate that modified ML and REML estimates (i.e., estimates of σ^2 and γ which treat the S_j as known) can be obtained reliably by Newton-Raphson, by finding the unique root of a convex function. The algorithm developed below is a generalization of an iteration proposed by Mandel and Paule (1970) for one-way random ANOVA, which is shown to be related to modified ML and modified REML in Vangel and Rukhin (1999) and Rukhin et al. (2000), respectively.

3 Modified ML for Multi-Subject fMRI Analyses

For simplicity, we restrict attention in this article to modified maximum-likelihood estimation; a similar derivation can be made for modified REML, though the details are somewhat more complex. For each voxel, we would like to estimate σ^2 and γ in (2), which we express in matrix form as

$$C = Z\gamma + \eta,$$

where $\eta \sim \mathrm{N}(0, \Sigma)$, with

$$\Sigma \equiv \sigma^2 I + \mathrm{diag}\,(S_1^2, \ldots, S_n^2).$$

Maximizing the likelihood for this model is easily seen to be equivalent to minimizing $|\Sigma|$ subject to

$$Q \equiv (C - Z\hat{\gamma})^T \Sigma^{-1} (C - Z\hat{\gamma}) = n,$$

where $\hat{\gamma}$ is the generalized least squares (GLS) estimate of γ

$$\hat{\gamma} = (Z^T \Sigma^{-1} Z)^{-1} Z^T \Sigma^{-1} C.$$

Denote the GLS projection ("hat") matrix by

$$H \equiv Z(Z^T \Sigma^{-1} Z)^{-1} Z^T \Sigma^{-1}.$$

The only unknown in the quadratic form Q is σ^2, so one can maximize the likelihood by solving

$$Q = r^T \Sigma^{-1} r = n,$$

where $r = (I - H)C$ is the GLS residual vector.

To show that Q is convex, we begin by noting that,

$$\frac{\mathrm{d}\,(Z^T \Sigma^{-1} Z)^{-1} (Z^T \Sigma^{-1} Z)}{\mathrm{d}\sigma^2} = \frac{\mathrm{d}\,I}{\mathrm{d}\sigma^2} = 0.$$

Thus, by the chain rule,

$$\begin{aligned}\frac{\mathrm{d}\,(Z^T \Sigma^{-1} Z)^{-1}}{\mathrm{d}\sigma^2} &= -(Z^T \Sigma^{-1} Z)^{-1} \frac{\mathrm{d}\,(Z^T \Sigma^{-1} Z)}{\mathrm{d}\sigma^2} (Z^T \Sigma^{-1} Z)^{-1} \\ &= (Z^T \Sigma^{-1} Z)^{-1} (Z^T \Sigma^{-2} Z)(Z^T \Sigma^{-1} Z)^{-1}\end{aligned}$$

A little manipulation leads to

$$\frac{\mathrm{d}\,Q}{\mathrm{d}\sigma^2} = r^T \Sigma^{-1} (H + H^T - I) \Sigma^{-1} r.$$

But it's easy to show (see Appendix A) that

$$r^T \Sigma^{-1} H = C^T (I - H)^T \Sigma^{-1} H = 0;$$

hence

$$\frac{\mathrm{d}\,Q}{\mathrm{d}\sigma^2} = -r^T \Sigma^{-2} r \leq 0,$$

and Q is monotone decreasing. Similarly,

$$\frac{\mathrm{d}^2\,Q}{\mathrm{d}\sigma^2} = r^T \Sigma^{-3} r \geq 0,$$

and thus Q is also a convex function of σ^2. Hence, the root $\hat{\sigma}^2$ is unique (when $Q(0) < n$, we set $\hat{\sigma}^2 = 0$).

4 Generalization

Next, we briefly consider the case of multiple variance components. Let

$$\Sigma = S^2 + \sum_{i=1}^{q} \sigma_i^2 V_i V_i^T,$$

where $S^2 \equiv \mathrm{diag}\,(S_1^2, \ldots, S_n^2)$, and let Q, r, and H denote the exponent of the likelihood, the GLS residual vector, and the GLS "hat" matrix, respectively. A straightforward calculation (see Appendix B for details) shows that

$$\frac{\partial H}{\partial \sigma_i^2} = -HV_iV_i^TV^{-1}(I-H),$$

and thus

$$\begin{aligned}\frac{\partial Q}{\partial \sigma_i^2} &= r^T\Sigma^{-1}\left[V_iV_i^TH^T + HV_iV_i^T - V_iV_i^T\right]\Sigma^{-1}r \\ &= -r^TV_iV_i\Sigma^{-1}r \\ &= -\|V_i^T\Sigma^{-1}r\|^2 \leq 0.\end{aligned}$$

Taking second derivatives, we can show that Q is convex in each σ_i^2. However, the computational value of this result is questionable because, unlike the single variance component case, for each set of $\{\sigma_1^2, \ldots, \sigma_q^2\}$ simultaneously satisfying the constraint $Q = n$, one must minimize $|\Sigma|$ in order to obtain ML estimates.

Appendix: Mathematical Details

A: Single Variance Component

First, let $V = S + \sigma^2 I$, and

$$Q \equiv (y - X\hat{\gamma})^TV^{-1}(y - X\hat{\gamma}).$$

It's easy to see that

$$\frac{\partial V^{-1}}{\partial \sigma^2} = -V^{-1}\frac{\partial V}{\partial \sigma^2}V^{-1} = -V^{-2};$$

hence

$$\frac{\partial (X^TV^{-1}X)^{-1}}{\partial \sigma^2} = +(X^TV^{-1}X)^{-1}(X^TV^{-2}X)(X^TV^{-1}X)^{-1}.$$

Denote the hat matrix by

$$H \equiv X(X^TV^{-1}X)^{-1}X^TV^{-1},$$

and note that

$$\begin{aligned}\frac{\partial H}{\partial \sigma^2} &= X\frac{\partial (X^TV^{-1}X)^{-1}}{\partial \sigma^2}X^TV^{-1} + (X^TV^{-1}X)^{-1}X^T\frac{\partial V^{-1}}{\partial \sigma^2} \\ &= \left[X(X^TV^{-1}X)^{-1}X^TV^{-1}\right]\left[V^{-1}X(X^TV^{-1}X)^{-1}X^TV^{-1} - V^{-1}\right] \\ &= \left[X(X^TV^{-1}X)^{-1}X^TV^{-1}\right]V^{-1}\left[X(X^TV^{-1}X)^{-1}X^TV^{-1} - I\right] \\ &= HV^{-1}(H-I) = -HV^{-1}(I-H).\end{aligned}$$

Using the above expression for the derivative of H, we have

$$\begin{aligned}\frac{\partial Q}{\partial \sigma^2} &= y^T \frac{\partial (I-H)^T}{\partial \sigma^2} V^{-1}(I-H)y + y^T (I-H)^T \frac{\partial V^{-1}}{\partial \sigma^2}(I-H)y \\ &\quad + y^T(I-H)^T V^{-1} \frac{\partial (I-H)}{\partial \sigma^2} y \\ &= y^T(I-H)^T V^{-1} H^T V^{-1}(I-H)y - y^T(I-H)^T V^{-2}(I-H)y \\ &\quad + y^T (I-H)^T V^{-1} H V^{-1}(I-H)y \\ &= r^T(V^{-1}H^T V^{-1} - V^{-1} + V^{-1}HV^{-1})r \\ &= r^T V^{-1}(H + H^T - I)V^{-1} r.\end{aligned}$$

But

$$(I-H)^T V^{-1} H = H^T V^{-1}(I-H) = 0;$$

so

$$\frac{\partial Q}{\partial \sigma^2} = -r^T V^{-2} r \leq 0.$$

B: Generalization

Now consider the more general covariance matrix V, denoted

$$V = S + \sum_i \sigma_i^2 V_i V_i^2.$$

Following the pattern of the above calculations, we have

$$\frac{\partial V^{-1}}{\partial \sigma_i^2} = -V^{-1}\frac{\partial V}{\partial \sigma_i^2} V^{-1} = -V^{-1} V_i V_i^T V^{-1};$$

$$\frac{\partial (X^T V^{-1} X)^{-1}}{\partial \sigma_i^2} = +(X^T V^{-1} X)^{-1}(X^T V^{-1} V_i V_i^T V^{-1})(X^T V^{-1} X)^{-1};$$

$$\begin{aligned}\frac{\partial H}{\partial \sigma_i^2} &= X \frac{\partial (X^T V^{-1} X)^{-1}}{\partial \sigma_i^2} X^T V^{-1} - X(X^T V^{-1} X)^{-1} X^T V^{-1} V_i V_i^T V^{-1} \\ &= X(X^T V^{-1} X)^{-1} X^T V^{-1} V_i V_i^T V^{-1} X (X^T V^{-1} X)^{-1} X^T V^{-1} - \\ &\quad X(X^T V^{-1} X)^{-1} X^T V^{-1} V_i V_i^T V^{-1} \\ &= H V_i V_i^T V^{-1}(H - I) = -H V_i V_i^T V^{-1}(I-H);\end{aligned}$$

$$\begin{aligned}\frac{\partial Q}{\partial \sigma_i^2} &= y^T \frac{\partial (I-H^T)}{\partial \sigma_i^2}\left[V^{-1}(I-H)y\right] + y^T(I-H)^T \frac{\partial V^{-1}}{\partial \sigma_i^2}(I-H)y + \\ &\quad y^T(I-H)^T V^{-1} \frac{\partial (I-H)}{\partial \sigma_i^2} y \\ &= r^T V^{-1}\left[V_i V_i^T H^T + H V_i V_i^T - V_i V_i^T\right] V^{-1} r \\ &= -r^T V^{-1} V_i V_i^T V^{-1} r = -\|V_i V^{-1} r\|^2 \leq 0.\end{aligned}$$

The second derivative of Q with respect to σ_i^2 and σ_j^2 is

$$\begin{aligned}\frac{\partial^2 Q}{\partial\sigma_i^2\partial\sigma_j^2} = & -y^T(I-H)^T V^{-1}V_jV_j^T H^T V^{-1}V_iV_i^T V^{-1}(I-H)y + \\ & y^T(I-H)^T V^{-1}V_jV_j^T V^{-1}V_iV_i^T V^{-1}(I-H)y + \\ & y^T(I-H)^T V^{-1}V_iV_i^T V^{-1}V_jV_j^T V^{-1}(I-H)y - \\ & y^T(I-H)^T V^{-1}V_iV_i^T V^{-1}HV_jV_j^T V^{-1}(I-H)y\end{aligned}$$

The first term equals zero, since

$$(I-H)^T V^{-1}V_jV_j^T H^T = (I-H^T)[(V^{-1}V_jV_j^T)H^T] = 0;$$

similarly, the fourth term is zero. Let W be the Hessian of Q. For any residual vector r, we see that

$$\begin{aligned}r^T W r &= \sum_{i=1}^{q}\sum_{j=1}^{q} r^T V^{-1}V_iV_i^T V^{-1}V_jV_j^T V^{-1}r \\ &= r^T\left[V^{-1}\left(\sum_{i=1}^{q} V_iV_i^T\right)V^{-1}\left(\sum_{j=1}^{q} V_jV_j^T\right)V^{-1}\right]r \\ &= r^T V^{-1}UV^{-1}UV^{-1}r \\ &= r^T V^{-1}UV^{-1/2}V^{-1/2}UV^{-1}r \\ &= \|V^{-1/2}UV^{-1}r\|^2 \geq 0,\end{aligned}$$

where

$$U \equiv \sum_{i=1}^{q} V_iV_i^T,$$

V^{-1}, and $V^{-1/2}$ are symmetric. Hence, Q is a monotone decreasing convex function of $\sigma_1^2, \ldots, \sigma_q^2$.

References

1. Mandel, J. and Paule, R. C. (1970). "Interlaboratory Evaluation of a Material with Unequal Numbers of Replicates," *Analytical Chemistry*, **42**, 1194–1197.
2. Rukhin, A. L., Biggerstaff, B. J. and Vangel, M. G. (2000). "Restricted Maximum Likelihood Estimation of a Common Mean and the Mandel-Paule Algorithm," *Journal of Statistical Planning and Inference*, **83**, 319–330.
3. Tagamets M.-A. and Horwitz, B. (2000). "A Model of Working Memory: Bridging the Gap Between Electrophysiology and Human Brain Imaging," *Neural Networks*, **13**, 941–952.
4. Vangel, M. G. and Rukhin, A. L. (1999). "Maximum-Likelihood Analysis for Heteroscedastic One-Way Random Effects ANOVA in Interlaboratory Studies," *Biometrics*, **55**, 302–313.

5. Worsley, K. J., Liao, C. H., Aston, J., Petre, V., Duncan, G. H., Morales, F., and Evans, A. C. (2002). "A General Statistical Analysis for fMRI Data," *NeuroImage*, **15**, 1–15.

Classifying the State of Parkinsonism by Using Electronic Force Platform Measures of Balance

Nicholas I. Bohnen[1], Marius G. Buliga[2], and Gregory M. Constantine[3]

[1] University of Pittsburgh, U.S.A.
nbohnen@pitt.edu
[2] University of Pittsburgh-Bradford, U.S.A.
buliga@pitt.edu
[3] University of Pittsburgh, U.S.A.
gmc@euler.math.pitt.edu

Abstract: Several measures of balance obtained from quiet stance on an electronic force platform are described. These measures were found to discriminate patients with Parkinson's disease (PD) from normal control subjects. First-degree relatives of patients with PD show greater variability on these measures. A primary goal is to develop sensitive measures that would be capable of identifying impaired balance in early stages of non-clinical PD. We developed a trinomial logistic model that classifies a subject as either normal, pre-parkinsonian, or parkinsonian taking as input the measures developed from the platform data.

1 A Description of Causes and Conditions Present in Parkinson's Disease

Parkinson's disease (PD) is a clinical syndrome consisting of a variable combination of symptoms of tremor, rigidity, postural imbalance and bradykinesia (Gelb and Gilman (1999), Quinn (1995)). The clinical features of PD result from degeneration of dopaminergic cells in the substantia nigra pars compacta and the ventral tegmental area, accompanied by the formation of Lewy bodies (Hughes (1997), Hughes et al. (1995)). The greater the neuronal loss in the substantia nigra, the lower the concentration of dopamine in the projection areas to the striatum, limbic regions, and frontal cortex in the brain. Langston and Koller noted that PD can be viewed as a disease having two phases. The first phase is a preclinical period that covers the period from disease inception to the time when the disease becomes symptomatic (Langston and Koller (1991)). The second phase represents the symptomatic period where the classical symptoms of PD such as bradykinesia, tremor and rigidity occur.

In this paper we focus on the development of measures of postural stiffness and motor dysfunction by making use of a Kistler electronic platform. There is preliminary evidence that some of these measures are significantly correlated with descriptive clinical assessments, such as those used in the Universal Parkinson's Disease Rating Scale (UPDRS), particularly the Motor Sub-scale. The platform measures are more objective measures than those offered by the UPDRS. They are inexpensive and can be easily done in a doctor's office. It would be particularly promising if these platform measure prove to be good covariates of the amount of dopamine in the brain as measured by a PET scan. This would provide an inexpensive means of correctly assessing the status of PD in preclinical cases. At this time we only have evidence that some of the platform measures are highly correlated with the scores on the peg board tests. These scores are, on the other hand, known to correlate well with the amount of dopamine in the brain. We hope to produce direct evidence of such correlation by carrying out PET and platform readings on patients in the future.

2 Postural Motor System Dynamic Modeling

The link between postural stability and PD has been probed by many researchers in the past (Bloem et al. (1998), Horak and Nashner (1992)). Chow et al. (1999) proposed a mechanical model of posture control from which an analytical form for the autocovariance function of the center of pressure (COP) motion was obtained. Later, a stiffness measure was derived from this model (Lauk et al. (1999)). The dynamic model that was adopted assumes that the body during quiet standing can be represented by a flexible string (polymer) with stiffness and damping. In addition, the model predicts the analytical form of the time-dependent correlations of COP displacements, from which a set of physiologically relevant parameters can be extracted. The autocovariance function is

$$a(t) = \sum_i (y_{i+t} - \mu)(y_i - \mu),$$

where the $y_i$are the mediolateral $y-$coordinates of the COP motion and μ is the mean of the process. For clarity of exposition we briefly reproduce some of the details. The body is assumed to be close to upright and that the combination of the destabilizing effects of gravity and the stabilizing effects of the imperfect control system are captured by a simple stochastic forcing term. This hypothesis is based on the observation that the dynamics of the COP obey a correlated random walk. The resulting equation is

$$\beta \frac{\partial^2}{\partial t^2} y(z,t) + \frac{\partial}{\partial t} y(z,t) = \nu \frac{\partial^2}{\partial z^2} y(z,t) - \alpha y(z,t) + \eta(z,t).$$

It describes the motion of a long rod or polymer that is elastically pinned to a single location and driven stochastically. Parameters β and α^{-1} have dimensions of time and ν has a dimension of length squared divided by time. Explicitly computing the Fourier transform, then inverting, gives in the time domain

$$\frac{d}{dt}a(t) = \frac{e^{-t/2\beta}}{2\sqrt{\nu\beta}} J_0\left(\frac{\sqrt{4\alpha\beta - 1}}{2\beta} t\right),$$

where J_0 is the zeroth-order Bessel function. For $4\alpha\beta < 1$, J_0 is replaced by the zeroth-order modified Bessel function I_0. From this biomechanical model, a "body stiffness" parameter $k = \alpha/\beta$ was derived.

Preliminary data from Boston University have shown that the COP-based postural stiffness measure k increases with more severe parkinsonian motor symptoms and correlates with UPDRS motor scores in PD patients; see Table 1 (Lauk et al. (1999)). These data indicate that this parameter not only measures stiffness but also bradykinesia and other motor impairments in PD. We extend this analysis with data from the University of Pittsburgh, and show that the discrimination between populations is particularly effective when the average residual to a smoothed version of the data and the rebound measures are used.

Table 1. Correlation coefficients between UPDRS measures and the postural stiffness measure.

Clinical measure	Kendall's τ correlation coefficients
Rigidity	0.48 $(P < 0.006)$
Bradykinesia	0.46 $(P < 0.008)$
Posture	0.60 $(P < 0.0005)$
Leg agility	0.52 $(P < 0.003)$
UPDRS motor score	0.49 $(P < 0.005)$

3 Data Driven Stochastic Analysis

Three populations were studied: parkinsonians, first-degree relatives of patients with PD, and normal controls. To account for possible differences due to age, subjects of comparable age were used across the groups. Several measures were used to study the differences between the three groups. Using the above-mentioned autocovariance and autocorrelation functions we found several marked differences between PD patients and normal control subjects enabling us to identify three significant traits of the autocorrelation curve on which measures of balance impairment are based. Parkinsonian curves are generally characterized by a precipitous initial drop, followed by rebounding efforts. By contrast, normal controls tend to exhibit gradual, essentially straight line, decay. First-degree relatives of patients with PD have greater between-subject variability indicating greater heterogeneity in this group. We developed and aim to utilize five numerical measures based on postural motor system modeling to characterize and quantify parkinsonian motor dysfunction. Some of these measures have been discussed in Constantine et al. (2001). Among the first-degree relatives of patients with PD we isolated two (out of four) who show features similar with the parkinsonian pattern of the autocorrelation curves in the absence of clinical parkinsonism. This finding and the observed increased heterogeneity in our group of first-degree relatives of patients with PD led to the hypothesis that this subgroup of apparently normal persons may be at risk of developing PD.

Thus far it seems that the statistics that best discriminate between the three groups are found in the residuals of the COP trajectories. The stiffness measure, discussed in the previous section, highlights some differences between the three populations. However, a purely statistical analysis of the residuals in the (mediolateral) x-coordinate of the trajectory, obtained after smoothing the series over two-second intervals, yields an even better separation between the groups. It is consistent with the stiffness measure but the statistics have a much stronger level of significance.

Specifically, we register the COP motion of a subject for two minutes at 50 readings per second; we repeat the process 5 times on the same subject. On each person we therefore have 5 COP time series, and we focus on the x-coordinate of the 5 series only. Data on each individual consists, therefore, of 5 time series of the x-coordinates of the COP motion. (In a few cases data was missing or was misrecorded due to operator or machine error. In such cases we have fewer than 5 series per individual.) Each series is smoothed over intervals of 2 seconds, that is, we average 100 consecutive readings across the series; the residual vector is, by definition, the difference between the original series and the smoothed series. We view the smoother series as a trend. The trend cannot be modeled formally in any traditional sense, since two series on the same individual can look very dissimilar in terms of trend. But the residuals show significant consistency, if the smoothing is done over the same time length. It is these residuals that we are taking interest in.

One of the simplest statistics is the average squared residual. By this we understand, for a given time series, the squared norm of the residual vector divided by its length. The average residual r_i for for subject i is simply the mean of the average residuals of the (usually) five time series associated with subject i, and s_i denotes the standard deviation of the statistic r_i. For each of the three groups we then compute $\bar{r}$, the average of the r_i's in that group, as well as the standard deviation s of the $\bar{r}$ of the group. We summarize the results on the average residuals in Table 2. Inspection of the data shows that the variance in the average residual visibly varies between groups (and much less between subjects of the same group). A formal test rejects the hypothesis of equality of variances between groups (the p-value is less than 0.0001). Even the most conservative approach (using always the larger estimate of the variance among two groups) yields the result that the parkinsonians have, on average, the average residual significantly greater than each of the other two groups (p-values of less than 0.0001 in both cases, using a Gaussian test).

Table 2. Residual summaries for the three groups.

	Number of Subjects	Average Squared Residual (ASR)	Standard Deviation of ASR
Parkinsonians	26	14.93	1.05
Relatives	4	9.34	0.74
Normal controls	10	3.68	0.18

Nonparametric tests offer similar conclusions. A Wilcoxon rank test finds that the median of the Parkinsonian average residual is significantly different from the other two groups, but the Blood Relatives and Normal Controls do not have median average residuals that are significantly different. These comparisons were also performed after taking away a smoothed trend over time intervals of five seconds, rather than two, and the results did not show any dramatic qualitative change.

Table 3 below displays summary information on the correlation of the average residual with some clinical UPDR scores. For purposes of comparison we focus on the same variables used in Table 1 for the stiffness measure. As in the case of the stiffness measure, foot agility shows the highest correlation, with bradykinesia and UPDRS motor both at 58%.

Table 3. Spearman correlations between UPDRS measures and the average squared residual.

Clinical measure	**Spearman correlation coefficient**
Rigidity	0.58 ($P < 0.0009$)
Bradykinesia	0.55 ($P < 0.0010$)
Posture	0.63 ($P < 0.0001$)
Foot agility (right)	0.52 ($P < 0.0002$)
Foot agility (left)	0.68 ($P < 0.0001$)
UPDRS motor score	0.58 ($P < 0.0006$)

We turn now to some of the other measures that we investigated. The data indicate differences in the rate of decay of the autocovariance between the parkinsonians and normal controls. In order to study these rates we fitted a simple exponential decay function. More complicated models were tried, but they offered no substantial gains to the qualitative understanding of the decay rates. Over a time interval of 30 seconds we fit the exponential family

$$A(t) = ae^{-bt}.$$

The parameter a is simply the variance of the time series of the mediolateral COP coordinate (which we call mediolateral noise), while b is the rate of decay. We used the Splus statistical package to fit this model to the data. The fit yields the least squares estimates of the rate and intercept. For a given subject we then obtain an estimate of the variance from the (at most 5) repeated platform readings. The variances are dependent upon the individual. When categorized by presence or absence of PD we obtain an average decay rate of 14.9 with a standard error of 1.3 for PD patients, and 8.6 with a standard error of 1.1 for normals; by standard error we always understand the standard deviation of the estimate of the parameter under discussion. A formal test for equality of the two population means rejects the hypothesis that the means are equal in favor of the alternative that the parkinsonians have a significantly higher rate of decay of the autocovariance function; the p-value is less than 0.0001

With regard to the mediolateral noise a of the model, the parkinsonians on average have mediolateral noise equal to 56.5 with a standard error of 7.6 while the normal controls register 17.5 with an standard error of 5.3. The conclusion is that the parkinsonians produce much greater noise in the mediolateral movement than normal subjects. An additional statistic, with potential clinical use, is the significant Spearman correlation of 0.51 that exists between the mediolateral noise and the number of falls that the subject experiences.

A measure of how much a person rebounds while trying to keep balance under quiet standing may be measured by the arc length of the autocovariance function per unit time. A long arc indicates significant rebounding efforts, whereas a short arc length is likely to be associated with autocovariance close to a straight line. The later is easily associated with absence of balance impairment. The rebounds, when present, have irregular structure with no evident periodicity. It appears that the arc length of the autocovariance function offers the best opportunity to numerically quantify this effect. We computed the arc length by normalizing the two axes to a same average increment, then summed the square roots of the sum of squares of the differenced time and autocovariance series; it is the usual formula for arc length. The rebound measure (or arc length of the autocovariance function) has a significant Spearman correlations with all the clinical variables listed in Table 3, and of about the same magnitude (plus or minus 10%). It has a Spearman correlation of 49.3% with the number of falls. Not unexpectedly the rebound measure and the average residual are highly correlated. The rebound measure has, however, the advantage of not being dependent on any smoothing.

Using the five platform measures constructed above and the UPDR clinical scores as input variables, we are in the process of constructing a logistic model having three categories as output for a subject under study: normal, pre-parkinsonian and parkinsonian. This trinomial logistic model assigns probabilities (the sum of which is 1) that a subject falls in each of the three categories and classifies the person within the category that carries the highest probability as estimated from data. The statistical packages Splus and SPSS have been used to analyze the data. We only give here the resulting (tentative and preliminary) classification. It should be observed that the true state of nature is not fully known in this study, particularly with regard to the relatives of parkinsonians. Of the 26 parkinsonians 6 were misclassified as normal. This misclassification is due to the fact that, though clinically known to have PD, the 6 subjects do not manifest balance problems. The model classified two out of the four relatives of parkinsonians to be pre-parkinsonian. This is consistent with other type of analyses of the data, as well as medical opinion based on clinical evaluation – though not on PET scans, and shows that the trinomial model seems reliable in this respect. Only one of the 10 normal subjects has been misclassified as parkinsonian. The logistic is as much a classification tool as it is a predictive model; we intend to explore its later feature with regard to the blood relatives of parkinsonians in future studies.

References

1. Bloem, B. R., Beckley, D. J., van Hilten, B. J., and Roos, R. A. (1998). "Clinimetrics of Postural Instability in Parkinson's Disease," *Journal of Neurology*, **245**, 669–673.
2. Chow, C. C., Lauk, M., and Collins, J. J. (1999). "The Dynamics of Quasi-Static Posture Control," *Human Movement Science*, **18**, 725–740.
3. Constantine, G., Chow, C. C., and Bohnen, N. (2001). "Assessing Postural Rigidity from Quiet Stance in Patients with Parkinson's Disease," *Bulletin of the International Statistical Institute*, Tome LIX, Book 2, pp. 147–159.
4. Gelb, D. J., Oliver, E., and Gilman, S. (1999). "Diagnostic Criteria for Parkinson Disease," *Archives of Neurology*, **56**, 33–39.
5. Horak, F. B., Nutt, J. G., and Nashner, L. M. (1992). "Postural Inflexibility in Parkinsonian Subjects," *Journal of Neurological Science*, **111**, 46–58.
6. Hughes, A. J. (1997). "Clinicopathological Aspects of Parkinson's Disease," *European Neurology*, **38** (Supplement 2), 13–20.
7. Hughes, M. A., Schenkman, M. L., Chandler, J. M., and Studenski, S. A. (1995). "Postural Responses to Platform Perturbation: Kinematics and Electromyography," *Clinical Biomechanics*, **10**, 318–322.
8. Langston, J. W., and Koller, W. C. (1991). "The Next Frontier in Parkinson's Disease: Presymptomatic Detection," *Neurology*, **41** (Supplement 2), 8–13.
9. Lauk, M., Chow, C. C., Lipsitz, L. A., Mitchell, S. L., Collins, J. J. (1999). "Assessing Muscle Stiffness from Quiet Stance in Parkinson's Disease," *Muscle & Nerve*, **22**, 635–639.
10. Quinn, N. (1995). "Parkinsonism-Recognition and Differential Diagnosis," *British Medical Journal*, **310**, 447–452.

Subject Filtering for Passive Biometric Monitoring

Vahan Grigoryan, Donald Chiarulli, and Milos Hauskrecht

University of Pittsburgh, U.S.A.
{vahan, don, milos}@cs.pitt.edu

Abstract: Biometric data can provide useful information about the person's overall wellness. However, the invasiveness of the data collection process often prevents their wider exploitation. To alleviate this difficulty we are developing a biometric monitoring system that relies on nonintrusive biological traits such as speech and gait. We report on the development of the pattern recognition module of the system that is used to filter out nonsubject data. Our system builds upon a number of signal processing and statistical machine learning techniques to process and filter the data, including, Principal Component Analysis for feature reduction, the Naive Bayes classifier for the gait analysis, and the Mixture of Gaussian classifiers for the voice analysis. The system achieves high accuracy in filtering non-subject data, more specifically, 84% accuracy on the gait channel and 98% accuracy on the voice signal. These results allow us to generate sufficiently accurate data streams for health monitoring purposes.

1 Introduction

This research is a part of the "Nursebot Project" which aims to develop a mobile robotic assistant that enables elderly people who are at risk of institutionalization to maintain independence for as long as possible. The goal of this part of the project is to monitor their wellness, detect any relevant change, and report it to the health care professional. Some people are sensitive about intrusion into their life, therefore, we would like to collect the data inconspicuously. The passive monitoring of wellness will give a better idea of a patient's condition to doctors and nurses.

People have always used biological traits, such as voice, face, and gait. to recognize each other. Biometrics emerged as an automated method of identifying individuals or verifying the identity of a person based on distinctive physiological or behavioral characteristics. It is natural to extend biometric analysis systems so that they assess a person's wellness by his/her behavioral and/or physiological traits. The non-intrusion constraint limits our choice of biometric traits mainly to behavioral ones. Our research develops solutions based on two of them: voice and gait.

Passive biometric monitoring in a real-world environment raises one important problem. Data collected by the sensors will include readings from all individuals who enter or leave the environment and will not always be generated by our target subject. Thus, it is very important to filter the data so that only the target subject is monitored and "biometric noise" from other individuals is rejected.

The problem of filtering of non-subject data is related to the problem of machine recognition of human subjects, but there are several important differences. First, we can tolerate a large number of "true-reject" errors. That is, because we deal with a long term monitoring of the subject, and low effective sample rate is not an issue for our system. Second, the sensors are placed in the environment in which we expect the presence of a rather limited number of people, e.g. family, friends, and caregivers. That puts an upper bound to a number of people our system detects besides the subject.

The filtering system described in this paper uses data from three sensors: two microphones and an accelerometer. One of the microphones and the accelerometer are used to collect data about the person's gait, and the other microphone is used to monitor vocalizations. The analysis consists of three steps: (1) feature extraction and reduction, (2) learning of discriminatory patterns and (3) filtering. In the first stage, the dimensionality of the data is reduced to a reasonable size that facilitates further analysis. In the learning stage the features are used to extract discriminatory patterns from labeled signal samples. The patterns use information from all three sensors. Filtering of the signal exploits the patterns learned and applies them to the continuous stream of data to identify the target subject.

In the following section we describe the underlying model and methods used in our system. Next we present the results of experiments with filtering of subject data. Finally, we give the summary in Sect. 4.

2 Model Description

Using gait and voice data, we present the proposed model.

2.1 Gait Analysis

Data Acquisition and Feature Extraction

Our system analyzes gait data collected from a piezoelectronic accelerometer and a microphone at sampling rate of 20KHz. The most significant footstep for each pair of "raw" signals is extracted by detecting the largest peak and taking $N = 10000$ data points in its neighborhood. Further processing is done in spectral domain. We take discrete Fourier Transform of the signal, then we use an ideal lowpass filter with a cutoff frequency of 4KHz.

Since working with 2000 features per sample would be computationally hard, we next have to reduce our feature dimensionality. One of the widely used dimensionality reduction methods is Principal Component Analysis (PCA). PCA performs linear transformation that aligns the transformed axis with the directions of maximum variance (Jolliffe, 2002). Principal components are eigenvectors of the covariance matrix of samples, taken in decreasing order of corresponding eigenvalues, i. e. the first principal component is an eigenvector corresponding to the largest eigenvalue of the (sample) covariance matrix. The first few dimensions of PCA transformed data contain most of information about the data. We keep the first 30 features for each of the samples as our main features for classification purposes.

Classification and Fusion

We use the Naive Bayes model to separate the main subject from the rest (Domingos and Pazzani, 1997). We compute the posterior probability of the subject given the feature vector $\mathbf{x}$,

$$P(\omega_i|\mathbf{x}) = \frac{p(\mathbf{x}|\omega_i)P(\omega_i)}{p(\mathbf{x})}, \tag{1}$$

and use it to discriminate between the subject class and the impostor class. The conditional density function $p(\mathbf{x}|\omega_i)$ is modeled by a multivariate normal density. We make the *naive* assumption that features are independent given the class, thus

$$p(\mathbf{x}|\omega_i) = p(x_1|\omega_i)p(x_2|\omega_i)\dots p(x_n|\omega_i). \tag{2}$$

We apply the maximum likelihood principle (Duda et al., 2001) to estimate the parameters of density functions.

The above mentioned data processing has been done for samples from each channel (vibration from accelerometer and audio from microphone) independently from the other channel. The central issue of this research is to combine data collected from different sensors (Brunelli and Falavigna, 1995; Hong et al., 1999) in order to obtain a better model of the patient's condition.

We build a logistic regression model (Duda et al., 2001) for the fusion of vibration and audio data characterizing the gait. The model uses a set of adaptive weights that determine the importance of audio and vibration signals. The results from the Naive Bayes model are supplied as four inputs to a sigmoidal unit. We employ the online gradient decent approach for weight optimization (Haykin, 1999):

$$\mathbf{w}_{k+1} = \mathbf{w}_k + \rho_k(y_k - f(\mathbf{w}_k, \mathbf{a}_k))\mathbf{a}_k, \tag{3}$$

where $\mathbf{w}_k$ is the weight vector, $\mathbf{a}_k$ is the input vector, y_k is the desired output, and ρ is the parameter that scales the gradient update.

2.2 Voice Analysis

Cepstral feature extraction

Speech spectrum is one of the best known characteristics of a speaker (Atal, 1976). Therefore we proceed with frame-based spectral analysis as described in Reynolds and Rose (1995). We build the spectrogram of the speech signal by taking the short-time Fourier Transform with a Hamming window of length 25.6 ms ($N = 512$). Next we apply mel-scaled filterbank (Stevens and Volkmann, 1940) of 29 overlapping triangular filters to the spectogram magnitude. We obtain the cepstral coefficients $c_m(n)$ by taking the discrete cosine transform of the logarithm of the filterbank output. The cosine transform helps to decorrelate the data, and thus reduces dimensionality. Finally, we form our feature vector from 12 cepstral coefficients. This process is repeated every 12.8 ms, producing about 78 feature vectors per second.

Gaussian Mixture Model

Human speech is a complex audio signal, and due to phonetic diversity it would be extremely hard if not impossible to come up with a simple parametric density model that effectively characterizes the speaker. So it is natural to describe it as a mixture of several density of functions. Gaussian Mixture Model was shown to be quite successful in solving speaker and speech recognition tasks (Reynolds and Rose, 1995; Gopinath, 1998).

The density function of the Gaussian mixture with m components is given by

$$p(\mathbf{x}|\theta) = \sum_{m=1}^{M} w_m f(\mathbf{x}|\boldsymbol{\mu}_m, \Sigma_m), \tag{4}$$

where $\mathbf{x}$ is a feature vector, w_m's denote the *mixing weights* and $f(\mathbf{x}|\boldsymbol{\mu}_m, \Sigma_m)$ are multivariate Gaussians. The parameter θ consists of weights, means and covariances of all component densities.

We use the training data for the target speaker to estimate the mean vectors, weights, and component densities for his/her model. In our model each Gaussian component has a diagonal covariance matrix. We proceed with parameter estimation using the Maximum Likelihood principle. Direct computation of parameters is not possible due to their nonlinearity. Therefore, we estimate the parameters iteratively using the Expectation Maximization (EM) algorithm (Dempster et al., 1977).

Identification is performed by using the Bayes rule and comparing the posterior probabilities of the mixture model for the target person with the mixture model for the rest of the subjects. The details about our experimental data and preliminary results are discussed in the next section.

3 Experimental Results

We conducted our gait identification experiments on data collected from 22 people. For each person there are 10 audio and vibration recordings, collected in 10 different sessions. However for the target person there are 50 recording.

Based on the signal to noise and classification analysis of window length, we set the length of our window to $N = 10000$. The mean signal to noise ratio averaged over the window is equal 2.49 dB for vibration signal and 5.67 dB for audio signal.

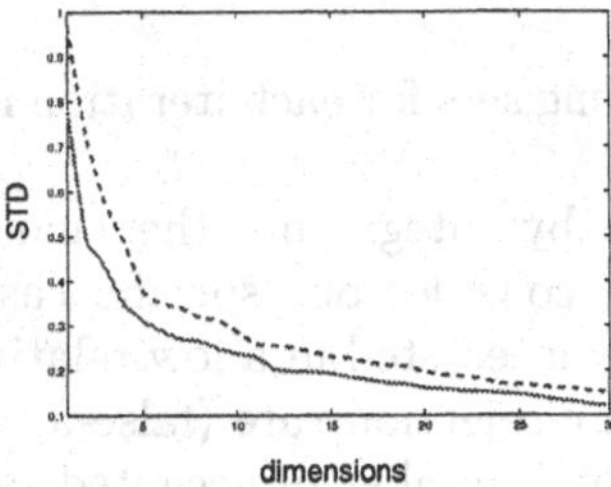

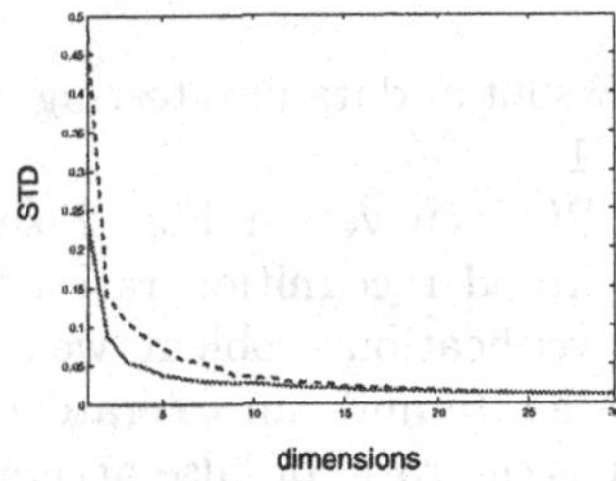

Fig. 1. PCA analysis of impostor and target data. Vibration signal is on the left, audio signal is on the right. The solid line is the standard deviation per dimension for the target subject, the dashed line is the standard deviation per dimension for non-target subjects.

The impostor model in our system is based on data determined not to be from the target subject. We made a preliminary statistical analysis in order to justify the choice of our impostor model. We performed PCA on 50 samples from the target subject and on 50 samples from five non-target subjects. As can be seen from Fig. 1, the PCA transformed data for the mixture of subjects displays more variability than the data for a single subject.

Table 1. Averaged confusion matrix of gait recognition by integrated system of audio and video channels.

		Actual	
		Target	Impostor
Prediction	Accept	4.44%	1.28%
	Reject	14.79%	79.49%

Using combined data from audio and vibration channels, we could identify the target person by his/her gait with about 84% accuracy. The averaged confusion matrix of person recognition by gait based on 30 iterations, and

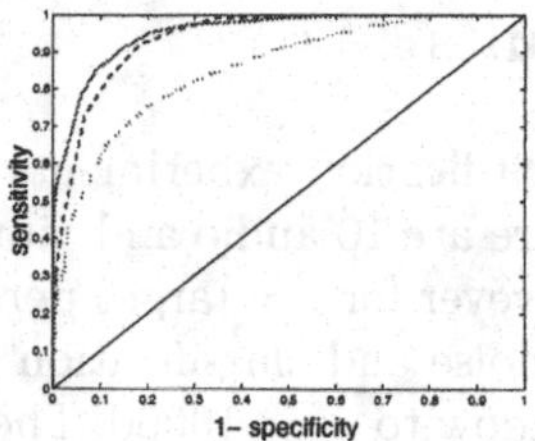

Fig. 2. ROC curves: The solid line is the integrated classifier, the dashed line is the vibration channel only, and the dotted line is the audio channel.

30%-70% split of data into testing and training sets for each iteration is shown in Table 1.

The ROC curves in Fig. 2 show that by integrating the channels we have improved recognition rates. Since we consider our specific case to be a strong verification problem, we are mainly interested in a low relative false-acceptance rate and can tolerate a high false-rejection rate (false-acceptance rate equals the ratio of false-accepts to a total number of accepted samples). That is, because we are conducting long term monitoring, we have access to a very large amount of subject data. Therefore, we can reject a lot of subject data as long as we keep some (in this case about one-fifth). However we would like to include as few non-subject features in our training set as possible.

The preliminary results show a somewhat high relative false-accept rate of 22.38%. This can be explained by the considerably small amount of testing data. In this case only one $(0.0128 * 78 = 0.998)$ falsely accepted feature greatly impacts relative false accept rate. We expect the false-accept rate to drop significantly once we collect a larger body of data and the voice channel is integrated with the gait subsystem.

Voice recognition was performed on speech data collected from 7 people. Each recording is about 1 minute long. We used 10 seconds of each recording for training purposes, and we tested our model on the remaining parts.

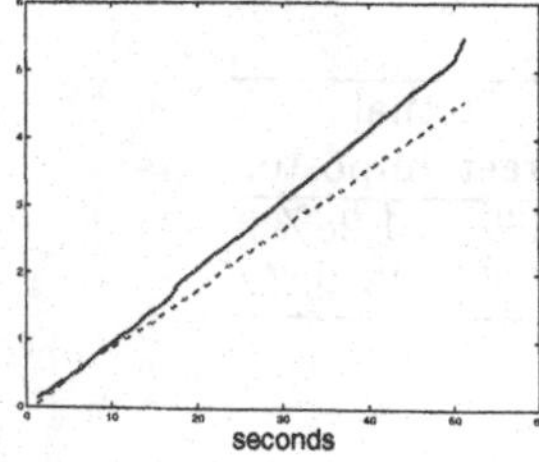

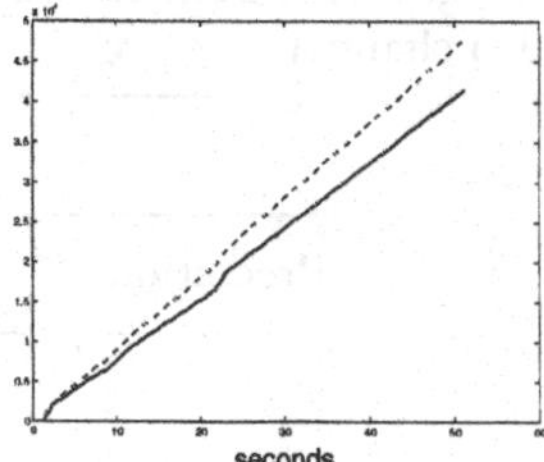

Fig. 3. Posterior probabilities computed with target subject's model (solid line) and the impostor model (dashed line) for the target subject's test data (left) and impostor's test data (right)

It can be seen from Fig. 3 that we are able to verify our target subject with about 10 seconds of speech data. As it was expected, the longer speech sample we are given the more reliable is the authentication. The speech was recorded in a relatively noise-free environment. Because of the low number of subjects and the controlled conditions, person identification using Gaussian Mixture Model was near perfect (over 98% accuracy). We used a mixture of five Gaussians in our subject model. Figure 4 shows the projections of those models into 3D space.

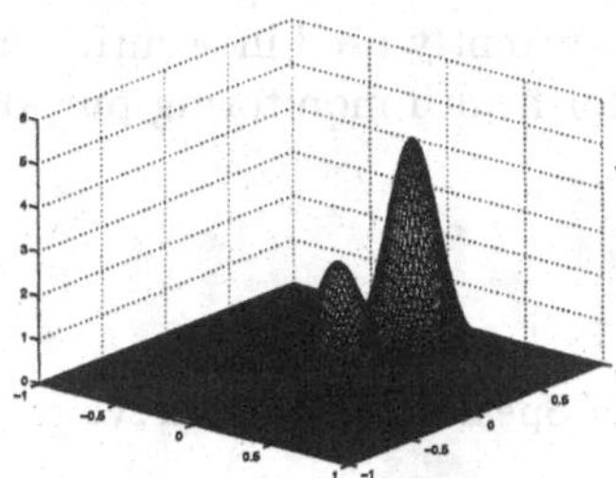

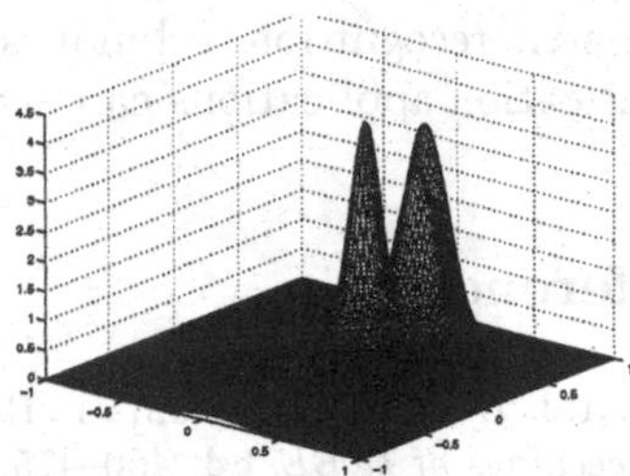

Fig. 4. Projections of twelve-dimensional mixtures of Gaussians into 3D space. The target model is on the left, and the impostor model is on the right.

In general, the accuracy results deteriorate with the number of people in the environment and the background noise. However, in an eldercare environment, the universe of individuals likely to come in contact with the subject is limited, typically consisting of family members and a small population of caregivers. Therefore, good accuracy results in our experiments are likely to be reproduced in real-world settings.

4 Summary and Future Work

We have built subject filtering module for our multimodal system for biometric analysis that relies on data from two audio and a vibration channel. We have shown that strong person verification can be performed using multimodal biometric system based on voice and gait. Our gait analysis subsystem indicates that the performance of the system improves by implementing information fusion of audio and vibration channels.

We introduced a novel approach in the gait recognition, namely the one based on audio and vibration of the foot impact with the floor. The preliminary results show that it is informative enough for our verification task.

The recognition accuracy of the voice channel was very high, though it could have been a result of a small data set and low-noise conditions during data acquisition. Thus we can cautiously expect high accuracy once we integrate it with the gait analysis subsystem.

Our models can effectively be used for the final stage of the research which is the passive monitoring of wellness. One of the approaches we are working on is to compare the current model state with the state which was archived a fixed time period ago. The model state is defined as a metric in the domain of parameters of both subsystems.

The preliminary results encourage further research in the multimodal biometric data fusion for recognition and monitoring. Current computational power at hand allows us to improve existing biometric recognition approaches by collecting biometric data through alternative channels, as we have done with audio- and vibration-based gait analysis. Finally, many of the advanced biometric recognition techniques which are currently used in security and authentication applications can also be used for health monitoring purposes.

References

1. Atal, B. (1976). "Automatic Recognition of Speakers from Their Voices," *Proceedings of IEEE*, **64**, 460–475.
2. Brunelli, R. and Falavigna, D. (1995). "Person Identification Using Multiple Cues," *IEEE Transactions on Pattern Analysis and Machine Intelligence*, **17**, 955-966.
3. Dempster, A. P., Laird, N. M., and Rubin, D. B. (1977). "Maximum Likelihood from Incomplete Data Via the EM Algorithm," *Journal of Royal Statistical Society*, **39**, 1–38.
4. Domingos, P. and Pazzani, M. (1997) "Beyond Independence: Conditions for the Optimality of the Simple Bayesian Classifier," *Machine Learning*, **29**, 103–130.
5. Duda, R. O., Hart, P. E., and Stork, D. G. (2001). *Pattern Classification*, Wiley, New York, 2 ed.
6. Gopinath, R. A. (1998). "Maximum Likelihood Modeling with Gaussian Distributions for Classification," *Proceedings of the International Conference on Acoustics, Speech, and Signal Processing*, **2**, 661–664.
7. Haykin, S. (1999). *Neural Networks: A Comprehensive Foundation*, 2nd ed., Prentice Hall, Upper Saddle River.
8. Hong, L., Jain, A. K., and Pankanti, S. (1999). "Can Multibiometrics Improve Performance?," in *Proceedings of AutoID'99: IEEE Workshop on Automated ID Technologies*, pp. 59–64.
9. Jolliffe, I. T. (2002) *Principal Component Analysis*. Springer, New York, 2 ed.
10. Reynolds, D. A. and Rose, R. C. (1995). "Robust Text-Independent Speaker Identification Using Gaussian Mixture Speaker Models," *IEEE Transactions on Speech and Audio Processing*, **3**, 72–82.
11. Stevens, S. S. and Volkmann, J. (1940). "The Relation of Pitch of Frequency: A Revised Scale," *American Journal of Psychology*, **53**, 329–353.

Part VI

Text Mining

Mining Massive Text Data and Developing Tracking Statistics

Daniel R. Jeske[1] and Regina Y. Liu[2]

[1] University of California at Riverside, U.S.A.
daniel.jeske@ucr.edu
[2] Rutgers University, U.S.A.
rliu@stat.rutgers.edu

Abstract: This paper outlines a systematic data mining procedure for exploring large free-style text datasets to discover useful features and develop tracking statistics, generally referred to as performance measures or risk indicators. The procedure includes text mining, risk analysis, classification for error measurements and nonparametric multivariate analysis. Two aviation safety report repositories *PTRS* from the FAA and *AAS* from the NTSB will be used to illustrate applications of our research to aviation risk management and general decision-support systems. Some specific text analysis methodologies and tracking statistics will be discussed. Approaches to incorporating misclassified data or error measurements into tracking statistics will be discussed as well.

1 Introduction

The recent advances in computing and data acquisition technologies have made the collection of massive amounts of data a routine practice in many fields. Besides the voluminous size, the types of data are also often less traditional. They may be textual, image, functional data, or high-dimensional data without specified models. Statisticians face increasingly the task of analyzing such massive non-standard datasets.

This paper outlines a systematic data mining procedure for some types of large free-style textual report datasets. New data extracting and tracking methodologies are developed using text analysis. Some procedures for constructing and tracking performance measures (PMs) or risk indicators (RIs) are proposed for general quality assurance or risk management programs. The goal of this paper is to develop a comprehensive statistical data mining scheme for text data which should have a broad applicability to many fields.

Using aviation safety as the main focus, two aviation safety report repositories *PTRS* (Program Tracking and Reporting Subsystem) from the FAA

(Federal Aviation Administration) and *AAS* (Aviation Accident Statistics) from the NTSB (National Transportation Safety Board) will be used to illustrate problem statements as well as applications throughout the paper. Although most examples here are drawn from aviation safety data, the proposed statistical data mining procedure can be a vital element of the decision support system for general quality assurance programs in all domains, including financial, engineering, medical, manufacturing and service.

The paper is organized as follows: Section 2 describes briefly the *PTRS* database and the related challenges in the mining of massive text data. Section 3 contains some approaches in text classification and a general principle for constructing tracking statistics based on the classification outcomes. Using the target hazard "The pilot failed to recognize and mitigate ice conditions", Sections 4 and 5 provide a detailed account of our mining procedure from filtering millions of PTRS reports, building text classifiers, constructing risk indicators, to, finally, developing tracking methodologies for the proposed risk indicator. In addition, several simulation studies are used to illustrate the properties of our proposed procedure. The results show that our procedure is quite effective.

2 Massive Text Data and Statistical Challenges

Massive streaming data are pervasive in many fields and there is an urgent need for effective data mining tools. To be specific, we use the FAA in the aviation domain as an example of where new challenges in statistics are confronted by massive data. We stress that their problems and solutions should be applicable to many other different sectors.

One of the primary responsibilities of the FAA is monitoring and regulating the security and safety of air transportation. To ensure compliance with federal aviation regulations, the FAA regularly performs surveillance inspections on aviation entities such as air carriers, and flight training schools. These inspection activities are documented in several FAA databases. Most FAA databases contain massive numerical data of measurements as well as textual data in the form of fixed-format or free-style word reports. It is hoped that, with proper analyses, these data should help the FAA identify emerging patterns of aviation risk, and oversee more effectively aviation operations. Many statistical methods have been applied to aviation safety analysis, but the applications so far have focused mostly on the analysis of numerical data in the context of reliability. The textual data in the massive detailed reports provide another rich source of aviation safety information. They should be systematically extracted, organized, and then used to help manage aviation risk.

We use the FAA *PTRS* database to motivate our approach. There are about a million *PTRS* reports per year. In each report, the inspector: 1) identifies the inspected objects, and the types and areas of inspections performed,

2) records his inspection activities and findings in a free-style write-up, and 3) assigns an opinion-code to rate the overall outcome of the inspection. The choices for opinion-codes are "U" (unacceptable), "P" (potential problem) and "I" (informational). U or P are considered unfavorable ratings, and I is considered favorable. The proportion of the unfavorable reports of a given entity, say an air carrier, over a period of time is used as a performance measure of that carrier. This performance measure helps the FAA determine enforcement decisions and future inspection plans for carriers. Using bootstrap and data depth, several rigorous tracking and thresholding schemes for monitoring the performance measures have been proposed, see e.g. Liu (2003), Cheng, et al. (2000) and Liu et al. (1999).

The tracking of unfavorable proportions of *PTRS* reports provides a quick summary, but it leaves untapped the rich detail findings in the reports. To help identify emerging safety trends or possible root causes for adverse events, it would be valuable to have a comprehensive statistical mining procedure which can systematically parse the reports and extract information pertinent to the risk management process. Several important statistical issues thus arise:

a) *Extracting relevant features from a sea of reports*;
b) *Constructing a PM (or a RI) as a tractable statistic*;
c) *Derive inference and tracking methods for the proposed PM (RI)*;
d) *Assessing the validity and the reliability of the proposed PM (RI).*

We briefly address here the first three issues. The last generally requires validation from large scale real data, which is discussed in the full project report by Jeske and Liu (2003).

3 Data Mining with Text Analysis

3.1 Develop Training Samples From and For Text Databases

Statistical data mining is the exploration of a large dataset by automatic means with the purpose of discovering meaningful patters or useful features. For textual data, there are additional steps required in the mining process. Namely, screening the data to better align it with subject matter topics of interest and transforming the data to more suitable computational forms.

The topics of interest are partially driven by the owners of the data and the entity responsible for using the data for process improvement. In the context of risk management, the topics might reflect a list of potential hazards that were constructed from classical techniques such as probabilistic safety assessment (PSA) [11] or failure mode and effects analysis (FMEA) [13]

Each topic of interest is mapped to a set of keywords that would be likely to appear in a text report which addresses the topic. The keywords are then used to filter the text reports into a set of candidates that are potentially relevant to the topic. Identifying the keywords is an important step since it reduces the number of reports to be considered in the analysis. If no filtering was done whatsoever, the sensitivity of the ensuing analysis tools such as classifiers would suffer. On the other hand, if the filter is too narrow, then the accuracy of the analysis tools or classifiers will suffer.

Next, the filtered set of reports is classified into two or more disjoint categories that could represent different inferential conclusions about the topic of interest. For example, one category might correspond to a conclusion that a particular event occurred while a second category might correspond to the conclusion that it did not occur. The classification step is usually conducted by a subject matter expert (SME) on the data source. To reduce the effect of possible subjectivity bias in a SME, a consensus classification from two or more SMEs could be used.

The filtered reports with their assigned classes are then saved as the training sample for the purpose of developing a classifier that can classify new reports without the aid of the SMEs. Text classification is a special case of general classification or model selection. We briefly describe this subject below. More complete details can be found in Liu et al (2002).

3.2 Text Classification

Text classification (or text categorization) plays an important role in information retrieval, machine learning, and "computer-aided diagnosis" in medical fields. The most well known text classification method is perhaps the "*naive Bayes classifier*", as studied in, for example, Spiegelhalter and Knill-Jones (1984), Lewis (1998), and Hastie et al. (2001). There are at least three basic variations of this classifier: the independent binary model, the multinomial model and the Poisson model. They have been applied in Liu et al (2002) to study the reliability of the assignment of opinion-codes in *PTRS* reports. The approaches used there can be modified and applied to perform the task of classifying "FAILURE", "SUCCESS" and "SKIP" reports as described in Section 4 pertaining to the monitoring of specific aviation hazards.

Specifically, the task in Liu et al (2002) is to classify each report to exactly one of m disjoint *classes*, $\{C_1, C_2, \cdots, C_m\}$. (In the case of *PTRS*, $m = 3$, indicating P, U or I.) Each report needs to be transformed into a mathematical expression suitable for manipulation in a probability framework. In our case, we express a report as a vector indexed by a set of words. This set generally contains the words used across all classes, and is referred to as *the bag of words.* To streamline the bag of words, we can preprocess reports by stemming the words, namely replacing words by their roots, e.g. replacing "leaks", "leaked", "leaking" by "leak". The preprocessing often also includes removing non-informative words, also called "stopword", e.g. "the", "there", etc. Assume that there are V words in *the bag of words.* The notation V denotes both the size and (more loosely) the ordered set of all the words in the bag, i.e., $V = \{w_1, w_2, \cdots, w_V\}$ where w_i represents the i-th word in the bag. A report is expressed as a set of random variables as

$D \equiv (X_1, \cdots, X_V)$. Here X_i indicates how the i-th word in the bag of words is represented in the report D. With these notations, the Bayes rule can be expressed as follows: $Pr(C = k|D) = \frac{Pr(C=k)}{Pr(D)} Pr(D|C = k)$. The so-called naive Bayes classifier is derived from the above Bayes rule and the additional assumption that $X_1, \cdots, X_V$ are conditionally independent given C. By assuming different probability distributions for X_i's, we eventually obtain different classification models. For example, X_i assumes binary values $\{0, 1\}$ in the independent binary model, and count-values in the Poisson and the multinomial models. The multinomial model is obtained by fixing the length of the report in the Poisson model. In the simplest case of $m = 2$ (e.g. I (favorable) v.s. PU (unfavorable) in *PTRS*), report D is assigned to class 1 if $\log Pr(C = 1|D)/1 - Pr(C = 1|D) > 0$. The logarithm form is used for computational efficiency and for its link to the so-called *weight of evidence*.

In the independent binary model, with $p_{jk} = P(X_j = 1|C = k)$, we have

$$\log \frac{Pr(C = 1|D)}{1 - Pr(C = 1|D)} = \log \frac{Pr(C=1)}{1-Pr(C=1)} + \sum_{j=1}^{V} \log \frac{(1-p_{j1})}{(1-p_{j2})} + \sum_{j=1}^{V} x_j \log \frac{p_{j1}(1-p_{j2})}{p_{j2}(1-p_{j1})}.$$

In the Poisson model, we have

$$\log \frac{Pr(C = 1|D)}{1 - Pr(C = 1|D)} = \log \frac{Pr(C = 1)}{1 - Pr(C = 1)} + \sum_{j=1}^{V} (\lambda_{2j} - \lambda_{1j}) + \sum_{j=1}^{V} x_j \log \frac{\lambda_{1j}}{\lambda_{2j}}.$$

Here $\lambda_{kj} = E(X_j|C = k)$, which can be estimated by $\hat{\lambda}_{kj} = \frac{\sum_{i=1}^{N} X_{j(i)} I\{C_{(i)}=k\}}{\sum_{i=1}^{N} I\{C_{(i)}=k\}}$, where N is the total number of reports in the training sample, and the i-th report with its class is denoted by $(X_{1(i)}, \cdots, X_{V(i)}, C_{(i)})$. In the multinomial model, we have

$$\log \frac{Pr(C = 1|D)}{1 - Pr(C = 1|D)} = \log \frac{Pr(C=1)}{1-Pr(C=1)} + \log \frac{Pr(\sum_j x_j|C=1)}{Pr(\sum_j x_j|C=2)} + \sum_{j=1}^{V} x_j \log \frac{\lambda_{1j}/\sum_k \lambda_{1k}}{\lambda_{2j}/\sum_k \lambda_{2k}}.$$

The terms on the right side of the formulas above can all be estimated from the training sample.

3.3 Construct Tracking Statistics and Tracking Methods

Once a process is set up to extract features from text reports and classify each into the mutually exclusive categories that represent conclusions pertinent to the topic of interest, the problem of making inferences from the classifications must be confronted. A well-defined tracking statistic that concretely measures the level of a suitable attribute and can detect a change of its target level must be constructed.

Constructing the tracking statistic is not as straightforward as it might seem. Consider, for example, the relatively simple context where the classification results in conclusions that either a particular event occurred or it did not occur. Interest in this case would be on the frequency of the event and how that varies over time. It would seem that one could utilize the predicted occurrences of the event based on the classification outcomes to construct a classical p-chart for the frequency of the event. The pitfall here is that the classification outcomes may be incorrect, and therefore using them as if they were precise to infer the event frequency is faulty. It is well-known (e.g., Bross (1954) and Fleiss (2003)) that misclassification rates, even when they are small, can lead to significant bias in frequency estimates. Thus, an adjusted procedure that accounts for the fallibility of the classifier used in the classification step is required. Tracking classification errors, especially in the context of machine learning and information retrieval, has attracted much attention lately, and numerous proposals have been put forth to address this issue. For example, there are annual competitions of *TDT* (Topic Detection and Tracking) Technology sponsored by NIST, and of *SIGIR* (Special Interest Group on Information Retrieval) sponsored by ACM.

It is not possible to define a general tracking statistic that applies to all data mining applications. It will depend quite heavily on both the topic of interest as well as the categories defined in the classification step. Our example on the analysis of the PTRS reports that follows in the next two sections will illustrate the important features of the process one must go through, to both define the tracking statistic and also derive the tracking methodology.

4 Example: A Text-Based Classifier

4.1 Context

Returning to the previously introduced FAA context, we consider the topic of interest to be the hazard "Pilot failure to recognize and mitigate ice conditions." This hazard is often identified in the AAS from NTSB as one of the leading causes of aviation accidents. In what follows, we work through the details of extracting a training sample and developing a classifier. In the next section, we construct a tracking statistic and develop a tracking methodology.

4.2 Training Sample

Our training sample was developed from all the *PTRS* reports that were collected in 1998, about 1.2 million in total. We filtered the reports using the following keywords: ice, icing, de-ice, de-icing, and anti-ice. As a result of our filter, we were left with 3,760 *PTRS* reports. We then elicited the opinion of two FAA subject matter experts to read these reports and place them into one of the three respective populations. The three populations correspond to

"FAILURE", the pilot failed to recognize and mitigate ice conditions, "SUCCESS" the pilot did not fail to recognize and mitigate ice conditions, and "SKIP" to indicate this comment is not pertinent to a context where the pilot's ability to recognize and mitigate ice conditions was tested. An example of the latter would be a report that included reference to the word "ice" in connection with ice cubes or ice trays. The SME classification resulted in $m_1 = 61$ reports in "FAILURE", $m_2 = 1,030$ reports in "SUCCESS" and $m_3 = 2,669$ reports in "SKIP". The processing of the training sample of *PTRS* reports is outlined in Figure 1.

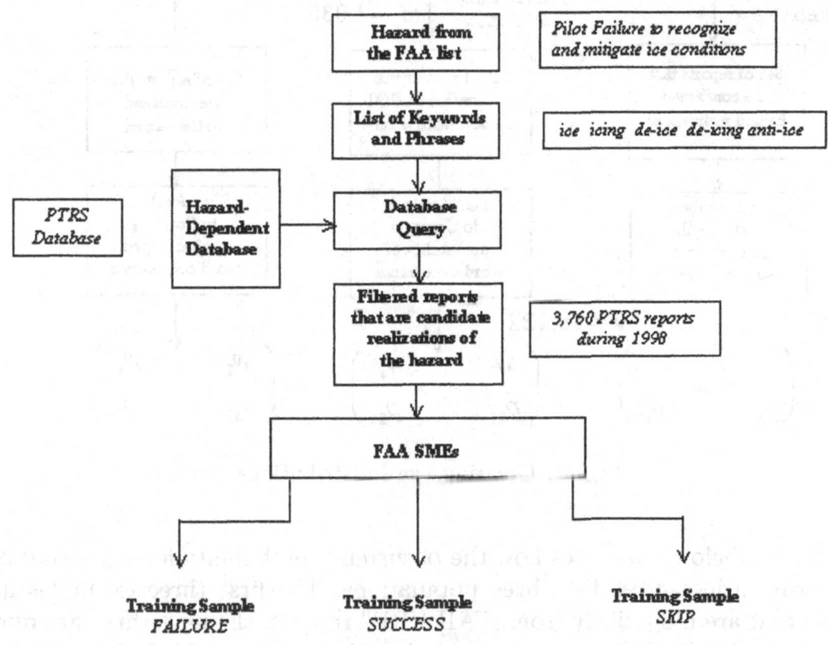

Fig. 1. Processing of *PTRS* training data set.

4.3 Developing the Classifier

Next, the set of 3,760 reports was read and a bag of $v = 16,122$ words was created. We denote the bag of words by $\{w_j\}_{j=1}^{v}$. The samples of reports within each of the three populations were then used to estimate the (marginal) probability that each of the words appears in a (filtered) report. We denote these probabilities respectively by $\{p_{1j}\}_{j=1}^{v}$, $\{p_{2j}\}_{j=1}^{v}$ and $\{p_{3j}\}_{j=1}^{v}$, following the binary approach mentioned in Section 3. In what follows, we shall assume the sample sizes within each of the three populations is large enough that the statistical error of the estimates is negligible. Figure 2 summarizes the analysis described thus far. As examples of some of the words that appear in the bag of words, and also for a subsequent example we shall use, we note that $w_{3229} = accumulation$, $w_{6258} = de-ice$, $w_{12002} = pilot$, $w_{14066} = snow$, $w_{15915} = wing$.

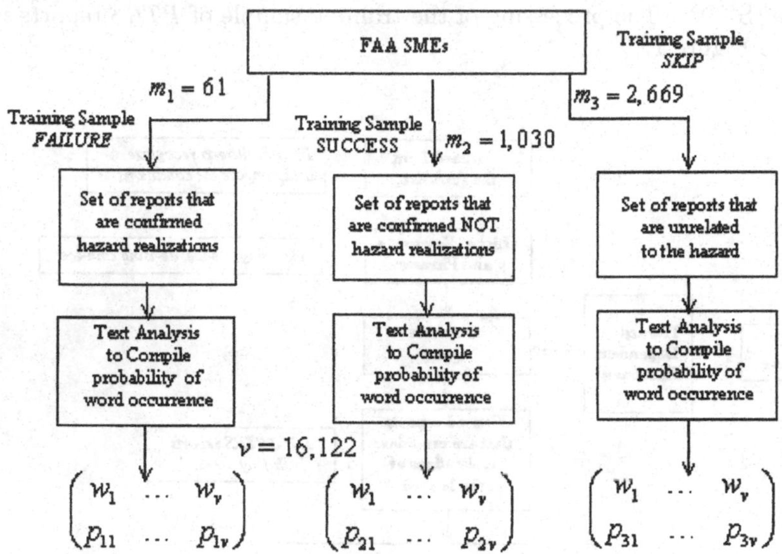

Fig. 2. Creating word distributions.

Table 1 below illustrates how the occurrence probability for a selected set of words varies across the three populations. The first three examples are words that are more likely from "FAILURE" reports, the next three are more likely from "SUCCESS" reports and the last three are more likely from "SKIP" reports.

The effectiveness of our classifier is predicated on the premise that many of the words are correlated to reports from a particular population. Words that are equally likely in all three populations have no discriminatory power. On the other hand, words whose appearance in a report makes it more likely the report is describing one of the three populations have potential to steer the classifier toward making correct predictions.

Suppose a new *PTRS* report has survived the initial filter of keywords. We desire to place it into one of the three populations. Let $\mathbf{X} = (X_1, \ldots, X_v)$ denote the binary vector whose i-th coordinate is unity (zero) if w_i appears (or does not appear) in the report. Note that prior to observing $\mathbf{X}$, we have the empirical probability (based on the training sample obtained from the 1998 *PTRS* reports) that the report belongs to each of the three populations is given

Table 1. Example word probabilities for each population.

WORD	FAILURE	SUCCESS	SKIP
aircraft	.68	.33	.22
wing	.54	.26	.07
pilot	.54	.14	.05
maintenance	.07	.16	.08
inspection	.09	.14	.09
ramp	.07	.10	.05
procedure	.07	.10	.15
fluid	.04	.07	.10
temperature	.07	.05	.08

by: $Pr(FAILURE) = 1.6\%$, $Pr(SUCCESS) = 27.4\%$ and $Pr(SKIP) = 71\%$. Under the assumption that words appear in the report independently, it follows that the posterior conditional probabilities (given **X**) that the report belongs to each of the three populations are proportional to

$$\begin{aligned} Pr(FAILURE|\mathbf{X}) &\propto m_1 \prod_{j=1}^{v} p_{1j}^{X_j}(1-p_{1j})^{1-X_j} \\ Pr(SUCCESS|\mathbf{X}) &\propto m_2 \prod_{j=1}^{v} p_{2j}^{X_j}(1-p_{2j})^{1-X_j} \\ Pr(SKIP|\mathbf{X}) &\propto m_3 \prod_{j=1}^{v} p_{3j}^{X_j}(1-p_{3j})^{1-X_j}. \end{aligned}$$

Normalizing these expressions so that they sum to unity gives the explicit posterior distribution for which population the report belongs to. Our classifier predicts the report belongs to the population that has the largest posterior probability.

4.4 Applying the Classifier

To illustrate the calculations associated with the classifier, consider the following hypothetical report that survived the keyword filter:

> *Flight crew had to be prompted for de-icing. Pilot was unaware that the wings and tail had approximately 1.5 inch accumulation of snow. Pilot failed to perform a pre flight check prior to flight until prompted by the inspector.*

The coding of this report sets the following indices in **X** to be unity, and the rest of the indices are zero: 7843, 5979, 8436, 15035, 4377, 12420, 7928, 6258, 12002, 15747, 15335, 14897, 14901, 15915, 3713, 14734, 8436, 3876, 409, 476, 3229, 11387, 14066, 12002, 7609, 15035, 11899, 3014, 1221, 7843, 5356, 12325, 15035, 7843, 15429, 12420, 4824 and 9132. Note that these indices map one-to-one to the words that appear in the report.

Using the probabilities $\{p_{1j}\}_{j=1}^{v}$, $\{p_{2j}\}_{j=1}^{v}$ and $\{p_{3j}\}_{j=1}^{v}$, with the values $m_1 = 61$, $m_2 = 1,030$ and $m_3 = 2,669$, it follows that $Pr(FAILURE|\mathbf{X}) =$

99.89%, $Pr(SUCCESS|\mathbf{X}) = .04\%$ and $Pr(SKIP|\mathbf{X}) = .07\%$. Consequently, the classifier would predict this report belongs to the "FAILURE" population, implying the pilot did indeed fail to recognize and mitigate ice conditions.

4.5 Accuracy of the Classifier

To assess the accuracy of the classifier we applied the classifier to each of the 3,760 reports in the training sample. Table 2 below shows the frequencies and conditional fractions of correct and incorrect classifications.

Table 2. Classification results.

Classified Population	True Population FAILURE	SUCCESS	SKIP
FAILURE	50 82%	2 .2%	4 .2%
SUCCESS	6 9.8%	733 75%	262 9.8%
SKIP	5 8.2%	255 24.8%	2403 90%

Although the classifier has reasonably high rates of correct classification for each population, the misclassification rates are not negligible. These misclassifications need be dealt with when we infer risk levels from the frequency of reports that get classified into the "FAILURE" population.

5 Example: Tracking Statistic and Tracking Methodology

5.1 A Tracking Statistic

We now turn our attention to developing a tracking statistic and tracking methodology for the ice hazard. Define three events E_1, E_2 and E_3, respectively, to be the event of a filtered *PTRS* report reflects that a pilot was confronted with ice conditions and failed to carry out his/her responsibilities, that a pilot was confronted with ice conditions and successfully carried out his/her responsibilities, and that a pilot was not confronted with ice conditions. Let $\boldsymbol{alpha} = (\alpha_1, \alpha_2, \alpha_3)$, where $\alpha_i = Pr(E_i), i = 1, 2, 3$,

are the corresponding (unknown) probabilities of the three events, and $\theta(\boldsymbol{\alpha}) = \alpha_1/(\alpha_1 + \alpha_2)$. The parameter $\theta(\boldsymbol{\alpha})$ represents the conditional probability that a filtered *PTRS* report reflects that the pilot fails to recognize and mitigate ice conditions given that his/her ability to do so is tested. High values of $\theta(\boldsymbol{\alpha})$ would be indicative of a hazardous condition and would prompt the FAA to consider remediation actions such as increasing pilot awareness of proper procedures.

If the events E_1, E_2 and E_3 were directly observable, standard techniques could be used to construct a control chart for $\theta(\boldsymbol{\alpha})$. For example, at periodic intervals a sample of reports $X_1, \ldots, X_n$ could be classified as E_1, E_2 or E_3 resulting in an observation $\mathbf{N} = (N_1, N_2, N_3)$ for the count in each event. Obviously, $\mathbf{N}$ has a multinomial distribution with parameters n and $\boldsymbol{\alpha}$, and it can easily be shown that the conditional distribution of N_1, given $N_1 + N_2$, is binomial with parameters $N_1 + N_2$ and $\theta(\boldsymbol{\alpha})$. An appropriate tracking statistic for $\theta(\boldsymbol{alpha})$ would be $U = N_1/(N_1 + N_2)$. Approaches for constructing a p-chart for $\theta(\boldsymbol{\alpha})$ based on $\boldsymbol{alpha}$ are well known. For example, following the arguments in Clopper and Pearson (1934) we show that $L(\boldsymbol{\alpha}) = N_1/[N_1 + N_2 F_{2(N_2+1),2N_1;\gamma}]$ is a $100(1-\gamma)\%$ lower confidence bound for $\theta(\boldsymbol{\alpha})$. Here $F_{\nu_1,\nu_2;\gamma}$ is the upper γ percentile of an F-distribution with numerator and denominator degrees of freedom equal to ν_1 and ν_2, respectively.

In our context, the events E_1, E_2 and E_3 are not observable, but instead are indirectly inferred from the results of a fallible text-based classifier (cf. Section 4). The misclassification rates of the classifier can be organized into a 3×3 matrix $\mathbf{A} = [a_{ij}]$ where a_{ij} is the probability the outcome is classified as E_i, given that it is actually E_j. If the classifier were perfect, $\mathbf{A}$ would simply be an identity matrix. Otherwise, $\mathbf{A}$ is a general matrix whose columns represent discrete probability distributions. We refer to $\mathbf{A}$ as the *proficiency matrix* for the classifier. Running the imperfect classifier on $X_1, \ldots, X_n$ produces an observation $\mathbf{S} = (S_1, S_2, S_3)$ which has a multinomial distribution with parameters n and $\boldsymbol{\beta} = \mathbf{A}\boldsymbol{\alpha}$. Clearly, using the statistic $V = S_1/(S_1 + S_2)$ as a risk indicator for $\theta(\boldsymbol{\alpha})$ is not appropriate since it intends to estimate $\theta(\boldsymbol{\beta}) = \beta_1/(\beta_1 + \beta_2)$ rather than $\theta(\boldsymbol{\alpha})$. In general, $\theta(\boldsymbol{\beta}) \neq \theta(\boldsymbol{\alpha})$ except for some special cases of $\mathbf{A}$ (e.g. $\mathbf{A}$ is the identity matrix).

The effect of simply neglecting unknown misclassifications rates on the estimate of $\boldsymbol{\alpha}$ [and hence $\theta(\boldsymbol{\alpha})$] was first discussed in Bross (1954) for the case of four categories where the categories constituted the populations of a 2×2 contingency table. It was noted that the bias in the estimate obtained by ignoring the misclassification rates can be substantial, even when the misclassification rates are small. Specifically, the bias problem can be conveniently illustrated with the proficiency matrix of the classifier expressed as

$$\mathbf{A} = \begin{bmatrix} a_{11} & 1 - a_{22} \\ 1 - a_{11} & a_{22} \end{bmatrix}.$$

Here a_{11} and a_{22} are the probabilities of correct classification, given the actual outcome was E_1 and $E_2 \equiv E_1^c$, respectively. The classification outcome $\mathbf{S} = (S_1, S_2)$ can be reduced to simply S_1 since $S_2 = n - S_1$. For this particular case, $\theta(\boldsymbol{\alpha})$ and $\theta(\boldsymbol{\beta})$ respectively reduce to simply α_1 and $\beta_1 \equiv a_{11}\alpha_1 + (1 - a_{22})(1 - \alpha_1)$. If the misclassification rates were ignored, then S_1/n would be used as an estimate of α_1. Clearly, depending on the magnitude of a_{11} and a_{22} there could be appreciable bias in the estimator.

As one might anticipate, the inference for $\theta(\boldsymbol{\alpha})$ based on $\mathbf{S} = (S_1, S_2, S_3)$ through $\theta(\boldsymbol{\beta})$ is not straightforward. For a preset type I error γ, let H denote the event $\{\theta(\boldsymbol{\beta}) \geq L(\mathbf{S})\}$. It follows that

$$Pr(H) \equiv P[\theta(\boldsymbol{\beta}) \geq L(\mathbf{S})] = 1 - \gamma.$$

It can be shown that H is equivalent to the event

$$\{\beta_1[1 - L(\mathbf{S})] - \beta_2 L(\mathbf{S}) \geq 0\}.$$

Using the relationship $\boldsymbol{\beta} = \mathbf{A}\boldsymbol{\alpha}$, it follows that H is equivalent to the event $\{[a_{11} - (a_{11} + a_{21})L(\mathbf{S})]\alpha_1 + [a_{12} - (a_{12} + a_{22})L(\mathbf{S})]\alpha_2 + [a_{13} - (a_{13} + a_{23})L(\mathbf{S})]\alpha_3 \geq 0\}$. Dividing this expression by $(\alpha_1 + \alpha_2)$ and then isolating $\theta(\boldsymbol{\alpha})$, we can show that H is equivalent to the following event

$$\left[\theta(\boldsymbol{\alpha}) \geq \frac{[(a_{13} + a_{23})L(\mathbf{S}) - a_{13}] \times [\alpha_3/(1 - \alpha_3)] + [(a_{12} + a_{22})L(\mathbf{S}) - a_{12}]}{[a_{11} - (a_{11} + a_{21})L(\mathbf{S})] - [a_{12} - (a_{12} + a_{22})L(\mathbf{S})]}\right].$$

For convenience, let

$$B(\alpha_3, \mathbf{A}\ , L(\mathbf{S})) \equiv \frac{[(a_{13} + a_{23})L(\mathbf{S}) - a_{13}] \times [\alpha_3/(1 - \alpha_3)] + [(a_{12} + a_{22})L(\mathbf{S}) - a_{12}]}{[a_{11} - (a_{11} + a_{21})L(\mathbf{S})] - [a_{12} - (a_{12} + a_{22})L(\mathbf{S})]}.$$

Except for the fact that α_3 and $\mathbf{A}$ are unknown, $B(\alpha_3, \mathbf{A}, L(\mathbf{S}))$ would be a valid lower $(1 - \gamma)$ confidence bound for $\theta(\boldsymbol{\alpha})$. Determining the *best way* to proceed from here is part of our on-going research. However, one practical approach when the training data set is sufficiently large is to replace $\mathbf{A}$ by an estimator, $\hat{\mathbf{A}}$, obtained from a cross-validation analysis on the training dataset and to replace α_3 by the third components of $\hat{\boldsymbol{\alpha}} = \hat{\mathbf{A}}^{-1}\hat{\boldsymbol{\beta}}$. The result is an approximate lower $100(1-\gamma)\%$ confidence bound for $\theta(\boldsymbol{\alpha})$. The tracking statistic, or risk indicator, can now formally be defined as $RI = B[\hat{\alpha}_3, \hat{\mathbf{A}}, L(\mathbf{S})]/\theta_0$, where θ_0 is a target value for $\theta(\boldsymbol{\alpha})$. The condition $RI > 1$ implies θ_0 is smaller than the (approximate) lower confidence bound, and therefore a size γ test of the hypothesis $H_0 : \theta(\boldsymbol{\alpha}) = \theta_0$ versus $H_a : \theta(\boldsymbol{\alpha}) > \theta_0$ would be rejected. That is, $RI > 1$ is equivalent to the evidence that $\theta(\boldsymbol{\alpha})$ has increased above the target value θ_0.

5.2 Sensitivity of Tracking Statistics

A natural question to ask next is how sensitive is RI to changes in the value of $\theta(\boldsymbol{\alpha})$. In particular, as $\theta(\boldsymbol{\alpha})$ increases beyond θ_0 we would hope that RI reacts quickly and that the probability $RI > 1$ also increases quickly. Figure 3 demonstrates the sensitivity by graphing $Pr(RI > 1)$ versus θ.

Here the function $Pr(RI > 1)$ was estimated by simulating 1000 observations of $\mathbf{S} = (S_1, S_2, S_3)$ and calculating the fraction of observations that

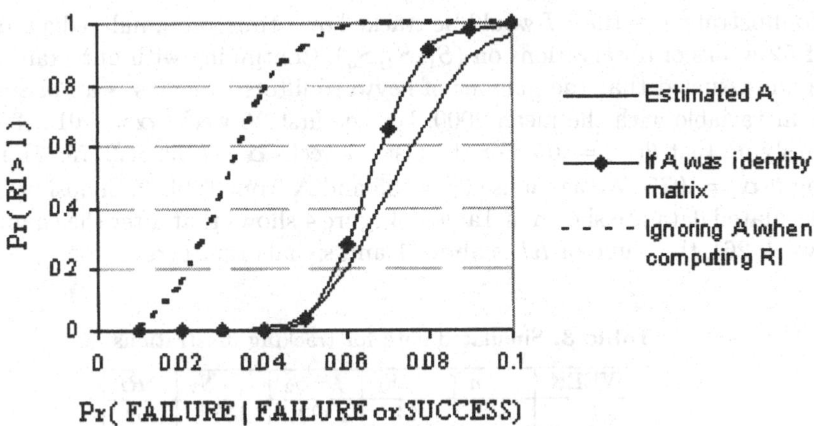

Fig. 3. Sensitivity of the risk indicator.

produce the event $RI > 1$. A Poisson distribution with the mean 2000 was used to simulate n, the number of filtered *PTRS* reports. Observations for $\mathbf{S} = (S_1, S_2, S_3)$ were then obtained by sampling from a multinomial distribution with parameters n and $\boldsymbol{\beta} = \mathbf{A}\boldsymbol{\alpha}$, where $\alpha_3 = .7$ and (α_1, α_2) are such that $\alpha_1 + \alpha_2 = .3$ and $\theta(\boldsymbol{\alpha}) \in \{.01, .02, \ldots, .1\}$. Each observation was then used to calculate RI with $\theta_0 = .05$.

The solid curve in Figure 3 is the case where we have used $\hat{\mathbf{A}}$ from Table 2 as though it were the true $\mathbf{A}$. We used $\gamma = .05$ to make $Pr(RI > 1|\theta = \theta_0) = .05$, but we can see that the probability quickly increases toward unity as θ increases beyond θ_0. The curve overlaid with points in Figure 3 corresponds to the case where $\mathbf{A}$ is the identity matrix, which would be appropriate if the classifier was perfect. Comparisons with the solid curve illustrate the diminished sensitivity of RI when the classifier makes errors. Clearly, the comparison shows it is important for the classifier to be as accurate as possible.

The dotted curve in Figure 3 is a different type of sensitivity study. In this case, we used $\hat{\mathbf{A}}$ from Table 2 when generating the observations (S_1, S_2, S_3), but we naively assumed that $\mathbf{A}$ was the identity when calculating RI. The purpose of this analysis was to investigate what would happen if we simply neglected (or were unaware of) the classification errors when computing RI. As can be seen from Figure 3, the result is a significant increase in type-I error. Obviously, naively assuming the classifier is perfect, when it is not, will lead to many false alarms. This shows that it is critical that our RI accounts for classification errors through the use of $\mathbf{A}$.

5.3 Tracking Methodology

To illustrate how the RI would be tracked over time, we simulated a sequence of 52 weeks of observations on (S_1, S_2, S_3). Continuing with our example, we again assumed that the number of keyword filtered reports is a Poisson random variable with the mean 2000. For the first 26 weeks $\boldsymbol{\alpha} = (.015, .285, .7)$, implying that $\theta(\boldsymbol{\alpha}) = .05$. For the last 26 weeks $\boldsymbol{\alpha} = (.0225, .2775, .7)$, implying $\theta(\boldsymbol{\alpha}) = .075$. We again used $\gamma = .05$ and $\hat{\mathbf{A}}$ from Table 2. Snapshots of the simulated data are shown in Table 3. Figure 4 shows that after the changeover (week 26), the value of RI is above 1 and signals that $\theta(\boldsymbol{\alpha}) > .05$.

Table 3. Simulated data for tracking illustrations.

WEEK	n	S_1	S_2	S_3	RI
1	1925	43	499	1383	.52
2	1992	34	472	1486	.22
.	.	.	.	.	.
26	2024	112	473	1439	.52
27	2059	70	510	1479	1.31
28	1995	64	483	1448	1.23
.	.	.	.	.	.
52	2036	64	511	1461	1.13

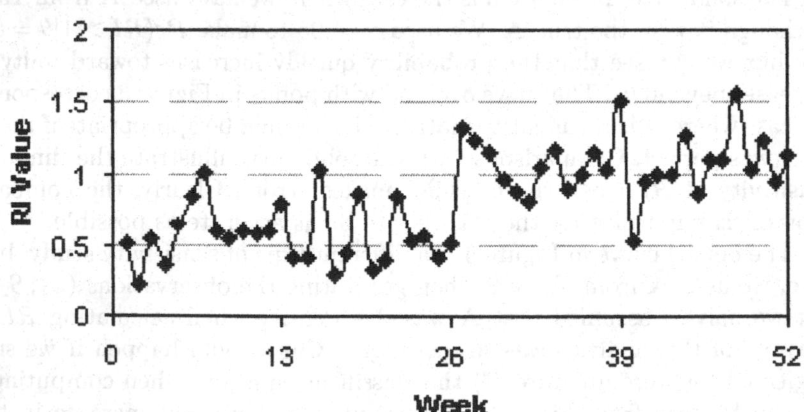

Fig. 4. Simulated RI values for tracking illustration.

6 Further Developments

The text classification approaches discussed in this paper can be developed further to improve the performance of the classifiers. To begin with, we may consider building the bag of words by including some feature selections. We plan to explore the following feature selections: 1) setting thresholds for the required minimum word frequencies or selecting suitable χ^2 values as thresholds to reduce the size of the bag of words, 2) combining highly positively correlated words into phrases as features, and 3) assigning higher weights to more relevant words in the subject, for example, certain pejorative words in $PTRS$ reports which appear to have strong indication of unfavorable outcomes.

In addition to the three approaches for text classification described in Section 3, other approaches such as the boosting and the SVM (support vector machines) methods have met with some success in information retrieval (see for example Hastie et al. (2001)). It would be interesting to see if these two methods can improve our data mining procedure.

In this paper we have constructed the tracking statistic RI and developed an inference procedure under the multinomial framework. Another direction is to consider tracking statistics based on m_1 under the framework of a non-stationary Poisson process change point problem.

Finally, we plan to search for approaches that can account for misclassifications more accurately in the inference stage, including formulating conservative confidence bounds for the tracking statistics.

Acknowledgments

This research is supported in part by grants from the *National Science Foundation*, the *National Security Agency*, and the *Federal Aviation Administration*. The authors thank Ms. Lixia Pei and Ms. Qi Xia for their computing assistance. The discussion on aviation safety in this paper reflects the views of the authors, who are solely responsible for the accuracy of the analysis results presented herein, and does not necessarily reflect the official view or policy of the FAA. The dataset used in this paper has been partially masked in order to protect confidentiality.

References

1. Bross, I. (1954). "Misclassification in 2×2 Tables," *Biometrics*, **10**, 478–486.
2. Cheng, A., Liu, R. and Luxhøj, J. (2000). "Monitoring Multivariate Aviation Safety Data by Data Depth: Control Charts and Threshold Systems," *IIE Transactions on Operations Engineering*, **32**, 861–872.
3. Clopper, C., and Pearson, E. (1934). "The Use of Confidence or Fiducial Limits Illustrated in the Case of the Binomial," *Biometrika*, **26**, 404–413.

4. Fleiss, J. L. (2003). *Statistical Methods for Rates and Proportions*, John Wiley & Sons, New York.
5. Jeske, D., and Liu, R. (2003). "Measuring Risk or Performance from a Sea of Text Data," Technical Report, Dept. of Statistics, Rutgers University.
6. Hastie, T., Tibshirani, R., and Friedman, J. (2001). *The Elements of Statistical Learning, Data Mining, Inference, and Prediction*, Springer, New York.
7. Lewis, D. (1998). "Naive (Bayes) at Forty: The Independence Assumption in Information Retrieval," in *ECML '98: Tenth European Conference on Machine Learning*, pp. 4–15.
8. Liu, R. (2003). "BootQC—Bootstrap for a Robust Analysis of Aviation Safety Data," in *Developments in Robust Statistics*, eds. R. Dutter et al., Heidelberg:Springer, pp. 246–258.
9. Liu, R., Madigan, D., and Eheramendy, S. (2002). "Text Classification for Mining Massive Aviation Inspection Report Data," in *Statistical Data Analysis Based on L_1 Norm and Related Methods*, ed. Y. Dodge, Birkhäuser, pp. 379–392.
10. Liu, R., Parelius, M., and Singh, K. (1999). "Multivariate Analysis by Data Depth: Descriptive Statistics, Graphics and Inference (with discussion)," *Annals of Statistics*, **27**, 783–858.
11. International Atomic Energy Agency, (1992). *Probabilistic Safety Assessment*, Safety Reports Safety Series, **75**.
12. Spiegelhalter, D., and Knill-Jones, R. (1984). "Statistical and Knowledge Based Approaches to Clinical Decision Support Systems, with an Application in Gastroenterology (with discussion)," *Journal of the Royal Statistical Society, Series A*, **147**, 35–77.
13. US MIL-STD-1629. *Failure Mode and Effects Analysis*. National Technical Information Service, Springfield, VA.

Contributions of Textual Data Analysis to Text Retrieval

Simona Balbi and Emilio Di Meglio

University of Naples, Italy
{sb,edimegli}@unina.it

Abstract: The aim of this paper is to show how Textual Data Analysis techniques, developed in Europe under the influence of the Analyse Multidimensionelle des Données School, can improve performance of the LSI retrieval method. A first improvement can be obtained by properly considering the data contained in a lexical table. LSI is based on Euclidean distance, which is not adequate for frequency data. By using the chi-squared metric, on which Correspondence Analysis is based, significant improvements can be achieved. Further improvements can be obtained by considering external information such as keywords, authors, etc. Here an approach to text retrieval with external information based on PLS regression is shown. The suggested strategies are applied in text retrieval experiments on medical journal abstracts.

1 Introduction

The development of Text Mining has been strictly connected with Computer Science and Computational Linguistics. This paper aims at showing how Textual Data Analysis techniques, mainly developed in Europe under the influence of the Analyse Multidimensionelle des Données School, can offer useful tools for knowledge extraction from documents, enhancing a statistical viewpoint. First of all, a deep investigation of the data structure can be helpful in choosing the optimal strategy to be applied in a specific context. Here we show how the introduction in Text Mining procedures of this perspective can give effective results. In the paper, we will consider a widely used tool in Text Retrieval, the Latent Semantic Indexing, showing how it is strictly connected with some assumptions on data and relations among words, not completely acceptable. LSI has been proposed as a statistical tool and many improvements and proposals have been introduced in the last few years. The algebraic tool underlying LSI is the Singular Value Decomposition, which is the core of most multivariate Data Analysis techniques. A crucial point is the nature of the LSI basic matrix: the document-by-term matrix, built according to the bag-of-words encoding. We will show how retrieval results can be improved by considering the matrix to be analyzed as a contingency table. In the following, a discussion related to the choice of a proper metric and weighting system will be presented. Additionally we will show how results obtained in a Textual Data Analysis framework can be useful for dealing with the problem of synonyms and homographs. Results can be additionally improved when we introduce external information on documents (e.g. keywords) by means of PLS method.

2 Latent Semantic Indexing

Latent Semantic Indexing (LSI), introduced by Deerwester et al. (Deerwester et al., 1990) is a Text Retrieval technique, which "tries to overcome the deficiencies of term matching retrieval by treating the unreliability of observed term-document association data as a statistical problem". The algebraic tool is the Singular Value Decomposition (SVD) (Eckart and Young, 1936) on which most multivariate techniques are based (Greenacre, 1984).

Let **A** be a rectangular matrix (n, p) with $n > p$. For sake of simplicity we consider **A** to be of rank p. By SVD **A** can be decomposed into the product of three matrices: $\mathbf{A} = \mathbf{U}\mathbf{\Lambda}\mathbf{V}'$ where $\mathbf{\Lambda}$ (p, p) is a diagonal matrix of the positive numbers λ_α's $(\alpha = 1, 2, \ldots, p)$ called singular values, arranged in decreasing order, **U** (n, p) and **V** (p, p) are orthonormalized matrices, having in columns the left and right singular vectors, respectively.

As $(\mathbf{U}'\mathbf{U}) = (\mathbf{V}'\mathbf{V}) = \mathbf{I}$, the left singular vectors form a p-dimensional orthonormal basis for the columns of **A** in a n-dimensional space and the right singular vectors form an orthonormal basis for the rows of **A** in a p-dimensional space.

SVD allows the best (in the sense of least squares) approximation of **A**, by a lower rank matrix, obtained by multiplying only the first $k << p$ components of **U**, $\mathbf{\Lambda}$, **V**.

LSI computes the SVD of the document-by-term matrix **F** (D, W) which general term $f_{d_x w}$ is the frequency of term w $(w = 1, \ldots, W)$ in document x $(x = 1, \ldots, D)$ according to the bag-of-word encoding (Manning and Schütze, 1999). In Textual Data Analysis **F** is named "lexical table". LSI aims at extracting the hidden semantic structures, determined by term co-occurrence patterns. The retrieval technique consists in projecting queries and documents in a k-dimensional subspace with "latent" semantic dimensions determined using SVD. Documents resulting closest to the query are retrieved. The power of the tool is that, in the latent subspace, a query and a document can be close even if they don't share any term (Manning and Schütze, 1999), as long as the terms are semantically similar. The position in space is therefore a *semantic index* (Deerwester et al., 1990).

The choice of k is crucial: it should be large enough to model the association structure of the data but not too large, for avoiding model noise. In general, no less than 100 dimensions are retained, the number usually selected in most applications being between 150 and 200 (Dumais, 1993).

Despite its efficacy and simplicity, from a statistical point of view, LSI presents several problems. First of all, it is implicitly based on Euclidean distance which is not adequate for the count data collected in **F**: as documents have different lengths, in longer ones, a term may appear several times even if it does not have a big importance; furthermore, a frequent word is not always a meaningful word, as sometimes concepts are conveyed by rarer words. LSI, for its construction, treats frequencies as intensities penalizing, in this way, short documents and rare terms. In literature, these problems are solved by normalizing document vectors and by adopting an appropriate (most of the times subjective) weighting scheme. LSI results greatly depend on the chosen weighting system. In an Analyse des Données framework, by considering **F** as a contingency table, we can find a data driven solution, thanks to Correspondence Analysis (Lebart et al., 1984).

3 Metrics for Text Retrieval

What in LSI literature are considered as weighting strategies can be faced focusing attention on the choice of a proper metric in computing distances among documents.

Our aim is to investigate the role of the metrics adopted in retrieval techniques and to propose the use of a proper one to improve retrieval performances.

All statistical and machine learning algorithms are in fact based on the concepts of distance or dissimilarity between objects. While for numerical data these concepts are easy to model and sometimes are even intuitive or innate, for texts everything is extremely more difficult. A human being when reading different texts is generally able to formulate a judgment on their similarity, based on their meaning. Text Retrieval systems try to mimic this human process. LSI suggests to approximate meanings with semantic contexts and force the use of distance models to measure semantic similarity with a huge degree of simplification.

4 Latent Semantic Correspondence Indexing

LSI in its canonic formulation applies SVD, that is really designed for normally distributed data, not for count data. This problem may be addressed by choosing a proper metric and a proper weighting system before applying SVD.

Correspondence Analysis (CA) is one of the most effective methods for visualizing the semantic associations in lexical tables (Lebart et al., 1998). CA is, in fact, the most suitable technique to deal with large contingency tables in an exploratory framework. Therefore, for Text Retrieval purposes, it could be a solution to all the drawbacks related to the use of Euclidean metric. CA is based on chi-square metric, which is a weighted Euclidean metric. It derives its name from Chi-square statistic χ^2 to which it is related. Chi-square distance measures the distance among profiles, i.e. conditional distributions of rows (documents) on columns (terms) and vice versa. Chi square distance between two w-dimensional document profiles $\mathbf{f_x}$ and $\mathbf{f_y}$ is given by:

$$d_{\chi^2}(\mathbf{f_x}, \mathbf{f_y}) = \sum_{i=1}^{w} \frac{1}{f_{\cdot w}} \left(\frac{f_{d_x w}}{f_{d_x \cdot}} - \frac{f_{d_y w}}{f_{d_y \cdot}} \right)^2 \tag{1}$$

where

$$f_{d_x \cdot} = \sum_{w=1}^{W} f_{d_x w} \quad \text{and} \quad f_{d_y \cdot} = \sum_{w=1}^{W} f_{d_y w} \tag{2}$$

using the matrix formulation

$$d_{\chi^2}(\mathbf{f_x}, \mathbf{f_y}) = (\mathbf{f_x} - \mathbf{f_y})^T \mathbf{D_w}^{-1} (\mathbf{f_x} - \mathbf{f_y}) \tag{3}$$

where $\mathbf{D_w}^{-1}$ is a diagonal matrix containing the marginal distributions of words. This distance, as said, is a weighted Euclidean distance, with the weights being the inverses of the expected relative frequencies i.e. the marginal term distribution. When comparing two term profiles, the weights will be the inverses of relative frequency of documents in the diagonal matrix $\mathbf{D_d}^{-1}$.

In this way the geometry of the row profiles (documents conditional distributions) is directly related to the one of column profiles (terms conditional distributions), hence the name of Correspondence Analysis.

Chi-squared distance has many important properties for textual data analysis. Documents are transformed into profiles, this allows one to compare documents with different length. Furthermore the weighting given by the inverse of relative frequency of terms allows one to not penalize rarer words. This peculiarity of chi-square distance makes it more respondent to the nature of textual data.

The chi-squared distance has an important property called the distributional equivalence. This property allows one to aggregate two columns (or rows) having the same profile without changing the distances between rows (or columns). This is useful when dealing with synonymy and disambiguation problems. Moreover, the latter problems can be addressed by bootstrap strategies for Correspondence Analysis of lexical tables (Balbi, 1995).

4.1 Retrieval Strategy

Here we propose the use of chi-square metric for text retrieval with Latent Semantic Indexing. This approach is equivalent to using Correspondence Analysis for building the latent factors on which retrieval is performed (Di Meglio, 2003). The retrieval strategy is the following:

- Correspondence Analysis is performed on the lexical table.
- A proper number of dimensions is selected, usually not less than 100.
- A query is projected in the latent space as supplementary element.
- Cosine similarity among the query and all the documents are calculated in the latent space and the n closest documents are retrieved.

We call this strategy Latent Semantic Correspondence Indexing (LSCI) as CA can be defined in terms of a Generalized Singular Value Decomposition (GSVD) (Greenacre, 1984). The generalization consists in imposing different normalization constraints both on right and left singular vectors. GSVD of previously introduced matrix $\mathbf{A}$ can be expressed as:

$$\mathbf{A} = \mathbf{U}^*\mathbf{\Lambda}^*\mathbf{V}'^* \tag{4}$$

where the columns of $\mathbf{U}^*$ and $\mathbf{V}'^*$ are orthonormalized as follows:

$$\mathbf{U}'\mathbf{\Omega}\mathbf{U} = \mathbf{V}'\mathbf{\Xi}\mathbf{V} = \mathbf{I}. \tag{5}$$

The $\mathbf{\Omega}$ (n, n) and $\mathbf{\Xi}$ (p, p) are given positive-definite symmetric matrices. The columns of $\mathbf{U}^*$ and $\mathbf{V}^*$ are still orthonormal bases for the columns and the rows of $\mathbf{A}$, but the metrics imposed in the n- and p-dimensional spaces are now weighted Euclidean metrics defined by $\mathbf{\Omega}$ and $\mathbf{\Xi}$ respectively. In CA $\mathbf{\Omega}$ and $\mathbf{\Xi}$ are respectively $\mathbf{D_w}^{-1}$ and $\mathbf{D_d}^{-1}$. In Textual Data Analysis, in specific applicative contexts it has been proposed to use (Balbi, 1995) a variant of CA, namely Non Symmetrical CA (Lauro and D'Ambra, 1984), when we just want to normalize documents with respect to their different lengths. The corresponding retrieval strategy will be based on a GSVD with the following orthonormalizing constraints:

$$\mathbf{U}'\mathbf{U} = \mathbf{V}'\mathbf{D_d}^{-1}\mathbf{V} = \mathbf{I}. \tag{6}$$

It is useful to point out that there is no metric that is absolutely better than other ones in all cases. There will reasonably be different solutions for different problems.

5 Text Retrieval with External Information

In text repositories, in addition to documents, we usually find information often discarded by commonly used Text Retrieval strategies. This external information, if properly considered, could drastically improve performances. A human user, when assessing the similarity between two documents or the relevance of a document uses also external information to support his/her decision.

This information can be explicit (titles, authors, keywords, classifiers, headers) or implicit (collocation, source, time and occasion of issue etc.).

At this respect a strategy for the analysis of lexical tables taking into account external information has been proposed (Amato et al., 2004). The methodological framework is given by causal models: two groups of variables are considered: the first group of variables, arranged in the lexical table $\mathbf{F}$; and the second group, $\mathbf{Y}$, that can be formed by the vocabulary of the external information, arranged as an indicator matrix where 1 indicates the presence of the information and 0 the absence.

The matrix $\mathbf{F}^*$ is obtained by weighting matrix $\mathbf{F}$ by marginal distributions of rows and columns so to consider chi-square metric. The modeling of the non symmetrical relationship between $\mathbf{F}^*$ and $\mathbf{Y}$ and the dimensionality reduction are jointly achieved by means of Partial Least Squares Regression (PLSR) (Wold et al., 1984).

The PLSR Retrieval strategy, here presented, performs retrieval in the subspace spanned by the columns of matrix $\mathbf{Y}$, in which the units (documents) of matrix $\mathbf{F}^*$ are projected.

6 PLS Regression

PLS Regression has been introduced by Svante Wold et al. (Wold et al., 1984) in order to model the non symmetrical relationship between two groups of variables with the aim of maximizing predictive power of the model and to cope with multicollinearity among variables.

Let r be the rank of $\mathbf{F}^*$; we define $\mathbf{F^*}_0 = \mathbf{F}^*$ and $\mathbf{Y}_0 = \mathbf{Y}$. First pair of PLS components $\mathbf{t}_1 = \mathbf{F^*}_0\mathbf{w}_1$ and $\mathbf{u}_1 = \mathbf{Y}_0\mathbf{c}_1$ are such that

$$\begin{cases} \max\limits_{\mathbf{w}_1,\mathbf{c}_1} \operatorname{cov}(\mathbf{F^*}_0\mathbf{w}_1, \mathbf{Y}_0\mathbf{c}_1) \\ \mathbf{w}_1'\mathbf{w}_1 = 1 \\ \mathbf{c}_1'\mathbf{c}_1 = 1 \end{cases}$$

where $\operatorname{cov}(\cdot,\cdot)$ stands for covariance. We now denote residual matrix $\mathbf{F^*}_1 = \mathbf{F^*}_0 - \mathbf{t}_1\mathbf{p}_1$ and $\mathbf{Y}_1 = \mathbf{Y} - \mathbf{t}_1\mathbf{c}_1$, where $\mathbf{p}_1 = \mathbf{F^*}_0'\mathbf{t}_1/\mathbf{t}'\mathbf{t}_1$ and $\mathbf{c}_1 = \mathbf{Y}'\mathbf{t}_1/\mathbf{t}'\mathbf{t}_1$. The second pair of PLS components $\mathbf{t}_2 = \mathbf{F^*}_1\mathbf{w}_2$ and $\mathbf{u}_2 = \mathbf{Y}_1\mathbf{c}_2$ are such that

$$\begin{cases} \max\limits_{\mathbf{w}_2,\mathbf{c}_2} \operatorname{cov}(\mathbf{F^*}_1\mathbf{w}_2, \mathbf{Y}_1\mathbf{c}_2) \\ \mathbf{w}_2'\mathbf{w}_2 = 1 \\ \mathbf{c}_2'\mathbf{c}_2 = 1 \\ \mathbf{w}_1\mathbf{F^*}_0'\mathbf{F^*}_1\mathbf{w}_2 = 0. \end{cases}$$

The last constraint in the above system ensures $\mathbf{t}_1$ and $\mathbf{t}_2$ to be orthogonal to each other. A generic pair h of PLS component is given by solving

$$\begin{cases} \max\limits_{\mathbf{w}_h,\mathbf{c}_h} \operatorname{cov}(\mathbf{F^*}_{h-1}\mathbf{w}_h, \mathbf{Y}_{h-1}\mathbf{c}_h) \\ \mathbf{w}_h'\mathbf{w}_h = 1 \\ \mathbf{c}_h'\mathbf{c}_h = 1 \\ \mathbf{w}_h'\mathbf{F^*}_{h-1}'\mathbf{F^*}_{j-1}\mathbf{w}_j = 0, \forall j < h. \end{cases}$$

The columns of matrix $\mathbf{W}_{(h)}$, $\mathbf{w}_1, \mathbf{w}_2, \ldots, \mathbf{w}_h$, give PLS components $\mathbf{t}$ by means of residual matrix $\mathbf{F}^*_{h-1}$; in order to compute the $\mathbf{t}$'s by means of original matrix $\mathbf{F}^*$, we use a transformation of $\mathbf{W}_{(h)}$:

$$\tilde{\mathbf{W}}_{(h)} = \mathbf{W}_{(h)} \left(\mathbf{P}'_{(h)}\mathbf{W}_{(h)}\right)^{-1}.$$

At each step $h = 1, 2, \ldots, r$, PLS regression maximizes covariance between components of residuals matrices $\mathbf{F}^*_h$ and $\mathbf{Y}_h$.We can see PLS regression as a compromise between canonical correlation analysis (maximum correlation between $\mathbf{t}_h$ and $\mathbf{u}_h$) and OLS regression on principal component analysis (maximum variance of $\mathbf{t}_h$ and $\mathbf{u}_h$).

7 PLS Retrieval Strategy

As described in the previous section, the first step of PLS performs a SVD of $\mathbf{F}^{*\prime}\mathbf{Y}$. Being $\mathbf{Y}$ an indicator matrix, non zero elements of $\mathbf{F}^{*\prime}\mathbf{Y}$ represent co–presence of keywords and terms.

The proposed retrieval strategy is carried out in three steps:

- PLS Regression of $\mathbf{F}^*$ on $\mathbf{Y}$; computation of PLS components ($\mathbf{T}$) and selection of relevant components by means of the Q^2 index (Tenenhaus, 1998).
- Projection of query vectors $\mathbf{v}_q$, $q = 1, 2, \ldots,$ number of queries on the built subspace; this is performed by applying the following formula:

$$\mathbf{z}_q = \mathbf{v}_q\tilde{\mathbf{W}} \tag{7}$$

  where h is the selected number of components and $\mathbf{z}_q$ is a row vector of h elements.
- Retrieval of relevant documents. This step is done by calculating the cosine between the projected query $\mathbf{z}_q$ and all projections of documents; for each query q, the distances d_{qi} obtained are sorted in ascending order and, the first k documents are retrieved as the most relevant to query q, according to the number of documents required by the user.

8 Application to OHSUMED data

The proposed strategies have been applied to a dataset extracted from the OHSUMED collection compiled by William Hersh (OHSUMED is available from ftp://medir.ohsu.edu in the directory /pub/ohsumed). This collection consists of medical journal abstracts. For each abstract, the author, keywords, and journal title are provided.

We have selected a subset of 963 documents with relative keywords and have used keywords as external information. Ten queries have been built and relevance of documents to these queries has been assessed by three independent judges. LSCI and PLS retrieval strategy have been compared with classical LSI. Performance has been measured with precision index that ranges between 0 and 1. Precision measures the proportion of documents that the system got right. Precision has been calculated, in order to take into account the rankings, at different *cutoff* points, that is, considering different numbers of retrieved documents. Usual cutoff points are 5, 10, 20 documents. We have used cutoff 1,2,...,10. For PLS retrieval 36 components have been selected using Cross Validation. For LSI and LSCI 79 components have been selected according to the criterion of explicated inertia decay.

In Figure 1 the precision plots of LSI and LSCI are shown.

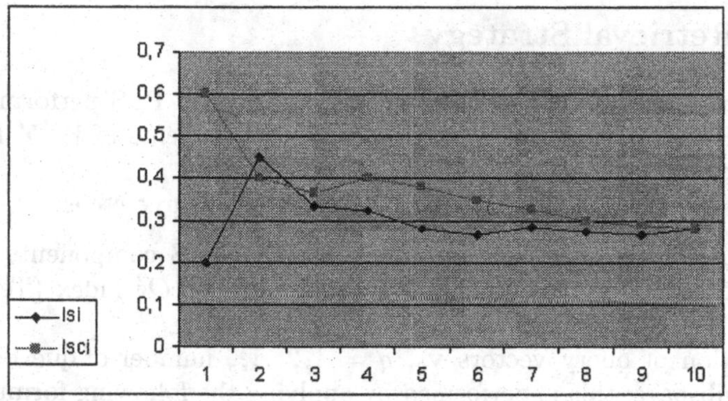

Fig. 1. Average Precision plot of LSI and LSCI compared on ten queries using 1,...,10 cutoff points.

LSCI significantly outperforms LSI, especially at low cutoff points. In particular, after a deeper examination of queries and retrieved documents it appears that LSI tends to give higher rank to documents in which the words used in the query have high occurrence and tends to prefer longer documents. With LSCI there is a significant gain in precision due to the proper consideration of document length and word frequencies. Furthermore in queries where a frequent and a rare but characterizing word were together LSI retrieved documents containing only the high frequency word and therefore not relevant to the query.

In Figure 2 the precision plots of LSCI and PLS retrieval are shown.

In some cases PLS retrieval strategy performed slightly better than LSCI, in other ones equally. To a deeper exam of queries and retrieved documents it results that PLS retrieved the same documents of LSCI but also some documents more similar to the query in terms of *meaning*, even if they did not share any word with the query. This happens because also keywords are

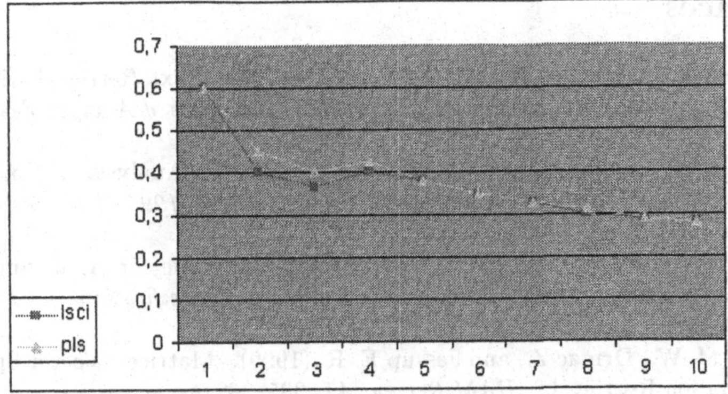

Fig. 2. Average Precision plots of LSCI and PLS for ten queries using 1,...,10 cutoff points.

taken into account. However further investigation is needed to see in which cases this strategy is more adequate.

9 Conclusions

In this paper new strategies for Text Retrieval have been proposed, by introducing an *Analyse Multidimensionelle des Données* viewpoint. As retrieval problems can be addressed in a geometric framework, the importance of choosing a proper metric with respect to the nature of the data has been stressed. Latent Semantic Indexing has been re-interpreted in this perspective, and a weighted Euclidean distance has been proposed. Namely Latent Semantic Correspondence Indexing has been suggested, basing retrieval on chi-square distance, which characterizes one of the most successful contribution of *Analyse Multidimensionelle des Données School*, i.e. Correspondence Analysis. In the paper we have shown how the use of this metric has reduced the LSI drawbacks of penalizing shorter documents and overestimating more frequent terms. The basic idea is that the document-by-term matrix is a contingency table and it has to be processed having it in mind. Further developments can be achieved referring to Correspondence Analysis on lexical tables wide literature. We are mainly interested to deeper investigate how results proposed for dealing with disambiguation and synonyms (e.g. bootstrap stability regions for lemmas and terms) can be introduced in a retrieval procedure. A second issue considered in the paper is the possibility of dealing with meta-information available both on documents and on terms. In the paper results obtained by PLS regression have been shown, but other data analysis methods (Balbi, Giordano, 2001) dealing with two or more sets of variables can be profitably investigated.

References

1. Amato, S., Di Meglio, E., and Guerra M. (2004). "Text Retrieval with External Information," to appear in *JADT 2004, Journées d'Analyse des Données Textuelles.*
2. Balbi, S. (1995). "Non-Symmetrical Correspondence Analysis of Textual Data and Confidence Regions for Graphical Forms," *JADT 1995, Journées d'Analyse des Données Textuelles*, **2**, 5–12.
3. Balbi, S., Giordano G. (2001). "A Factorial Technique for Analyzing Textual Data with External Information," in *Advances in Classification and Data Analysis*, Springer, pp. 169–176.
4. Berry, M. W., Drmac Z., and Jessup E. R. (1999). "Matrices, Vector Spaces and Information Retrieval," *SIAM Review*, **41**, 335–362.
5. Deerwester, S., Dumais, S., Furnas G., Landauer, T., and Harshman, R. (1990). "Indexing by Latent Semantic Analysis," *Journal of the American Society for Information Science*, **41**, 391–407.
6. Di Meglio, E. (2003). "Improving Text Retrieval with Latent Semantic Indexing using Correspondence Analysis," *Atti del Convegno Intermedio SIS 2003, CD Contributed Papers.*
7. Dumais, S. T. (1993). "Latent Semantic Analysis (lsi) and trec2," in *Second Text REtrieval Conference (TREC2)*, pp. 105–115.
8. Eckart C., and Young, G. (1936). "The Approximation of One Matrix by Another of Lower Rank," *Psychometrika*, **1**, 211–218.
9. Greenacre, M. J. (1984). *Theory and application of correspondence analysis*, Academic Press, London.
10. Lauro, C., and D'Ambra, L. (1984). "L'Analyse Non-Symetrique des Correspondances," *Data Analysis and Informatics*, **3**, 433–446.
11. Lebart, L., Morineau, A., and Warwick K. (1984). *Multivariate Descriptive Statistical Analysis*, John Wiley, New York.
12. Lebart, L., Salem, A., and Berry, L. (1998). *Exploring Textual Data.* Kluwer, Amsterdam.
13. Manning C. D., and Schütze, H. (1999). *Foundations of Statistical Natural Language Processing*, MIT Press, Cambridge.
14. Tenenhaus, M. (1998). *La Régression PLS, Theorie et Pratique.* Éditions Technip, Paris.
15. Wold S., Rube R., Wold H., and Dunn W. (1984). "The Collinearity Problem in Linear Regression. The PLS Approach to Generalized Inverses," *SIAM Journal of Scientific and Statistical Computing*, **5**, 735–743.

Automated Resolution of Noisy Bibliographic References

Markus Demleitner[1,2], Michael Kurtz[2], Alberto Accomazzi[2], Günther Eichhorn[2], Carolyn S. Grant[2], Steven S. Murray[2]

[1] Universität Heidelberg, Germany
msdemlei@cl.uni-heidelberg.de
[2] Harvard-Smithsonian Center for Astrophysics, U.S.A.
kurtz@cfa.harvard.edu

Abstract: We describe a system used by the NASA Astrophysics Data System to identify bibliographic references obtained from scanned article pages by OCR methods with records in a bibliographic database. We analyze the process generating the noisy references and conclude that the three-step procedure of correcting the OCR results, parsing the corrected string and matching it against the database provides unsatisfactory results. Instead, we propose a method that allows a controlled merging of correction, parsing and matching, inspired by dependency grammars. We also report on the effectiveness of various heuristics that we have employed to improve recall.

1 Introduction

The importance of linking scholarly publications to each other has received increasing attention with the growing availability of such materials in electronic form (see, e.g., van de Sompel, 1999). The use of citations is probably the most straightforward approach to generate such links.

However, most publications and authors still do not give machine readable publication identifiers like DOIs in their reference sections. The automatic generation of links from references therefore is a challenge even for recent literature. Bergmark (2000), Lawrence et al. (1999) and Claivaz et al. (2001) investigate methods to solve this problem under a record linkage point of view.

For historical literature, the situation is even worse in that not even the "clean" reference strings as intended by the authors are usually available. In 1999, the NASA Astrophysics Data System (ADS, see Kurtz et al., 2000) began to gather reference sections from scans of astronomical literature and subsequently processed them with OCR software. This has yielded about three million references (Demleitner et al., 1999), many of them with severe recognition errors. We will call these references *noisy*, whereas references that were wrong in the original publication will be denoted *dangling*. Noisy references show the entire spectrum of classic OCR errors in addition to the usual variations in citation style. Consider the following examples:

> Bidelman, W. P. 1951, Ap. J. "3, 304; Contr. McDonald Obs., No. 199.
> Eggen, 0. J. 195oa, Ap.J. III, 414; Contr. Lick Obs., Series II, No. 27.
> —195ob, ibid. 112, 141; ibid., No. 30.
> Huist, H. C. van de. 1950, Astrophys. J. 112,1.
> 8tro~mgren, B. 1956, Astron. J. 61, 45.
> Morando, B. 1963, "Recherches sur les orbites de resonance, "in Proceedings of t he First International Symposium on the Use of Artilicial Satellites for Geodesy , Washington, D. C. (North- Holland Publishing Company, Amsterdam, 1963), p. 42.

While our situation was worse than the one solved by the record linkage approaches cited above, we had the advantage of being able to restate the problem into a classification problem, since we were only interested in resolving references to publications contained in the ADS' abstract database—or decide that the target of the reference is not in the ADS. This is basically a classification problem in which there are (currently) 3.5 million categories.

A method to solve this problem was recently developed by Takasu (2003) using Hidden Markov Models to both parse and match noisy references (Takasu calls them "erroneous"). While his approach is very different from ours, we believe the ideas behind and our experiences with our resolver may benefit other groups also facing the problem of resolution of noisy references.

In the remainder of this paper, we will first state the problem in a rather general setting, then discuss the basic ideas of our approach in this framework, describe the heuristics we used to improve resolution rates and their effectiveness and finally discuss the performance of our system in the real world.

2 Statement of the Problem

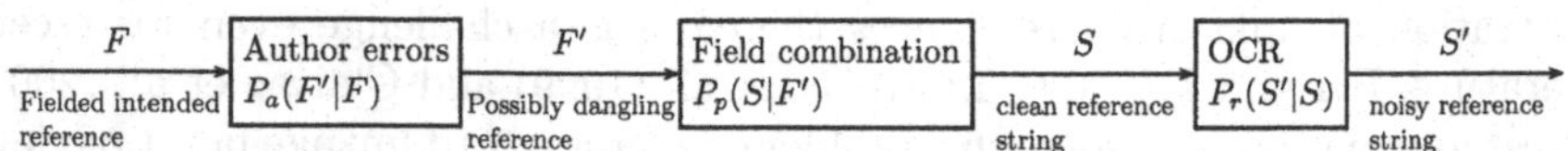

Fig. 1. A noisy channel model for references obtained from OCR. F and F' are a tuple-valued random variables, S and S' are string-valued random variables.

Fig. 1 shows a noisy channel model for the generation of a noisy reference from an original reference that corresponds to an entry in a bibliographic database. In principle, the resolving problem is obtaining

$$\underset{F}{\operatorname{argmax}} P_m(F' \mid F)\, P_p(S \mid F')\, P_r(S' \mid S), \quad S \in \Sigma^*, F' \in (\Sigma^*)^{n_f} \tag{1}$$

for a given noisy reference S'. Here, Σ is the base alphabet (in our case, we normalize everything to 7-bit ASCII) and n_f is the number of fields in a bibliographic record. The domain of random variable F is the database plus the special value $\emptyset$ for references that are missing from the data base but nevertheless valid.

The straightforward approach of modeling each distribution mentioned above separately and trying to compute (1) from back to front will not work very well. To see why, let us briefly examine each element in the channel.

Under a typical model for an OCR system, $P_r(S' \mid S)$ will have many likely S for any S', since references do not follow common language models and are hard to model in general because of mixed languages and (as text goes) high entropy. To give an example, the sequence "L1" will have a very low probability in normal text, but, depending on the reference syntax employed by authors, could occur in up to 2.5% of the references in our sample (it is actually found in 1.7% of the OCRed strings).

In contrast, the "parsing" distribution $P_p(S \mid F')$ is sharply peaked at few values. Although reference syntax is much less uniform than one might wish, even regular grammars can cope with a large portion of the references, avoiding ambiguity altogether. Even if the situation is not so simple in the presence of titles or with monographs and conferences, the number of interpretations for a given value of S with nonvanishing likelihood will be in the tens.

In the matching step modeled by $P_m(F' \mid F)$, we have a similar situation. For journal references, ambiguity is very low indeed, and even for books this record linkage problem is harmless with $P_m(F' \mid F)$ sharply peaked on at worst a few dozen F. The main complication here is detecting the case $F = \emptyset$.

So, while P_m and P_p have quite low conditional entropies, the one of P_r is very high. This is unfortunate, because in computing (1) one would generate many S only to throw them away when computing P_p or P_m.

In this light, an attempt to resolve noisy references along the lines of Accomazzi et al. (1999)'s suggestion for clean references—which boils down to computing $\operatorname{argmax}_F P_m(F \mid \operatorname{argmax}_{F'} P_p(F' | S))$—is bound to fail when extended to noisy references.

It is clear that there have to be better ways since the conditional entropy of $P(F \mid S')$ is rather low, as can be seen from the fact that a human can usually tell very quickly what the correct interpretation for even a very noisy reference is, at least when equipped with a bibliographic search engine like the ADS itself.

Takasu (2003) describes how Dual and Variable-length output Hidden Markov Models can be used to model a combined conditional distribution $P_{p,r}(F' \mid S')$, thus exploiting that many likely values of S will not parse well and therefore have a low combined probability. The idea of combining distributions is instrumental to our approach as well.

3 Our Approach

One foundation of our resolver comes from dependency grammars (Heringer, 1993) in natural language processing, which are based on the observation that given the "head" of a (natural language) phrase (say, a verb), certain "slots" need to be filled (e.g., eat will usually have to be complemented with something that eats and something that is eaten).

In the domain of reference resolving, the equivalent of a phrase is the reference. As the head of this phrase, we chose the publication source, i.e., a journal or conference name, a book title, a hint that a given publication is a Ph.D. thesis or a preprint. This was done for three reasons. Firstly, it is easy to robustly extract this information from references in our domain, secondly, there are relatively few possible heads (disregarding monographs), and thirdly, the publication source governs the grammar of the entire reference.

For example, in addition to the publication year and authors references to most journals need a volume and a page , while a Ph.D. thesis is complemented by a name of an institution, and reports or documents from the ArXiv preprint servers may just take a single number.

Let us for now assume that references follow the regular expression *Author+ Year Rest*, where Rest contains a mixture of alphabetic and numeric characters, and a title is not given for parts of article collections – in astronomy, almost all references follow this grammar. A simple regular expression can identify the year with very close to 100% recall and precision even in noisy references, yielding a robust fielding of the reference.

To find the head as defined above, we simply collect all alphabetic characters from the Rest. The remaining numeric information, i.e., all sequences of digits separated by non-digits, are the fillers required by the head. This exploits that fillers are almost always numeric and avoids dependency on syntactic markers like commas that are very prone to misrecognition. Heads that have non-numeric fillers (mostly theses and monographs) receive special treatment.

This head is matched against an authority file that maps N_t full titles and common abbreviations for the sources known to the ADS to a "bibstem" (cf. Grant et al., 2000). We select the n-best matching of these, where $n = 5$ proved a good choice. To assess the quality of a match, a string edit distance suffices. The one we use is

$$1 - \frac{(\Delta(a,h) - |a|)L(a,h)}{|h|},$$

where a and h are a string from the authority file and the head, respectively, $\Delta(a,h)$ denotes the number of matching trigrams from h that are found in a, $L(a,h)$ is the plain Levenshtein distance (Levenshtein, 1966) and $|.|$ is the length of the string. The worst-case runtime of this procedure is $O(|h| \max(|a|) N_t \log N_t)$, but since we compute trigram similarities first and compute Levenshtein distances only for those a having at least half as many trigrams in common with h as the best matching a, typical run time will be of order $O(|h|^2 \log |h|)$.

This corresponds to maximizing $P_{p,r}((\ldots, source, \ldots) \mid S')$, i.e., we derive a distribution on publication sources directly from the noisy reference. The conditional entropy of this distribution is relatively low, because there are few possible sources (order 10^4) and the edit distance induces a sharply peaked distribution.

For each bibstem, the number of slots and their interpretation is known (actually, we have an exception list and normally assume two slots, volume and page), and we can simply match the slots with the fillers or give educated guesses on insertion or deletion errors based on our knowledge of the fillers expected. In the noisy channel model, this corresponds to greedily evaluating $P_{p,r}(F' \mid S', (\ldots, source, \ldots))$. While in principle, the distribution would have a rather high conditional entropy (e.g., many readings for the numerals would have to be taken into account), it turns out that most of these complications can be accounted for in the matching step, alleviating the need to actually produce multiple F', even more so since parsing errors frequently resemble errors made by authors in assembling their references, which are modeled in P_a.

If filling the slots with the available fillers is not possible, the next best head is tried, otherwise, we have a complete fielded record f' that can be matched against the database using a P_m to be discussed shortly. If this matching is successful, the resolution process stops, otherwise, the next best head is tried.

The matching has to be a fast operation since it is potentially tried many times. Fortunately, the bibliographic identifiers (bibcodes, see Grant et al., 2000) used by the ADS are, for serials, computable from the record in constant time, and thus, matching requires a simple table lookup, taking $O(\log N_r)$ time for N_r records we have to match against.

Due to the construction of bibcodes, the plain bibcode match only checks the first character of the first authors' last name. The numbers below show that the entropy of references with respect to the distribution implied by our algorithm is so low that this shortcoming does not impact precision noticeably – put another way, the likelihood that OCR errors conspire to produce a valid reference is very small even without using most of the information from the author field.

The core resolving process typically runs in $O(\log N_r |h|^2 \ln |h|)$ time. On a 1400 MHz Athlon XP machine, a python script implementing this resolves about 100 references per second and already catches more than 84% of the total resolvable references in our set of 3,027,801 noisy references.

3.1 Reference Matching

For journals for which the database can be assumed complete $P_m(F \mid F')$ is nontrivial, i.e., different from $\delta_{F,F'}$. The single most important ingredient is a mapping from volume numbers to publication years and vice versa, because even if one field is wrong because of either OCR or author errors, the other can be reconstructed. We also scan the surrounding page range (authors surprisingly frequently use the last page of an article) and try swapping adjacent digits in the page number. Finally, we try special sections of journals (usually letter pages). The definition of this matching implies that $P_m(F = f \mid F' = f') = 0$ if f and f' differ in more than one field.

While these rules are somewhat ad hoc, they are also straightforward and probably would not profit from learning. They alone account for 8% of the successfully resolved references without further source string manipulation.

When any of these rules are applied, the authors given in the reference are matched against those in the data base using a tailored string edit distance. It is computed by deleting initials, first names and common non-author phrases (currently "and", "et", and "al") and then evaluating

$$\mathit{fault} = \sum_{w' \in A'} \min_{w \in A} L(w', w),$$

where L is the Levenshtein distance with all weights one and A and A' the author last names for the paper in the database and from the reference, respectively. The edit distance then is $d_a = 1 - \mathit{fault}/\mathit{limit}$, where limit is given by allowing 2 errors for each word shorter than 5 characters, 3 errors for each word shorter than 10 characters and 4 errors otherwise. This reflects that OCR language models do much better on longer words than on shorter ones, even if they come from non-English languages. Unless we have reason to be stricter (usually with monographs), we accept a match if $d_a > 0$.

If, after all string manipulations described below have not yielded a match, we relax P_m for all sources and also try to match identifiers with a different first author (in case the author order is wrong), scan a page range of plausible mis-spellings and try identifiers with different qualifiers—this is necessary if there is more than one article mapping to the same bibcode on one page, for details see Grant et al. (2000). Only after this were 7.8% of the total resolved references accepted. We have not attempted to ascertain how many of these references were dangling in the original publication.

3.2 Monographs and Theses

The procedures described above are useful for serials and article collections of all kinds. Two kinds of publications have to be treated differently.

As mentioned above, theses have alphabetic fillers. Thus, we use keyword spotting (a hand-tailored regular expression for possible readings of "Thesis") to identify the head within the rest. Together with the first character of the author's last name and the publication year, we select a set of candidates and match authors and granting institutions analogous to the author matching procedure described above.

Monographs are completely outside this kind of handling. For them, a set of candidates is selected based on the first character of the author name and the publication year, and authors and titles are matched. Since this is a very time-consuming procedure, it is only attempted if the resolving to serials failed.

Note that using authors as heads as is basically done with monographs would probably most closely mimic the techniques of human librarians. However, given the fragility of author names both in the OCR process and in transliteration, we doubt that a low-entropy distribution would result from doing so.

4 Heuristics

Takasu (2003) conjectured that the comparatively unsatisfactory performance of his method could be significantly improved through the use of a set of heuristics. We find that the same is true for our approach. Almost 16% of the total resolved papers only become resolvable by the algorithm outlined above after some heuristic manipulations are performed on the noisy reference.

We apply a sequence of such manipulations ordered according to their "daringness" and re-resolve after each manipulation. These manipulations—typically regular-expression based string operations—model a noisy channel, but of course it would be very hard to write down its governing distribution. Still, it may be useful to see what heuristics had what payoff.

In a first step, we correct the most frequently misrecognized abbreviations based on regular expressions for the errors. We concentrate on abbreviations because misrecognitions in longer words usually do not confuse our matching algorithm. While better models may have a higher payoff, our method only contributes 0.6% of the total resolved references.

The second step is more effective at 1.7% of the total resolved references. We code rules about common misreadings of numerals in a set of regular expressions, including substituting numerals at the beginning of the reference using a unigram model for OCR errors, fixing numerals within the reference string using a hand-crafted bigram model and joining single digits to a preceding group to make up for blank insertion errors.

At 4.9% of the total still more effective are transformations on the alphabetic part behind the year, including attempts to remove additional specifications (e.g., "English Translation"), and mostly very domain-specific operations with the purpose of increasing the conformity of journal specifications with the authority information used by the source matcher. The most important measure here, however, is handling very short publication names ("AJ") that are particularly hard for the OCR. From these experiences we believe a learning system will have to have a special mode for short heads.

The last fixing step is dissecting the source specification along separators (we use commas and colons) and try using the part that yields the best match against the authority file as the new head. This usually removes bibliographic information primarily in references to conference proceedings. 0.9% of the total resolved references become resolvable after this. Note that this step would be more important if we had to frequently deal with title removal.

Further, less interesting, heuristics are applied to bring references into the format required by the resolver including title removal (for astronomy references, this is rarely needed), or to reconstruct references that refer to other reference's parts, or to split reference lines containing two or more references. This last task only applies to the rare entries consisting of two separate references listed together by the author. The resolver makes no attempt to discover errors in line joining that were made earlier in the processing chain.

5 Application

Our dataset from OCR currently contains 3,027,801 references (some 10^4 of which actually consist of non-reference material misclassified by the reference cutting engine). Of these, 2,552,229 (or about 84%) could be resolved to records in the database.

In order to assess recall and precision of the system described here, we created a subset of 852 references by selecting each reference with a probability of 0.00025, which yielded 118 references that were not resolved and 734 that were resolved. We then manually resolved each selected reference, correcting dangling references as best we could. Thus, the following numbers compare the resolver's $P(F \mid S')$ with a human's $P(F \mid S')$.

The result was that two of the 734 resolved records were incorrectly resolved. In both cases, the correct record was not in the ADS, which illustrates that the $F = \emptyset$ problem dominates the issue of precision. Of the non-resolved records, 94 were not in our database, while 23 were, though six of these were marked doubtful by the human resolvers. Counting doubtful cases as errors, we thus have a precision of more than 99% and a recall of about 97%. Of the 17 definite false negatives, 7 are severely dangling or excessively noisy references to journals, while 6 are references to conference proceedings and the rest monographs.

Note that it is highly unlikely that any of the drawn references were ever inspected during the development of the heuristics. Still, one might question if evaluating the resolver with data that at least might have been used to "train" it is justified. Since during development we mainly inspected resolving failures rather than possibly incorrectly resolved references, we would expect the fact the we did not hold back pristine reference data for evaluation purposes to impact recall more than precision.

For journal literature between 1981 and 1998, we also compared the resolver result with data purchased from ISI's science citation index (see http://www.isinet.com/). Randomly selecting 1% of the articles covered by ISI and removing references to sources outside the ISI sample, we had 10832 citing-cited pairs, of which 311 were missing in the OCR sample and 1151 were missing from ISI.

A manual examination of the citing-cited pairs missing from the OCR sample revealed that 112 were really attributable to the resolver, 107 were due to incorrect reconstructions of reference lines, and 86 references were missed because the references were not found by the reference zone identification.

Of the references apparently missing from ISI, 2 were due to resolver errors (actually, in one case the OCR conspired to produce an almost valid reference to a wrong paper, in the second case, incorrect line joining resulted in two references that were mangled into a valid one), and less than 20% were dangling references that ISI did not correct, but were clearly identifiable nevertheless. We have not attempted to identify why the other (correct) pairs were missing from our ISI sample; most problems probably were introduced during the necessarily conservative matchup between records from ISI and the ADS, and possibly in the selection of our data set from ISI's data base.

For journal articles (others are, for the most part, not available from ISI), we can thus state a recall of 99% and a precision of 99.9% for our resolver and a recall of about 97% for the complete system.

6 Discussion

In this paper we contend that robust interpretation of bibliographic references, as required when resolving references obtained by current OCR techniques, should integrate as much information obtainable from a set of known publications as possible even in parsing and not delay incorporating this information to a "matching" or linkage phase.

Our approach has been inspired by dependency grammars, in which a head of a phrase governs the interpretation of the remaining elements. For (noisy) references, it is advantageous to use the name or type of the publication as head. The existence of bibliographic identifiers that are for most references easily computable from fielded records has been instrumental for the performance of our system.

While we believe some of the rather ad hoc string manipulations and edit distances employed by our current system can and should be substituted by sound and learning algorithms, it seems evident to us that a certain degree of domain-specific knowledge (most notably, a mapping between publication dates and volumes) is very important for robust resolving.

The system discussed here has been in continuous use at the ADS for the past four years, for noisy references from OCR as well as for references from digital sources. The ADS in turn is arguably the most important bibliographic tool in astronomy and astrophysics. The fact that the ADS has received very few complaints concerning the accuracy of its citations backs the estimates of recall and precision given above.

Acknowledgement

We wish to thank Regina Weineck for help in the generation of validation data. The NASA Astrophysics Data System is funded by NASA Grant NCC5-189.

References

1. Accomazzi, A., Eichhorn, G., Kurtz, M., Grant, C., and Murray, S. (1999). "The ADS Bibliographic Reference Resolver," in *Astronomical Data Analysis Software and Systems VIII*, eds. R. L. Plante and D. A. Roberts, Vol. 172 of *ASP Conference Series*, pp. 291–294.
2. Bergmark, D. (2000). "Automatic Extraction of Reference Linking Information from Online Documents," Technical Report TR 2000-1821, Computer Science Department, Cornell University.
3. Claivaz, J.-B., Meur, J.-Y. L., and Robinson, N. (2001). "From Fulltext Documents to Structured Citations: CERN's Automated Solution," *HEP Libraries Webzine* 5 (http://doc.cern.ch/heplw/5/papers/2/).
4. Demleitner, M., Accomazzi, A., Eichhorn, G., Grant, C. S., Kurtz, M. J., and Murray, S. S. (1999). "Looking at 3,000,000 Referencenes Without Growing Grey Hair," *Bulletin of the American Astronomical Society*, **31**, 1496.
5. Grant, C. S., Accomazzi, A., Eichhorn, G., Kurtz, M. J., and Murray, S. S. (2000). "The NASA Astrophysics Data System: Data holdings," *Astronomy and Astrophysics Supplement*, **143**, 111–135.
6. Heringer, H. J. (1993). "Dependency Syntax—Basic Ideas and the Classical Model," in *Syntax—An International Handbook of Contemporary Research, volume 1*, eds J. Jacobs, A. von Stechow, W. Sternefeld, and T. Venneman, Berlin: Walter de Gruyter, pp. 298–316.
7. Kurtz, M. J., Eichhorn, G., Accomazzi, A., Grant, C. S., Murray, S. S., and Watson, J. M. (2000). "The NASA Astrophysics Data System: Overview," *Astronomy and Astrophysics Supplement* **143**, 41–59.
8. Lawrence, S., Giles, C. L., and Bollacker, K. (1999). "Digital Libraries and Autonomous Citation Indexing," *IEEE Computer*, **32**, 67–71.
9. Levenshtein, V. I. (1966). "Binary Codes Capable of Correcting Deletions, Insertions and Reversals," *Soviet Physics Doklady*, **10**, 707–710.
10. Takasu, A. (2003). "Bibliographic Attribute Extraction from Erroneous References Based on a Statistical Model," in *Proceedings of the Third ACM/IEEE-CS Joint Conference on Digital Libraries*, pp. 49–60.
11. van de Sompel, H. V. and Hochstenbach, P. (1999). "Reference Linking in a Hybrid Library Environment," *D-Lib Magazine* 5(4).

Choosing the Right Bigrams for Information Retrieval

Maojin Jiang, Eric Jensen, Steve Beitzel, and Shlomo Argamon

Information Retrieval Laboratory & Laboratory of Linguistic Cognition,
Illinois Institute of Technology, U.S.A.
{jianmao,ej,steve, argamon}@ir.iit.edu

Abstract: After more than 30 years of research in information retrieval, the dominant paradigm remains the "bag-of-words," in which query terms are considered independent of their coocurrences with each other. Although there has been some work on incorporating phrases or other syntactic information into IR, such attempts have given modest and inconsistent improvements, at best. This paper is a first step at investigating more deeply the question of using bigrams for information retrieval. Our results indicate that only certain kinds of bigrams are likely to aid retrieval. We used linear regression methods on data from TREC 6, 7, and 8 to identify which bigrams are able to help retrieval at all. Our characterization was then tested through retrieval experiments using our information retrieval engine, AIRE, which implements many standard ranking functions and retrieval utilities.

1 Introduction

For the most part, information retrieval (IR) has traditionally viewed queries and documents as bags of words ((Salton et al., 1975), treating each term as independent of all other terms. Despite the obvious shortcomings of this approach, in that a great deal of language's meaning is carried in the co-occurrence and order of words, the "bag-of-words" (BOW) approach is still dominant, after more than 30 years of IR research. There are several reasons for this. One is that, with sufficiently sophisticated term-weighting, BOW works surprisingly well. Furthermore, users appreciate the 'convenience' of just throwing a set of relevant keywords to create a query; without a convincing improvement in results, users are unlikely to spend time thinking about the structure of the query. And third, work at incorporating phrases or other syntactic information into IR systems has given modest and inconsistent improvement, at best.

This paper is a first step at investigating more deeply the question of using *phrases* in IR. Use of phrases typically means using term *bigrams* (sequential pairs) in addition to *unigrams* (individual terms). Previous work on using query bigrams for retrieval has given modest improvements, and often highly inconsistent performance (as we describe in more detail below). Our hypothesis is that only certain kinds of bigrams are likely to aid retrieval; by identifying the class of 'good bigrams', we hope to improve retrieval effectiveness by using only the good bigrams in the retrieval process. Surprisingly, there have apparently not been any studies on this question previously. We first compared 'super-optimal' retrieval effectiveness with and without bigrams for the Ad-Hoc Retrieval tracks of TREC 6, 7, and 8, and studied the ranking of the documents produced by our learner in order to identify where we expect bigrams to be at all helpful. A coarse characterization is that Classifier-Thing bigrams ought to be helpful in most cases (though there are other useful bigrams as well). We test this characterization through retrieval experiments using our information retrieval engine, AIRE, which implements many standard ranking functions and retrieval utilities (Chowdhury et al., 2000).

2 Prior Work

The many attempts at integrating phrases, whether they be linguistic or statistical, into existing retrieval frameworks have shown at best disappointingly small improvements over the simple bag of words model. This is in contrast with many natural language processing tasks in which context around a word has been shown to significantly improve effectiveness (speech recognition, part-of-speech tagging, etc.). However, in addition to the intuitive motivation that phrases should aid retrieval effectiveness, interactive work with users manually selecting phrases to expand their queries has suggested that the addition of certain phrases can significantly improve average precision (Smeaton and Kelledy, 1998). There are two typical explanations for the failure of phrases to improve effectiveness of ad-hoc information retrieval. First, incorporating phrase frequencies with word frequencies when ranking documents is a challenge due to their differing distributions. Second, it is difficult to determine which query phrases will improve performance and which will degrade it. In addition to these practical issues, incorporating phrases into existing IR models is often difficult to formally justify as the words composing them are naturally correlated with each other, violating the independence assumptions on which many models are based.

Most IR ranking functions, including the relatively new language modeling approaches, can be shown to be similar in that they rank documents via a linear combination of term (word or phrase) weights (Hiemstra and Vries, 2000). Much work has been devoted to combining phrases with terms inside of the same model (Strzalkowski, 1999). In order to compensate for the vastly greater rarity of phrases than terms across the collection (typically resulting in much larger term weights), these approaches often discount the weights of phrases for all queries by a heuristically-set constant factor. Recent work has shown that dynamically computing phrase weights based on query length can be as effective as static weights empirically tuned and tested on the same query set (Chowdhury, 2001). Studies incorporating context into language models for information retrieval typically interpolate the conditional probability of each query term given the previous one with its unigram probability, performing no phrase selection. Although intuitive, this gives no significant improvement over baseline unigram models and often yields unintuitive optimal interpolation parameters, with bigrams having only minimal weight (Jiang et al., 2004; Song and Kroft 1999; Miller et al., 1999; Hiemstra, 2001).

Previous approaches for selecting phrases have been either statistically or syntactically motivated. Mitra selected only those phrases that appear at least 25 times in the corpus for inclusion in the vector-space model and saw no significant improvement (Mitra et al., 1997). Turpin further examined these results, trying many permutations of topics with varying length and phrase selection techniques, and also could find no significant improvement from statistical phrases (Turpin and Moffat, 1999). Attempts to incorporate syntactic phrases date to the beginning of information retrieval itself (Salton, 1968). In a recent study, Voorhees analyzes the consistent failure to produce improvement of many attempts to integrate NLP techniques with the statistical methods widely used by document retrieval systems (Voorhees, 1999). She observed that these studies often produce inconsistent results, e.g. Fagan (1987); quite often there is improvement for some topics and a reduction in effectiveness for others. Arampatzis and colleagues proposed a framework for information retrieval that incorporates linguistically selected phrases (Arampatzis et al., 198l; Arampatzis, 2000). They found that exploiting co-occurrence of noun-phrases that contain query terms could improve recall, but precision dropped significantly. Zhai, et. al., selected noun phrases where any ambiguity is resolved through the statistical addition of structure and found improvements in precision for some topics, but damaged performance on others (Zhai, 1997). Narita and Ogawa also examined the use of noun phrases for ad-hoc retrieval and saw no significant improvement in overall average precision (Narita and Ogawa, 2000). Lewis and Croft clustered syntactic phrases to group redundant phrases in an attempt to mediate the phrase sparseness problem, but found only small improvements in ad-hoc retrieval (Lewis and Croft, 1990). Kraaij and Pohlmann experimented with both statistical and syntactic phrases and found that neither significantly improved effectiveness, and often performed equivalently (Kraaij and Pohlmann, 1998).

Text categorization often employs machine learning algorithms using features mined from unstructured text. Similarly to most IR ranking algorithms, many learning algorithms employ a linear combination of weighted feature values. Although integration of phrase features has been slightly more effective in categorization than ad-hoc retrieval, improvements are still disappointingly low. Koster and Seutter compared several combinations of head-modifier phrases with a word-only baseline and found that providing phrase features to the learning algorithm did not improve effectiveness in text categorization (Koster and Seutter, 2003).

3 Methodology

In order to differentiate between different bigrams for their possible usefulness in information retrieval, we constructed an experiment to compare unigram and bigram retrieval under "more optimal than optimal" conditions, with the additional goal of doing so in a system-independent fashion. We constructed a 'pseudo-ranking function' for each query by performing linear regression from a set of query-dependent parameters of each document (described below) to the values 0 or 1, depending on whether or not the document was prejudged to be relevant to that document (we used the TREC 6, 7, and 8 queries and relevance judgements). The ranking thus produced can then be evaluated on the document set (which was used to compute the regression function) for precision. Comparison of the resultant document rankings between using just unigrams or using unigrams and bigrams thus gives an optimistic measure of the potential contribution of bigrams to the retrieval process.

Our methodology is as follows. Given a document d and query q, we compute a set of unigram parameters $u_i = f(q_i, d)$, one for each word in the query, as well as a set of bigram parameters $b_i = f(q_i - 1, q_i, d)$, one for each bigram in the query. Given this representation, and assuming a particular query, each document in the collection is then represented by either a unigram vector, $U_d = [u_1 \ldots u_n]$, or a bigram vector, $B_d = [u_1, \ldots, u_n, b_2, \ldots, b_n]$. Note that we only considered bigrams appearing 25 times or more in the collection, as done in prior statistical phrasing approaches (Mitra et al., 1997). We take all relevant documents for the query along with 3 times as many top-ranked non-relevant documents to produce a document set C and then compute the following two weight vectors minimizing the sum-of-squares difference between weight-vector dot-products and the binary relevance judgements R_d:

$$w_u = \text{argmin}_w \sum_{d \in C} (w^T U_d - R_d)^2 \tag{1}$$

$$w_b = \text{argmin}_w \sum_{d \in C} (w^T B_d - R_d)^2 \tag{2}$$

Note that the vectors have different dimensions. Each such weight vector can then be used to rank all the documents in the collection by their 'estimated relevance' to the query; a higher dot-product indicates more likely relevance. This use of linear regression is meant to simulate, on a coarse scale, the action of a 'typical' IR system, whose ranking functions can be formulated as nearly a linear function of parameters of query word occurrences in target documents (see Hiemstra and Vries, 2000).

For generality, we used three different methods of computing the parameters. First was to use raw count of the number of each n-gram occurring in the given document (**cnt**). The second method was to use a Dirichlet-smoothed unigram language model (with the μ parameter set to 3000 as recommended in Zhai and Lafferty, 2001) for single words, and a maximum likelihood bigram model for phrases to get a 'probability' of the term given the document (as used in language modeling), which we term here *prob*. And third was a logarithmically scaled inverse probability (to avoid log(0)), termed *log*, computed as $\log(1 - prob)$. Retrieval effectiveness was measured using two standard techniques: average precision which averages precision at 11 points from 0% to 100% recall, and R-precision which is the retrieval precision for the top r documents, where r is the total number of relevant documents for the query. The potential improvement of using bigrams together with unigrams was measured by relative precision improvement, I_prec, defined as $I_{prec} = (prec_b - prec_u)/prec_u$. A query was considered bigram-good if I_{prec} for the query was non-negative for all three parameter types under both effectiveness metrics, and positive for at least one parameter type under each effectiveness metric; a query is bigram-bad if I_{prec} was negative for at least one type under each metric and not positive for any; otherwise, a query is considered bigram-neutral.

4 Results

Table 1 shows the bigram-good queries from TRECs 6, 7, and 8, with their I_{prec} values for different parameters, while Tables 2 and 3 show the bigram-bad and bigram-neutral queries respectively. An examination of the queries in Table 1 reveals that many of the queries contain a bigram whose first word is a Classifier for the second, which is a Thing (and the head of a nominal phrase). These are functional roles within a nominal group structure, as analyzed in Systemic Functional Linguistics (Halliday, 1994); a Classifier is a nominal modifier which effectively narrows the domain of reference to a subcategory of the category indicated by the nominal head. For example, "airport" in the phrase "airport security" (contrast with "national security"). Not all modifiers are classifiers, however; for example, "tight" in "tight security" is an Epithet, describing an attribute of the Thing, as shown by the fact that it can be intensified ("very tight security") and can be used to modify a variety of subtypes (i.e., we can have "tight airport security" as well as "tight national security"). The few queries without Classifier-Thing bigrams are all special cases, for which individual explanations can be easily found why two of the words would appear in the same irrelevant document, but only together in a relevant document. For example "Iran" and "Iraq", since the are in the same region, may tend to be mentioned in the same articles about the Middle East, even ones not about relations between the countries; however, when they are mentioned in succession, the likelihood of relevance to cooperative relations between the countries is much higher.

Table 1. Bigram-good selected queries from TREC 6, 7, and 8. Columns give Iprec for different measures: $P(cnt)$ for average precision on **cnt**, $R(cnt)$ for R-precision on **cnt**, and so forth. Maximum I_{prec} is boldfaced for each query, as are "Classifier-Thing" bigrams.

P(cnt)	**P(log)**	**P(prob)**	**R(cnt)**	**R(log)**	**R(prob)**	**Query terms**
0.24%	**0.75%**	0.05%	2.21%	**6.60%**	0.00%	Int'l **Organized Crime**
0.03%	3.60%	**3.77%**	0.00%	28.57%	**33.31%**	**End. Species** (Mamm.)
0.92%	0.76%	0.01%	2.90%	**5.73%**	0.00%	African **Civ. Deaths**
1.85%	9.40%	**10.36%**	5.13%	19.49%	**22.50%**	**Mag-Lev**-Maglev
1.65%	0.05%	0.00%	**16.65%**	0.00%	0.00%	**Marine Veg.**
11.96%	5.66%	5.66%	**12.51%**	0.00%	0.00%	**Unsolicited Faxes**
5.05%	1.54%	0.12%	**22.86%**	4.62%	0.00%	Women in Parliaments
5.72%	2.58%	2.41%	**6.46%**	0.00%	0.00%	**Ferry Sinkings**
7.69%	0.00%	0.00%	**14.28%**	0.00%	0.00%	Pope Beatifications
2.84%	**7.85%**	4.78%	2.49%	**7.32%**	2.32%	Iran-Iraq Cooperation
2.20%	1.65%	1.83%	4.44%	**6.38%**	**6.38%**	**World Bank** Criticism
0.15%	0.41%	**0.82%**	0.00%	**2.08%**	**2.08%**	**Income Tax Evasion**
0.00%	**3.33%**	**3.33%**	0.00%	**9.09%**	**9.09%**	**Black Bear** Attacks
9.87%	0.00%	0.00%	**25.00%**	0.00%	0.00%	Alzheimer's **Drug Treat.**
0.49%	**4.87%**	0.37%	0.00%	**4.65%**	0.00%	**Airport Security**
0.34%	**0.50%**	0.22%	**2.99%**	0.00%	0.00%	**Police Deaths**
1.60%	**1.66%**	0.72%	**2.32%**	2.26%	0.00%	**Educational Standards**
0.00%	**1.19%**	0.00%	0.00%	**9.38%**	0.00%	**British Chunnel** impact
6.64%	3.88%	2.70%	**34.34%**	10.06%	2.32%	**territ. waters** dispute
44.29%	33.41%	26.68%	**41.17%**	32.35%	21.63%	**blood-alcohol** fatalities
0.64%	**2.29%**	1.36%	**4.54%**	0.00%	**4.54%**	**mutual fund** predictors
2.27%	0.33%	0.33%	**2.94%**	0.00%	0.00%	**El Nino**
0.00%	**5.34%**	**5.34%**	0.00%	**16.68%**	**16.68%**	**anorex. nerv.** bulimia
0.70%	**2.75%**	2.18%	2.78%	0.00%	**2.86%**	**Native American** casino
5.88%	**6.43%**	2.27%	**12.90%**	12.50%	0.00%	**World Court**
1.38%	0.24%	0.25%	**14.82%**	3.70%	3.70%	**cigar smoking**
15.19%	7.93%	5.59%	**14.29%**	6.99%	4.56%	**space station** moon
1.27%	0.77%	0.56%	**2.38%**	0.00%	0.00%	**hybrid fuel** cars
3.32%	1.73%	1.34%	**4.88%**	2.45%	2.45%	**sick building** syndrome
0.82%	0.07%	0.07%	**2.10%**	0.00%	0.00%	Ireland, **peace talks**
9.73%	8.36%	8.36%	**20.01%**	**20.01%**	**20.01%**	**Parkinson's disease**
16.42%	10.07%	10.23%	**41.95%**	25.00%	25.00%	**tropical storms**
5.99%	1.83%	1.83%	**12.52%**	2.29%	2.29%	**airport security**
0.00%	**1.94%**	**1.94%**	0.00%	**2.13%**	**2.13%**	**steel production**
10.67%	1.53%	1.55%	**25.63%**	0.00%	0.00%	drugs, **Golden Triangle**
4.17%	8.33%	8.33%	**20.00%**	**20.00%**	**20.00%**	**killer bee** attacks
0.00%	**0.58%**	**0.58%**	0.00%	**2.05%**	**2.05%**	tourism, increase
16.06%	8.06%	8.06%	**13.32%**	9.67%	9.67%	**child labor**

An examination of Table 2 allows us to refine this hypothesis somewhat. Even though each of the bigram-bad queries contains a Classifier-Thing bigram, such bigrams are not central to the meaning of the query. To understand this, consider first the query "Legionnaire's disease". It is highly unlikely that any document in the collection contains the word "Legionnaire" while not being about this disease. Similarly for "Schengen" or "obesity". In the case of "encryption equipment export", we find that "encryption export" is also an excellent query. So to be more precise, we believe that queries that contain Classifier-Thing bigrams that contrast with other Classifiers for the same Thing in the corpus will be useful bigrams for retrieval. We validated this method by examining retrieval performance with only words, all phrases, and only our list of (hand-chosen) Classifer-Thing phrases when using a common, highly effective retrieval strategy, Robertson's probabilistic model BM25 (Robertson et al., 1995). Phrases were weighted such that their scores counted for only .25 of terms' scores. When using the list, phrases not appearing in our list of relevant phrases did not contribute any weight to a document. We used a hand-tailored set of conflation classes for stemming (Xu and Croft, 1998) and the 342-word stop list from Cornell's SMART system (ftp://cs.cornell.edu/pub/smart). These results are summarized in Table 3.

Table 2. Bigram-bad queries from TREC 6, 7, and 8. Columns give I_{prec} for different measures: P(cnt) for average precision on cnt, R(cnt) for R-precision on cnt, and so forth. Lowest I_{prec} is boldfaced for each query, as are "Classifier-Thing" bigrams.

P(cnt)	*P(log)*	*P(prob)*	*R(cnt)*	*R(log)*	*R(prob)*	Query terms
-1.16%	**-2.05%**	0.00%	0.00%	**-4.00%**	0.00%	**encrypt. equip.** export
-3.55%	-2.02%	-2.02%	**-16.66%**	0.00%	0.00%	obesity **medical trtmt.**
0.00%	0.00%	**-61.54%**	0.00%	0.00%	**-80.01%**	**Schengen agreement**
-1.49%	**-1.50%**	**-1.50%**	**-2.05%**	-1.99%	-1.99%	**ind. waste disposal**
-6.38%	-2.49%	-2.49%	**-18.18%**	-9.09%	-9.09%	**Legionnaires' disease**

Table 3. Bigram improvement for average precision and R-precision, using BM25 retrieval. Averages and standard deviations are shown for bigram-good, bigram-bad, and all queries in TRECs 6, 7, and 8.

Query Type	**Measure**	**min**	**max**	**avg**	**stderr**
good	avg. prec.	-70%	2827%	**113%**	74%
good	R-prec	-100%	400%	**12%**	11%
bad	avg. prec.	-30%	400%	**74%**	81%
bad	R-prec	-13%	20%	**1.5%**	5.2%
all	avg. prec.	-82%	2827%	**42%**	23%
all	R-prec	-100%	400%	**5.3%**	4.0%

These results clearly confirm that the set of queries singled out by our 'overly optimal' linear regression technique as where bigrams may possible be useful, indeed get higher levels of retrieval improvement when using bigrams. The results for bigram-bad queries, however, are misleading, since the strongly positive results are due to a single query, "industrial waste disposal", while all other bad queries give neutral or negative effect from using bigrams in retrieval. Indeed, this query fits our proposed pattern of "Classifer-Thing" bigrams, containing two of them.

5 Discussion and Future Work

We have proposed a system-independent methodology for determining which bigrams are likely to be useful for retrieval, and have validated the methodology by showing that those queries our method shows to be good candidates for bigram use indeed get higher improvements from using bigrams than other queries. We examined the phrases in the queries that improved and concluded that an important characteristic of "good" bigrams (for retrieval purposes) is that they are "Classifier-Thing" pairs, in which the first word effectively selects for a subclass of the type referred to by the second word. At the same time, there are a few other interesting types of bigrams which are more difficult to characterize directly in this way. Future work will include devising and evaluating methods for automatically determining the good bigrams without the use of relevance judgments, as well as incorporating such selective bigram use in our retrieval system.

References

1. Arampatzis, A. T., T. P. van der Weide, C. H. A. Koster and v. Bommel (1998). "Phrase-based Information Retrieval." *Information Processing and Management*, **34**. 693-707.
2. Arampatzis, A. T., T. P. van der Weide, C. H. A. Koster and v. Bommel (2000). *An Evaluation of Linguistically-motivated Indexing Schemes.* BCSIRSG '2000.
3. Chowdhury, A., S. Beitzel, E. Jensen, M. Saelee, D. Grossman and O.Frieder (2000). *IIT-TREC-9 - Entity Based Feedback with Fusion.* Ninth Annual Text Retrieval Conference, NIST.
4. Chowdhury, A. (2001). *Adaptive Phrase Weighting.* International Symposium on Information Systems and Engineering (ISE 2001).
5. Cornell Cornell University - SMART - ftp://cs.cornell.edu/pub/smart.
6. Fagan, J. (1987). *Automatic phrase indexing for document retrieval.* 10th annual international ACM SIGIR conference on Research and development in information retrieval (SIGIR'87), New Orleans, Louisiana.
7. Halliday, M. A. K. (1994). *An Introduction to Functional Grammar.* London, Edward Arnold.

8. Hiemstra, D. and A. d. Vries (2000). Relating the new language models of information retrieval to the traditional retrieval models, Centre for Telematics and Information Technology.
9. Hiemstra, D. (2001). *Using language models for information retrieval, Center for Telematics and Information Technology*: 164.
10. Jiang, M., E. Jensen, S. Beitzel and S. Argamon (2004). *Effective Use of Phrases in Language Modeling to Improve Information Retrieval.* 2004 Symposium on AI & Math Special Session on Intelligent Text Processing, Florida.
11. Koster, C. H. A. and M. Seutter (2003). *Taming Wild Phrases.* ECIR'03.
12. Kraaij, W. and R. Pohlmann (1998). *Comparing the effect of syntactic vs. statistical phrase index strategies for dutch.* 2nd European Conference on Research and Advanced Technology for Digital Libraries (ECDL'98).
13. Lewis and Croft (1990). *Term Clustering of Syntactic Phrases. 13th ACM Conference on Research and Development in Information Retrieval* (SIGIR'90).
14. Miller, D. R. H., T. Leek and R. M. Schwartz (1999). *A hidden Markov model information retrieval system.* 22nd ACM Conference on Research and Development in Information Retrieval (SIGIR'99).
15. Mitra, M., C. Buckley, A. Singhal and C. Cardie (1997). *An Analysis of Statistical and Syntactic Phrases.* 5th International Conference Recherche d'Information Assistee par Ordinateur (RIAO'97).
16. Narita, M. and Y. Ogawa (2000). *The use of phrases from query texts in information retrieval. 23rd ACM Conference on Research and Development in Information Retrieval* (SIGIR'00).
17. Robertson, S. E., S. Walker, M. M. Beaulieu, M. Gatford and A. Payne (1995). *Okapi at TREC-4.* 4th Annual Text Retrieval Conference (TREC-4), NIST, Gaithersburg, MD.
18. Salton, G. (1968). *Automatic information organization and retrieval.* New York, McGraw-Hill.
19. Salton, G., C. S. Yang and A. Wong (1975). "A Vector-Space Model for Automatic Indexing." *Communications of the ACM* **18** (11): 613-620.
20. Smeaton, A. F. and F. Kelledy (1998). *User-chosen phrases in interactive query formulation for information retrieval.* 20th BCS-IRSG Colloquium, Springer-Verlag Electronic Workshops in Computing.
21. Song, F. and W. B. Croft (1999). *A general language model for information retrieval.* Eighth International Conference on Information and Knowledge Management (CIKM'99).
22. Strzalkowski, T. (1999). *Natural Language Information Retrieval*, Kluwer Academic Publishers.
23. Turpin, A. and A. Moffat (1999). *Statistical phrases for Vector-Space information retrieval.* 22nd ACM Conference on Research and Development in Information Retrieval (SIGIR'99).
24. Voorhees, E. (1999). *Natural Language Processing and Information Retrieval.* Information Extraction: Towards Scalable, Adaptable Systems (SCIE'99), New York, Springer.
25. Xu, J. and B. Croft (1998). "Corpus-based Stemming using co-occurrence of word variants." *ACM Transactions on Information Systems* **16** (1): 61-81.
26. Zhai, C., X. Tong, N. Milic-Frayling and D. A. Evans (1997). *Evaluation of syntactic phrase indexing - CLARIT NLP track report.* The Fifth Text Retrieval Conference (TREC-5), NIST Special Publication.

27. Zhai, C. and J. Lafferty (2001). *A Study of Smoothing Methods for Language Models Applied to ad-hoc Information Retrieval.* 24th ACM Conference on Research & Development in Information Retrieval, New Orleans, LA, ACM Press.

A Mixture Clustering Model for Pseudo Feedback in Information Retrieval

Tao Tao and ChengXiang Zhai

University of Illinois at Urbana-Champaign, U.S.A.
{taotao, czhai}@cs.uiuc.edu

Abstract: In this paper, we present a new mixture model for performing pseudo feedback for information retrieval. The basic idea is to treat the words in each feedback document as observations from a two-component multinomial mixture model, where one component is a topic model anchored to the original query model through a prior and the other is fixed to some background word distribution. We estimate the topic model based on the feedback documents and use it as a new query model for ranking documents.

1 Introduction

Information Retrieval (IR) refers to retrieving relevant documents from a large document database according to a user-submitted query, and is among the most useful technologies to overcome information overload. Indeed, search capabilities are becoming more and more popular in virtually all kinds of information management applications.

Given a query, a retrieval system would typically estimate a relevance value for each document with respect to this query, and rank the documents in the descending order of relevance. Over the decades, many different retrieval models have been proposed and tested, including vector space models, probabilistic models, and logic-based models (Sparck Jones and Willet, 1997). As a special family of probabilistic models, the language modeling approaches have attracted much attention recently due to their statistical foundation and empirical effectiveness (Ponte and Croft, 1998; Croft and Lafferty, 2003).

A particular effective retrieval model based on statistical language models is the Kullback-Leibler (KL) divergence unigram retrieval model proposed and studied in Lafferty and Zhai (2001) and Zhai and Lafferty (2001a). The basic idea of this model is to measure the relevance value of a document with respect to a query by the Kullback-Leibler divergence between the corresponding query model and the document model. Thus the retrieval task essentially boils down to estimating a query unigram model (unigram language model is just a multinomial word distribution) and a set of document unigram language models. The retrieval accuracy is largely affected by how good the estimated query and document models are. In this paper, we study how to improve the query model estimation through fitting a mixture model to some number of top ranked documents, which are retrieved by the original query itself. We present a new mixture model that extends and improves an existing mixture feedback model and addresses its two deficiencies. We study parameter estimation for this mixture model, and evaluate the model on a document set with $160,000$ news article documents and 50 queries. The results show that using the new mixture model not only significantly improves the retrieval performance over using the original query model, but also performs better than the old mixture model.

The rest of the paper is organized as follows: First, in Section 2, we provide some details about the KL-divergence retrieval formula as background for understanding the mixture problem estimation. We then present our mixture model and its estimation in Section 3. Finally, experiment results are presented in Section 4.

2 The Kullback-Leibler Divergence Retrieval Model

The basic idea of the KL-divergence model is to score a document with respect to a query based on the KL-divergence between an estimated document model and an estimated query model. Given two probability mass functions $p(x)$ and $q(x)$, the Kullback-Leibler divergence (or relative entropy) between p and q, denoted $D(p||q)$, is defined as

$$D(p||q) = \sum_x p(x) \log \frac{p(x)}{q(x)}.$$

Now, assume that a query $\mathbf{q}$ is obtained as a sample from a unigram language model, i.e., a multinomial word distribution) $p(\mathbf{q} \,|\, \theta_Q)$ with parameters θ_Q. Similarly, assume that a document $\mathbf{d}$ is generated by a model $p(\mathbf{d} \,|\, \theta_D)$ with parameters θ_D. If $\widehat{\theta}_Q$ and $\widehat{\theta}_D$ are the estimated query and document language models respectively, then the relevance value of $\mathbf{d}$ with respect to $\mathbf{q}$ can be measured by $D(\widehat{\theta}_Q||\widehat{\theta}_D)$.

The KL-divergence model contains three independent components: (1) the query model $\widehat{\theta}_Q$; (2) the document model $\widehat{\theta}_D$; and (3) the KL-divergence function. (See Fig. 1 for an illustration.) Given that we fix the KL-divergence function, the whole retrieval problem essentially boils down to the problem of accurately estimating a query model and a set of document models.

The simplest generative model of a document is just the unigram language model θ_D, a multinomial distribution. Usually a smoothing method is applied to avoid overfitting (Zhai and Lafferty, 2001b). The simplest generative model for a query is also just a unigram language model, which can be estimated

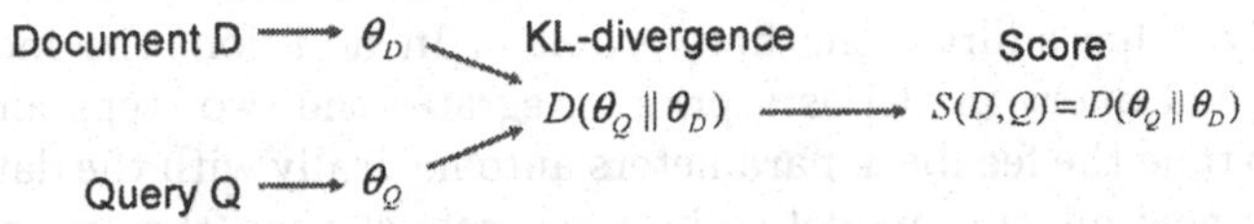

Fig. 1. The KL-divergence Retrieval Model

as the relative frequency of the words in the query. Generally, a query is too short to estimate a query model accurately. A general heuristic approach used in information retrieval is the so-called "pseudo feedback". The basic idea is to assume a small number of top-ranked documents from an initial retrieval result to be relevant, and use them to refine the query model. Presumably, a relevant document can provide a lot of information about what a user is interested in, thus can be expected to help improve the estimated query model. Even though not all the top-ranked documents are actually relevant, we can expect some of them to be relevant and those non-relevant ones are also similar to a relevant document. For this reason, pseudo feedback in general leads to improvement of average retrieval accuracy.

In Zhai and Lafferty (2001a), a general two-step pseudo feedback procedure is proposed, in which we first estimate a feedback topic model $\hat{\Theta}_F$ based on a set of feedback documents (e.g., top 5 documents) F, and then update the original query model $\hat{\Theta}_Q$ through heuristically interpolating $\hat{\Theta}_Q$ with $\hat{\Theta}_F$ to obtain a new query model $\theta_{Q'}$ i.e., $\hat{\Theta}_{Q'} = (1-\alpha)\Theta_Q + \alpha\hat{\Theta}_F$, where $\alpha \in [0,1]$ is a parameter to control the influence of feedback.

Two specific methods are proposed in Zhai and Lafferty (2001a) to estimate the feedback model Θ_F, one being based on a mixture model and one on divergence minimization. Although both methods have been shown to be quite effective, the separation of the original query model from the estimation of the feedback model makes it hard to automatically tune the feedback parameters. More specifically, the separation causes two problems: (1) It makes it hard to discriminate the feedback documents when estimating the feedback model. Presumably, we should trust the top ranked documents more than the lowly ranked ones. But without involving the original query model, it is difficult to implement this intuition in a principled way. Without implementing this intuition, the feedback performance will be very sensitive to the number of documents to use for pseudo feedback. (2) It is difficult to automatically tune the interpolation coefficient, since this parameter is now outside our feedback model. In this paper, we extend this work and develop a new mixture model that will incorporate the original query model as a prior when estimating the feedback model. In essence, we perform *biased clustering* of words in the feedback documents with one cluster "anchored" to our query model and the other to more general vocabulary. A key novel feature of the new mixture model is that it does *not* assume that all the feedback documents have the same amount of relevance information to contribute to the new query model, which presumably helps address the first problem. In addition, the incorporation of the original query model as a prior integrates the two steps and makes it possible to tune the feedback parameters automatically with the data. We thus expect the new mixture model to be more robust than the original mixture model proposed in Zhai and Lafferty (2001a).

3 A Mixture Clustering Model for Pseudo Feedback

In this section, we present our new mixture model in detail. We first define the following notations. Here Q is a query and C is the set of all documents in the whole collection, i.e., document database. An d $D = \{d_1, ..., d_k\}$ is a set of documents as feedback. We use w and d to represent an individual word and document and $c(w, d)$ ($c(w, Q)$) to mean the count of word w in document d (query Q).

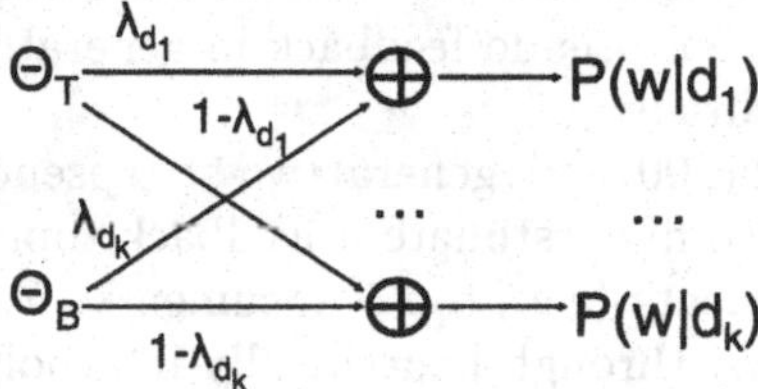

Fig. 2. Mixture model for pseudo feedback.

Our general idea is to regard the original (current) query model θ_Q as inducing a prior on the true query model θ_T, $p(\theta_T|\theta_Q)$, and view the feedback documents D as providing new evidence about the true query model. We then use Bayesian estimation to obtain a (presumably better) query model θ_T.

$$\hat{\theta}_T = \arg\max_{\theta_T} p(D|\theta_T)p(\theta_T|\theta_Q). \tag{1}$$

The feedback document sampling model is a mixture generative model for the feedback documents, where each document is assumed to be "generated" from a two-component unigram mixture model $P(w|d_i)$, one being the topic language model θ_T , which intends to capture the relevance information in the feedback documents, and one being a background language model θ_B capturing the general English usage and any distracting non-relevant information. Intuitively, we are assuming that a feedback document is "written" by sampling words in such a way that we sometimes draw words according to θ_T and sometimes according to θ_B. The *document-dependent* mixing weight parameter $\lambda_d \in [0, 1]$ determines how often we would sample a word using the topic model θ_T. In effect, this model allows us to perform a biased clustering of the words in D where one cluster is anchored to the query model while the other to general background vocabuary. The model is illustrated in Fig. 2.

According to this mixture model, the log-likelihood for the feedback documents is

$$L(\Lambda|D) = \sum_{i=1}^{k} \sum_{w \in V} c(w, d_i) \log(\lambda_{d_i} p(w|\theta_T) + (1 - \lambda_{d_i}) p(w|\theta_B)),$$

where $\Lambda = (\theta_T, \theta_B, \lambda_1, ..., \lambda_k)$ is all the parameters and V is the vocabulary.

To regulate the mixture model, we will fix the background model θ_B to some unigram language model estimated using all the documents in the collection C, since most of them are non-relevant. We thus only need to estimate θ_T and λ_{d_i}'s. θ_T is meant to be our new (presumably improved) query model, and λ_{d_i}'s are meant to model the amount of relevant information in each document and thus allow us to discount feedback documents appropriately. To incorporate the original query model, we use it to define a Dirichlet conjugate prior for θ_T, and estimate θ_B and λ_{d_i}'s using the Maximum A Posterior (MAP) estimator. We will also put a conjugate prior (a beta distribution) on the λ_{d_i}'s, which encodes our prior belief of the amount of relevant information in each feedback document.

The MAP estimate can be implemented using the standard EM algorithm with some slight modification to the M-step to incorporate the prior pseudo counts (Dempster et al., 1977), leading to the following updating formulas:

$$Z_{w,d} = \frac{\lambda_d^{(n)} p^{(n)}(w|\theta_T)}{\lambda_d^{(n)} p^{(n)}(w|\theta_T) + (1 - \lambda_d^{(n)}) p(w|\theta_B)}, \tag{2}$$

$$\lambda_d^{(n+1)} = \frac{\mu \lambda_{prior} + \sum_{w \in V} c(w, d) Z_{w,d}}{\mu + \sum_{w \in V} c(w, d)}, \tag{3}$$

$$p^{(n+1)}(w|\theta_T) = \frac{\sigma k p(w|\theta_Q) + \sum_{d \in D} c(w, d) Z_{w,d}}{\sigma k + \sum_{w' \in V} \sum_{d \in D} c(w', d) Z_{w',d}}, \tag{4}$$

where λ_{prior} is the mean of the beta prior for λ_d, $p(w|\theta_Q)$ is the original query model (defining the Dirichlet prior mean), and σ and μ are our confidence on λ_{prior} and the original query model prior (*i.e.*, prior equivalent sample size), respectively. Note that k is the number of feedback documents, and we parameterize the confidence on the query model prior with σk so that σ can be interpreted as the equivalent sample size relative to each document.

On the surface, it appears that we now have more parameters to set than in the old model. However, all the parameters can be set in a meaningful way, and with appropriate regulation, we can hope the model not to be sensitive to the setting of all parameters.

First, σ encodes our confidence on the original query model, corresponding to the expected amount of feedback. It can be interpreted as the "equivalent sample size" of our prior as compared with one *single* feedback document. Thus if σ is set to 10, the original query model would influence the estimated query model as much as a *completely* relevant document with $10 \times k$ words. This setting is found to be optimal in all our experiments.

Second, λ_{prior} corresponds to our prior of how much relevance information is in each document. A smaller λ_{prior} would cause a more discriminative topic model to be estimated, since with a very small λ, only the rarest words in a document will be taken as from the topic model. The influence of this prior is controlled by the confidence parameter μ. A larger μ would cause all the documents to have nearly identical λ's, whereas a smaller μ would allow us to discount different feedback documents more aggressively and differently. A smaller μ would also make the performance insensitive to λ_{prior}, since the prior would be weak. As will be discussed later, the experiment results do show that a smaller μ is indeed beneficial.

While this model appears to be similar to the model proposed in Zhai and Lafferty (2001a), there are two important differences:

(1) In the old mixture model proposed in Zhai and Lafferty (2001a), we pool all the feedback documents together, and have a single mixture model for the "concatenated feedback document", whereas in our new model, each document has a *separate* mixture model, which allows us to model the different amount of relevant information in each document. As a result, we can discount documents with little relevant information in a principled way.

(2) In the old mixture model, we do not consider the original query model when estimating the mixture model parameters, whereas in the new model, we use a Maximum A Posterior (MAP) estimator and use the original query model to define a conjugate prior for the topic language model θ_T. Although, in effect, this also results in a linear interpolation between the original query model and the feedback document model, the interpolation coefficient is dynamic and the query model can regulate the estimation of the feedback model, making the estimate more robust against shifting to a distracting topic in the feedback document set.

These two differences allow the new model to address the above-mentioned two problems with the old mixture model. Note that if we put an infinitely strong prior on all the λ_i's, and we do not use the original query model as a prior, we will recover the old model proposed in Zhai and Lafferty (2001a) as a special case.

4 The Experiments

In this section, we present some experiment results with the proposed mixture model. Since the purpose of the mixture model is to estimate a potentially better query model θ_T by exploiting biased clustering of words in the feedback documents, we evaluate the effectiveness of our model and parameter estimation based on the retrieval performance from using the estimated query model θ_T.

4.1 Experiment Design

We use the Associated Press (AP) data available through TREC Voorhees and Harman (2001) as our document database, which has 164597 news articles. We use TREC topics 101 – 150 as our experiment queries (Voorhees and Harman, 2001). On average, each topic has about 100 relevant documents. We use the standard average precision measure to evaluate retrieval performance (Baeza-Yates and Ribeiro-Neto, 1999); the average precision is a single number measure for a ranking result.

4.2 Experimental Results

This section reports on three kinds of effects that were studed in the designed experiments.

Influence of λ

The first research question we want to answer is whether the flexibility of allowing each document to have a different relevance parameter λ actually leads to a more accurate estimate of the query model. This question can be answered by varying the parameter μ while fixing all the other parameters.

As discussed in Section 3, the parameter μ is our confidence on the prior λ_{prior}. The larger μ is, the more we trust the prior. When μ goes to infinity, we essentially fix the λ of each document to a constant value λ_{prior}. On the other hand, when μ is set to zero, the model has maximum flexibility to allow each document to have a different λ. Therefore, by changing the value of λ, we can see how such flexibility affects the retrieval performance of the estimated query model. To exclude the influence of other parameters, we set $\sigma = 0$, which is equivalent to ignoring the query model prior entirely, thus the estimated query model is entirely based on the feedback documents.

The results are shown in Fig. 3, where the x-axis is different μ in log scale and the y-axis is the mean average precision over all the 50 topics. The two curves in the figure correspond to using 100 and 300 feedback documents, respectively.

From the results in Fig. 3, we see clearly that the performance drops as μ increases. Since a larger μ means less flexibility in estimating a different λ for each document, we can conclude from these results that allowing each document to have a potentially different λ – a feature of our new mixture model as compared with the old model proposed in Zhai and Lafferty (2001a)

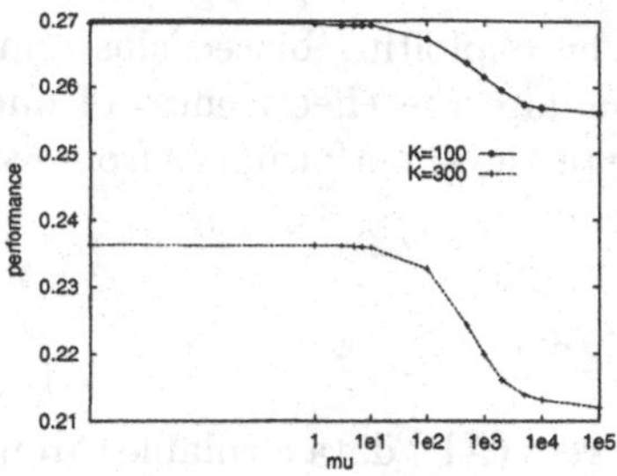

Fig. 3. Influence of μ .

– indeed helps improve performance. Intuitively, this also makes sense, since with a small μ, the EM algorithm has more flexibility to estimate a potentially different λ for each document, which, in effect, achieves a weighting of each document when pooling the word counts to estimate the new query model. When μ is large, we do not have this flexibility, and *all* feedback documents are treated equally, which is not reasonable because not all the feedback documents are relevant. This is especially true when we use a large number of documents for feedback. These results are quite encouraging, as it suggests that we can simply set $\mu = 0$ and the model will be insensitive to the prior λ_{prior}. Compared with the old mixture model, this is a significant advantage, as in the old model, we must manually tune the parameter λ to optimize the retrieval performance (Zhai and Lafferty, 2001a).

Influence of query prior

The second question we want to answer is whether our treatment of the original query model as a prior has any advantages over the heuristic interpolation of the original query model with a feedback model as in Zhai and Lafferty (2001a). This question can be answered by varying the parameter σ while fixing λ (to 0.9 and μ as infinity in our experiments).

Since σ reflects our confidence on the query model prior, it essentially controls how much weight we put on the original query model when mixing it with the new relevance information from the feedback document. Setting $\sigma = 0$ would ignore the original query model completely, while setting σ to a very large number would, in effect, turn off feedback and our estimated new query model would be precisely the original query model. One possible advantage of treating the original query model as a prior is that it allows a flexible interpolation in the sense that different queries may have a different interpolation coefficient, depending on how much relevance information exists in the feedback documents. This means that the optimal setting of σ can be expected to be more *stable* than that of the interpolation coefficient in the old mixture model.

Fig. 4 (left) shows the results of varying σ. We see that: (1) The optimal performance is usually achieved when σ is somewhere not too small and not too large, suggesting that a good balance between query prior and feedback relevant model is necessary to achieve optimal performance. (2) The optimal setting of σ appears to be insensitive to the number of documents used for feedback.

We also plotted how the performance is affected by the interpolation coefficient in the old mixture model in Fig. 4 (right). The two plots have similar patterns. Theoretically, when σ goes to 0, it is equivalent to that α goes to 1, when both methods perform worst. However, our method tends to be more flat/stable when σ increases than the old model when α goes to 0.

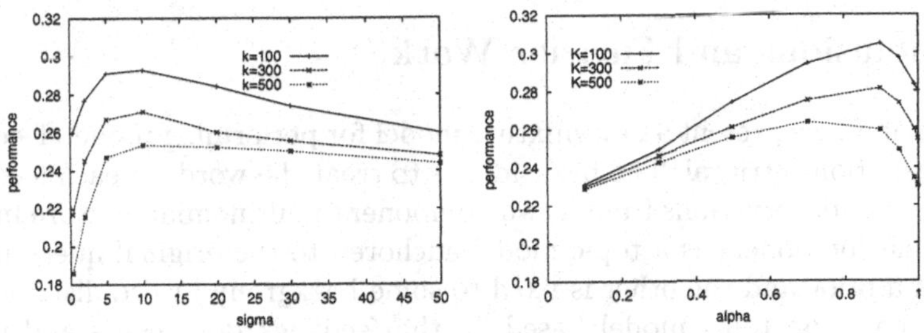

Fig. 4. Influence of σ for the new mixture model (left) and α for the old mixture model .

Sensitivity on the number of feedback documents

Finally, we examine the sensitivity of performance to the number of feedback document. For this purpose, we control σ and μ and vary the number of feedback documents. The results are plotted in Fig. 5 (left), where μ is set to infinity and λ is set to 0.9). For comparison,we also plot similar results from using the old mixture model in Fig. 5(right), where λ is set to 0.9. We see that in both figures, the performance is least sensitive to the number of documents when the original query model has the largest weight (σ = 50 for the new model and α = 0.1 for the old model), but their absolute retrieval performance is not good, as we barely update the query model with the feedback documents. As we do more feedback, we see that the sensitivity pattern appears to be similar for both our new model and the old model. This suggests that while we allow each document to have a different λ, it does not penalize the low-ranked documents sufficiently to ensure the estimated model to be mainly based on the top ranked documents. This can also be seen from the fact that the performance tends to peak around using 50 documents for all parameter settings and for both models. That is, the number of documents to use is still the major parameter to set empirically.

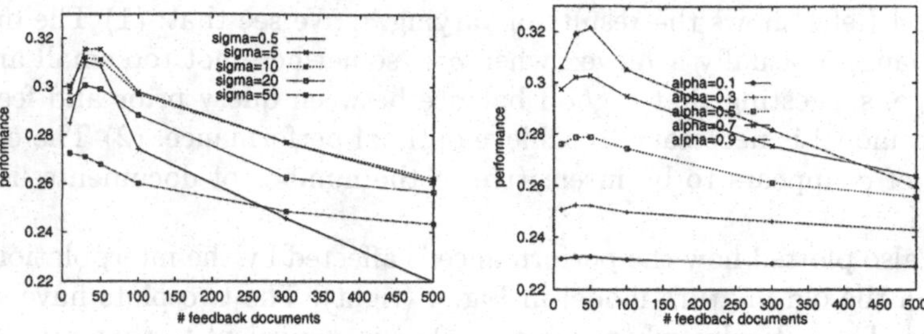

Fig. 5. Precision of using different number of feedback documents for new model (left) and old model(right).

5 Conclusions and Further Work

In this paper, we present a new mixture model for performing pseudo feedback for information retrieval. The basic idea is to treat the words in each feedback document as observations from a two-component multinomial mixture model, where one component is a topic model anchored to the original query model through a prior and the other is fixed to some background word distribution. We estimate the topic model based on the feedback documents and use it as a new query model for ranking documents. This new model extends and improves a similar existing mixture model in two ways: (1) It allows each feedback document to have a different mixing parameter, which is shown to improve retrieval performance in our experiments. (2) It incorporates the original query model into the mixture model as a prior on the topic model, which is a more principled way of updating the query model than the heuristic interpolation used in the old mixture model. Our model can be regarded as performing a "biased clustering" of words in the feedback documents.

There are several directions for further extending the work presented here. First, we need to test the model with more data sets to see if the patterns reported here are general patterns of the model. Second, the high sensitivity to the number of feedback documents remains an unsolved issue. It is very important to further improve the mixture model and the estimation methods to make it more robust against the change in the number of feedback documents. One possibility is to let the EM algorithm start with the original query model and *very conservatively* "grow" the topic model by incorporating the relevance information from the feedback documents. As long as we grow the topic model *"slowly"* and maintain a discrimination among documents based on relevance, the estimation can be expected to be more robust against the number of feedback documents. The growth of the topic model can be controlled by the two prior confidence parameters (for the topic model prior and the mixing weight prior). So one heuristic way for regulating the EM algorithm is to *dynamically* change these confidence parameters.

References

1. Baeza-Yates, R. A., Ribeiro-Neto, B. A. (1999). *Modern Information Retrieval*, Addison-Wesley, New York.
2. Croft, W. B., and Lafferty, J.(2003). *Language Modeling and Information Retrieval*, Kluwer Academic Publishers.
3. Dempster, A. P., Laird,N. M., and Rubin, D. B. (1977). "Maximum Likelihood from Incomplete Data Via the EM Algorithm, *Journal of the Royal Statistical Society, Series B*, **39**, 1–38.
4. Lafferty, J., and Zhai, C. (2001). "Document Language Models, Query Models, and Risk Minimization for Information Retrieval," in *Proceedings of SIGIR'01*, 111–119.
5. Ponte, J., and Croft, W. B. (1998). "A Language Modeling Approach to Information Retrieval," in *Proceedings of the ACM SIGIR'98*, 275–281.
6. Sparck-Jones, K., and Willet, P. (1997). *Readings in Information Retrieval*, Morgan Kaufmann Publishers.
7. Voorhees E., and Harman, D. (2001). *Proceedings of Text REtrieval Conference (TREC1-9)*. NIST Special Publications.
8. Zhai, C., and Lafferty, J.(2001). "Model-Based Feedback in the KL-Divergence Retrieval Model," in *Proceedings of Tenth International Conference on Information and Knowledge Management.*
9. Zhai, C., and Lafferty, J. (2001). "A Study of Smoothing Methods for Language Models Applied to Ad Hoc Information Retrieval," *Proceedings of SIGIR'01*, 334–342.

Analysis of Cross-Language Open-Ended Questions Through MFACT

Mónica Bécue[1], Jérôme Pagès[2], and Campo-Elías Pardo[3]

[1] Universitat Politècnica de Catalunya, Spain
monica.becue@upc.es
[2] Institut Nationales Supérieur de Formation Agro-Alimentaire, France
jerome.pages@agrorennes.educagri.fr
[3] Universidad Nacional de Colombia, Colombia
cepardot@unal.edu.co

Abstract: International surveys lead to multilingual open-ended responses. By grouping the answers for the same categories from different countries, sets of comparable category-documents are obtained. The methodology here presented, called multiple factor analysis of contingency tables (MFACT), provides a representation of all of the documents in a common reference space, on the one hand, and of all of the words in a common reference space, on the other hand; these both spaces are related by transition formulae. This methodology allows a direct generalized canonical analysis approach to analyzing multiple contingency tables as well as for keeping correspondence analysis-like features. It works from the raw data, without any previous translation. An example, extracted from a large international survey in four countries, illustrates the potential of this approach.

1 Introduction

One of the reference methodologies to analyze open-ended questions is correspondence analysis (CA) (Lebart et al., 1998), as applied to individual lexical tables (individual answers × word tables) or to aggregated lexical tables (category-documents × word tables). These are built up by gathering the answers of individuals belonging to the same category (e.g. young women, etc.).

International surveys lead one to deal with cross-language open-ended questions. A solution could be to translate all of the answers into one of the languages, but this presents two different drawbacks. First, it is costly. Second, important features and nuances can be destroyed by translation.

The methodology that we propose, multiple factor analysis for contingency tables (MFACT) (Bécue and Pagès, 2004), tackles all of the responses without any translation, operating from the various aggregated lexical tables, one for each country, which can be juxtaposed row-wise when using the same categories. The goal consists of analyzing this multiple contingency table in order to describe the categories from an international point of view but also from the point of view of each country, looking for structures common to all the countries or specific to only some of them. MFACT, an extension of multiple factor analysis (MFA), can be seen as a particular multicanonical method.

Section 2 shows the close connection existing between MFA and Carroll's generalized canonical correlation analysis. In Section 3, after introducing the notation (Section 3.1), CA is presented as a particular principal component analysis (Section 3.2) and the main properties of MFACT as applied to lexical tables are described (Sections 3.3 and 3.4). Section 4 offers some results obtained from an international survey.

2 MFA as a Multicanonical Analysis

Among multicanonical methods, Carroll's generalized canonical correlation analysis (Carroll, 1968) and multiple factor analysis MFA (Escofier and Pagès, 1998) similar strategies. Both methods deal with a multiple table of individual×quantitative variables $\mathbf{X}$ of order $I \times J$, where the variables are divided into groups K_t containing the variables $v_{j,t}$ (for $t = 1, \ldots, T$; $j = 1, \ldots, J_t$; $\sum_{t=1}^{T} J_t = J$)), and search for a series of S uncorrelated latent general variables, z_s that are related as much as possible to the T groups K_t of variables. Then, for each general variable z_s, they look for their representatives in every group, called canonical variables, which are linear combinations of the variables of the group having the maximum relationship with the corresponding general variable. The difference between these methods comes from their measures of the relationship between a variable and a group of variables.

In Carroll's generalized canonical correlation analysis, the relationship between a quantitative variable z and the set of variables of group K_t is the cosine of the angle between z and the subspace generated by the variables of this group. In MFA (Pagès and Tenenhaus, 2001), the relationship between a quantitative variable z and the set of variables of group K_t is the weighted total inertia of the variables of this group in the direction of z as given by:

$$\mathcal{L}_g(z, K_t) = \sum_{j=1}^{J_t} m_t \mathrm{Corr}^2(z, v_{j,t}) \tag{1}$$

with $m_t = 1/\lambda_1^t$ for λ_1^t the first eigenvalue of the separate principal component analysis of group K_t. The weights m_t balance the influence of the groups of variables in the determination of the first general variable. Using this relationship measure, the general variables z_s are defined by maximizing $\sum_t \mathcal{L}_g(z_s, K_t)$ subject to the constraints $\mathrm{Var}(z_s) = 1$ and $\mathrm{Corr}(z_s, z_t) = 0 \,\forall\, t \neq s$.

Both methods can also be seen as principal component analysis with specific metrics. The general variables are the standardized principal components.

Carroll's generalized canonical correlation analysis can also be performed as a PCA applied to the global table $\mathbf{X}$, using as the metric the block diagonal matrix composed of the inverses of the variance-covariance matrices internal to every group K_t. In the case of MFA, from reexpressing $\mathcal{L}_g(z_s, K_t)$ and $\sum_t \mathcal{L}_g(z_s, K_t)$ respectively as

$$\mathcal{L}_g(z_s, K_t) = \frac{1}{I^2}\mathbf{z}_s'\mathbf{X}_t\mathbf{M}_t\mathbf{X}_t'\mathbf{z}_s, \quad \sum_t \mathcal{L}_g(z_s, K_t) = \frac{1}{I^2}\mathbf{z}'_s\mathbf{XMX}'\mathbf{z}_s$$

it can be deduced that the set of variables z_s are the standardized principal components ($\mathbf{z}_s = \mathbf{F}_s/\sqrt{\lambda_s}$) of the global table $\mathbf{X}$ using matrix $\mathbf{M}$ as weights for columns (and as the metric in the space of individuals). The $\mathbf{M}$ is the diagonal matrix of order $J \times J$, composed by T diagonal submatrices, of order $J_t \times J_t$, with term m_t repeated J_t times (Pagès and Tenenhaus, 2001).

3 MFACT

This section provides the technical details needed to apply MFACT to cross-language survey data.

3.1 Notation

When considering only one country, a lexical table $\mathbf{X}$, of order $I \times J$, is built up. Its general term f_{ij} is the relative number of occurrences of the word j, $j = 1, \ldots, J$, in all of the answers in category i, $i = 1, \ldots, I$, so $\sum_{ij} f_{ij} = 1$. And $\mathbf{D}_I$ is the diagonal matrix with general term $f_{i\cdot} = \sum_j f_{ij}$, $i = 1, \ldots, I$. The $\mathbf{D}_J$ is the diagonal matrix with general term $f_{\cdot j} = \sum_i f_{ij}$, $j = 1, \ldots, J$. When dealing with several countries, there are T lexical tables $\mathbf{X}_t$, of order $I \times J_t$, built up and juxtaposed row-wise to form the global table $\mathbf{X}_G$ of dimension $I \times J$. The general term f_{ijt} is the proportion, in table t for $t = 1, \ldots, T$, with which category i is associated with word j ($j = 1, \ldots, J_t$; $\sum_t J_t = J$) so that $\sum_{ijt} f_{ijt} = 1$.

We denote the row margin of table $\mathbf{X}_G$ as $f_{i\cdot\cdot} = \sum_{jt} f_{ijt}$ and the column margin of table $\mathbf{X}_G$ as $f_{\cdot jt} = \sum_i f_{ijt}$. The row margin of table t, as a subtable of table $\mathbf{X}_G$, is $f_{i\cdot t} = \sum_j f_{ijt}$, and the sum of the terms of table t inside table $\mathbf{X}_G$ is $f_{\cdot\cdot t} = \sum_{ij} f_{ijt}$. Then $\mathbf{D}_{I_T}$ is the diagonal matrix with general term $f_{i\cdot\cdot}$ and $\mathbf{D}_{J_T}$ is the diagonal matrix with general term $f_{\cdot jt}$.

3.2 CA as a Principal Component Analysis

To apply classical CA to table $\mathbf{X}$ is equivalent to performing a principal component analysis (cf. Escofier and Pagès, 1998, pp. 95-97) on the table $\mathbf{W}$ whose general term is given by

$$w_{ij} = \frac{f_{ij} - f_{i\cdot}f_{\cdot j}}{f_{i\cdot}f_{\cdot j}}, \tag{2}$$

using $\mathbf{D}_I$ as the row weights and metric in the column space, and $\mathbf{D}_J$ as the column weights and metric in the row space.

3.3 MFACT as a Specific PCA

MFACT applied to table $\mathbf{X}_G$ consists in a PCA on the table $\mathbf{Y}$ whose general term is given by

$$y_{ijt} = \frac{f_{ijt} - \left(\frac{f_{i\cdot t}}{f_{\cdot\cdot t}}\right) f_{\cdot jt}}{f_{i\cdot\cdot} f_{\cdot jt}} = \frac{1}{f_{i\cdot\cdot}} \left[\frac{f_{ijt}}{f_{\cdot jt}} - \frac{f_{i\cdot t}}{f_{\cdot\cdot t}} \right], \tag{3}$$

using $\mathbf{D}_{I_T}$ as the row weights and metric in the column space and $\mathbf{D}_{J_T}$ as the column weights and metric in the row space.

The global principal components are $\mathbf{F}_s = \lambda_s{}^{-1} \sum_t \mathbf{Y}_t \mathbf{D}_{J_t} \mathbf{Y'}_t \mathbf{D}_{I_T} \mathbf{F}_s$. The general variables are the standardized global principal components $\mathbf{z}_s = \mathbf{F}_s / \sqrt{\lambda_s}$. The canonical components $\mathbf{F}_s^t$ associated with the global principal components $\mathbf{F}_s$ in each group t are defined from $\mathbf{F}_s = \sum_t \mathbf{F}_s^t$ so that $\mathbf{F}_s^t = \lambda_s{}^{-1} \mathbf{Y}_t \mathbf{D}_{J_t} \mathbf{Y'}_t \mathbf{D}_{I_T} \mathbf{F}_s$.

3.4 Application of MFACT to Cross-Language Surveys

Global and Partial Documents. All of the answers corresponding to category i for $i = 1, \ldots, I$ over the different countries, form the global category-document i, characterized through the coordinates given by (4). The weighting by $1/\sqrt{\lambda_1^t}$ balances the importance of each country in the global document.

$$\frac{f_{ijt} - \left(\frac{f_{i\cdot t}}{f_{\cdot\cdot t}}\right) f_{\cdot jt}}{f_{i\cdot\cdot} f_{\cdot jt} \sqrt{\lambda_1^t}} = \frac{1}{\sqrt{\lambda_1^t} f_{i\cdot\cdot}} \left[\frac{f_{ijt}}{f_{\cdot jt}} - \frac{f_{i\cdot t}}{f_{\cdot\cdot t}} \right] \quad t = 1, \ldots, T; j = 1, \ldots, J_t. \tag{4}$$

The *partial* document i^t consists in the whole of the answers of category i but only in country t. Its coordinates are those given by (4) restricted to t.

MFACT analyzes the global-document$\times$words table and defines distances between global documents and between words. In MFACT, each partial document i^t is considered as a supplementary row by completing the columns j, r ($r \neq t$) by zeroes and projecting onto the global axes. In this way, the representations of the partial documents and of the global documents (or average documents) are superimposed. Thus, the relative positions of the separate documents corresponding to a same global document can be studied.

Distances Between Global Documents. The squared distance between documents i and l, calculated from coordinates given in (4), is:

$$d^2(i,l) = \left[\sum_t \frac{1}{\lambda_1^t} \sum_{j \in J_t} \left(\frac{f_{ijt}}{f_{i\cdot\cdot}} - \frac{f_{ljt}}{f_{l\cdot\cdot}}\right)^2 \frac{1}{f_{\cdot jt}}\right] - \left[\sum_t \frac{1}{\lambda_1^t f_{\cdot\cdot t}} \left(\frac{f_{i\cdot t}}{f_{i\cdot\cdot}} - \frac{f_{l\cdot t}}{f_{l\cdot\cdot}}\right)^2\right].$$

Here, disregarding weighting by the inverse of the first eigenvalue, the first term corresponds to the distance between profiles i and l in the CA of the juxtaposed tables. The second term corresponds to the distance between profiles i and l in the CA of the table containing the sums by row and by subtable. And the general term $i \cdot t$ in this table denotes the sum over j for row i in table t. We see here how this last table is neutralized by recentering each subtable on its own margins.

Distances Between Words. The squared distance between word j (belonging to table t) and word k (belonging to table r) is given below:

$$d^2(j \in t, k \in r) = \sum_i \frac{1}{f_{i\cdot\cdot}} \left[\left(\frac{f_{ijt}}{f_{\cdot jt}} - \frac{f_{ikr}}{f_{\cdot kr}}\right) - \left(\frac{f_{i\cdot t}}{f_{\cdot\cdot t}} - \frac{f_{i\cdot r}}{f_{\cdot\cdot r}}\right)\right]^2. \tag{5}$$

Case 1: the words belong to a same table ($t = r$). The proximity between two words is interpreted in terms of resemblance between profiles, as in CA.
Case 2: the words belong to different tables ($t \neq r$). Equation (5) shows how the differences between word profiles are relativized by the differences between average profiles.

Distributional Equivalence Property. The distance between words and between documents induced by MFACT conserves the distributional equivalence property. It preserves the fact that, as in CA applied to one lexical table, gathering synonyms (in terms of a synonym dictionary) changes neither the distances between words nor the distances between documents when they have the same profiles. But such gathering does change these distances if the synonym profiles are different. In that case one might avoid this data transformation and claims for operating without any translation which could collapse words with different profiles into a unique column-word.

Transition Formula for Documents Among Words. The relation giving (along the s-axis) the coordinate $F_s(i)$ of global document i from the coordinates $\{G_s(j,t): j = 1,\ldots,J_t; t = 1,\ldots,T\}$ of the words is:

$$F_s(i) = \frac{1}{\sqrt{\lambda_s}} \sum_t \frac{1}{\lambda_1^t} \frac{f_{i\cdot t}}{f_{i\cdot\cdot}} \left[\sum_{j \in J_t} \frac{f_{ijt}}{f_{i\cdot t}} G_s(j,t)\right]. \tag{6}$$

Except for a constant, each category-document lies in the centroid of the words associated with this document. Globally, a document is attracted by the words with which it is associated.

Transition Formula for Partial Documents Among Words. The superimposed representation of the partial documents benefits from CA properties. In particular, these partial representations can be related to word representation by means of a "restricted" transition formula:

$$F_s^t(i) = \frac{1}{\sqrt{\lambda_s}} \frac{f_{i\cdot t}}{f_{i\cdot\cdot}} \left[\sum_{j \in J_t} \frac{f_{ijt}}{f_{i\cdot t}} \frac{G_s(j,t)}{\lambda_1^t} \right].$$

In the graph superimposing partial representations (see Fig. 3 in Section 4), the coordinates of the partial documents are dilated by the coefficient T (number of tables). Thus, a global document point is located in the centroid of the corresponding partial document points.

Transition Formula for Words Among Documents. The expression (along the s-axis) for the coordinate $G_s(j,t)$ of word j,t from the coordinates $\{F_s(i), i{=}1,\ldots,I\}$ of documents is:

$$G_s(j,t) = \frac{1}{\sqrt{\lambda_s}} \left[\sum_i \left(\frac{f_{ijt}}{f_{\cdot jt}} - \frac{f_{i\cdot t}}{f_{\cdot\cdot t}} \right) F_s(i) \right].$$

As the coefficient of $F_s(i)$ can be negative, the words are not in the centroid of the documents except when the document weights are the same in all the tables. This coefficient measures the discrepancy between the profile of words j,t and the column margin of table t. A word is attracted (or repelled) by documents that are more (or less) associated with it than if there were independence between documents and words in table t.

4 Example

The data are extracted from a large international survey (Hayashi et al., 1992). People from four countries (Great Britain, France, Italy, Japan) were asked several closed questions and the open-ended question: *"What is the most important thing to you in life?"* was also considered. The Japanese answers are romanized.

In each country, the free answers are grouped into 18 category-documents by crossing gender (male, female), age (into three categories: 18-34, 35-44, 55 and over) and education level (into three categories: low, medium and high). Then, for each country, from the count of words in the whole answers, the lexical table arises by crossing the 18 documents and the most frequent words. Only the words used at least 20 times are kept.

4.1 Results Obtained From MFACT

Visualization of the Global Documents. The visualization of the documents obtained by MFACT is given by Fig. 1. On this figure, the six trajectories for gender and age are drawn; they show a rather regular structure, a compromise between the representations that would have been offered by the separate CA. Age increases along the first axis, and the second axis opposes the genders. The categories with the high education degree have, on the first axis, coordinates which correspond to younger people with lower degrees.

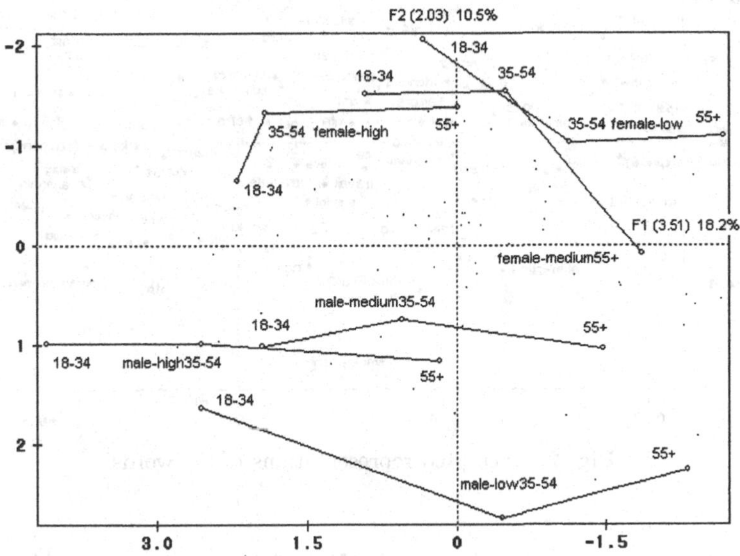

Fig. 1. Representation of the global documents.

Visualization of the Words. Figure 2 shows an excerpt of the representation of the words. We can see, for example, that the word *husband* and its translation in French (*mari*) and Japanese (*shuzin* and *otto*) tend to be quoted in the same categories.

Superimposed Representation of the Partial Documents. In order to compare the structures induced on the documents by the four sets of words, we superimpose the global description of the documents and those induced by each country (partial documents). We can interpret the relative positions of partial documents of a same country: for example, Fig. 3 suggests that males and females in the 35-54 age interval, whatever the qualifications, almost do not differ in Italy. We can also interpret the relative positions of partial documents corresponding to a same global document; Fig. 3 suggests that males in the 35-54 age interval with high education degree or with only medium degree

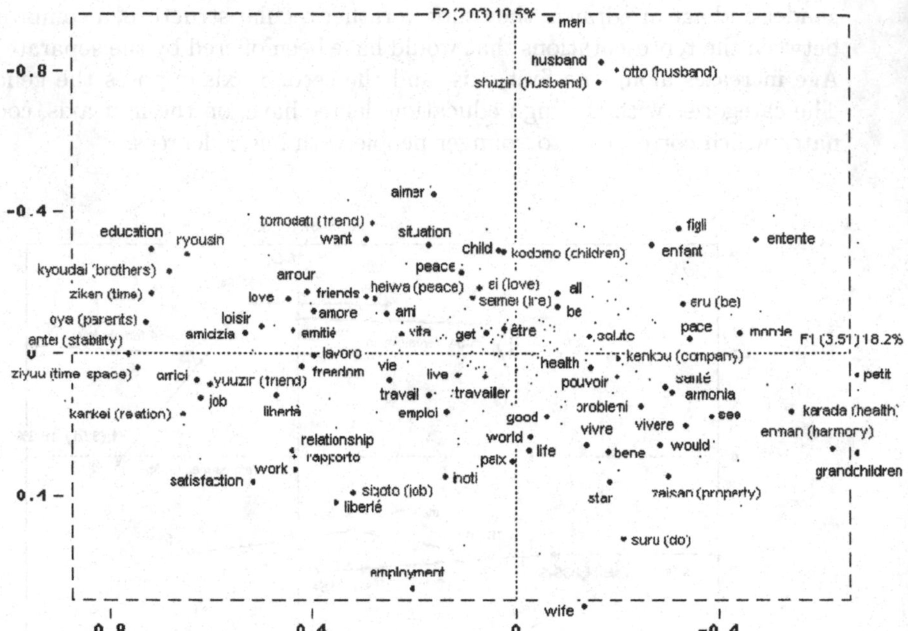

Fig. 2. Excerpted representations of the words.

use almost the same vocabulary in the United Kingdom but greatly differ in Japan.

5 Conclusion

MFACT allows one to adopt a direct multicanonical approach to analyze multiple contingency table. Its application to cross-language aggregated lexical tables presents interesting properties such as to the ability to locate all of the words in the same representation space, on the one hand, and all the documents in the same representation space, on the other hand, with both spaces being linked through transition formulae. So the similarities between documents can be interpreted in terms of semantics and the similarities between words in terms of user profiles.

Acknowledgements

This work has been supported by the European project NEMIS (IST-2001-37574), by the Spanish Science and Technology Ministery (SEC2001-2581-C02-02) and by a grant from National University of Colombia - Bogotá. We

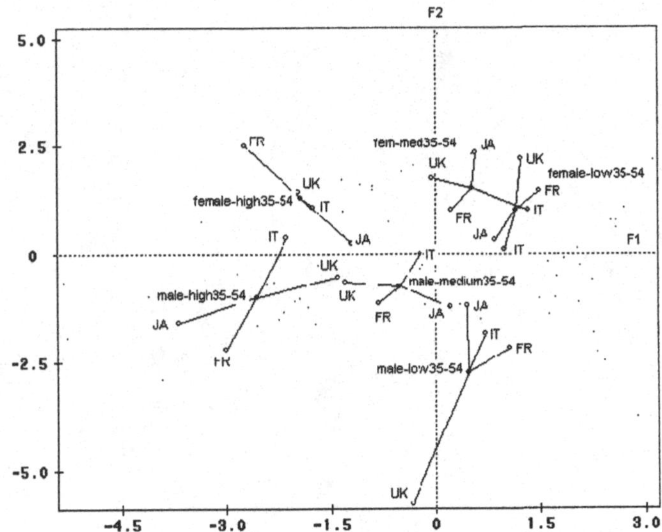

Fig. 3. Excerpts of the superimposed representation: Global and partial documents corresponding to all the categories between 35 and 54 years old.

also thank Profesor Ludovic Lebart for his help in acquiring the dataset used in Section 4.

References

1. Bécue, M., and Pagès, J. (2004). "A Rrincipal Axes Method for Comparing Multiple Contingency Tables: MFACT," *Computational Statistics & Data Analysis* (in press, available online in Science Direct).
2. Carroll, J. D. (1968). "Generalization of Canonical Correlation Analysis to Three or More Sets of Variables," *Proceedings of the 76th Convention of the American Psychology Association*, **3**, 227–228.
3. Escofier, B., and Pagès, J. (1998). *Analyses Factorielles Simples et Multiples. Objectifs, Méthodes et Interprétation*, 3rd ed., Dunod, Paris.
4. Hayashi, C., Suzuki, T., and Sasaki, M. (1992). *Data Analysis for Social Comparative Research: International Perspective*, North Holland.
5. Lebart, L., Salem, A., and Berry, E. (1998). *Exploring Textual Data*, Kluwer, Dordrecht.
6. Pagès, J., and Tenenhaus, M. (2001). "Multiple Factor Analysis Combined With PLS Path Modelling. Application to the Analysis of Relationships Between Physicochemical Variables, Sensory Profiles and hedonic Judgements," *Chemometrics and Intelligent Laboratory Systems*, **58**, 261–273.

Inferring User's Information Context from User Profiles and Concept Hierarchies

Ahu Sieg, Bamshad Mobasher, and Robin Burke

DePaul University, U.S.A.
{asieg,mobasher,rburke}@cs.depaul.edu

Abstract: The critical elements that make up a user's information context include the user profiles that reveal long-term interests and trends, the short-term information need as might be expressed in a query, and the semantic knowledge about the domain being investigated. The next generation of intelligent information agents, that can seamlessly integrate these elements into a single framework, are enabled to effectively locate and provide the most appropriate results for users' information needs. In this paper we present one such framework for contextualized information access. We model the problem in the context of our client-side Web agent ARCH (Adaptive Retrieval based on Concept Hierarchies). In ARCH, the user profiles are generated using an unsupervised document clustering technique. These profiles, in turn, are used to automatically learn the semantic context of user's information need from a domain-specific concept hierarchy. Our experimental results show that implicit measures of user interests, combined with the semantic knowledge embedded in a concept hierarchy, can be used effectively to infer the user context and improve the results of information retrieval.

1 Introduction

The heterogeneity and the lack of structure of the information sources on the World Wide Web, such as hypertext documents, make automated discovery, organization, and management of Web-based information difficult. Despite great advances in Web-based information retrieval technologies, the user interactions with Web search engines can generally be characterized as one size fits all (Allan et al., 2003). This is mainly due to the fact that current systems provide no mechanisms for the representation of user preferences and the semantic context of the domain or the task at hand. Indeed, contextual retrieval has been identified as a long-term challenge in information retrieval. Allan et al. (2003) define it as follows. *Contextual retrieval: Combine search technolo-*

gies and knowledge about query and user context into a single framework in order to provide the most appropriate answer for a user's information needs.

In most information retrieval applications, the burden is placed on the users to formulate effective queries which represent their true search intent. Typical users find this task quite difficult: research confirms that the queries submitted to search engines by Web users are relatively short and are usually limited to less than three keywords (Spink et al., 2002). As a result, the user's search experience is often unsatisfactory.

In previous work we have presented our client-side Web agent ARCH (Adaptive Retrieval based on Concept Hierarchies) (Parent et al., 2001; Sieg et al., 2003). ARCH allows the user to interact with a concept classification hierarchy and uses the results of this interaction to derive an explicit user context for each query session. This user context is represented in the form of an enhance query which can be used for Web search. The goal of the system is, thus, to close the gap between the initial representation of the user's information need and the actual intent for the search. Unlike traditional approaches, ARCH assists users in the creation of an effective query prior to the initial search task.

Various forms of query enhancement have long been a research topic in information retrieval, from relevance feedback (Buckley et al., 1997) to incremental query refinement (Allan, 1996; Eguchi, 2000) to query expansion based on lexical variants such as synonyms (Miller, 1997). Synonym-based query expansion could be considered a primitive form of the application of domain knowledge. However, without a mechanism to disambiguate the sense of the user's query, mere synonym expansion does not tend to improve precision. A number of researchers have explored intelligent Web agents that learn about user's interests in Web-based information access (Boley et al., 1999; Joachims et al., 1997; Lieberman, 1997). All of this work depends on elicitation of user interests and preference. To lessen the requirement for user interaction, lately the attention of the research community has been drawn to explore how various implicit measures of user interests can be used in information retrieval and filtering applications (Dumais et al., 2003; Kelly and J. Teevan, 2003). These approaches, while taking into account the user behavior, do not consider the domain knowledge that can be used as an additional source for disambiguating the context.

In this paper we extend ARCH to provide a more integrated framework for contextualized information access which combines automatically learned user profiles and the semantic knowledge of the domain represented by the concept hierarchy. Our specific goal is to reduce or eliminate the need for explicit user interaction by utilizing the user profiles, while still maintaining the explicit representation of the semantic knowledge as an integral part of the framework. To this end, we use unsupervised document clustering and other text mining techniques for the derivation of user profiles based in past actions. We, then, use these profiles, in lieu of explicit user interaction, to derive the user context from the concept hierarchy. Our experimental results show that our integrated approach does, indeed, result in substantial gains in retrieval precision, without sacrificing recall.

2 Inferring User Context for Information Access

Our main goal is to create a unified model of user information goals through the seamless integration of semantic knowledge with automatically learned user profiles. In this section we discuss our approaches for the derivation of user profiles from document clusters and for learning an aggregate representation of the domain ontology in the form of a concept taxonomy. We then discuss how these two sources of information can be used for contextualized information access and retrieval.

2.1 Derivation of User Profiles from Document Clusters

The profiling component of ARCH attempts to learn a model of user behavior through the passive observation of user's information access activity (including browsing and searching) over time. Other implicit measures of user interest such as dwell time, click through, and user activities like annotation, printing, and purchasing can also be used to develop predictive models for a variety of purpose (Dumais et al., 2003). Through this observation, ARCH collects a set of documents in which the user has shown interest. Several factors, including the frequency of visits to a page, the amount of time spent on the page, and other user actions such as bookmarking a page are used as bases for heuristics that are employed by the system to automatically collect these documents without user intervention.

Once enough documents have been collected as part of the profile generation, a clustering algorithm is used to cluster the documents into semantically related categories based on a vector similarity measure. Each document is represented as a term vector. For computing the term weights extracted from content, the system employs a standard function of the term frequency and inverse document frequency (tf.idf) (Salton and McGill, 1983; Frakes and Baeza-Yates, 1992). Our method for the generation of topical profiles is similar to the concept indexing method (Karypis and Han, 2000). Individual profiles are obtained by computing the centroid vector of each of the document clusters produced by the clustering algorithm. Specifically, given a document collection D and a document cluster $C \subseteq D$, we construct a profile pr_c as a set of term-weight pairs:

$$pr_c = \{\langle t, weight(t, pr_c)\rangle \,|weight(t, pr_c) \geq \mu\}.$$

In the above equation, the significance weight, *weight(t,pr_c)*, of the term t within the profile pr_c is computed as follows:

$$weight(t, pr_c) = \frac{1}{|C|} \cdot \sum_{d \in C} w(t, d).$$

In the above formula, $w(t, d)$ is the weight of term t in the document vector d. The threshold μ is used to filter out terms which are not significant within each profile. Each profile is represented as a vector in the original n-dimensional space of terms, where n is the number of unique terms in the global dictionary.

2.2 Representation of Domain Knowledge

To support the users with the task of searching on the Web, ARCH exploits a concept classification hierarchy. The Web is home to Web concept hierarchies, collections of documents labeled with conceptual labels and related to each other in a hierarchical arrangement. The most well known of these is Yahoo (http://www.yahoo.com), which has a multi-level hierarchy covering the full breadth of the topics found on the Web. ARCH uses the domain knowledge inherent in Yahoo and allows the users to interact with the concept hierarchy to explicitly provide user context for each of their query sessions.

ARCH includes an offline component which allows the system to learn a concept classification hierarchy which is then maintained in the system in aggregate form. The system maintains this aggregate representation by pre-computing a weighted term vector for each node in the hierarchy which represents the centroid of all documents and subcategories indexed under that node.

Let's consider a specific node n in the concept hierarchy and assume this node contains, D_n, a collection of individual documents, and, S_n, a set of subconcepts. The term vector for the node n is computed as follows:

$$T_n = \left[\left(\sum_{d \in D_n} T_d \right) / |D_n| + \sum_{s \in S_n} T_s \right] / (|S_n| + 1).$$

In the above formula, T_d is the weighted term vector which represents an individual document d indexed under node n and T_s is the term vector which represents the subconcept s of node n. Note that a term vector is calculated for each indexed document under a concept. The term vectors for the indexed documents are added to get a single term vector which represents the average. This term vector is added to the term vectors for the subconcepts to calculate the final average for the concept.

A global dictionary of terms is created by performing standard information retrieval text preprocessing methods. A stop list is used to remove high frequency, but semantically non-relevant terms from the content. Porter's stemming algorithm (Porter, 1980) is utilized to reduce words to their stems. Term weights are computed, as before, based on the tf.idf measure.

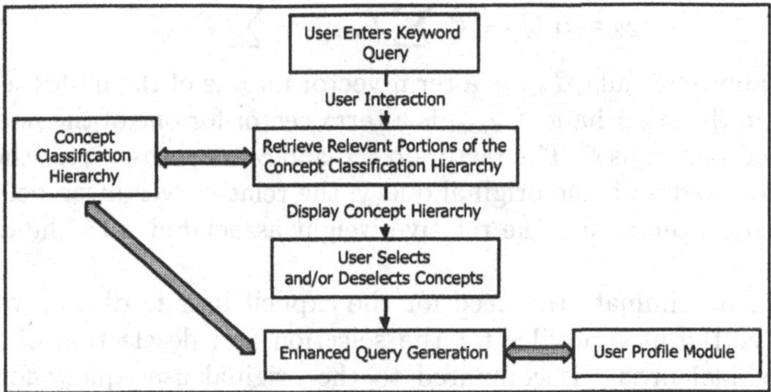

Fig. 1. Query enhancement mechanism in ARCH.

2.3 Utilizing User Context for Web Search

As noted earlier, once enough documents have been collected for profiling, these documents go through a process which clusters them into semantically related categories. The documents are preprocessed and converted into n-dimensional term vectors by computing the tf.idf weights for each term, where n is the total number of unique terms in the global dictionary. It should be noted that the global dictionary contains all unique terms in both the profile documents as well as those used in the aggregate representation of the concepts in the hierarchy. This allows us to use a clustering application, which performs k-means clustering, to partition the document set into groups of similar documents based on a measure of vector similarity. Individual profiles, each representing a topic category, are computed based on the centroid of the document clusters. As a result, each profile is represented as a term vector and the results of our computations are maintained in an XML document.

Our previous work on ARCH focused on an interactive approach for assisting the user in formulating an effective search query. To initiate the query generation process, the user enters a keyword query. The system matches the term vectors representing each node in the concept hierarchy with the list of keywords typed by the user. Those nodes which exceed a similarity threshold are displayed to the user, along with other adjacent nodes. These nodes are considered to be the matching nodes in the concept hierarchy. Once the relevant portions of the hierarchy are displayed, the user interface allows the user to provide explicit feedback by selecting those categories which are relevant to the intended query and to deselect those categories which are not relevant. The query enhancement mechanism is displayed in Figure 1.

We employ a variant of Rocchio's method (1971) for relevance feedback to generate the enhanced query. The pre-computed term vectors associated with each node in the hierarchy are used to enhance the original query, Q_1 as follows:

$$Q_2 = \alpha.Q_1 + \beta.\sum T_{sel} - \gamma.\sum T_{desel}.$$

In the above formula, T_{sel} is a term vector for one of the nodes selected by the user. On the other hand, T_{desel} is a term vector for one of the nodes which is deselected by the user. The factors α, β, and γ are respectively the relative weight associated with the original query, the relative weight associated with the selected concepts, and the relative weight associated with the deselected concepts.

In order to eliminate the need for the explicit user feedback, we alternatively utilize the user profiles for the selection and deselection of concepts. Each individual profile is compared to the original user query for similarity. Those profiles which satisfy a similarity threshold are then compared to the matching nodes in the concept hierarchy. Note that the matching nodes include those nodes which originally exceeded a similarity threshold when compared to the user's original keyword query. While comparing these nodes to the appropriate user profiles, each node is assigned a similarity score. Once all of the appropriate nodes are processed, the node with the highest similarity score is used for automatic selection. The nodes with relatively low similarity scores are used for automatic deselection.

3 Experiments with User Profiles

Our previous work provides a detailed summary of our evaluation results for query enhancement in ARCH based on concept hierarchies (Sieg et al., 2004). To-date, however, query modification in ARCH has involved the manual selection and deselection of concepts. Our current approach allows us to utilize the information stored in the user profiles for the automatic selection and deselection of concepts in the concept hierarchy in order to automatically determine user's context for the original keyword search query.

Since the queries of average Web users tend to be short and ambiguous (Spink et al., 2002), the search keywords we use in our experiments are intentionally chosen to be ambiguous. For each of our keyword queries, several search scenarios were created with the intention of solving the problem of effective discovery of user context. Our keyword queries and search scenarios are displayed in Table 1. We measure the effectiveness of query enhancement in terms of precision and recall.

For our experiments, a one-time learning of the concept hierarchy is necessary to build the aggregate representation of the concept hierarchy in our system. In addition, two sets of user profiles are created with the intention of having each set represent different user interests. The contents of the user profiles are depicted in Table 2.

For evaluation purposes, 10 documents are collected for each word sense of our predetermined keywords which are intentionally chosen to be ambiguous. As an example, for the keyword query *python*, a total of 30 documents are collected where 10 documents relate to the *snake* sense of the word *python*, 10 documents provide information about *Python* as a *programming language*, and the rest of the documents discuss the comedy group *Monty Python*.

Table 1. Example keyword queries and corresponding search scenarios.

# of Term(s)	Query	Signal	Noise
1	bat	buying a baseball bat	information on bat mammal
1	hardware	home hardware and tools	upgrading computer hardware
1	python	python as a snake	Monty Python; Python prog. language
2	baseball bat	buying a baseball bat	information on bat mammal
2	home hardware	home hardware and tools	upgrading computer hardware
2	python snake	python as a snake	Monty Python; Python prog. language

Depending on the search scenario, each document in our collection can be treated as a signal or a noise document. The signal documents are those documents that should be ranked high in the search results. The noise documents are those documents that should be ranked low or excluded from the search results. In order to create an index for the signal and noise documents, a term frequency and inverse document frequency (tf.idf) weight is computed for each term in the document collection using the global dictionary of the concept hierarchy.

Table 2. User interests and corresponding user profiles.

User Profiles	User Interest
Set 1	buying a baseball bat
Set 1	home hardware and tools
Set 1	information about a pet python
Set 2	information on bat as a mammal
Set 2	upgrading computer hardware
Set 2	Python programming language

As depicted in Table 1, our keyword queries are used to run a number of search scenarios. The first set of keyword queries contain only one term and include the following: *bat*, *bug*, *hardware*, *mouse*, and *python*. For example, in order to evaluate the search results when the single keyword *bat* is typed by the user as the search query, one scenario assumes that the user is interested in *buying a baseball bat*. In this case, our user is represented by the first set of user profiles. The documents that are relevant to the *baseball* sense of the word *bat* are treated as signal documents whereas the documents that are related to the *bat mammal* are treated as noise documents.

The second set of queries contain two terms and include the following: *baseball bat*, *bat mammal*, *bug spy*, *hardware computer*, *hardware tools*, *hardware upgrade*, *mouse computer*, and *python snake*. For example, in the case of a user typing *bug spy* as the search query, our search scenario assumes the user's intent for the query is to find information about the *surveillance* sense of the word *bug* as opposed to the *software programming* or the *insect* senses.

In the case of enhanced query search, we use the query that is generated by ARCH. Based on our search scenarios, the user profiles are utilized to automatically select and/or deselect certain concepts in the hierarchy for the generation of the enhanced query.

Our evaluation methodology is as follows. We use the system to perform a simple query search and an enhanced query search for each of our keyword queries. In the case of simple query search, a term vector is built using the original keyword(s) in the query text. Removal of stop words and stemming is utilized. Each term in the original query is assigned a weight of 1.0. The search results are retrieved from the signal and noise document collection by using a cosine similarity measure for matching. The similarity scores are normalized so that the best matching document always has a score of a 100%. This allows us to apply certain thresholds to the similarity scores. For each of our search scenarios, we calculate the precision and recall at similarity thresholds of 0% to 100%.

As mentioned above, each search scenario assumes that the user has a specific goal for the search. The user's context is derived from the information stored in the user profiles. Based on the user's intent for the query and the search results, we calculate the precision and recall metrics for our keyword searches. For each of our search scenarios, the precision and recall metrics are calculated at each 10 point interval between a similarity threshold of 0% and a similarity threshold of 100%.

In order to compare the simple query search results with the enhanced query search results, we have created separate precision and recall graphs for each of our search scenarios. In the case of the simple query search, precision is expected to improve as more terms are added to the query. Our evaluation results verify that precision is higher for the simple query search when using multiple keywords than performing a simple query search using a single keyword.

Figure 2, shows the average precision and recall of the autoamtically enahnced queries in comparison with with simple queries using one and two keywords. These results were obtained by averaging precision and recall values over all the search scenarios described above. These results show that enhancing the query based on the user's search context improves the effectiveness of the search queries, especially in a typical case when relatively short queries are used. We see two types of improvement in the search results using the enhanced query in ARCH. From the user's perspective, precision is improved

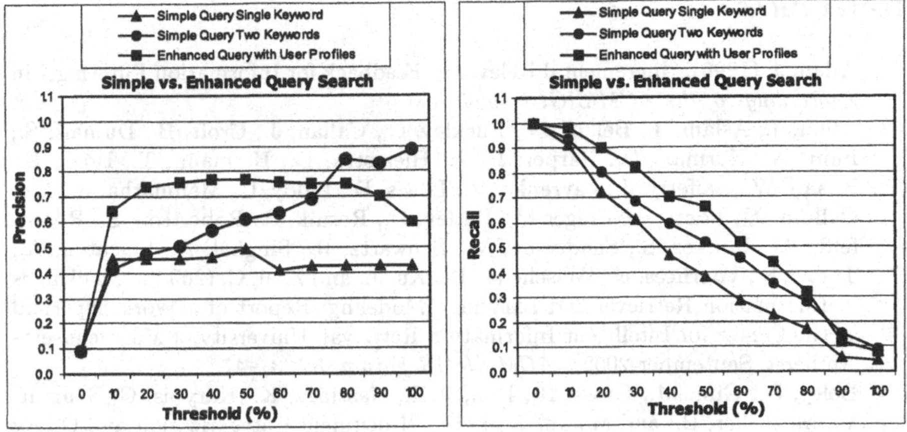

Fig. 2. Avg. precision and recall: Enhanced Query v. Simple Query Search.

since ambiguous query terms are disambiguated by the enhanced query. In addition, when comparing single keyword queries to the enhanced query, we see better recall in the search results since additional query terms, obtained from the concept hierarchy, retrieve documents that would not be retrieved by using only the original keyword query.

4 Conclusions and Outlook

We have presented a framework for the integration of user profiles in ARCH with semantic knowledge represented by a concept hierarchy. We have shown that the information from the user profiles can be successfully utilized to replace the selection and/or deselection of concepts in a domain-specific concept hierarchy. Our experiments also show that we able to create effective user profiles by using clustering techniques. The Web documents that are of interest to the user are divided into clusters for user profiling. The user profiles that are derived from these document clusters accurately represent user interests and user context. This allows for the automatic generation of an enhanced query which retrieves much better search results than a user's poorly designed keyword query.

For future work, we plan to extend the underlying representation of concepts in our framework from unstructured term-vector representation to an ontology-based object-oriented representation which takes into account relationships among objects based on their properties and attributes. This will enable information access and discovery based on a more structured representation of Web information resources, as well as the integration of information access with semantic inference mechanisms.

References

1. Allan, J. (1996). "Incremental Relevance Feedback for Information Filtering," in *Proceedings of the ACM SIGIR 1996.*
2. Allan, J., Aslam, J., Belkin, N., Buckley, C., Callan, J., Croft, B., Dumais, S., Fuhr, N., Harman, D., Harper, D. J., Hiemstra, D., Hofmann, T., Hovy, E., Kraaij, W., Lafferty, J., Lavrenko, V., Lewis, D., Liddy, L., Manmatha, R., McCallum, A., Ponte, J., Prager, J., Radev, D., Resnik, P., Robertson, S., Rosenfeld, R. , Roukos, S., Sanderson, M., Schwartz, R., Singhal, A., Smeaton, A., Turtle, H., Voorhees, E., Weischedel, R., Xu, J., and Zhai, C. (2003). "Challenges in Information Retrieval and Language Modeling: Report of a Workshop Held at the Center for Intelligent Information Retrieval, University of Massachusetts Amherst, September 2002," *ACM SIGIR Forum*, **37**, 31–47.
3. Boley, D., Gini, M., Gross, R., Han, E.H., Hastings, K., Karypis, G., Kumar, V., Mobasher, B., and Moore, J. (1999). "Document Categorization and Query Generation on the World Wide Web Using WebACE," *Artificial Intelligence Review*, **13:5-6**, 365–391.
4. Buckley, C., Salton, G., and Allan, J. (1994). "The Effect of Adding Relevance Information in a Relevance Feedback Environment," in *Proceedings of the ACM SIGIR1994.*
5. Dumais, S., Joachims, T., Bharat, K., and Weigend, A. (2003). "SIGIR 2003 Workshop Report: Implicit Measures of User Interests and Preferences," *ACM SIGIR Forum*, Fall, **37:2**.
6. Eguchi, K. (2000). "Incremental Query Expansion Using Local Information of Clusters," in *Proceedings of the 4th World Multiconference on Systemics, Cybernetics and Informatics (SCI 2000).*
7. Frakes, W. B. and Baeza-Yates, R. (1992). *Information Retrieval: Data Structures and Algorithms*, Prentice Hall, Englewood Cliffs, NJ.
8. Joachims, T., Freitag, D., and Mitchell, T. (1997). "WebWatcher: A Tour Guide for the World Wide Web," in *Proceedings of the Fifteenth International Joint Conference on Artificial Intelligence*, Nagoya, Japan.
9. Karypis, G., and Han, E. H. (2000). "Concept Indexing: A Fast Dimensionality Reduction Algorithm with Applications to Document Retrieval and Categorization," in *Proceedings of the 9th ACM International Conference on Information and Knowledge Management (CIKM'2000)*, McLean, VA.
10. Kelly, D., and Teevan, J. (2003)."Implicit Feedback for Inferring User Preference: A Bibliography," *ACM SIGIR Forum*, Fall, **37:2**.
11. Lieberman, H. (1997). "Autonomous Interface Agents," in *Proceedings of the ACM Conference on Computers and Human Interface (CHI-97)*, Atlanta, GA.
12. Miller, G. (1997). "WORDNET: An Online Lexical Database," *International Journal of Lexicography*, **3:4**.
13. Parent, S., Mobasher, B., and Lytinen, S. (2001). "An Adaptive Agent for Web Exploration Based on Concept Hierarchies," in *Proceedings of the Ninth International Conference on Human Computer Interaction*, New Orleans, LA.
14. Porter, M. F. (1980). "An Algorithm for Suffix Stripping," *Program*, **14:3**, 130-137.
15. Rocchio, J. (1971). "Relevance Feedback in Information Retrieval," in *The SMART Retrieval System: Experiments in Automatic Document Processing*, ed. G. Salton, Prentice Hall, pp. 313–323.

16. Salton, G., and McGill, M. J. (1983). *Introduction to Modern Information Retrieval*, McGraw-Hill, New York.
17. Sieg, A., Mobasher, B., Lytinen, S., and Burke, R. (2003). "Concept Based Query Enhancement in the ARCH Search Agent," in *Proceedings of the 4th International Conference on Internet Computing*, Las Vegas, NV.
18. Sieg, A., Mobasher, B., Lytinen, S., and Burke, R. (2004). "Using Concept Hierarchies to Enhance User Queries in Web-based Information Retrieval," in *Proceedings of the IASTED International Conference on Artificial Intelligence and Applications*, Innsbruck, Austria.
19. Spink, A., Ozmutlu, H.C., Ozmutlu, S., and Jansen, B. J. (2002). "U.S. Versus European Web Searching Trends," in *Proceedings of the ACM SIGIR Fall 2002.*

Database Selection for Longer Queries

Wensheng Wu[1], Clement Yu[2], and Weiyi Meng[3]

[1] University of Illinois at Urbana-Champaign, USA
wwu2@uiuc.edu
[2] University of Illinois at Chicago, USA
yu@cs.uic.edu
[3] State University of New York at Binghamton, USA
meng@cs.binghamton.edu

1 Introduction

Given the enormous amount of information now available on the Web, search engines have become the indispensable tools for people to find desired information from the Web. These search engines can be classified into two broad categories by the extent of their coverage. In the first category, we have the general-purpose search engines, such as Google and Yahoo, which have been attempting to index the *whole* Web and provide a search capability for *all* Web documents. Unfortunately, these *centralized* search engines suffer from several serious limitations such as the poor scalability and the difficulty in maintaining the freshness of their contents (Hawking and Thistlewaite, 1999).

In the second category, we have the hundreds and thousands of search engines on confined domains which include the pervasive organization-level search engines and a large number of specialty search engines, such as CiteSeer (a technical report search engine) and mwsearch.com (a search engine for medical information), to name just a few (http://www.SearchEngineWatch.com). Since each of these *local* search engines focuses on a much smaller portion of the Web, they are more scalable than the general-purpose search engines and it is much easier to keep their index data up to date. In this paper, we consider the *metasearch engine* approach, a highly scalable alternative to provide the search capability for the entire Web.

A metasearch engine is a system that supports unified access to multiple local search engines. It does not maintain its own index on Web documents but a sophisticated metasearch engine often maintains characteristic information about each underlying local search engine in order to provide better service. There are several serious challenges to implement an effective and efficient metasearch engine. Among the main challenges, the *database selection problem* is to identify, for a given user query, the local search engines that are likely to contain useful documents for the query. The *collection fusion problem* is to retrieve documents from selected databases and then merge these documents with the objective of listing more useful documents ahead of less useful ones. A good metasearch engine should have the retrieval effectiveness close to that as if all documents were in a single database while minimizing the access cost.

In Yu et al. (2001, 1999) an approach was introduced to perform database selection and collection fusion (see Section 2 for more information). However, the approach works well only for typical Internet queries which are known to be short. It has been found that better search effectiveness can often be achieved when additional terms are added to the initial queries through query expansion or relevance feedback (Kwok and Chan, 1998; Sugiura and Etzioni, 2000; Xu and Callan, 1998). The resulting queries are usually much longer than the initial queries.

In this paper, we propose a new method (Section 3) to construct database representatives and to decide which databases to select for a given query when the query may be long. One critical difference from the earlier approaches is that the dependencies of words in documents are *captured* in the database representatives. Usually, the dependencies are limited to phrases, especially noun phrases. In spite of the restrictions, the problem seems difficult to conquer. One approach is to employ a probabilistic parser to identify phrases, as exemplified by Lima and Pedersen (1999). Given the extreme varieties of vocabularies in the Web, accuracies may suffer significantly as words from specialized domains may not satisfy ordinary syntax rules. Another approach is to consider enumeration of all possible triplets or quadruplets of terms. Given the huge number of possible terms, this approach is unlikely to be feasible either.

In Xu and Callan (1998) and Xu and Croft (1999), experimental results were given to demonstrate that it was possible to retrieve documents in distributed environments with essentially the same effectiveness as if all data were at one site. However, the results in Xu and Callan (1998) depend on a *training collection* which has similar coverage of subject matters and terms as the collection of databases to be searched. In the Internet environment where data are highly heterogeneous, it is unclear whether such a training collection can in fact be constructed. Xu and Croft (1999) relies on the properly clustering of the documents. In the Internet environment, it is not clear whether it is feasible to cluster large collections and to perform re-clustering for dynamic changes. Please see Meng et al. (2001) for a more comprehensive review of other work in the metasearch engine and distributed information retrieval area.

2 A Framework for Database Selection and Collection Fusion

A query in this paper is simply a set of words submitted by a user. It is transformed into a vector of *terms* with *weights* (Salton and McGill, 1983), where a term is essentially a content word and the dimension of the vector is the number of all distinct terms. The weight of a term typically depends on two factors: tf (term frequency) and idf (inverse document frequency) (Salton and McGill, 1983). A document is similarly transformed into a vector with weights. The similarity between a query and a document, denoted by sim(q, d), can be measured by the dot product of their respective vectors. Often, the vectors are normalized by division with their lengths such that the similarity values obtained are between 0 and 1. The corresponding weights in normalized vectors are called *normalized weights.* The similarity function with such a normalization is known as the Cosine function (Salton and McGill, 1983). When the idf of each term is computed based on the global document frequency of the term (i.e., the number of documents containing the term across *all* databases), it is called global idf (or gidf) and the computed similarities are global similarities.

We now review a framework for database selection and collection fusion which was first introduced in Yu et al. (2001) and Yu et al. (1999). Suppose a user is interested in retrieving the m most similar documents for a query q from N databases $D_1, D_2, \ldots, D_N$, where m is any positive integer. This framework can be summarized into one definition on optimal database ranking, a necessary and sufficient condition for ranking databases optimally and an algorithm for integrated database selection and collection fusion based on ranked databases.

Definition 1. *A set of N databases is said to be optimally ranked in the order $[D_1, D_2, ..., D_N]$ with respect to a given query q if for every positive integer m, there exists a k such that $D_1, D_2, ..., D_k$ contain the m most similar documents and each D_i, $1 \leq i \leq k$, contains at least one of the m most similar documents.*

Note that the ordering of the databases with respect to a query and a given similarity function may be different from their ordering with respect to the same query but with a different similarity function. However, the following proposition holds for any similarity functions.

Proposition 1. *(Yu et al., 2001.) Databases $D_1, D_2, ..., D_N$ are optimally ranked in the order $[D_1, D_2, ..., D_N]$ with respect to a given query q if and only if $msim(q, D_1) > msim(q, D_2) > ... > msim(q, D_N)$, where $msim(q, D_i)$ is the global similarity of the most similar document in database D_i with the query q.* □

After the databases have been ordered, a merging algorithm, known as OptDocRetrv, was developed to perform database selection and collection fusion (Yu et al., 2001, Yu et al.,1999). This algorithm is sketched as follows. Suppose the first s databases have been selected (s is 2 initially). Each of these selected search engines returns the actual global similarity of the most similar document to the metasearch engine which computes the minimum, denoted *min_sim*, of these s values. Each of the s search engines then returns to the metasearch engine those documents whose global similarities are greater than or equal to *min_ sim*. Note that at most m documents from each search engine need to be returned to the metasearch engine. If m or more documents have been returned from the s search engines, then they are sorted in descending order of similarity and the first m documents are returned to the user. Otherwise, the next database in the determined order will be selected and the above process is repeated until at least a total m documents are returned to the user.

3 Ranking Databases with Reduced Document Vectors

In this section, we propose our new method for database selection based on the framework described in Section 3. A key step is to estimate the global similarity of the most similar document in each database for any given query. We present a new type of database representative, which we believe is more capable of handling longer queries in estimating the similarity of the most similar document than existing approaches.

Consider a term t_i and a local database D_j. Let $\text{mnw}_{i,j}$ and $\text{anw}_{i,j}$ be the *maximum normalized weight* and the *average normalized weight* of t_i over all documents in D_j, respectively. Suppose a query q is represented by vector $(q_1 * \text{gidf}_1, \ldots, q_n * \text{gidf}_n)$, where q_i and gidf_i are the tf and the global idf of term t_i in query q, respectively. Then the global similarity of the most similar document of database D_j with respect to q can be estimated by Yu et al. (2002):

$$\max_{1 \le i \le n} \{q_i * \text{gidf}_i * \text{mnw}_{i,j} + \sum_{k=1, k \ne i}^{n} q_k * \text{gidf}_k * \text{anw}_{k,j}\}/|q|. \quad (1)$$

The intuition for having this estimate can be described as follows. The most similar document in a database is likely to have the maximum normalized weight on one of the query terms, say term t_i. This yields the first half of the above expression within the braces. For each of the other query terms, the document takes the average normalized value. This yields the second half. Then, the maximum is taken over all i, since the most similar document may have the maximum normalized weight on any one of the n query terms.

The reason that equation (1) can be inaccurate is explained as follows. Consider a query having term t and a set of other terms T. Formula (1) would use the maximum normalized weight of term t and the average normalized weights of the terms in T. It was observed in Meng et al. (2002) that the average normalized weight of a term is usually one to two orders of magnitude smaller than the maximum normalized weight, because the average is computed over all documents in the database, including those that do not contain the term. For queries with 2 or 3 terms, the inaccuracy is tolerable as the maximum normalized weight is usually much larger than other weights. However, for queries with more terms, the problem becomes more serious.

3.1 A New Type of Representative

One can observe that, in the above discussion, if the document d (having the maximum normalized weight of a query term) itself were kept in the database representative, then the precise similarity between d and the query would be calculated, and as a result, there would be no need to estimate this similarity. (Note, however, this document may not necessarily be the most similar document to the query in that database.) Based on this observation, we propose the following representative for a database.

Let $T(D)$ denote the set of terms that appear in database D. For each term t in $T(D)$, let $d(t)$ be the set of documents in D that have the *maximum normalized weight* on t across all documents in D. Although it is possible that $d(t)$ could contain more than one document, in practice $d(t)$ usually contains just a single document. For ease of discussion, we assume that $d(t)$ contains exactly one document and $d(t)$ denotes this document. Since $d(t)$ is a document, it usually contains many terms, many of which are somewhat unrelated to t. We consider only terms that are likely to form phrases with t. It is well known that components of a phrase usually occur within 3 words apart. Thus, any term t_1 in which all occurrences of t_1 in d are more than 3 words apart from any occurrence of t in d is removed. This forms a reduced document $d'(t)$. Now the new representative of database D can be defined as

$$Rep(D) = \{(t, d'(t)) | t \in T(D)\} \tag{2}$$

In other words, for each distinct term in the database, the representative contains the term as well as the reduced document that has the maximum normalized weight of the term.

3.2 Estimation of the Similarity of the Most Similar Document

Based on this database representative, the similarity of the most similar document can be estimated as follows. Suppose q is a query with k terms $(t_1, ..., t_k)$. For each term t in the query, if t appears in the database, then document $d'(t)$ can be identified in the database representative and the similarity between q and $d'(t)$ can be computed. If t does not appear in the database, then t is not used in the estimation process for this database. The similarity of the most similar document in the database can be estimated to be the largest similarity between q and $d(t_i)$, $1 \le i \le k$, that is:

$$msim(q, D) = \max_{1 \le i \le k \wedge t_i \in T(D)} \{sim(q, d'(t_i))\}. \tag{3}$$

Note that $msim(q, D)$ as computed by the above formula may not be 100% accurate. This is because (a) the reduced vectors $d'(t)$ are used instead of the original document vectors $d(t)$ and (b) equation (2) considers only those documents that have the maximum normalized weight for at least one query term.

It is possible that a document in D does not have the maximum normalized weight for any query term but its similarity with the query is higher than that produced by equation (2). In this case, the similarity produced by (2) won't be the same as $msim(D, q)$. Our experimental results (see Section 4) indicate that (2) is reasonably accurate in obtaining the similarity of the most similar document in a database.

3.3 Integration of New Representatives

To achieve storage and computational efficiencies, instead of keeping a separate representative for each database, a single integrated representative for all databases is constructed (Wu et al., 2001). Suppose the metasearch engine is designed to search no more than r search engines for any given query (a small r, say 30, is likely to be sufficient for most users if relevant search engines can be selected. In the Internet environment, most users examine a small number of documents, say no more than 30 documents per query.). If this is the case, it will be sufficient to store, for each term, the r reduced document vectors from different databases, that have the overall r largest maximum normalized weights and the corresponding database identifiers in the representative.

3.4 Capturing Additional 2-Term Phrases

When equation (2) is applied to our integrated representative to estimate the similarity of the most similar document for each of the r most promising databases, there are potential inaccuracies. These inaccuracies can be due to (1) not all meaningful phrases are captured by our representative, i.e., certain phrases are not in any of our reduced document vectors; (2) although a phrase is in our representative, not all of the r highest maximum normalized weights for that term are kept in our representative.

To provide partial remedy to these situations, we provide the following process to identify additional *2-term phrases*, where the two terms occur in adjacent locations in a query. Let two such terms be t_i and t_j. For a database D there are two documents, one having the maximum normalized weight on t_i denoted by $S = (s_1, \ldots, s_i, \ldots, s_j, \ldots)$ and another document having the maximum normalized weight on t_j denoted by $R = (r_1, \ldots, r_i, \ldots, r_j, \ldots)$. For a document $d = (d_1, \ldots, d_i, \ldots, d_j, \ldots, d_m)$ in a database D, if $\max_{d \in D}\{gidf_i * d_i + gidf_j * d_j\} > \max\{gidf_i * s_i + gidf_j * s_j,\ gidf_i * r_i + gidf_j * r_j\}$, then the co-occurrences of t_i and t_j in d is very high (in fact higher than their co-occurrences in S and in R) and as a consequence, t_i and t_j will be considered as a *2-term phrase*. We then compute, for each such *2-term phrase*, its maximum normalized weight for each database. Then, only the top r maximum normalized weights together with the corresponding database IDs where these maximum normalized weights are achieved are stored. Thus, our integrated representative consists of (1) the top r reduced document vectors for each individual term, together with their database IDs and (2) the top r maximum normalized weights for each *2-term phrase* (which is constructed as described above) together with their database IDs.

Intuitively, a database selection method is effective if the most desired documents are contained in a relatively small number of databases selected by this method. In Section 4, we shall conduct experiments to evaluate the effectiveness of our method based on more rigorous measures. The proposition below shows that for any single-term query (which constitutes about 30% of all Internet queries: Jansen et al, 1998), the local databases selected by the integrated representative are guaranteed to contain the m most similar documents in all databases with respect to the query when $m \leq r$.

Proposition 2. *For any single-term query, if the number of documents desired by the user, m, is less than or equal to r — the number of documents stored in the integrated representative for the query term, then all the m most similar documents to the query are contained in the r local databases containing the r stored documents for the query term.* □

4 Experimental Results

In this section, we report some experimental results. 221 databases are used in our experiments. These databases are obtained from five document collections on TREC disks 4 & 5 created by NIST (National Institute of Standards and Technology of the US). The five collections are CR (Congressional Record of the 103rd Congress), FR (Federal Register 1994), FT (articles in Financial Times from 1992 to 1994), FBIS (articles via Foreign Broadcast Information Service) and LAT (randomly selected articles from 1989 & 1990 in Los Angeles Times). These collections are partitioned into 221 databases of various sizes ranging from 222 documents (about 2 MB) to 7,760 documents (about 20 MB). A total of about 555,000 documents (about 2 GB in size) are in these databases. There are slightly over 1 million distinct terms in these databases.

Two sets of experiments are conducted. In the first set of experiments, the Cosine similarity function is used and test queries are the 400 queries in the first 8 TREC conferences. A typical TREC query consists of three portions (i.e., *topic*, *description* and *narrative*). We used the topic portion of each query in the first set of experiments. The average length of a query is slightly over 4. In contrast, the average length of real Internet queries is only about 2.2 (Kirsch, 1998).

In this experiment, we use the following two measures to evaluate the performance of a method to search for the m most similar documents in a set of databases: (1) **cor_iden_doc**: The percentage of correctly identified documents, that is, the ratio of the number of documents retrieved among the m most similar documents over m. (2) **db_effort**: The database search effort is the ratio of the number of databases searched by the algorithm over the number of databases which contain one or more of the m most similar documents. The ratio can be both higher or lower than 1. Note that the first measure indicates effectiveness (quality) of retrieval while the second measure reflects efficiency of retrieval.

m	cor_iden_doc (%)			db_effort (%)		
	previous	new	add. phrases	previous	new	add. phrases
5	64.8	87.6	92.4	112.1	120.4	121.2
10	68.8	87.1	92.8	100.3	108.1	109.9
20	72.7	87.0	92.9	92.3	100.9	103.0
30	76.6	87.9	93.7	89.9	97.7	101.1

Table 1. Comparisons of previous and new integrated representatives by use of the cosine similarity function.

For a given set of queries, the measures reported in this paper are averaged over all queries in the set that contain at least one real term. The results obtained from the previous approach (Wu et al., 2001) and the new integrated representative approach using the cosine function are given in Table 1 where the *add. phrases* columns show the results with new representatives *and* additional 2-term phrases being captured as described in Section 3.4.

From the table, we can observe that the new integrated database representative gives much higher retrieval effectiveness on longer queries (as mentioned above, the average length of TREC queries is much larger than that of a typical Internet query). The percentage of correctly identified documents range from 64.8% to 76.6% when the previous integrated database representative is used; the corresponding figures for the new database representative (containing the reduced document vectors) are from 87.0% to 87.9%. When additional 2-term phrases are captured, the accuracy of retrieving the m most similar documents increases consistently over all m's, ranging from 4.8% to 5.9%. In both types of new representatives, the efficiencies of accessing databases vary from 97.7% to 121.2%. In other words, in order to retrieve most of the most similar documents, only 21.2% of additional databases need to be accessed.

In the second set of experiments, we utilize the human relevance assessments available from TREC to evaluate the effectiveness of our database selection algorithm and to further evaluate our methods on the Okapi similarity function (Robertson et al., 1998) which is known to be among the best performers in TREC competitions. The Okapi's formula is given as follows.

$$\sum_{t \in q} (\log \frac{P - n + .5}{n + .5}) * (\frac{(k_1 + 1)tf}{k_1((1-b) + b\frac{dl}{avgdl}) + tf}) * (\frac{(k_3 + 1)qtf}{k_3 + qtf}). \quad (4)$$

The first term in the summation can be regarded as *gidf* where P is the total number of documents in the global database (the global database logically

m	prec_ratio		db_effort	
	previous	new	previous	new
5	61.8%	98.3%	138.9%	134.3%
10	60.8%	94.9%	107.9%	117.5%
20	65.3%	93.6%	90.2%	105.6%
30	65.1%	95.2%	79.6%	100.8%

Table 2. Comparisons of previous and new representatives using the Okapi similarity function on *long* queries

contains data from all local databases but physically it does not exist), and n is the number of documents in the global database which contain term t. The second and the third term correspond to the document term weight and the query term weight respectively. Note that tf and qtf are the document and query term frequency of term t, respectively, dl is the length of the document and $avgdl$ is the average length of documents. Note also that k_1, b and k_3 are 3 empirical constants and the summation is taken over all terms in query q.

The test queries are the 50 queries from TREC-6 ad hoc tasks (Voorhees and Harman, 1997). Both the title and description portions of the queries are used, the average number of terms per query is about 12 which is much longer than that in the first set of experiments, and none of the new queries has less than 5 terms. In this set of experiments, we also gauge the performance of our method based on the ratio of the average precision of the m documents retrieved by the metasearch engine to the average precision of the m documents retrieved as if all documents were placed in a single database. This new measure is denoted as **prec_ratio**.

The result is shown in Table 2. The new representative utilizes both 2-term and 3-term phrases in the queries. From the table it can be observed that the new representative permits a highly effective retrieval of documents from selected databases on longer queries with *prec_ratio* improved from 60.8-65.3% with the previous representative to 93.6-98.3% with the new representative. This indicates that the same effectiveness can be achieved as that of the retrieval from a centralized database with new representatives.

5 Concluding Remarks

Being able to accurately estimate the similarity of the most similar document in a database for a given query is critical in order to rank databases optimally. Previous solutions were designed to estimate the desired similarity for short queries. In this paper, we proposed a new type of database representative that is more suitable to handle longer queries. The information we use to construct this type of database representative is drastically different from previously proposed approaches. The main difference is that the new representative is better at capturing the dependencies of words in documents. As a result, it can produce more accurate estimates for longer queries. Our experimental results using the TREC collection indicated that the new approach can yield high retrieval effectiveness while maintaining high scalability.

References

1. Hawking, D. and Thistlewaite, P. (1999). "Methods for Information Server Selection," *ACM TOIS*, **17**.
2. Jansen, B., Spink, A., Bateman, J., and Saracevic, T. (1998). "Real Life Information Retrieval: A Study of User Queries on the Web," *ACM SIGIR Forum*, **32**.
3. Kirsch, S. (1998). "The Future of Internet Search: Infoseek's Experiences Searching the Internet," *ACM SIGIR Forum*, **32**, 3–7.
4. Kwok, K., and Chan, M. (1998). "Improving Two-Stage Ad-Hoc Retrieval for Short Queries," *ACM SIGIR*.
5. Lima, E., and Pedersen, J. "Phrases Recognition and Expansion for Short, Precision-based Queries on a Query Log," *SIGIR*.
6. Meng, W., Wu, Z., Yu, C., and Li, Z. (2001). "A Highly Scalable and Effective Method for Metasearch," *ACM TOIS*.
7. Meng, W., Yu, C., and Liu, K. (2002). "Building Effective and Efficient Metasearch Engines," *ACM Computing Surveys*, **34**, 48–84.
8. Robertson, S., Walker, S., and Beaulieu, M. (1998). "Okapi at TREC-7: automatic ad hoc, filtering, VLC and interactive track," *TREC-7*.
9. Salton, G., and McGill, M. (1983). *Introduction to Modern Information Retrieval*, New York: McCraw-Hill.
10. http://www.SearchEngineWatch.com.
11. Sugiura, A., and Etzioni, O. (2000). "Query Routing for Web Search Engines: Architecture and Experiments," *WWW9 Conference*.
12. Voorhees, E., and Harman, D. (1997). "Overview of the Sixth Text REtrieval Conference," *TREC-6*.
13. Wu, Z., Meng, W., Yu, C., and Li, Z. (2001). "Towards a Highly-Scalable and Effective Metasearch Engine," *WWW10*, Hong Kong.
14. Xu, J., and Callan, J (1998). "Effective Retrieval with Distributed Collections," *SIGIR*.
15. Xu, J., and Croft, B. (1999). "Cluster-based Language Models for Distributed Retrieval", *ACM SIGIR*.
16. Yu, C., Liu, K., Meng, W., Wu, Z., and Rishe, N. (2002). "A Methodology for Retrieving Text Documents from Multiple Databases," *IEEE TKDE*, **14**, 1347–1361.
17. Yu, C., Meng, W., Liu, K., Wu, W., and Rishe, N. (1999). "Efficient and Effective Metasearch for a Large Number of Text Databases," *CIKM'99*.
18. Yu, C., Meng, W., Wu, W., and Liu, K. (2001). "Efficient and Effective Metasearch for Text Databases Incorporating Linkages among Documents," *SIGMOD'01*.

Part VII

Contingency Tables and Missing Data

An Overview of Collapsibility

Stefano De Cantis and Antonino M. Oliveri

Università di Palermo, Italy
decantis,oliveri@unipa.it

Abstract: Collapsing over variables is a necessary procedure in much empirical research. Consequences are yet not always properly evaluated. In this paper, different definitions of collapsibility (simple, strict, strong, etc.) and corresponding necessary and sufficient conditions are reviewed and evaluated. We point out the relevance and limitations of the main contributions within a unifying interpretative framework. We deem such work to be useful since the debate on the topic has often developed in terms that are neither focused nor clear.

1 Introduction

In their daily work, researchers are obliged to take into account only a limited number of variables, and must neglect (collapse over) others that are potentially influential. Without control on all theoretically relevant dimensions (variables), every statistical analysis can be biased, perhaps only approximately, but it is difficult to foresee the direction of the bias.

In the context of categorical data analysis, it is possible to say a multiway table contingency table is *collapsible* if all *relevant information* about its structure is preserved in a lower-dimension table obtained by marginalizing over one or more variables, by pooling two or more categories, or by grouping statistical units at some level.

The debate on collapsibility and related phenomena started at the beginning of the century, when paradoxes emerged from the analysis of statistical relations among three categorical variables (Yule, 1903). During the last decades, the debate on collapsibility has greatly developed, even if not always linearly but rather by means of disputations of previous results. This makes it useful to have an overview on the topic.

From different circumstances, we identify three kinds of collapsing (De Cantis and Oliveri, 2000):

(1) Collapsing over variables: this refers to the marginalization of the conjoint distribution of an n-vector of variables over a subset of them.
(2) Collapsing over the categories of a variable: this refers to the aggregation of the levels of a factor and to related effects on the relations among variables.
(3) Collapsing over units: this can be found within multilevel data structures, when "aggregations" are made by attaching to higher level units the mean value of lower level variables. Even the elementary operation of frequency counting derives from collapsing on i.i.d. units.

Types 1 and 2 are clearly characterized in literature; problems deriving from Type 3 have not yet been directly related to the others.

In this paper we discuss collapsing over variables. According to some authors, all kinds of collapsing can be reduced, at least formally, to it. We refer to Bishop (1971) and Davis (1987) with regard to collapsing the levels of a factor and to Vaccina (1996) with regard to collapsing over units. In Section 2 we discuss the earlier formalizations of problems related to collapsing multiway tables and the first explicit definition of collapsibility (Bishop, 1971). We also report Whittemore's (strict) collapsibility (1978). In Section 3 we give the definition of strong collapsibility (with particular reference to the odds ratio and to the relative risk), and a generalization to any measure of association is reported. Section 4 addresses collapsibility of the parameters in linear and generalized linear regression models. Finally, some conclusions are drawn. Throughout the text, we report and compare necessary and sufficient conditions corresponding to the different definitions of collapsibility.

2 Earlier Definitions, Whittemore's Strict Collapsibility

Up to the end of the 1980s, collapsing and collapsibility were almost exclusively linked to the development of categorical data analysis. Yule (1903) was certainly one of the first to identify the paradoxes generated by collapsing operations, considering *"... fallacies that may be caused by the mixing of distinct records"*. Soon after, contributions were made by Bartlett (1935), Norton (1945), and Lancaster (1951), who investigated different order interactions in $2 \times 2 \times 2$ and higher tables; these give a logical premise for collapsibility. It is due to Simpson (1951) that the understanding that in a three-way contingency table the "...vanishing of second order interaction does not necessarily justify the mechanical procedure of forming the three component 2×2 tables...," thus underlining the confusion between conditions for collapsing and the absence of a second order interaction. Further contributions focused on testing the hypothesis of no interaction in multi-way contingency tables (Roy and Kastenbaum, 1955; Kastenbaum and Lamphiear, 1959; Darroch, 1962; Lewis, 1962; Plackett, 1962). In a milestone paper, Birch (1963) finally defined interactions in three-way and higher contingency tables as *certain linear combinations* of the logarithms of the expected frequencies and discussed maximum likelihood estimations for multiway tables.

The term "collapsibility" seems to have been introduced by Bishop (1971). The author distinguished between collapsing over variables and over levels of a factor, and wondered: under what conditions

> [S]hould all the variables be included or should the table be collapsed by omitting some variables? Should all the elementary cells be retained or should the table be condensed by reducing the number of categories for some variables?

In later work Bishop, in cooperation with Fienberg and Holland, discussed collapsibility within the unifying framework of log-linear models (Bishop et al., 1975): let A,B,C, be three categorical variables and m_{ijk} $i = 1, ..., I$, $j = 1, ..., J$, $k = 1, ..., K$ be the expected frequencies in the ijkth cell of a three-way contingency table. Let m_{ij} be the expected frequencies in the ijth cell of a table collapsed over the third variable (C). The saturated log-linear models for the three-way and two-way tables are, respectively:

$$\log(m_{ijk}) = \theta + \theta_i^A + \theta_j^B + \theta_k^C + \theta_{ij}^{AB} + \theta_{ik}^{AC} + \theta_{jk}^{BC} + \theta_{ijk}^{ABC} \; \forall \, i, j, k$$

$$\log(m_{ij}) = \lambda + \lambda_i^A + \lambda_j^B + \lambda_{ij}^{AB} \; \forall \, i, j$$

where the θ and λ terms are constrained to identify the models (the θ and λ terms sum to zero over each subscript). In general, θ terms are different from λ terms. Thus, if in a rectangular three-way table $\theta_{ij}^{AB} = \lambda_{ij}^{AB}$ for all i, j, then variable C is *collapsible* with respect to the two-factor effect between A and B (Bishop et al., 1975). The authors extended their definition to tables of higher dimensions:

> [W]e say that the variables we sum over are collapsible with respect to specific u-terms [theta terms in our symbology] when the parameters of the specified u-terms in the original array are identical to those of the same u-terms [lambda terms] in the corresponding log-linear model for the reduced array.

Such definitions do not give any condition on higher interaction parameters (i.e., θ_{ijk}^{ABC}). On this subject Whittemore (1978) pointed out that in a three-way table the absence of the second order interaction is not necessary for collapsibility:

> [V]anishing of 3-factor interaction neither implies nor is implied by collapsibility over a factor with respect to the set of remaining factors.

In the same paper she reported an example for which $\theta_{ijk}^{ABC} \neq 0$ even though $\theta_{ij}^{AB} = \lambda_{ij}^{AB}$, $\theta_{ik}^{AC} = \lambda_{ik}^{AC}$, and $\theta_{jk}^{BC} = \lambda_{jk}^{BC}$. Nevertheless,

> [I]t is clear that information about the structure of ... the table is lost by collapsing the table over any one of its three factors. This ... suggests that tables should be collapsed in this way only if the three-factor interaction is zero.

The absence of a second order interaction implied a different definition of collapsibility, which she called *strict collapsibility*: a three dimensional table is said *strictly* collapsible over a factor C with respect to the remaining factors if

(1) $\theta_{ij}^{AB} = \lambda_{ij}^{AB}$; and
(2) $\theta_{ijk}^{ABC} = 0$.

In the same paper, Whittemore extended her definition of strict collapsibility to n-dimensional tables.

After having introduced the definitions of collapsibility, we now discuss necessary and sufficient conditions to collapse. In their book, Bishop et al. (1975) asserted: "in a rectangular three-dimensional table a variable is collapsible with respect to the interaction between the other two variables if and only if it is at least conditionally independent of one of the other two variables given the third." That is: the table is collapsible over C if $\theta_{ijk}^{ABC} = 0$ and either $\theta_{ij}^{AC} = 0$ or $\theta_{ik}^{AC} = 0$ or both. The conditions given by Bishop et al. appear to be too restrictive. Whittemore (1978) gave examples that contradict the theorem. In particular, the condition that the two factor terms (first order parameters) be equal is not necessary for $2 \times 2 \times k$ tables nor for higher ones, but is only sufficient. In contrast to Bishop et al., Whittemore gave necessary and sufficient conditions for strict collapsibility, consistent with her definition of the property.

A different approach was proposed by Asmussen and Edwards (1983), Wermuth and Lauritzen (1983), Lauritzen and Wermuth (1989), Madigan and Mosurski (1990), and Frydemberg (1990), who defined collapsibility with direct reference to probabilistic structures characterizing hierarchical log-linear or decomposable (graphical) models (for a comparison between Asmussen and Edwards' collapsibility and Whittemore's, see Davis, 1986).

3 Strong Collapsibility

Let n_{ijk} denote the entry at level $i = 1, 2$ of variable A, $j = 1, 2$ of B, and $k = 1, 2, .., K$ of C and let n_{ij} denote the frequencies in the table summing over the K categories of C (so that $n_{ij} = \sum_{k=1}^{K} n_{ijk}$). We assume the relationship of interest is that between variable A and B and that A is a response variable. We use $OR_k = (n_{11k}n_{22k})/(n_{12k}n_{21k})$ and $OR = (n_{11}n_{22})/(n_{12}n_{21})$ as general notation for the conditional and marginal odds ratios.

Strict collapsibility occurs when $OR = OR_k$ for all $k, = 1, 2, ..., K$. When this condition is satisfied, the second-order interaction vanishes and, in addition, the conditional association between the first two variables can be studied in the corresponding 2×2 marginal table. In a $2 \times 2 \times 2$ table, $OR = OR_1 = OR_2$ corresponds to the conditional independence of A and C given B ($A \perp C \mid B$) or of B and C given A ($B \perp C \mid A$). Nevertheless, in

$2 \times 2 \times K$ tables ($K > 2$), $OR = OR_k$ for $k = 1, 2, ..., K$ is not necessary for strict collapsibility, as shown by Shapiro (1982). This author was the first to note that although conditional independence is not required to collapse over all of the (three or more) categories of a variable, it is still necessary if we want to combine arbitrary subsets of categories, that is to *partially* collapse the table. Strict collapsibility was defined with respect to the K categories of the third variable, but if some of these categories are modified, for instance by pooling some of them, then strict collapsibility can be lost. This leads to a "stronger" definition introduced by Ducharme and Lepage (1986):

> a table that remains strictly collapsible no matter how the categories of the third variables are pooled together, that is no matter how it is partially collapsed, will be called strongly collapsible.

In a strongly collapsible table, the structure of association between A and B is totally independent of the levels of the third variable C. Notice also that, for $K = 2$, strong and strict collapsibility coincide. In their work Ducharme and Lepage wrote:

> A $2 \times 2 \times K$ contingency table is strongly collapsible over K if and only if one of the following three conditions is satisfied for all i, j and k

where, in our notation, the conditions are:

(1) $m_{ijk} = n_{ij+}m_{+jk}/m_{+j+}$, that is $B \perp C \mid A$;
(2) $m_{ijk} = n_{ij+}m_{i+k}/m_{+j+}$, that is $A \perp C \mid B$;
(3) $m_{ijk} = n_{ij+}/m_{++k}$, that is $C \perp (A, B)$.

the subscript "+" denotes the sum over the index it replaces. In terms of the parameters of a log-linear model, the conditions of the theorem reduce to $\theta_{jk}^{BC} = 0$, or $\theta_{ik}^{AC} = 0$, or both; hence, each of these conditions can be tested by standard methods developed for log-linear models. Note that the conditions of the theorem were once thought by Bishop et al. (1975) to be necessary and sufficient for their own definition of collapsibility.

Ducharme and Lepage observed also that if $OR = \prod_{k=1}^{K} OR_k$, some authors (Aickin, 1983) want to collapse the table on the ground that the loss of information is negligible if the variance of the OR_k is small, or would in any case be outweighed by the benefits of the dimension reduction. In this case the table can be called *pseudo-collapsible.*

Ducharme and Lepage derived tests to verify the conditions of strict and pseudo-collapsibility. In particular, they derived a closed form Wald's test of strict collapsibility against an unconstrained alternative; such a test is different from those proposed by Whittemore's conditional likelihood ratio test (1978) and from Greenland and Mickey's closed form conditional test (1988) based on the comparison of the strictly collapsible model against the more general model of odds ratio homogeneity (no three-way log-linear interaction).

Ducharme and Lepage's definition of collapsibility seems to be a property of a table. Following contributions stressed, on the contrary, the fact that a table can be collapsible with respect to a particular measure of association but not another. In very general terms, a measure of association between variables A and B can be said to be strictly collapsible over C if it is constant across the conditional sub-tables and this constant value equals the value obtained from the marginal table (Greenland, 1998). Similarly, a measure of association can be said to be strongly collapsible if it remains strictly collapsible no matter how the categories of the background variable are pooled together.

In 1987 Wermuth elicited different conditions for the odds ratio and the relative risk, which we now recognize as strict collapsibility conditions. Using the expression "lack of a moderating effect" as a result of a long-standing debate in the social sciences, Zedeck (1971) gave a definition corresponding to Whittemore's strict collapsibility and related necessary and sufficient conditions for the case of $2 \times 2 \times 2$ tables. Wermuth's conditions for (strict) collapsibility of the odds ratio are the same as Ducharme and Lepage's conditions for strong collapsibility; for the relative risk they are: $A \perp C \mid B$ or $B \perp C$. They hold only if results are strongly consistent (i.e., if all partial relative risks are equal). Wermuth showed also that collapsibility of the relative risk does not imply collapsibility of odds ratios (nor holds the contrary). Like Bishop et al. (1975), Wermuth's conditions for collapsibility seem to be incoherent with previous definitions. Such incoherence is probably due to the fact that she focused on $2 \times 2 \times 2$ tables (for which, as already said, strict and strong collapsibility overlap).

Geng (1992) considered Wermuth's necessary and sufficient conditions for the strong collapsibility of the odds ratio and the relative risk. In his Theorem 3 he wrote:

> [I]n $I \times J \times K$ tables assume that $B \perp C$. Then the (partial) relative risks ... are consistent over C ... if and only if $[B \perp C \mid A]$.

Using the example given by Wermuth (1987) it is yet easy to point out that even if (i) $B \perp C$ and (ii) relative risks are strongly consistent, then $B \perp C \mid A$ does not hold. In other words, given $B \perp C$, $B \perp C \mid A$ implies strongly consistent relative risks, but not vice-versa. It seems evident that Geng's conditions for strong collapsibility of the relative risk: (i) $A \perp C \mid B$, (ii) $B \perp C$ and $B \perp C \mid A$, (iii) $(A, B) \perp C$ are only sufficient but not necessary. This contradicts his conclusion that

> we find that necessary and sufficient conditions for relative risks are stronger than those for odds ratios i.e. if the relative risks are strongly collapsible than odds ratios are also strongly collapsible.

4 Collapsibility in Regression Models

Wermuth (1987) pointed out that "... relative risks behave similarly to regression coefficient in bivariate normal regression." In the case that the partial regression coefficient differs from zero, necessary and sufficient conditions for the collapsibility of the regression coefficient are similar to those for the relative risk. This intuition was fully developed in a following work (Wermuth, 1989). Following Wermuth's definition, let us assume a homogeneous linear dependence of Y on X in terms of regression coefficients. Let the model be defined in the following terms:

$$\begin{aligned} \mathrm{E}(Y \mid X = x, C = C_k) &= \theta_0(C_k) + \theta_1 x \\ \mathrm{Var}(Y \mid X = x, C = C_k) &= \alpha(x) \\ \mathrm{E}(X \mid C = C_k) &= \mu_k \\ \mathrm{Var}(Y \mid C = C_k) &= \beta \\ \Pr[C = C_k] &= p_i > 0 \end{aligned}$$

where Y is a continuous response, X and C are a continuous influence variable and a discrete moderator factor, respectively, with C_k being the kth level for $k = 1, 2, ..., K$. The homogeneous regression coefficient θ_1 is collapsible over C if it coincides with the marginal regression coefficient λ_1 defined as:

$$\mathrm{E}(Y \mid X = x) = \lambda_0 + \lambda_1 x.$$

The following conditions for collapsibility are defined under the assumption of a normal distribution for Y given X and C, and a normal distribution for X given C, giving a saturated homogeneous conditional Gaussian (CG) distribution for Y, X, and C ("saturated" since constraints are imposed on the interaction terms to ensure their uniqueness; see Lauritzen and Wermuth, 1989). In the described parallel regression model:

(1) A necessary and sufficient condition for collapsibility of the homogeneous regression coefficient over C is: $\mathrm{Cov}(\theta_0(C_k), \mu_k) = 0$.

(2) A sufficient condition for no moderating effect of C on the linear dependence of Y on X is that the parallel regressions are also coincident or that the means of the influence variable X coincide for all levels of C.

Geng and Asano (1993), referring to Wermuth's results, announced a theorem asserting that, in a parallel regression model for Y on X and C, the regression coefficients are strongly collapsible over C if and only if (i) $\theta_0(Ck) = \theta_0(Ck')$ for $k \neq k'$ or (ii) C is independent of Y. It seems that their conditions were wrongly referring to strong collapsibility since they correspond to those proposed by Wermuth for the "lack of a moderating effect" that we recognize as strict collapsibility. Wermuth (1989) finally demonstrated that if a parallel regression model for Y on X and C derives from a homogeneous CG distribution, and if $X \perp C \mid Y$, the three following statements are equivalent:

(i) the variable C has no moderating effect on the linear dependence of Y on X; (ii) $Y \perp C \mid X$ or $Y \perp X \mid C$; (iii) $X \perp C$.

Previous definitions and conditions can easily be extended to a more general regression model (Greenland and Maldonado, 1994; Greenland, 1998).

Consider a generalized linear model for the regression of Y on X and Z:

$$E(Y \mid X = x, Z = z) = \theta_0 + \theta_1 x + \theta_2 z,$$

where Y, X, and Z are single variables (or vectors), either qualitative or quantitative. The regression coefficient θ_1 is collapsible over Z if $\theta_1 = \lambda_1$ in the regression model omitting Z:

$$E(Y \mid X = x) = \lambda_0 + \lambda_1 x.$$

Even if the full model is correct, the collapsed model can have a different functional form that does not adequately fit to data. Greenland (1998) says:

> One way around this dilemma (and the fact that neither of the full and collapsed models is likely to be exactly correct) is to define the model parameters as the asymptotic means of the maximum likelihood estimators. These means are well defined and interpretable even if the models are not correct.

Such solutions have been used to construct collapsibility tests and confidence intervals for logistic regression, log-linear hazard models, and other generalized linear models, on the basis of a generalization of Hausman's test (Hausman, 1978) for omitted covariates in ordinary least squares linear regression (Greenland and Maldonado, 1994). Necessary and sufficient conditions to collapse parameters within logistic regression models are also discussed by Guo and Geng (1995). They are, not surprisingly, the same as those given for the odds ratio, since a logistic regression coefficient is essentially an odds ratio for one unit of change in a continuous variable.

5 Conclusions

In this paper we reconstructed the essential terms of the debate on collapsing over variables. We followed mainly the development of different versions of collapsibility and secondarily the historical course of the contributions, trying to impose a coherent interpretative framework to the topic. We noted that starting from the parameters of log-linear models (and from related association measures), collapsibility extended as far as any measure of association and finally generalized to linear model parameters. We also noted that the consequences of an intuitive, simple, and inevitable procedure like collapsing over variables were studied only in the last decades and, at least at the beginning, referred just to categorical data analysis. Similar remarks can be made regarding other partially overlapping topics (the investigation of paradoxes, the definition of higher-order interactions for metric variables, the study of deviations from linearity) but the understanding of the intellectual history requires further investigation.

Not always did necessary and sufficient conditions proposed by some authors demonstrate coherency with related definitions. Such incoherence is frequently related to terminological confusions and inaccuracies, and we have tried to clarify those.

Many fields and boundaries still have to be investigated: the relations among different notions of collapsibility and with the concept of "confounding;" the paradoxes of multivariate analysis; the difficult extensions of different kinds of collapsibility to the case of metric variables and to the parameters of more complex models; the relevance of collapsing within the context of the methodology of research and the logic of experiments.

Acknowledgements

Although this paper is due to the common work of both authors, Sections 1 and 3 are attributable to A. M. Oliveri, Sections 2, 4 and 5 to S. De Cantis.

References

1. Aickin, M. (1983). *Linear Statistical Analysis of Discrete Data*, Wiley, New York.
2. Asmussen, S., and Edwards, D. (1983). "Collapsibility and Response Variables in Contingency Tables," *Biometrika*, **70** 567–578.
3. Bartlett, M.S. (1935). "Contingency Table Interactions," *Supplement to the Journal of the Royal Statistical Society, Series B*, **2**, 248–252.
4. Birch, M. W. (1963). "Maximum Likelihood in Three-Way Contingency Tables," *Journal of the Royal Statistical Society, Series B*, **25**, 220–233.
5. Bishop, Y. M. M. (1971). "Effects of Collapsing Multidimensional Contingency Tables," *Biometrics*, **27**, 545–562.
6. Bishop, Y. M. M., Fienberg, S. E., and Holland, P. W. (1975). *Discrete Multivariate Analysis: Theory and Practice*, MIT Press, Cambridge, Massachusetts.
7. Darroch, J. N. (1962). "Interactions in Multi-Factor Contingency Tables," *Journal of the Royal Statistical Society, Series B*, **24**, 251–263.
8. Davis, L. J. (1986). "Whittemore's Notion of Collapsibility in Multidimensional Contingency Tables," *Communications in Statistics, Part A - Theory and Methods*, **15**, 2541–2554.
9. Davis, L. J. (1987). "Partial Collapsibility in Multidimensional Tables," *Statistics & Probability Letters*, **5**, 129–134.
10. De Cantis, S., and Oliveri, A. (2000). "Collapsibility and Collapsing Multidimensional Contingency Tables: Perspectives and Implications," in *Data Analysis, Classification and Related Methods*, y of Multidimensional Contingency Tables," *Journal of the Royal Statistical Society, Series B*, **40**, 328–340.
11. Yule, G. U. (1903). "Notes on the Theory of Association of Attributes in Statistics," *Biometrika*, **2**, 121–134.

12. Zedeck, S. (1971). "Problems with the Use of Moderator Variables," *Psychological Bulletin*, **76**, 295–310.

Generalized Factor Analyses for Contingency Tables

François Bavaud

Université de Lausanne, France
Francois.Bavaud@imm.unil.ch

Abstract: Quotient dissimilarities constitute a broad aggregation-invariant family; among them, f-dissimilarities are Euclidean embeddable (Bavaud, 2002). We present a non-linear principal components analysis (NPA) applicable to any quotient dissimilarity, based upon the spectral decomposition of the central inertia. For f-dissimilarities, the same decomposition yields a non-linear correspondence analysis (NCA), permitting us to modulate as finely as wished the contributions of positive or negative deviations from independence. The resulting coordinates exactly reproduce the original dissimilarities between rows or between columns; however, Huygens's weak principle is generally violated, as measured by a quantity we call 'eccentricity'.

1 Introduction and Notation

Let n_{jk} be a $(J \times K)$ contingency table, with relative frequencies $f_{jk} := n_{jk}/n$. Marginal profiles (assumed strictly positive) are $\rho_j^* := n_{j\bullet}/n = f_{j\bullet}$ and $\rho_k := n_{\bullet k}/n = f_{\bullet k}$, where $n_{j\bullet} := \sum_{k\in K} n_{jk}$ are the row marginals, $n_{\bullet k} := \sum_{j\in J} n_{jk}$ are the column marginals, and $n := n_{\bullet\bullet}$ is the grand total. The *independence quotients* q_{jk} are the ratios of the observed counts to the expected counts under independence:

$$q_{jk} := \frac{n_{jk}\, n}{n_{j\bullet}\, n_{\bullet k}} = \frac{f_{jk}}{\rho_j^*\, \rho_k} \quad \text{with} \quad \sum_{j\in J} \rho_j^*\, q_{jk} = 1 \quad \forall k, \quad \sum_{k\in K} \rho_k\, q_{jk} = 1 \quad \forall j. \quad (1)$$

One has $q_{jk} = 1$ for all cells iff perfect independence holds. The chi-squared dissimilarity $D^{\chi}_{jj'}$ between rows j and j' expresses in terms of quotients as $D^{\chi}_{jj'} = \sum_k \rho_k\, (q_{jk} - q_{j'k})^2$.

Quotient dissimilarities are of the form $D_{jj'} := \sum_k \rho_k\, F(q_{jk}, q_{j'k})$, where $F(q,q') \geq 0$, $F(q,q') = F(q',q)$ and $F(q,q) = 0$. The *f-dissimilarities* are quotient dissimilarities with $F(q,q') = (f(q) - f(q'))^2$, whereas *g-dissimilarities* are quotient dissimilarities with $F(q,q') = (g(q) - g(q'))(q - q')$ (Bavaud,

2002). Quotient dissimilarities are aggregation-invariant, f-dissimilarities are (Euclidean) embeddable, that is representable as $D_{jj'} = \sum_l (x_{jl} - x_{j'l})^2$ (where x_{jl} is the coordinate of object j in dimension l), and g-dissimilarities obey Huygens's weak principle $I_1 = I_2$ where $I_1 := \sum_j \rho_j^* D_{jg}$ is the central inertia (here g is the average profile with associated quotient profile $g_k \equiv 1$—see equation (1)) and $I_2 := \frac{1}{2} \sum_{jj'} \rho_j^* \rho_{j'}^* D_{jj'}$ is the pair inertia (cf. Bavaud, 2002). Moreover, the only member common to both families is (up to a constant) the chi-square dissimilarity characterized by $F^{\chi}(q, q') = (q - q')^2$ (see Figure 1). But one cannot rule out a priori the possibility of discovering, besides the already identified g- and f-dissimilarities, a new family $F(q, q')$ that entails both properties.

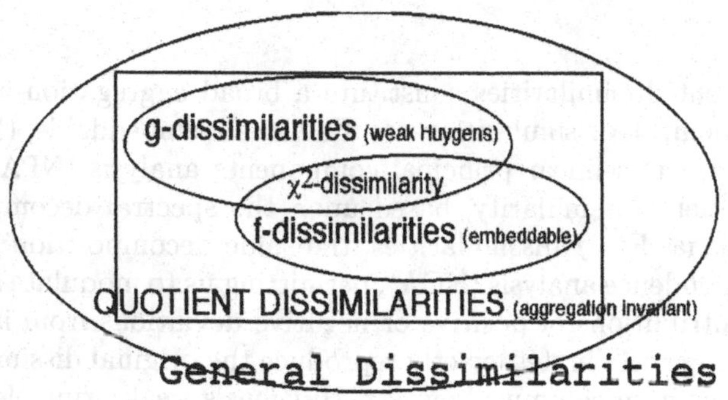

Fig. 1. Types of categorical dissimilarities under consideration.

Classical factorial correspondence analysis (FCA) consists in visualizing the rows (and columns) of the contingency table in a low-dimensional space, i.e., in representing row j by factorial coordinates $x_{j\alpha}$ (respectively $y_{k\alpha}$) such that $D^{\chi}_{jj'} = \sum_\alpha (x_{j\alpha} - x_{j'\alpha})^2$. The first dimensions $\alpha = 1, 2 \ldots$ are chosen to express a maximum proportion of the central inertia $I_1 = I_2 = \frac{1}{n}\chi^2$; in contrast, classical MDS seeks to maximize the low-dimensional representation of $\sum_j D_{jg}$, the total *unweighted* dispersion around g. Here χ^2 is the chi-square associated with the contingency table, measuring the total row/column dependence, and it is reconstructed by the sum $\sum_{\alpha=1}^{m} \lambda_\alpha$ (with $m = \min\{J - 1, K - 1\}$) of the eigenvalues of the associated spectral decomposition problem.

The same eigen-structure is also well-known to arise as the solution to a principal component analysis (PCA) applied on a particular $m_2 \times m_2$ variance-covariance matrix Γ with m_2 variables represented by the columns and $\text{Tr}(\Gamma) = I_1$.

In this paper we propose a generalized factor analysis for contingency tables, the *non-linear principal components analysis* (NPA), that applies to any *quotient* dissimilarity. As a factor-analytic method, NPA finds the projection hyperplanes that maximize the explained inertia, but one must choose which of I_1, I_2, I_1^* and I_2^* best defines inertia (starred notation denotes dual quantities obtained by row-column transposition; e.g., $n_{kj}^* = n_{jk}$ and $q_{kj}^* = q_{jk}$). In fact, $I_1 = I_1^*$ for quotient dissimilarities, since

$$I_1^* = \sum_k \rho_k D_{kg^*}^* = \sum_k \rho_k \sum_j \rho_j^* F(q_{kj}^*, 1) = \sum_j \rho_j^* \sum_k \rho_k F(q_{jk}, 1) = I_1,$$

while $I_2 = I_2^*$ $(=I_1 = I_1^*)$ for g-dissimilarities. In general, Huygens's weak principle is violated, which can be measured by the *eccentricity* ϵ and the *dual eccentricity* ϵ^* defined by $\epsilon := (I_1 - I_2)/I_2 = I_1/I_2 - 1$ and $\epsilon^* := (I_1^* - I_2^*)/I_2^* = I_1/I_2^* - 1$. In general, $\epsilon^* \neq \epsilon$. By construction, $\epsilon^* = \epsilon = 0$ for g-dissimilarities, while $\epsilon \geq 0$ and $\epsilon^* \geq 0$ for f-dissimilarities (see Section 3).

To preserve the rows-columns symmetry, we choose to define NPA as a low-dimensional projection of the *central inertia* I_1. The associated spectral decomposition yields factor-variable correlations or *loadings* representing the rows (and the columns) in the unit hypersphere (see Section 2). Moreover, when restricted to f-dissimilarities, the same procedure yields row (and column) *coordinates* defined by `coordinates` = `loadings` × `distance to the origin` (see equation 8 below), whose squared Euclidean distances restore the (embeddable) dissimilarities $D_{jj'}$, as expected. We call this procedure *non-linear factorial correspondence analysis* (NCA). Most of the usual properties of ordinary FCA are still valid, with a notable exception that corresponds to the non-vanishing eccentricities: the weighted average of row or column coordinates is generally not zero anymore (see Section 3).

The search for exotic, non-chi-squared dissimilarities that are endowed with attractive formal properties possesses a long tradition in the classification and data analysis community. Besides the Hellinger dissimilarity investigated by Escoffier (1978) and defined in our set-up as the f-dissimilarity $F(q, q') = (\sqrt{q} - \sqrt{q'})^2$, there is the logarithmic dissimilarity with $F(q, q') = (\ln q - \ln q')^2$ that occurs in the statistical analysis of compositional data (Aitchison and Greenacre (2002)) and the non-chi-squared dissimilarities $F(q, q') \neq (q - q')^2$ that allow one to distort and modulate the contributions of the profiles to the global measures of dependence, and to overweight or underweight, as finely as wished, the effect of attractions ($q > 1$) and/or repulsions ($q < 1$) (see Bavaud (2002) for additional examples). To that extent, the construction of factorial decompositions applied to exotic dissimilarities (NPA and NCA) constitutes a natural continuation of this tradition, aimed at visualizing the rows (and columns) in a way corresponding to the chosen distortion.

2 Non-Linear PCA for Quotient Dissimilarities (NPA)

The goal is to express $I_1 = I_1^*$ as the trace of some positive semi-definite (p.s.d.) $(J \times J)$ symmetric matrix Γ of components $\gamma_{jj'}$ that is interpretable as a variance-covariance matrix between variables $\{V_j\}_{j=1}^J$ associated to the J rows. Define the $(J \times K)$ matrix C with components

$$c_{jk} := \text{sgn}(q_{jk} - 1)\sqrt{\rho_j^* \, F(q_{jk}, 1)\, \rho_k}. \qquad (2)$$

Then, by construction, $\Gamma := CC'$ is p.s.d. It satisfies

$$\gamma_{jj} = \rho_j^* \sum_k \rho_k \, F(q_{jk}, 1) = \rho_j^* \, D_{jg} \qquad (3)$$

and $\text{Tr}(\Gamma) = I_1$. Decreasingly-ordered eigenvalues λ_α and associated eigenvectors $u_{j\alpha}$ (where $\alpha = 1, \ldots, m := \min(J, K)$) are obtained from the spectral decomposition $\Gamma = U\Lambda U'$ with U orthogonal and Λ diagonal, that is

$$\text{cov}(V_j, V_{j'}) = \gamma_{jj'} = \sum_{\alpha=1}^m \lambda_\alpha \, u_{j\alpha} \, u_{j'\alpha}$$

$$\sum_\alpha u_{j\alpha} \, u_{j'\alpha} = \delta_{jj'},$$

$$\sum_j u_{j\alpha} \, u_{j\beta} = \delta_{\alpha\beta}.$$

The term $\text{sgn}(q_{jk} - 1)$ in equation (2) insures that feature k contributes positively to $\text{cov}(V_j, V_{j'}) > 0$ iff quotients q_{jk} and $q_{j'k}$ are either both greater than 1 or both less than 1. By construction, the factors $F_\alpha := \sum_j V_j \, u_{j\alpha}$ are uncorrelated: $\text{cov}(F_\alpha, F_\beta) = \delta_{\alpha\beta} \, \lambda_\alpha$; moreover,

$$\text{cov}(V_j, F_\alpha) = \lambda_\alpha \, u_{j\alpha} \qquad s_{j\alpha} := \text{corr}(V_j, F_\alpha) = \frac{\sqrt{\lambda_\alpha}}{\sqrt{\gamma_{jj}}} \, u_{j\alpha}. \qquad (4)$$

As usual in PCA, the variables V_j can be represented by their *loadings* $s_{j\alpha}$ on the factors F_α (see Section 4). Loadings reproduce original correlations in that $\sum_\alpha s_{j\alpha} \, s_{j'\alpha} = \text{corr}(V_j, V_{j'})$. Also, the identities $\sum_\alpha s_{j\alpha}^2 = 1$ and $\sum_j \gamma_{jj} \, s_{j\alpha}^2 = \lambda_\alpha$ permit us to define the contributions of factors F_α to the proportion of explained variance of the variables V_j (communalities) and vice-versa.

The above NPA is applicable for *any* quotient dissimilarity D (provided $\gamma_{jj} > 0$ for all j), irrespective of its possible metric properties. In the chi-squared case, $\text{sgn}(q - 1)\sqrt{F(q, 1)} = q - 1$ and the vector $u_{jm} := \sqrt{\rho_j^*}$ is well-known to constitute a normalized eigenvector of Γ with associated trivial eigenvalue $\lambda_m = 0$; this property is false for quotient dissimilarities where $\lambda_m > 0$ in general.

The spectral decomposition applied to the $(K \times K)$ matrix $\Gamma^* := C'C = V\Lambda V'$ instead of to Γ yields a factorial representation of the column variables V_k^*, with *identical* eigenvalues λ_α and with normalized eigenvectors $v_{k\alpha}$ related to normalized eigenvectors $u_{j\alpha}$ of Γ by

$$v_\alpha = \frac{1}{\sqrt{\lambda_\alpha}} C' u_\alpha, \quad u_\alpha = \frac{1}{\sqrt{\lambda_\alpha}} C v_\alpha. \tag{5}$$

In summary, orthogonal matrices U and V and a diagonal Λ satisfy:

$$\begin{aligned} C &= U \sqrt{\Lambda} V', & C' &= V \sqrt{\Lambda} U', \\ \Gamma &= CC' = U \Lambda U', & \Gamma^* &= C'C = V \Lambda V'. \end{aligned} \tag{6}$$

3 Non-Linear FCA for f-Dissimilarities (NCA)

The f-dissimilarities obey $\operatorname{sgn}(q_{jk}-1)\sqrt{F(q_{jk},1)} = f(q_{jk}) - f(1)$. It is convenient to calibrate $f(q)$ (defined up to an affine transformation) so that $f(1)=1$. Moreover, if $f(q)$ is smooth enough, the choice $f'(1)=1$ ensures $f(q) = q - 1 + \kappa(q-1)^2 + \mathcal{O}((q-1)^3)$, where $\kappa := \frac{1}{2} f''(1)$ is the reference curvature (measured at the independence value $q=1$). One then has

$$\gamma_{jj'} = \sqrt{\rho_j^* \, \rho_{j'}^*} \sum_k \rho_k \, f(q_{jk}) \, f(q_{j'k}) = \sum_{\alpha=1}^{m} \lambda_\alpha \, u_{j\alpha} \, u_{j'\alpha}. \tag{7}$$

The NCA coordinates $x_{j\alpha}$ for row j (aimed at metrically embedding the categories) are obtained by multiplying the loadings $s_{j\alpha}$ in (4), which are used to represent the variables in the associated NPA, by the distance to the average profile $\sqrt{D_{jg}}$. In view of (3) and (4):

$$x_{j\alpha} := \sqrt{D_{jg}} \, s_{j\alpha} = \frac{\sqrt{\gamma_{jj}}}{\sqrt{\rho_j^*}} \, s_{j\alpha} = \frac{\sqrt{\lambda_\alpha}}{\sqrt{\rho_j^*}} \, u_{j\alpha}. \tag{8}$$

Using (7), the $x_{j\alpha}$ are Euclidean coordinates for objects $j \in J$:

$$\begin{aligned} \sum_\alpha (x_{j\alpha} - x_{j'\alpha})^2 &= \sum_{\alpha=1}^{m} \lambda_\alpha \left[\frac{u_{j\alpha}^2}{\rho_j^*} + \frac{u_{j'\alpha}^2}{\rho_{j'}^*} - 2 \frac{u_{j\alpha} u_{j'\alpha}}{\sqrt{\rho_j^* \rho_{j'}^*}} \right] \\ &= \frac{\gamma_{jj}}{\rho_j^*} + \frac{\gamma_{j'j'}}{\rho_{j'}^*} - 2 \frac{\gamma_{jj'}}{\sqrt{\rho_j^* \rho_{j'}^*}} \\ &= \sum_k \rho_k \left(f^2(q_{jk}) + f^2(q_{j'k}) - 2 f(q_{jk}) f(q_{j'k}) \right) \\ &= \sum_k \rho_k \left(f(q_{jk}) - f(q_{j'k}) \right)^2 \\ &= D_{jj'}. \end{aligned}$$

Proceeding analogously with columns leads to the represention of feature k in dimension α by the coordinate $y_{k\alpha}$, defined as

$$y_{k\alpha} := \frac{\sqrt{\lambda_\alpha}}{\sqrt{\rho_k}} \, v_{k\alpha} = \frac{\sqrt{\gamma_{kk}^*}}{\sqrt{\rho_k}} \, s_{k\alpha}^* = \sqrt{D_{k\rho^*}^*} \, s_{k\alpha}^*,$$

where $s^*_{k\alpha} = \text{corr}(V^*_k, F^*_k)$ is the corresponding column loading. Using (5) yields the transition formulas

$$y_{k\alpha} = \frac{1}{\sqrt{\lambda_\alpha}} \sum_{j \in J} \rho^*_j \, f(q_{jk}) \, x_{j\alpha} \qquad (9)$$

$$x_{j\alpha} = \frac{1}{\sqrt{\lambda_\alpha}} \sum_{k \in K} \rho_k \, f(q_{jk}) \, y_{k\alpha}.$$

3.1 High- Versus Low-Dimensional Coordinates

The formula $\sum_k \rho_k \, (f(q_{jk}) - f(q_{j'k}))^2 = D_{jj'}$ shows categories $j = 1, \ldots, J$ to be metrically embedded by the coordinates $x_{j\alpha}$ (a low-dimensional, factorial embedding) or equivalently by the coordinates $\tilde{x}_{jk} := \sqrt{\rho_k} \, f(q_{jk})$ (a high-dimensional, original embedding). The two systems of coordinates are linearly related by

$$x_{j\alpha} = \sum_k \sqrt{\rho_k} \, \tilde{x}_{jk}, \qquad \tilde{x}_{jk} = \sum_\alpha \sqrt{\rho_k} \, x_{j\alpha}. \qquad (10)$$

Thus $X = \tilde{X} \, V$, where V is a rotation. Similarly, the factorial column coordinates $Y = (y_{k\alpha})$ are related to the original column coordinates $\tilde{Y} = (\tilde{y}_{kj})$, where $\tilde{y}_{kj} := \sqrt{\rho^*_j} \, f(q_{jk})$, by $Y = \tilde{Y} \, U$ and $\tilde{Y} = Y \, U'$.

To see that V is a rotation, denote by Φ the $(J \times J)$ diagonal matrix containing the ρ^*_j. Then one has $X = \Phi^{-1} \, U \, \sqrt{\Lambda} = \Phi^{-1} \, C \, V = \tilde{X} \, V$, where the first equality follows from (8), the second follows from (7), and the third follows from the definition $\tilde{X} = \Phi^{-1} C$ (since $c_{jk} = \sqrt{\rho^*_j \, \rho_k} \, f(q_{jk}) = \sqrt{\rho^*_j} \, \tilde{x}_{jk}$).

As an application, consider a supplementary row a with quotient profile $a_k \geq 0$ obeying $\sum_k \rho_k \, a_k = 1$. Its factorial coordinates $x_{a\alpha}$ can be obtained from its original coordinates $\sqrt{\rho_k} \, f(a_k)$ by the transformation in equation (10), yielding $x_{a\alpha} = \sum_k \sqrt{\rho_k} \, f(a_k) \, v_{k\alpha}$. By construction, this satisfies

$$\sum_\alpha (x_{j\alpha} - x_{a\alpha})^2 = \sum_k \rho_k \, (f(q_{jk}) - f(a_k))^2 = D_{ja}.$$

In particular, the factorial coordinates of the average profile g with $g_k = 1 \; \forall \, k$ are $x_{g\alpha} = 0$, since $f(1) = 0$. As in usual CA, the average profile is represented at the origin.

3.2 Eccentricity

Although the coordinates $x_{g\alpha}$ of the average profile g are zero, the average components of the row coordinates $\bar{x}_\alpha := \sum_j \rho^*_j \, x_{j\alpha}$ are not, in general, zero. The square of their norm is instead

$$\sum_\alpha \bar{x}^2_\alpha = \sum_k \rho_k \, \bar{f}^2_k \text{ where } \bar{f}_k := \sum_j \rho^*_j \, f(q_{jk}).$$

The latter is directly related to the eccentricity ϵ (see Section 1), measuring the violation of Huygens's weak principle:

$$\begin{aligned} I_1 - I_2 &= \sum_j \rho_j^* D_{jg} - \frac{1}{2}\sum_{jj'} \rho_j^* \rho_{j'}^* D_{jj'} \\ &= \sum_{jk} \rho_j^* \rho_k f^2(q_{jk}) - \frac{1}{2}\sum_{jj'k} \rho_j^* \rho_{j'}^* \rho_k (f(q_{jk}) - f(q_{j'k}))^2 \\ &= \sum_{jj'k} \rho_j^* \rho_{j'}^* \rho_k f(q_{jk}) f(q_{j'k}) \\ &= \sum_k \rho_k \bar{f}_k^2 . \end{aligned}$$

In first approximation, eccentricities behave as $\epsilon \cong c\kappa^2$ and $\epsilon^* \cong c^*\kappa^2$ (where $\kappa := \frac{1}{2}f''(1)$ is the reference curvature and c and c^* are two constants), and thus they constitute a measure of distortion between the "exotic profile" $f(q)$ and the "classical profile" $f^{\chi}(q) = q - 1$.

4 An Example

Consider the *power dissimilarity* $f_\beta := \frac{1}{\beta}(q^\beta - 1)$ (with $\beta > 0$), such that $f(1) = 0$, $f'(1) = 1$, and $\kappa := \frac{1}{2}f''(1) = \frac{1}{2}(\beta - 1)$. The case $\beta = 1$ yields the chi-square dissimilarity; $\beta = 0.5$ yields the Hellinger dissimilarity. For the (4×4) contingency table in Table 1, Table 2 gives the matrices of squared distances between rows D_β and the columns D_β^* for the three cases $\beta = 1$, $\beta = 3$, and $\beta = 0.2$.

Figures 2-4 show the loadings $s_{j\alpha}$ and $s_{k\alpha}^*$ (lower case for NPA) lying inside the circle of unit radius, and the coordinates $x_{j\alpha}$ and $x_{k\alpha}^*$ (upper case for NCA) that reproduce the distances of Table 2. Loadings and coordinates are not on the same scale; e.g., the transformation $f(q) \to a\, f(q)$ sends $x_{j\alpha} \to a\, x_{j\alpha}$ but $s_{j\alpha}$ is unchanged. The figures show the common factorial structure associated with both NPA and NCA, making x_j and s_j parallel (as well as x_k^* and s_k^*). The proportion of explained variance for dimension α is λ_α / I_1.

Table 1. Cross counts n_{jk} of eye and hair color of 592 subjects (top), with associated quotients q_{jk} (bottom). Source: Snee (1974).

hair color k → eye color j ↘	black W	brunette X	red Y	blond Z	total	ρ^*
A = brown	68	119	26	7	220	.37
B = hazel	15	54	14	10	93	.16
C = green	5	29	14	16	64	.11
D = blue	20	84	17	94	215	.36
total	108	286	71	127	592	1
ρ	.18	.48	.12	.22	1	

hair color k → eye color j ↘	W	X	Y	Z
A	1.69	1.12	.99	.15
B	.88	1.20	1.26	.50
C	.43	.94	1.82	1.17
D	.51	.81	.66	2.04

Table 2. Squared distances for the power dissimilarity between the rows and between the columns, for $\beta = 1$, $\beta = 3$ and $\beta = 0.2$.

$D_1 =$

	A	B	C	D
A	0	.16	.61	1.08
B	.16	0	.20	.65
C	.61	.20	0	.34
D	1.08	.65	.34	0

$D_1^* =$

	W	X	Y	Z
W	0	.20	.43	1.82
X	.20	0	.10	.98
Y	.43	.10	0	1.09
Z	1.82	.98	1.09	0

$D_3 =$

	A	B	C	D
A	0	.37	.89	2.21
B	.37	0	.33	1.78
C	.89	.33	0	1.58
D	2.21	1.78	1.58	0

$D_3^* =$

	W	X	Y	Z
W	0	.53	1.09	3.81
X	.53	0	.34	2.67
Y	1.09	.34	0	3.04
Z	3.81	2.67	3.04	0

$D_{0.2} =$

	A	B	C	D
A	0	.28	1.04	1.51
B	.28	0	.27	.60
C	1.04	.27	0	.22
D	1.51	.60	.22	0

$D_{0.2}^* =$

	W	X	Y	Z
W	0	.21	.38	2.55
X	.21	0	.07	1.53
Y	.38	.07	0	1.56
Z	2.55	1.53	1.56	0

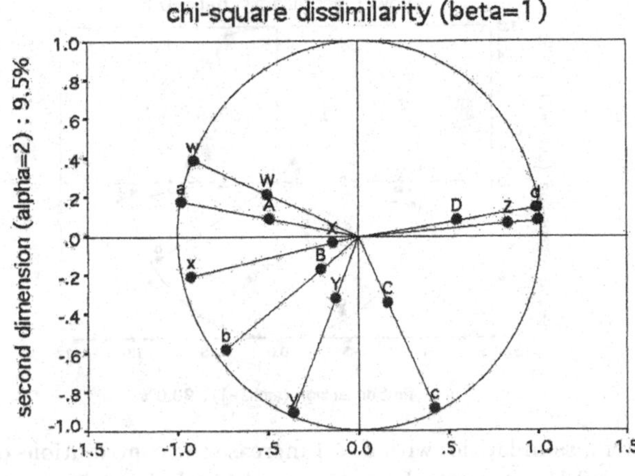

Fig. 2. NPA and NCA, with $I_1 = .23$ and eccentricities $\epsilon = \epsilon^* = 0$.

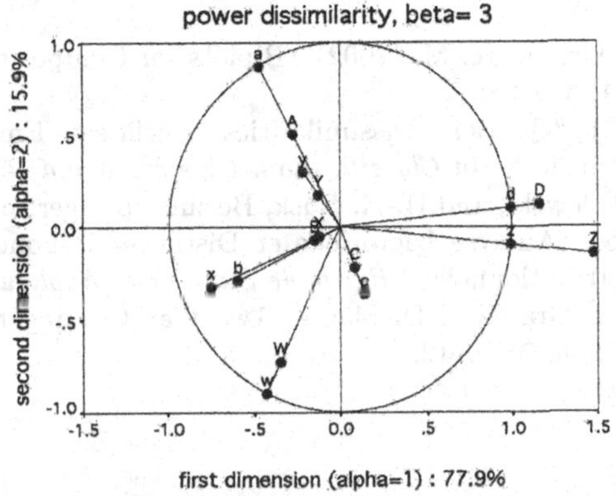

Fig. 3. Power dissimilarities with $\beta > 1$ increase the contributions of large quotients, namely $q_{DZ} = 2.04$. One gets $I_1 = .67$, $\epsilon = .28$ and $\epsilon^* = .13$.

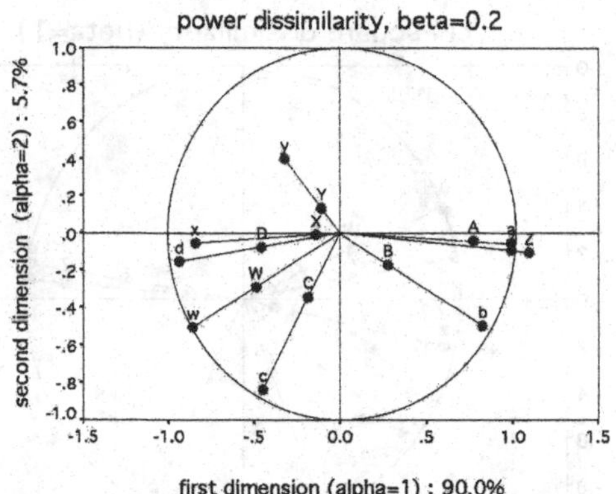

Fig. 4. Power dissimilarities with $\beta < 1$ increase the contributions of small quotients, namely $q_{AZ} = 0.15$. One gets $I_1 = .35$, $\epsilon = .12$ and $\epsilon^* = .05$.

References

1. Aitchison, J. and Greenacre, M. (2002). "Biplots for Compositional Data," *Applied Statistics*, **51**, 375–382.
2. Bavaud, F. (2002). "Quotient Dissimilarities, Euclidean Embeddability, and Huygens' Weak Principle," in *Classification, Clustering and Data Analysis*, eds. K. Jajuga, A. Sokolowski, and H.-H. Bock, Berlin: Springer, pp. 195–202.
3. Escofier, B. (1978). "Analyse Factorielle et Distances Répondant au Principe d'Équivalence Distributionnelle," *Revue de Statistique Appliquée*, **26**, 29–37.
4. Snee, R.D. (1974). "Graphical Display of Two-Way Contingency Tables," *The American Statistician*, **28**, 9–12.

A PLS Approach to Multiple Table Analysis

Michel Tenenhaus

HEC School of Management, France
tenenhaus@hec.fr

Abstract: A situation where J blocks of variables are observed on the same set of individuals is considered in this paper. A factor analysis logic is applied to tables instead of individuals. The latent variables of each block should explain their own block well and at the same time the latent variables of the same rank should be as positively correlated as possible. In the first part of the paper we describe the hierarchical PLS path model and review the fact that it allows one to recover the usual multiple table analysis methods. In the second part we suppose that the number of latent variables can be different from one block to another and that these latent variables are orthogonal. PLS regression and PLS path modeling are used for this situation. This approach is illustrated by an example from sensory analysis.

Introduction

We consider in this paper a situation where J blocks of variables $X_1, \ldots, X_J$ are observed on the same set of individuals. All the variables are supposed to be standardized. We can follow a factor analysis logic on tables instead of variables. In the first two sections of this presentation we suppose that each block X_j is multidimensional and is summarized by m latent variables plus a residual E_j. Each data table is decomposed into two parts: $X_j = t_{j1}p_{j1}^{'} + \cdots + t_{jm}p_{jm}^{'} + E_j$. The first part of the decomposition is $t_{j1}p_{j1}^{'} + \cdots + t_{jm}p_{jm}^{'}$. The latent variables $(t_{j1}, \ldots, t_{jm})$ should well explain the data table X_j and at the same time the latent variables of same rank h $(t_{1h}, \ldots, t_{Jh})$ should be as *positively* correlated as possible. The second part of the decomposition is the residual E_j which represents the part of X_j not related to the other block, i.e., the part specific to X_j.

The two-block case is considered in the first section. The J-block case is presented in Section two where we show that the PLS approach allows one to recover the usual methods for multiple table analysis. In the third section we suppose that the number of latent variables can be different from one bloc to another and that these latent variables are orthogonal. This last approach is illustrated by an example from sensory analysis in the last section.

1 The Two-Block Case

In the two-block case the first block X_1 plays the role of predictors and X_2 the one of responses. Orthogonality constraints are imposed on the X_1 latent variables $t_{11}, \ldots, t_{1m}$, but are optional on the X_2 latent variables $t_{21}, \ldots, t_{2m}$. The path model describing the two-block case is given in Fig. 1 (where the residual terms for the regression of t_{2h} on t_{1h} are not shown, as is the case for the other figures given in this text.

We denote by E_{1h} the residual of the regression of X_1 on the latent variables $t_{11}, \ldots, t_{1h}$ (with $E_{10} = X_1$). This way of constructing E_{1h} is called the deflation process. The blocks E_{2h} are defined in the same way if orthogonality constraints are imposed, and stay equal to X_2 otherwise.

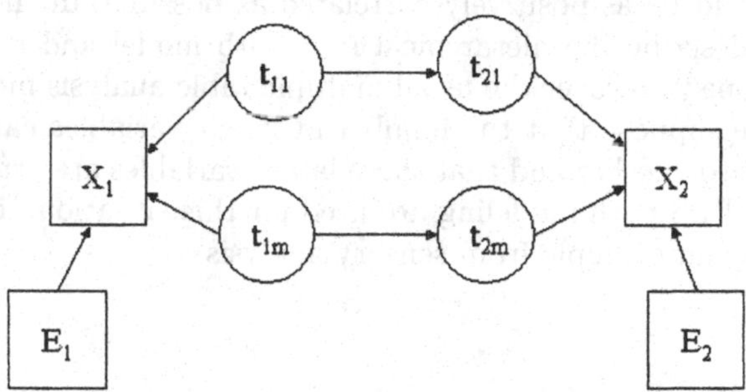

Fig. 1. Path model for the two-block case.

Each pair of latent variables (t_{1h}, t_{2h}) is obtained by considering the causal model where $E_{1,h-1}$ is the block of manifest variables related with t_{1h}, $E_{2,h-1}$ the one of manifest variables related with t_{2h}, and where t_{1h} is a predictor of t_{2h}. This causal model is drawn in Fig. 2.

We now describe the PLS algorithm for the two-block case. The latent variables are defined as $t_{1h} = E_{1,h-1}w_{1,h}$ and $t_{2h} = E_{2,h-1}w_{2h}$. The weights w_{jh} can be computed according to two modes: Mode A or B. For Mode A, simple regression is used:

$$w_{1h} \propto E'_{1,h-1}t_{2h} \text{ and } w_{2h} \propto E'_{2,h-1}t_{1h} \tag{1}$$

where $\propto$ means that the left term is equal to the right term up to a normalization. For Mode B, multiple regression is used:

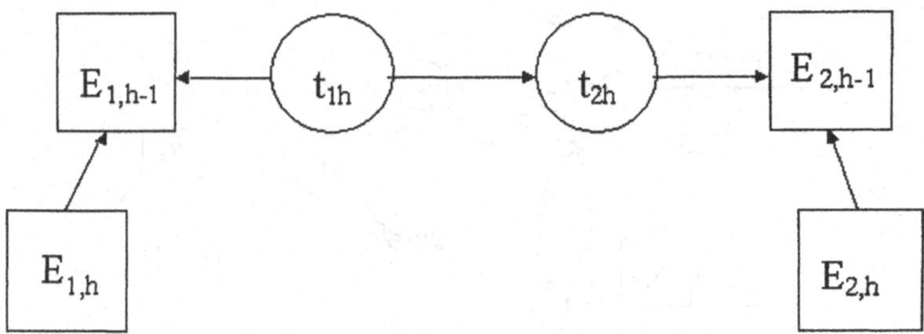

Fig. 2. Path model for the two-block case : Step h.

$$w_{1h} \propto (E_{1,h-1}^{'}E_{1,h-1})^{-1}E_{1,h-1}^{'}t_{2h}$$
$$w_{2h} \propto (E_{2,h-1}^{'}E_{2,h-1})^{-1}E_{2,h-1}^{'}t_{1h}.$$

The normalization depends upon the method used. For some methods w_{jh} is normalized to 1. For other methods the variance of t_{jh} is equal to 1.

The PLS algorithm is iterative. We begin with an arbitrary choice of weights w_{jh} and iterate until convergence using Mode A or B as selected. Inter-battery factor analysis (Tucker, 1958), PLS regression (Wold et al., 1983), redundancy analysis (Van den Wollenberg, 1977) and canonical correlation analysis (Hotelling, 1936) are special cases of the two-block PLS Path Modeling algorithm according to the options given in Table 1. More details about these results are given in Tenenhaus et al. (2004).

Table 1. The two block-case and the PLS algorithm.

Method	Mode for X_1	Mode for X_2	Deflation for X_1	Deflation for X_2
Inter-battery factor analysis	A	A	Yes	Yes
PLS Regression of X_2 on X_1	A	A	Yes	No
Redundancy Analysis of X_2 on X_1	B	A	Yes	No
Canonical Correlation Analysis	B	B	Yes	Yes

2 The J-Block Case: A Classical Approach

In the general case ($J > 2$) a super-block X_{J+1} that merges all the blocks X_j is introduced. This super-block is summarized by m latent variables $t_{J+1,1}, \ldots, t_{J+1,m}$, also called auxiliary variables. The causal model describing this situation is given in Fig. 3. This model corresponds to the hierarchical model proposed by Wold, 1982.

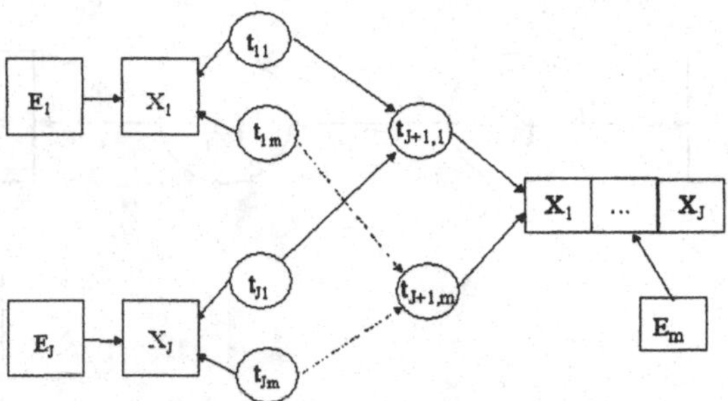

Fig. 3. Path model for the J-block case.

The latent variables $t_{j1}, \ldots, t_{jm}$ should explain their own block X_j well. At the same time, the latent variables of the same rank $(t_{1h}, \ldots, t_{Jh})$ and the auxiliary variable $t_{J+1,h}$ should be as positively correlated as possible. In the usual Multiple Table Analysis (MTA) methods, as in Horst (1961) and Carrol (1968) with generalized canonical correlation analysis, orthogonality constraints are imposed on the auxiliary variables $t_{J+1,h}$ but the latent variables t_{jh} related to block j have no orthogonality constraints. We define for the super-block X_{J+1} the sequence of blocks $E_{J+1,h}$ obtained by deflation. Figure 4 corresponds to step h.

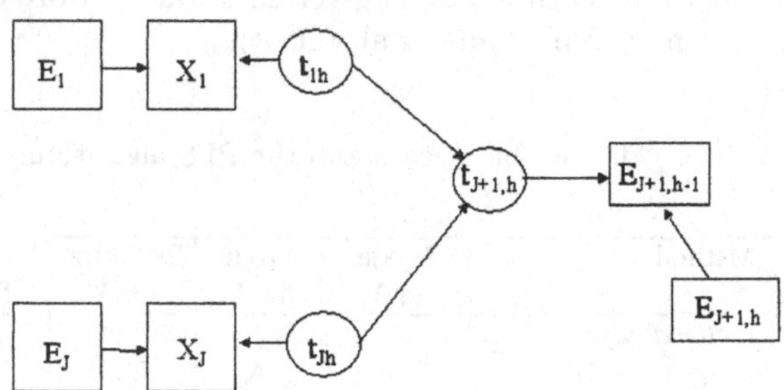

Fig. 4. Path model for the J-block case : Step h.

For computing the latent variables t_{jh} and the auxiliary variables $t_{J+1,h}$ we use the general PLS algorithm (Wold, 1985) defined as follows for step h of this specific application:

External Estimation:

Each block X_j is summarized by the latent variable $t_{jh} = X_j w_{jh}$.

The super-block $X_{J+1,h}$ is summarized by the latent variable $t_{J+1,h} = E_{J+1,h-1} w_{J+1,h}$.

Internal Estimation:

Each block X_j is also summarized by the latent variable $z_{jh} = e_{jh} t_{J+1,h}$, where e_{jh} is the sign of the correlation between t_{jh} and $t_{J+1,h}$. We will however choose $e_{jh} = +1$ and show that the correlation is then positive.

The super-block $E_{J+1,h-1}$ is summarized by the latent variable $z_{J+1,h} = \sum_{j=1}^{J} e_{J+1,j,h} t_{jh}$, where $e_{J+1,j,h} = 1$ when the centroid scheme is used, or the correlation between t_{jh} and $t_{J+1,h}$ for the factorial scheme, or the regression coefficient of t_{jh} in the regression of $t_{J+1,h}$ on $t_{1h}, \ldots, t_{Jh}$ for the path weighting scheme.

We can now describe the PLS algorithm for the J-block case. The weights w_{jh} can be computed according to two modes: Mode A or B. In Mode A simple regression is used:

$$w_{jh} \propto X_j' t_{J+1,h},\; j = 1 \text{ to } J, \text{ and } w_{J+1,h} \propto E_{J+1,h-1}' z_{J+1,h}. \tag{2}$$

For Mode B multiple regression is used:

$$\begin{aligned} w_{jh} &\propto (X_j' X_j)^{-1} X_j' t_{J+1,h},\quad j = 1 \text{ to } J, \\ w_{J+1,h} &\propto (E_{J+1,h-1}' E_{J+1,h-1})^{-1} E_{J+1,h-1}' z_{J+1,h}. \end{aligned} \tag{3}$$

As in the two-block case the normalization depends upon the method used. For some methods w_{jh} is of norm 1. For other methods the variance of t_{jh} is equal to 1.

It is now easy to check that the correlation between t_{jh} and $t_{J+1,h}$ is always positive: $t_{J+1,h}' t_{jh} = t_{J+1,h}' X_j w_{jh} \propto t_{J+1,h}' X_j X_j' t_{J+1,h} > 0$ when Mode A is used. The same result is obtained when Mode B is used.

The PLS algorithm can now be described. We begin with an arbitrary choice of weights w_{jh}. We get the external estimates of the latent variables, then the internal ones. Using equations (2) or (3) we get new weights. This procedure is iterated until convergence; convergence occurs almost always in practice, but has only been mathematically proven for the two-block case.

The various options of PLS Path Modeling (Mode A or B for external estimation; centroid, factorial or path weighting schemes for internal estimation) allow us to find again many methods for Multiple Table Analysis: generalized canonical analysis (Horst, 1961, and Carrol, 1968), multiple factor analysis (Escofier and Pagès, 1994), Lohmöller's split principal component analysis (1989), and Horst's maximum variance algorithm (1965). The links between PLS and these methods have been demonstrated in Lohmöller (1989) or Tenenhaus (1999) and studied in practical examples by Guinot et al. (2001) and Pagès and Tenenhaus (2001). These various methods are obtained by using the PLS algorithm according to the options described in Table 2. Only the super-block is deflated; the original blocks are not deflated.

2.1 Discussion of the Orthogonality Constraints

There is a great advantage from imposing orthogonality constraints only on the latent variables related to the super-block: no dimension limitation due to block sizes. If orthogonality constraints were imposed on the block latent variables, then the maximum m of latent variables would be the size of the smallest block. The super-block X_{J+1} is summarized by m orthogonal latent variables $t_{J+1,1}, \ldots, t_{J+1,m}$. Each block X_j is summarized by m latent variables $t_{j1}, \ldots, t_{jm}$. But these latent variables can be highly correlated and consequently do not reflect the real dimension of the block. In each block X_j the latent variables $t_{j1}, \ldots, t_{jm}$ represent the part of the block correlated with the other blocks. A principal component analysis of these latent variables gives the actual dimension of this part of X_j.

It may be preferrable to impose orthogonality on the latent variables of each block. But we have to remove the dimension limitation due to the smallest block. This situation is discussed in the next section.

Table 2. J-block case and PLS algorithm.

Scheme of calculation for the inner estimation	Mode of calculation for the outer estimation	
	A	*B*
Centroid	PLS Horst's generalized canonical correlation analysis	Horst's generalized canonical correlation analysis (SUMCOR criterion)
Factorial	PLS Carroll's generalized canonical correlation analysis	Carroll's generalized canonical correlation analysis
Path weighting scheme	- Lohmöller's split principal component analysis - Horst's maximum variance algorithm - Escofier & Pagès Multiple Factor Analysis	

No deflation on the original blocks, deflation on the super-block

3 The J-Block Case: New Perspectives

We will describe in this section a new approach that focuses more on the blocks than on the super-block. This approach is called PLS-MTA: a PLS approach to Multiple Table Analysis.

Suppose there are a variable number of common components in each block:

$$X_j = t_{j1}p'_{j1} + \ldots + t_{jm_j}p'_{jm_j} + E_j. \tag{4}$$

A two-step procedure is proposed to find these components.

Step 1. For each block X_j we define the super-block $X_{J+1,-j}$ obtained by merging all the other blocks X_i for $i \neq j$. For each j we carry out a PLS regression of $X_{J+1,-j}$ on X_j. Thus we obtain the PLS components $\tilde{t}_{j1}, ..., \tilde{t}_{jm_j}$ which represent the part of X_j related to the other blocks. The choice of the number m_j of components is determined by cross-validation.

Step 2. One of the procedures described in Table 2 is used on the blocks $\tilde{T}_j = \{\tilde{t}_{j1}, \ldots, \tilde{t}_{jm_j}\}$ for $h = 1$. We obtain the rank one components $t_{11}, \ldots, t_{J1}$ and $t_{J+1,1}$. Then, to obtain the next components, we only consider the blocks with $m_j > 1$. For these blocks we construct the residual $\tilde{T}_{j1}$ of the regression of $\tilde{T}_j$ on t_{j1}. An MTA is then applied on these blocks and we obtain the rank two components $t_{12}, \ldots, t_{J2}$ (for j with $m_j > 1$) and $t_{J+1,2}$. The components t_{1j} and t_{2j} are uncorrelated by construction, but the auxiliary variables $t_{J+1,1}$ and $t_{J+1,2}$ can be slightly correlated as we did not impose an orthogonality constraint on these components. These components are finally expressed in term of the original variables. This iterative search for components continues until the various m_j common components are found.

4 Application

Six French brands of orange juice were selected for study. Three products can be stored at room temperature (r.t.): Joker, Pampryl, and Tropicana. Three others must be refrigerated (refr.): Fruivita, Pampryl, and Tropicana. Table 3 provides an extract of the data. The first nine variables correspond to the physico-chemical data, the following seven to sensory assessments, and the last 96 variables represent marks of appreciation of the product given by students at ENSA, Rennes. These figures have already been used in Pagès and Tenenhaus (2001) to illustrate the connection between the multiple factorial analysis and the PLS approach.

A PLS regression has been applied to relate the set Y of judges to the set X_1 of physico-chemical variables and the set X_2 of sensory variables. In order to efficiently apply MTA on these data we have selected judges who are very positively correlated with the first PLS component or the second one. This set of 50 judges is the third set of variables X_3. The result of the PLS regression of X_3 on X_1 and X_2 is shown in Figure 5.

We now illustrate the PLS-MTA methodology described in Section 3 on these data.

Step 1. The PLS regressions of $[X_2, X_3]$ on X_1, $[X_1, X_3]$ on X_2, and $[X_1, X_2]$ on X_3 lead to, respectively, 2, 1, and 2 components when we decide to keep a component if it is both scientifically significant (Q^2 is positive) *and* interpretable. Then using the standardized PLS X-components, we define the physico-chemical block $\tilde{T}_1 = \{\tilde{t}_{11} = TPC1, \tilde{t}_{12} = TPC2\}$, the sensory block $\tilde{T}_2 = \{\tilde{t}_{21} = \mathit{TSENSO1}\}$, and the hedonic block $\tilde{T}_3 = \{\tilde{t}_{31} = TJ1, \tilde{t}_{32} = TJ2\}$.

Table 3. Extract from the orange juice data file.

	PAMPRYL r.t.	TROPICANA r.t.	FRUIVITA refr.	JOKER r.t.	TROPICANA refr.	PAMPRYL refr.
Glucose	25.32	17.33	23.65	32.42	22.70	27.16
Fructose	27.36	20.00	25.65	34.54	25.32	29.48
Saccharose	36.45	44.15	52.12	22.92	45.80	38.94
Sweetening power	89.95	82.55	102.22	90.71	94.87	96.51
pH before processing	3.59	3.89	3.85	3.60	3.82	3.68
pH after centrifugation	3.55	3.84	3.81	3.58	3.78	3.66
Titer	13.98	11.14	11.51	15.75	11.80	12.21
Citric acid	.84	.67	.69	.95	.71	.74
Vitamin C	43.44	32.70	37.00	36.60	39.50	27.00
Smell intensity	2.82	2.76	2.83	2.76	3.20	3.07
Odor typicity	2.53	2.82	2.88	2.59	3.02	2.73
Pulp	1.66	1.91	4.00	1.66	3.69	3.34
Taste intensity	3.46	3.23	3.45	3.37	3.12	3.54
Acidity	3.15	2.55	2.42	3.05	2.33	3.31
Bitterness	2.97	2.08	1.76	2.56	1.97	2.63
Sweetness	2.60	3.32	3.38	2.80	3.34	2.90
Judge 1	2.00	2.00	3.00	2.00	4.00	3.00
Judge 2	1.00	3.00	3.00	2.00	4.00	1.00
Judge 3	2.00	3.00	4.00	2.00	3.00	1.00
.						
.						
Judge 96	3.00	3.00	4.00	2.00	4.00	1.00

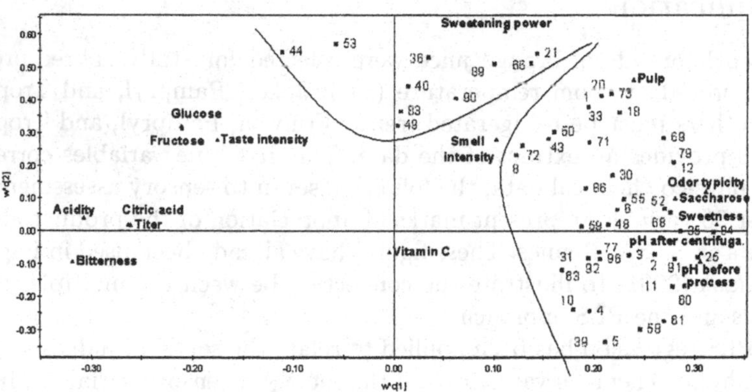

Fig. 5. PLS regression of the preferences of the 50 judges on the product descriptors.

Step 2. The PLS components being orthogonal, it is equivalent to use Mode A or B for the left part of the causal model given in Fig. 6 (PLS-Graph output, Chin, 2003). Due to the small number of observations Mode A has to be used for the right part of the causal model of Fig. 6. We use the centroid scheme for the internal estimation. As the signs of the PLS components are somewhat arbitrary, we have decided to change signs if necessary so that all the weights are positive. We give in Fig. 6 the MTA model for the first rank components and in Table 4 the correlations between the latent variables.

Table 4. Correlation between the rank 1 latent variables.

	Physico-chemical	Sensory	Hedonic	Global
Physico-chemical	1	.852	.911	.948
Sensory		1	.979	.972
Hedonic			1	.993
Global				1

In Fig. 6 the figures above the arrows are the correlation loadings and the figures in brackets below the arrows are the weights applied to the standardized variables. Correlations and weights are equal on the left side of the path model because the PLS components are uncorrelated.

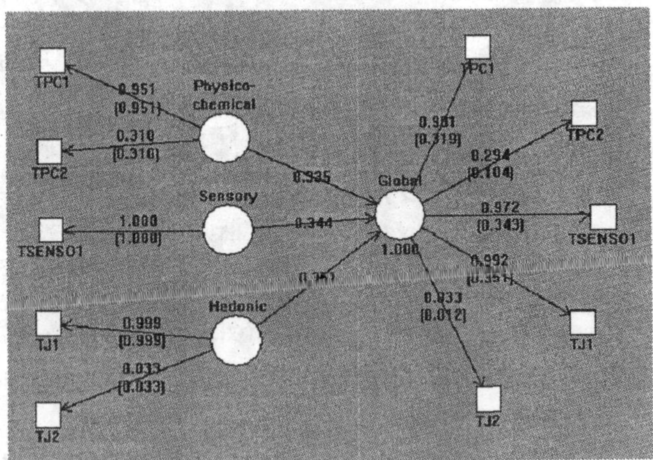

Fig. 6. Path model for the first-rank components (PLS–Graph output).

Rank one components are written as:

$$t_{11} = .951 \times TPC1 + .310 \times TPC2$$
$$t_{21} = TSENSO1$$
$$t_{31} = .999 \times TJ1 + .033 \times TJ2$$
$$t_{41} = .319 \times TPC1 + .104 \times TPC2 + .343 \times TSENSO + .351 \times TJ1 \\ + .012 \times TJ2$$

We note that the rank one components are highly correlated to the first PLS components *TPC1*, *TSENSO1*, and *TJ1*.

To obtain the rank two components we first regress

$$\tilde{T}_1 = \{\tilde{t}_{11} = TPC1,\ \tilde{t}_{12} = TPC2\} \text{ on } t_{11}$$
$$\tilde{T}_3 = \{\tilde{t}_{31} = TJ1,\ \tilde{t}_{32} = TJ2\} \text{ on } t_{31}.$$

Then the path model used for rank one components is used, after deletion of the sensory branch, on the standardized residual tables

$$\tilde{T}_{11} = \{\tilde{t}_{111} = TPC11,\ \tilde{t}_{121} = TPC21\}$$
$$\tilde{T}_{31} = \{\tilde{t}_{311} = TJ11,\ \tilde{t}_{321} = TJ21\}.$$

The results are given in Figure 7.

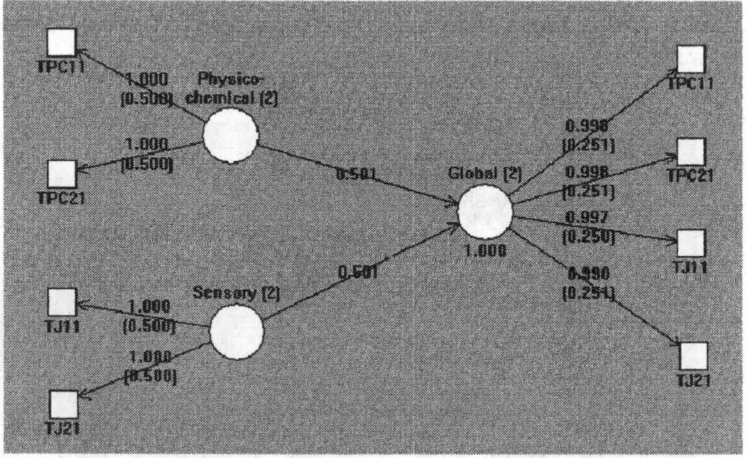

Fig. 7. Path model for the second-rank components in term of residuals.

It is more clear to express the rank two components in term of the original standardized variables. We get the following expressions:

$$t_{12} = -.311 \times TPC1 + .950 \times TPC2$$
$$t_{32} = -.042 \times TJ1 + .999 \times TJ2$$
$$t_{42} = -.148 \times TPC1 + .465 \times TPC2 - .025 \times TJ1 + .514 \times TJ2.$$

And the path model is redrawn in Figure 8.

In Table 5 we give the correlations between the rank-two components. The physico-chemical components of ranks one and two are uncorrelated by construction, as are the hedonic ones. The global components are also practically uncorrelated (r = -.004).

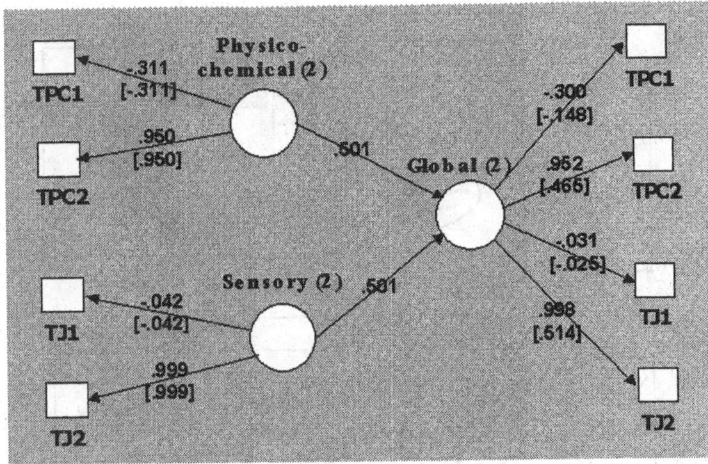

Fig. 8. Path model for the second-rank components in terms of the original variables.

Table 5. Correlations between rank two latent variables.

	Physico-Chemical	Hedonic	Global
Physico-Chemical	1	.992	.998
Hedonic		1	.998
Global			1

4.1 Communality for Manifest Variables and Blocks

Communality of a manifest variable is defined in factor analysis as the R-Squared value between the manifest variable and the latent variables. The average communality can be calculated for each block. These communalities are given in Table 6. We conclude that the latent variables of each block explain respectively 84.5, 67.7 and 67.0 % of their block.

5 Conclusions

PLS-MTA carries out a kind of principal component analysis on each block and on the super-block such that the components of same rank are as positively correlated as possible. This means that the interpretations of each block can be related. In Fig. 9 the physico-chemical, sensory and hedonic loadings with their own components are displayed, and the products are also displayed using the global components. Using the correlations of the physico-chemical, sensory, hedonic variables and the product dummy variables with the global components we get the complete representation of the data given in Fig. 10. The structure of this set of data is so strong that we obtain the same results as the ones given in Tenenhaus et al. (2004).

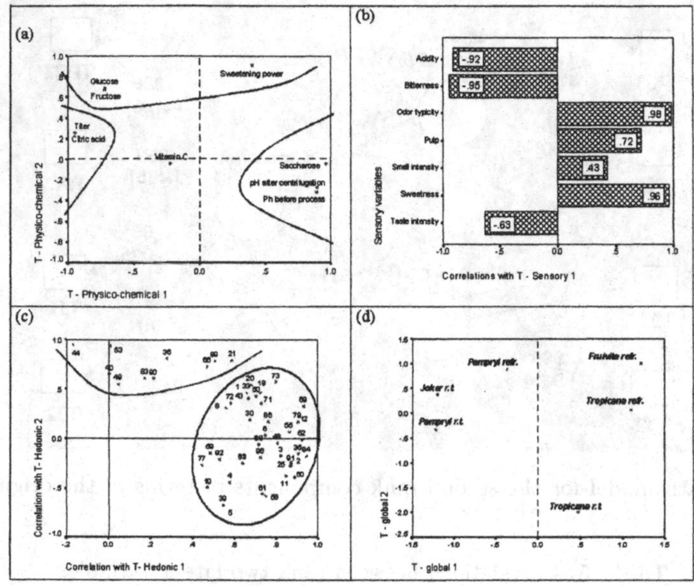

Fig. 9. Variables loadings (a, b,c) and product visualization in the global space (d).

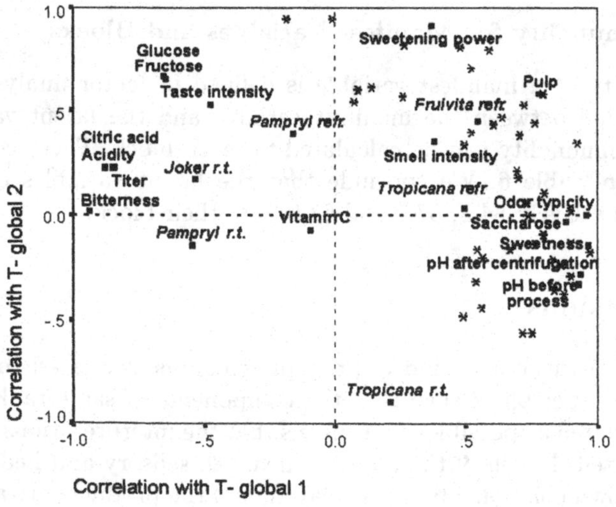

Fig. 10. Visualization of products, product descriptors and judges in the global space.

Table 6. MTA of the orange juice data: Communality.

Physico-Chemical	Communality	Sensory	Communality
Glucose	0.974	Smell intensity	0.186
Fructose	0.964	Odor typicity	0.962
Saccharose	0.933	Pulp	0.522
Sweetening power	0.984	Taste intensity	0.401
pH before processing	0.902	Acidity	0.842
pH after centrifugation	0.882	Bitterness	0.894
Titer	0.951	Sweeteness	0.927
Citric acid	0.958		
Vitamin C	0.050		
Average	*0.845*	*Average*	*0.677*

Hedonic	Communality	Hedonic	Communality	Hedonic	Communality
Judge 1	0.65	Judge 35	0.84	Judge 66	0.75
Judge 2	0.81	Judge 36	0.73	Judge 68	0.52
Judge 3	0.71	Judge 39	0.76	Judge 69	0.98
Judge 4	0.53	Judge 40	0.43	Judge 71	0.65
Judge 5	0.76	Judge 43	0.61	Judge 72	0.46
Judge 6	0.56	Judge 44	0.91	Judge 73	0.97
Judge 8	0.41	Judge 48	0.65	Judge 77	0.27
Judge 10	0.47	Judge 49	0.30	Judge 79	0.85
Judge 11	0.86	Judge 50	0.68	Judge 83	0.40
Judge 12	0.85	Judge 52	0.85	Judge 84	0.92
Judge 18	0.74	Judge 53	0.88	Judge 86	0.61
Judge 20	0.76	Judge 55	0.75	Judge 89	0.87
Judge 21	0.97	Judge 58	0.90	Judge 90	0.41
Judge 26	0.83	Judge 59	0.25	Judge 91	0.83
Judge 30	0.49	Judge 60	0.94	Judge 92	0.32
Judge 31	0.47	Judge 61	0.85	Judge 96	0.56
Judge 33	0.65	Judge 63	0.47		
Average	*0.67*				

References

1. Carrol, J. D. (1968). "A Generalization of Canonical Correlation Analysis to Three or More Sets of Variables. *Proceedings of the 76th Convention of the American Psychological Association*, 227–228.
2. Chin, W. W. (2003). *PLS-Graph User's Guide*, Technical Report, C.T. Bauer College of Business, University of Houston–Texas, USA.
3. Escofier, B., and Pagès, J. (1994). "Multiple Factor Analysis (AFMULT Package)" *Computational Statistics and Data Analysis*, **18**, 121-140.
4. Guinot, C., Latreille, J., and Tenenhaus, M. (2001). "PLS Path Modelling and Multiple Table Analysis: Application to the Cosmetic Habits of Women in Ile-de-France," *Chemometrics and Intelligent Laboratory Systems*, **58**, 247–259.
5. Horst, P. (1961). "Relations Among m Sets of Variables," *Psychometrika*, **26**, 126–149.
6. Horst, P. (1965). *Factor Analysis of Data Matrices*, Holt, Rinehart and Winston, New York.
7. Hotelling, H. (1936). "Relations Between Two Sets of Variates," *Biometrika*, **28**, 321–377.

8. Lohmöller, J. B. (1989). *Latent Variables Path Modeling with Partial Least Squares*, Physica–Verlag, Heidelberg.
9. agés, J., and Tenenhaus, M. (2001). "Multiple Factor Analysis Combined with PLS Path Modeling: Application to the Analysis of Relationships Between Physico-Chemical Variables, Sensory Profiles, and Hedonic Judgements," *Chemometrics and Intelligent Laboratory Systems*, **58**, 261–273.
10. Tenenhaus, M. (1999). "L'approche PLS," *Revue de Statistique Appliquée*, **47**, 5–40.
11. Tenenhaus, M., Esposito Vinzi, V., Chatelin, Y.M., and Lauro, C. (2004). "PLS Path Modeling," submitted to *Computational Statistics and Data Analysis.*
12. Tenenhaus, M., Pagès, J., and Guionot, C. (2004). "A PLS Methodology to Study Relationships Between Hedonic Judgements and Product Characteristics," submitted to *Food Quality and Preferences.*
13. Tucker, L. R. (1958). "An Inter-Battery Method of Factor Analysis," *Psychometrica*, **23**, 111–136.
14. Van den Wollenberg, A. L. (1977). "Redundancy Analysis: An Alternative for Canonical Correlation," *Psychometrika*, **42**, 207–219.
15. Wold, H. (1982). "Soft Modeling: The Basic Design and Some Extensions," in *Systems Under Indirect Observation, Part 2*, eds. K. Jöreskog and H. Wold, Amsterdam:North Holland, pp. 1–54.
16. Wold, H. (1985). "Partial Least Squares," in *Encyclopedia of Statistical Sciences*, eds. S. Kotz, N. Johnson, and C. Read, **6**, 581–591.
17. Wold, S., Martens, H., and Wold, H. (1983). "The Multivariate Calibration Problem in Chemistry Solved by the PLS Method," in *Proceedings of the Conference on Matrix Pencils*, eds. A. Ruhe, and B. Kagström, Lectures Notes in Mathematics, Heidelberg:Springer-Verlag, pp. 286–293.

Simultaneous Row and Column Partitioning in Several Contingency Tables

Vincent Loonis

Ecole Nationale de la Statistique et de l'Administration Economique, France
vloonis01@ensae.org

Abstract: This paper focuses on the simultaneous aggregation of modalities for more than two categorical variables. I propose to maximize an objective function closely similar to the criteria used in multivariate analysis. The algorithm I suggest is a greedy process which, at each step, merges the two most criterion-improving items in the nomenclature. As the solution is only *quasi-optimal*, I present a consolidation algorithm to improve on this solution, for a given number of clusters.

1 Introduction

Researchers in social sciences are often led to aggregate modalities in nomenclatures. In some cases, the nomenclature devised by the official statistical institutes to collect and encode data turns out to be ill-suited to the specific problem the researcher is interested in. For example, a sociologist wanting to study occupation of men in relation to social mobility and endogamy might provide two tables crossing occupations of men with occupations of their father and occupation of men with occupations of their wives. This sociologist may feel that the number of modalities for these occupations is too high and that some aggregation is needed. But he/she may be dissatisfied with the more aggregated levels available in the official nomenclature. The sociologist will then have, in this case, to simultaneously aggregate the modalities of 3 different variables. This article deals with the simultaneous grouping of modalities of several variables, at least one of which has a high number of modalities. To date, we know contributions to this problem only refer to the case of two variables.

In the framework of contingency table, Benzécri (1973) fixes the numbers of clusters and looks for the partitions of the two sets of modalities that maximize the Pearson chi-square. Gilula and Krieger (1983) study how the Pearson chi-square behaves when the table is reduced by aggregation. More recently

Ritschard, Zighed & Nicoloyannis (2001) have introduced a new methodology. Their algorithm successively seeks the optimal grouping of two rows or columns categories. They find both the number of groups and the joint partition of rows and columns of a contingency table that maximizes an association criteria. I present here a generalization to more than two variables. I suggest maximizing a weighted mean of different association criteria calculated on each contingency table. This formulation is similar to what is widely used in multivariate analysis.

The proposed algorithm is an iterative greedy process. At each step, the effect on the criteria of all possible merging of 2 modalities is calculated and the most effective merging is retained. As the solution is only *quasi-optimal*, I suggest to use a consolidation algorithm which will improve on this result, for a given number of clusters. See in annex, for a *SAS* macro implementing the approach. This article is composed of four sections. In Section 2 the formal framework and the notations are defined. The heuristic is described in Section 3. Section 4 deals with the consolidation algorithm. Finally, Section 5 discusses further developments.

2 Notation and Formal Framework

Let $X_i\,(i = 1, \ldots, S)$ be S qualitative variables. We are not interested in the variables themselves but in the sets of their modalities. Two different variables may have the same set of modalities (for example occupation of the son and occupation of his father) so that $M \leq S$ denotes the number of sets. Let m be one of these sets, p_m^0 the number of its modalities, and $\mathcal{P}_m$ a partition of these modalities. Let m_i the set for the variable i.

Assume we have data allowing to cross X_i with X_j generating a contingency table $T^{i,j}_{p^0_{m_i} \times p^0_{m_j}}$ with $p^0_{m_i}$ rows and $p^0_{m_j}$ columns. Let $\theta_{i,j} = \theta(T^{i,j}_{p^0_{m_i} \times p^0_{m_j}})$ denote a generic association criterion for table $T^{i,j}_{p^0_{m_i} \times p^0_{m_j}}$. Each couple (i, j) and each partition $(\mathcal{P}_{m_i}, \mathcal{P}_{m_j})$ define a contingency table $T(\mathcal{P}_{m_i}, \mathcal{P}_{m_j})$. The optimization general problem considered is the maximization of the criteria among the M partitions $\mathcal{P}_m$:

$$\underset{(\mathcal{P}_m)_{m=1}^M}{Max}\ \Theta \ = \ \underset{(\mathcal{P}_m)_{m=1}^M}{Max}\ (\sum_{i=1}^{S}\sum_{j=1}^{S} a_{ij}\theta(T(\mathcal{P}_{m_i}, \mathcal{P}_{m_j}))) \tag{1}$$

where $a_{i,j}$ are positive and such that $\sum_{i=1}^{S}\sum_{j=1}^{S} a_{i,j} = 1$.

The Θ criteria can be interpreted as a weighted mean of association measures between variables X_i. The weights have to be fixed by the statistician in relation to his study(see Section 3.3). The formulation of Θ is similar to what is widely used in multivariate analysis. Saporta (1988) points out that many well-known methods of multivariate analysis may be presented in terms of maximizing the sum of association measures between an unknown variable Y and several known variables $X_1, X_2 \cdots X_p$:

- When $Y, X_1, \cdots, X_p$ are numerical,

$$\max_Y \sum_{k=1}^{p} r^2(Y; X_k)$$

  leads to the first principal component in a principal component analysis (PCA), where r^2 is the square correlation coefficient.
- When Y is categorical and $X_1, \cdots, X_p$ numerical,

$$\max_Y \sum_{k=1}^{p} \eta^2(Y; X_k)$$

  leads to clusters analysis where η^2 is the square correlation ratio.
- When $X_1, \cdots, X_p$ are categorical Marcotorchino (1988) notes that the central partition problem, which consist in maximizing the number of agreements with p known partitions, may be set as

$$\max_Y \sum_{k=1}^{p} R(Y; X_k),$$

  where R is Rand's measure of association (1971).

Redundancy analysis, multiple correspondence analysis (MCA), and generalized canonical analysis lie within this framework too (Saporta, 1988). The criteria (1) obviously falls within the scope of this general approach.

The Θ criteria is a generalization of the criteria maximized by Ritschard, Zighed & Nicoloyannis (2001) in the special case of two variables. In our formulation they maximize:

$$\theta(T(\mathcal{P}_{m_1}, \mathcal{P}_{m_2})).$$

Our generalization, using a weighted mean, is more or less arbitrary but is very natural in the field of multivariate analysis. For example, such a generalization is used for Generalized Canonical Analysis.

3 The Heuristic

To describe the heuristic we begin with a general description of the algorithm, followed by specific algorithm details and an example.

3.1 The Algorithm

The heuristic is an iterative greedy process. At each step, the effect of the merging of two modalities on the criteria Θ is calculated, for all possible pair of modalities. The most improving "merging" is retained. Formally, the configuration $(\mathcal{P}_m^k)_{m=1}^M$, where $\mathcal{P}_m^k$ is a partition in p_m^k clusters for the set of modalities m obtained at step k. is the solution of:

$$\begin{cases} \max\limits_{(\mathcal{P}_m^k)_{m=1}^M} \Theta^k = \max\limits_{(\mathcal{P}_m^k)_{m=1}^M} \sum\limits_{i=1}^{S}\sum\limits_{j=1}^{S} a_{ij}\theta(\mathcal{P}_{m_i}^k, \mathcal{P}_{mj}^k) \\ \text{such that } \exists\, m_0^k \backslash \mathcal{P}_{m_0^k}^k \in \mathcal{P}_{m_0^k}^{(k-1)} \text{ and } \forall m \neq m_0^k : \mathcal{P}_m^k = \mathcal{P}_m^{k-1} \end{cases} \quad (2)$$

where $\mathcal{P}_{m_0^k}^{(k-1)}$ stands for the set of partitions resulting from the grouping of two clusters of the partition $\mathcal{P}_{m_0^k}^{k-1}$.

3.2 Choosing θ

Variables $X_1, \ldots, X_S$ can either be nominal or ordinal. The parameter θ has to be available for both kinds of variables. The choice is limited to the measures derived from the Pearson chi-square or the Rand index (1971).

The most common measure derived from the chi-square is Cramer's V. Studying his property relative to aggregation,Ritschard, Zighed & Nicoloyannis (2001) point out that Cramer's V could increase only when aggregating two modalities of the variable with the lowest number of modalities. This technical property will systematically favor the variable with the least number of modalities. I chose not to adopt this obviously biased measure.

I prefer to follow Milligan and Cooper (1986) and to adopt the Adjusted Rand Index (Hubert and Arabie, 1985) as my measure of agreement. These authors compare many different indices for measuring agreement between two variables with different numbers of clusters. They find that the adjusted Rand index is best adapted. Further developments should investigate the influence of the θ measure on the result of our procedure.

3.3 Example

Figure 1 shows how the algorithm performs in the following example. I want to find the most homogeneous grouping for the modalities of men's occupation according to their father's and wife occupations.
Let

- X_1 be the occupation of 333 3531 men according to the French labour survey

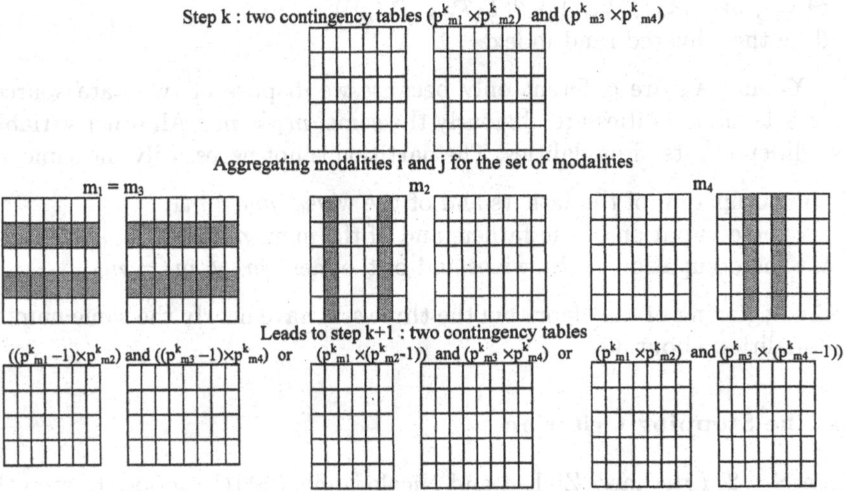

Fig. 1. Step $k+1$ of maximization algorithm for the example of Section 3.3.

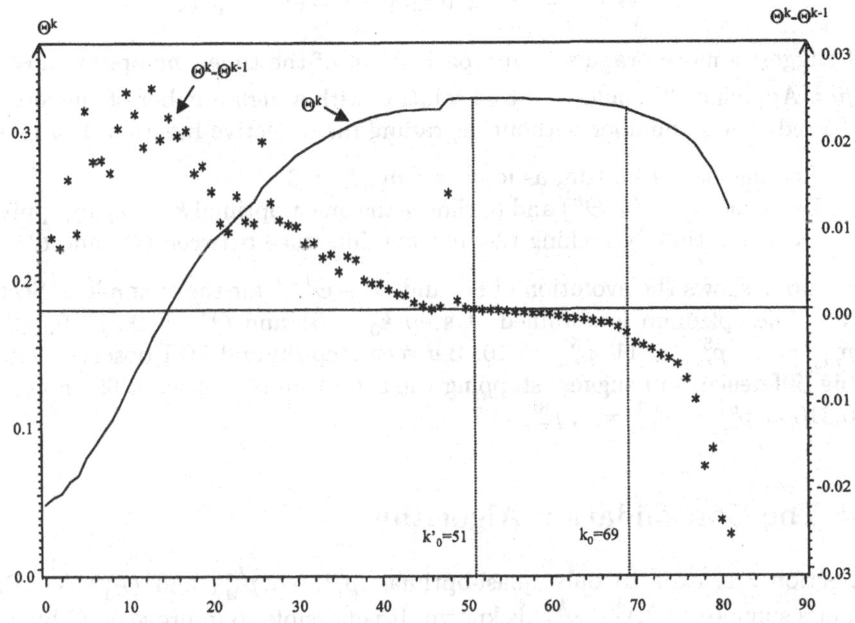

Fig. 2. Evolution of Θ^k and $\Theta^k - \Theta^{k-1}$ for the example of Section 3.3.

- X_2 be the occupation of their father
- X_3 be the occupation of 370 637 married men according to the French census
- X_4 be the occupation of their wife

- $\Theta = \frac{1}{2}(\theta(T(\mathcal{P}_{m_1}, \mathcal{P}_{m_2})) + \theta(T(\mathcal{P}_{m_3}, \mathcal{P}_{m_4})))$
- θ be the adjusted rand index.

The X_1 and X_3 are different only because we dispose of two data sources. Their sets of modalities are obviously the same, $m_1 = m_3$. All other variables have different sets of modalities. The partition is not necessarily the same for:

- the occupation of the fathers and of the wives, $m_2 \neq m_4$,
- for the occupation of the fathers and of the men, $m_2 \neq m_1 = m_3$,
- for the occupation of the wives and of the men, $m_4 \neq m_1 = m_3$.

At the beginning of the algorithm the three sets have nearly the same number of modalities, about 30.

3.4 The Stopping Criterion

When $S = 2$, Ritschard, Zighed and Nicoloyannis (2001) propose to stop the algorithm at the step k'_0 where:

$$\Theta^{k'_0+1} - \Theta^{k'_0} < 0 \text{ and } \Theta^{k'_0} - \Theta^{k'_0-1} \geq 0. \tag{3}$$

I suggest a more pragmatic approach. Most of the time, the optimum $\Theta^{k'_0}$ is *flat*. Applying (3) could lead to a solution with a high number of clusters $p_m^{k'_0}$. To reduce this number without degrading the objective function, I propose:

1 Let the algorithm run, as long as $\exists\, m \backslash p_m^k > 2$
2 Draw the curve (k, Θ^k) and to choose the quasi-optimal $k_0 \geq k'_0$ by applying a rule of thumb, seeking the first big difference between Θ^{k_0} and θ^{k_0+1}.

Figure 2 shows the evolution of Θ^k and $\Theta^k - \Theta^{k-1}$ for the example of Section 3.3. The optimum is obtained at step $k'_0 = 51$ and $\Theta^{51} = 0.31756$, $p_{m_1}^{51} = p_{m_3}^{51} = 14$, $p_{m_2}^{51} = 11$, $p_{m_4}^{51} = 10$. Between step 69 and 70 I observe the first big difference, so I suggest stopping the algorithm at step $k_0 = 69$ and $\Theta^{69} = 0.31006$, $p_{m_1}^{69} = p_{m_3}^{69} = 5$, $p_{m_2}^{69} = 7$, $p_{m_4}^{69} = 6$.

4 The Consolidation Algorithm

Section 3.1 leads to only quasi-optimal $(p_1^{k_0}, \cdots, p_M^{k_0})$ and $(\mathcal{P}_1^{k_0}, \cdots, \mathcal{P}_M^{k_0})$. Let's suppose $(p_1^{k_0}, \cdots, p_M^{k_0})$ is known. It is possible to improve on Θ by modifying $(\mathcal{P}_1^{k_0}, \cdots, \mathcal{P}_M^{k_0})$ with a consolidation algorithm. Our algorithm consists in transferring one modality at a time. At the first step, it considers, among all the M sets of modalities, the modality j and the corresponding set m^j whose transfer from its original cluster in partition $\mathcal{P}_{m^j}^{k_0}$ to another cluster of this partition maximizes the objective function Θ. Let Θ_1 be the new value of objective function; if $\Theta_1 > \Theta^{k_0}$ we validate the transfer. The algorithm goes on as long as it can find a transfer that improves the objective function.

4.1 Example

Let's consider the partition obtained at step 69 for the 3 sets of modalities of Section 3.3. Table 1 shows the 5 steps of the consolidation algorithm.

Table 1. Steps of the consolidation algorithm.

Step	m	modality	original cluster	final cluster	Θ
0					0.31006
1	m_2	12	4	3	0.31019
2	m_4	5	2	4	0.31025
3	m_2	7	4	5	0.31031
4	$m_1 = m_3$	4	3	2	0.31032
5	m_2	8	4	2	0.310324

During the first step, transferring the modality 12 for the set of modalities m_2 *(occupation of the fathers)* from cluster 4 to cluster 3 improves the objective function whose value is now 0.31019. No other transfer could have done better at this step. After five steps no transfer can be found to improve the objective function, at which point the algorithm stops.

5 Discussion

I propose a solution to the problem of the simultaneous grouping of rows and columns of several contingency tables. The method raises a number of questions that are subjects for future research and improvements.

- Does our procedure give close-to-optimal solutions?
- How can we introduce θ indicators adapted to the ordinal case?
- What can be said of asymmetric θ measures?
- What is the true impact of the numbers of rows and columns on the θ measure?
- How strongly is the solution dependent on θ?

Those questions will probably have to be answered by simulation, as was the case for $S = 2$ by Ritschard (2001).

6 Appendix

6.1 The Adjusted Rand Index

Let X_1, X_2 be two categorical variables with p, q different modalities. Let a be the number of pairs, among N observations, that are placed in the same modalities for X_1 and X_2, Let d be the number of pairs in the different modalities for X_1 and X_2. The Rand index(1971) is simply $2(a+d)/[N(N-1)]$. It can be interpreted as the proportion of agreement between X_1 and X_2.

A problem with the Rand index is that the expected value of the Rand Index of two random variables does not take a constant value (say zero). The adjusted Rand index proposed by Hubert and Arabie (1985) assumes the generalized hypergeometric distribution as the model of randomness. Let $N_{i,j}$ be the number of individuals with modality i of X_1 and j of X_2. Let $N_{i.}$ and $N_{.j}$ be the number of objects in state i respectively j.

The general form of an index with constant expected value is

$$\frac{\text{index - expected index}}{\text{maximum index - expected index}}.$$

Under the generalized hypergeometric model, it can be shown:

$$\theta = \frac{\sum_{i,j} C^2_{N_{i,j}} - [\sum_i C^2_{N_{i.}} \sum_j C^2_{N_{.j}}]/C^2_N}{\frac{1}{2}[\sum_i C^2_{N_{i.}} + \sum_j C^2_{N_{.j}}] - [\sum_i C^2_{N_{i.}} \sum_j C^2_{N_{.j}}]/C^2_N}.$$

6.2 *SAS* Program

A SAS program can be obtained from the author at the email address given at the beginning of this article. It performs the methodology presented in this article in the following case:

- θ is the Rand Adjusted Index
- $\forall (i,j) \neq (i',j') \backslash a_{i,j} a_{i',j'} \neq 0 : a_{i,j} = a_{i',j'}$

Acknowledgment

I am grateful to two anonymous referees for valuable comments on a previous version of the article.

References

1. Benzécri, J. P. (1973). *Analyse des Données. Tome 2: Analyse des Correspondences.* Dunod, Paris.
2. Gilula, Z. and Krieger, A. M. (1993). "The Decomposability and Monotonicity of Pearson's Chi-Square for Collapsed Contingency Tables with Applications," *Journal of the American Statistical Association*, **78**, 176–180.
3. Ritschard, G. Zighed, D. A. and Nicoloyannis, N. (2001). "Maximization de l'Association par Regroupement de Lignes ou de Colonnes d'un Tableau Croisé," *Revue Mathématiques Sciences Humaines*, **39**, 81–97.

4. Saporta, G. (1988). "About Maximal Analysis Association Criteria in Linear Analysis and in Cluster Analysis" in *Classification and Related Methods of Data Analysis*, ed. H.-H. Bock, North Holland.
5. Marcotorchino, F (1988). "Maximal Association as a Tool for Classification," in *Classification as a Tool of Research*, eds. W. Gaul, M. Schader, North Holland, pp. 275–288.
6. Rand, W. M. (1971). "Objective Criteria for the Evaluation of Clustering Methods," *Journal of the American Statistical Association*, **66**, 846–850.
7. Milligan, G. W. and Cooper, M. C. (1986). "A Study of the Comparability of External Criteria for Hierarchical Cluster Analysis," *Multivariate Behavorial Research*, **21**, 441–458.
8. Hubert, L. and Arabie, P. (1985). " Comparing Partitions," *Journal of Classication*, **2**, 193–218.
9. Ritschard, G. (2001). "Performance d'une heuristique d'agrégation optimale bidimensionnelle," *Extraction des Connaissances et Apprentissage*, **1**, 185–196.

Missing Data and Imputation Methods in Partition of Variables

Ana Lorga da Silva[1], Gilbert Saporta[2], and Helena Bacelar-Nicolau[3]

[1] Universidade Lusofona de Humanidades e Tecnologias, Portugal
ana.lorga@ulusofona.pt

[2] Statistics Department, CNAM, France
saporta@cnam.fr

[3] Lisbon University, Portugal
hbacelar@fpce.ul.pt

Abstract: We deal with the effect of missing data under a "Missing at Random Model" on classification of variables with non-hierarchical methods. The partitions are compared by the Rand index.

1 Introduction

The missing data problem in some classical hierarchical methods has been studied using the affinity coefficient (Bacelar-Nicolau, 2002) and the Bravais-Pearson correlation coefficient, e.g., in Silva, Saporta et al. (2001) and also in Silva et al. (2003), where we have been studying the missing data under a "Missing at Random Model" - MAR - as described for instance in Little and Rubin(2002), which we and other authors consider a more "realistic model" - which means that it occurs more often in the real situations - of missing data. Missing data can be found in data from marketing analysis and social sciences, among others.

So, when we do classification, we must be prepared to "interpret" the results. In most papers on missing data, researchers deal mainly with estimation of the parameters of the population such as mean, and standard deviation, among others, or in estimating regression models (this is frequent in Economics studies). Partition methods are sometimes used as a complement of hierarchical classification methods for choosing the best level where "cut the structure"; here we analyse the performance of one of those methods when missing data are present.

2 Methodology

The partition method we use in this work is composed of two algorithms: a hierarchical algorithm followed by the partitioning algorithm. To the best of our knowledge, no prior work about missing data nor imputation methods has been done for this method. Our approach is derived from Vigneau and Qannari(2003) and is closely related to principal components analysis. From one perspective, this approach consists in clustering variables around latent components. More precisely, the aim is to determine simultaneously k clusters of variables and k latent components so that the variables in each cluster are related to the corresponding latent component. This method leads us to choose the adequate number groups in a partition.

The Method: Assume that one has

- p variables measured on n objects - $x_1, x_2, ..., x_p$ (the variables are centered),
- K clusters of the p variables - $G_1, G_2, ..., G_k$ (comprising a partition wich we can design by P_1)
- K latent variables - $l_1, l_2, ..., l_k$ - associated with each of the K groups.
- The criterion $S = \sqrt{n}\sum_{k=1}^{K}\sum_{j=1}^{p}\delta_{kj}cov(x_j, l_k)$, under the constraint

  $$l_k.l_k' = 1$$

  where

  $$\delta_{kj} = \begin{cases} 1 & if\ x_j \in G_k \\ 0 & if\ x_j \notin G_k. \end{cases}$$

We optimize S rather than a criterion based on squared correlation because, for us, in many situations, the sign of the correlation coefficient makes sense (cf. Vigneau and Qannari, 2003): "p consumers are asked to rate their acceptability of n product. A negative covariance between the scores of two consumers emphasizes their different views of the products."

The partition algorithm used in this work is as follows:

i) Start with K groups obtained by a hierarchical cluster method (this hierarchical cluster method is based on the same criterion S described for the partition, as in Vigneau and Qannari (2003)).
ii) In cluster G_k $(k = 1, 2, ..., K)$, $l_k = \bar{x}_k / \sqrt{\bar{x}_k \bar{x}'_k}$ where $\bar{x}_k$ is the centroid of G_k, so that $\bar{x}_k = p_k^{-1}\sum_{j=1} x_{kj}$ for p_k the number of elements in G_k.
iii) Following Vigneau and Qannari (2003), "New clusters are formed by moving each variable to a new group if its covariance with the standardised centroid of this group is higher than any other standardised centroid."

2.1 The Imputation Methods

There are many strategies for imputation. In this work, we consider the folowing techniques:

a) the listwise method,
b) the NIPALS algorithm adapted to a regression method (as described in Silva et al. (2002) and Tenenhaus (1998)),
c) the EM imputation method,
d) an OLS (ordinary least squares) regression method, i.e., one estimates missing values by standard multiple regression, e.g., as described in Silva et al. (2002),
e) the PLS2 regression method used as an imputation method; PLS2 stands for a particular application of partial least squares regression where one has to predict simultaneously q variables (PLS or PLS1 stand for $q = 1$),
f) multiple imputation - (MI) - a Bayesian Method based on an OLS regression (Rubin, 1987).

we note that, usually, neither the PLS2 regression method nor NIPALS algorithm is used as an imputation method. The version of PLS2 we use here comes naturally from the NIPALS algorithm which has, as the main feature, the possibility of allowing us to work with missing data without suppressing observations that have missing data in some of the measured variables (and even without estimating the missing data). In the simulation studies, we shall deal with the case in which there is missing data on two of variables on which the observations are measured. For the MI imputation method, the results will be combined in two ways as described at Section 2.3

2.2 Missing Data and MAR

Missing data is said to be MAR (Missing at Random) if it can be written as:

$$\text{Prob}(M|X_{obs}, X_{miss}) = \text{Prob}(M|X_{obs}),$$

where

- X_{obs} represents the observed values of $X_{n \times p}$,
- X_{miss} represents the missing values of $X_{n \times p}$, and
- $M = [M_{ij}]$ is a missing data indicator:

$$M_{ij} = \begin{cases} 1 & \text{if } x_{ij} \text{ observed} \\ 0 & \text{if } x_{ij} \text{ missing.} \end{cases}$$

2.3 Multiple Imputation, Correlation Matrices, and Partitions

By using imputation methods m matrices $X^1, X^2, ..., X^m$ are obtained. In our experience, usually $m = 5$ is sufficient. It is necessary to combine these results in order to apply the partition method.

First Method: Combination of the Correlation Matrices (MIave).

i) First, we obtain $X^1, X^2, ..., X^m$ to which are associated m correlation matrices (R_k, $k = 1, ...m$).
ii) We determine the average of the m correlation matrices:

$$\overline{R} = m^{-1}\sum_{k=1}^{m} R_k.$$

iii) We apply the partition method to $\overline{R}$.

Second Method: Consensus Between the Partitions (MIcons).

With this method we try to establish a consensus between m partitions in order to find a representative partition. To compare the partitions we use the Rand index (see Saporta and Youness, 2002). This measures us the proportion of agreements between the partitions.

Suppose we have two partitions P_1, P_2 of p variables, with the same number of classes k. We will find four types of pairs:

- a, the number of pairs belonging simultaneously to the same classes of P_1 and P_2,
- b, the number of pairs belonging to different classes of P_1 but to the same of P_2,
- c, the number of pairs belonging to different classes of P_2 but to the same of class in P_1, and
- d, the number of pairs belonging to different classes of P_1 and P_2.

So we have:

A=a+d represents the total number of agreements
D=b+c represents the total number of discordances

and $A + D = p(p-1)/2$. The classical Rand's index is given then by the expression $I_R^* = 2A/p(p-1)$. But we will use the version modified by Marcotorchino:

$$I_R = n^{-2}\left[2\sum_{i=1}^{k}\sum_{j=1}^{k}(n_{ij})^2 - \sum_{i=1}^{k}(n_{i.})^2 - \sum_{j=1}^{k}(n_{.j})^2 + n^2\right]$$

where the n_{ij} are the elements of the contingency table crossing the two partitions, $n_i.$ is the row total and $n.j$ the column total.

In this paper we will deal with five variables and two partitions. In that case 0.5 is the expected value of Rand's index under the independence hypothesis.

We start with each of the m matrices $X^1, X^2, ..., X^m$. The methodology described previously is applied to each one, so that m partitions are obtained. We do a "consensus between the partitions" that consists of:

i) Determining if there are $n_i \in \{\frac{m}{2} + 1, \ldots, m\}$ partitions for which I_R=1 and those partitions are the representative, and also all equal, so that we find a representative partition;

ii) If the first condition is not satisfied, we reapply the imputation method with $m = 10$; then new partitions in the described conditions are searched. If they are not found, it means that there is no consensus between the partitions and no partition is representative of the ten partitions obtained.

3 Simulation Studies

In order to study the performance of imputation methods in the presence of missing data we use the modified Rand's index as described above. First, one hundred samples of each type of simulated data were generated from five multivariate normal populations (Saporta and Bacelar-Nicolau, 2001)), so $X_i \sim N(\mu_i, \Sigma_i)$, $i = 1, ..., 5$, (1000 observations, 5 variables) with ($\mu_1 = \mu_2 = \mu_3 = \mu_4 = \mu_5$). The values of the variance and co-variance matrices have been chosen in order to obtain specific hierarchical structures as shown below:

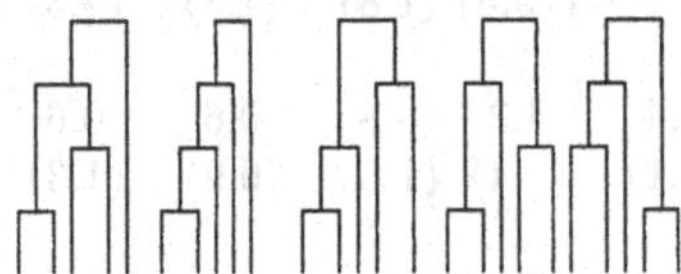

Fig. 1: The order of variables: x_1, x_2, x_3, x_4, x_5.

Here we use twenty-five matrices for each one of the five normal multivariate cases. The partition method gives one of the two following partitions:

i) $\{x_1, x_2, x_3\}$, $\{x_4, x_5\}$
ii) $\{x_1, x_2, x_3, x_4\}$, $\{x_5\}$.

Therefore, it performs quite well on the original structures.

For the missing data, we consider three different percentages: 10%, 15% and 20% of missing data (over the total of the data, i.e., each 1000×5 matrices). Missing data are estimated with the imputation methods described previously.

Then we evaluated the effect of missing data and the imputation methods on the partition method by comparing each obtained partition with the corresponding partition obtained with the original (complete) data. In the following tables, we present the results of the comparisons (where the first line represents the mean and the second line—in brackets—is the standard deviation).

Here $I_R = 1$, $I_R > 0,5$ and $I_R <= 0,5$, means:

- $I_R = 1$ the obtained partitions are the same
- $I_R > 0.5$ the obtained partitions are correlated
- $I_R \leq 0.5$ the obtained partitions are independent

Table 1. 10% of missing data

	listwise	EM	OLS	NIPALS	PLS	MIave	MIcons
$I_R = 1$	23.4	15	24.8	25	22.9	15	12.2
	(3.6)	(13.7)	(0.4)	(0)	(3.9)	(13.7)	(11.9)
$I_R > 0.5$	1.6	0.6	0.2	0	2.1	10	4
	(4)	(1.3)	(0.4)	(0)	(3.9)	(13.7)	(8.9)
$I_R <= 0.5$	0	9.4	0	0	0	0	8.8
	(0)	(12.9)	(0)	(0)	(0)	(0)	(2.2)

Table 2. 15% of missing data

	listwise	EM	OLS	NIPALS	PLS	MIave	MIcons
$I_R = 1$	21.6	15	24.2	23.8	19.6	14.2	16
	(7.1)	(13.5)	(1.8)	(1.3)	(9.3)	(13.1)	(12.5)
$I_R > 0.5$	3.4	4.2	0.8	0.6	0.6	6	0
	(7.1)	(9.4)	(1.8)	(0.9)	(1.3)	(10.7)	(0)
$I_R <= 0.5$	0	5.8	0	0.6	4.8	4.8	5
	(0)	(10.8)	(0)	(1.3)	(9.8)	(10.2)	(11.2)

Table 3. 20% of missing data

	listwise	EM	OLS	NIPALS	PLS	MIave	MIcons
$I_R = 1$	21	5.4	23.6	19.4	20.5	14.8	16
	(7.9)	(10.9)	(3.1)	(9.8)	(6.1)	(13.5)	(12.5)
$I_R > 0.5$	3.8	10	1.4	2.4	1.2	5.4	0
	(7.9)	(13.7)	(3.1)	(3.9)	(1.8)	(10.9)	(0)
$I_R <= 0.5$	0.2	9.8	0	3	2.3	4.8	9
	(0.4)	(13.4)	(0)	(6.2)	(6)	(10.7)	(12.5)

4 Conclusions

Surprisingly (as compared to previous results for hierarchical methods) multiple imputation does not perform well. The best results are obtained with the OLS regression method and the NIPALS algorithm as an imputation method. On the whole, we can say that the OLS regression method performs better than the others but not significantly better.

This study shows that the partition method we have analysed to help us in finding the "best" partition in a hierarchical classification does not perform well when missing data are present and so we are using imputation methods. A probabilistic approach based on the affinity coefficient for finding the best "cut-off" appears to be a good solution.

Acknowledgements

This work has been partially supported by the Franco-Portuguese Scientific Programme "Modeles Statistiques pour le Data Mining" MSPLLDM-542-B2 (Embassy of France and Portuguese Ministry of Science and Superior Education - GRICES) co-directed by H. Bacelar-Nicolau and G. Saporta and the Multivariate Data Analysis research team of CEAUL/FCUL directed by H. Bacelar-Nicolau.

References

1. Bacelar-Nicolau, H. (2002). "On the Generalised Affinity Coefficient for Complex Data," *Byocybernetics and Biomedical Engineering*, **22**, 1, 31–42.
2. Little, R. J. A., and Rubin, D. B. (2002). *Statistical Analysis with Missing Data*, John Wiley and Sons, New York.
3. Rubin, D. B. (1987). *Multiple Imputation for Nonresponse in Surveys*, John Wiley and Sons, New York.
4. Saporta, G., and Youness, G. (2002). "Comparing Two Partitions: Some Proposals and Experiments," in *Proceedings in Computational Statistics*, eds. W. Hardle and B. Ronz, Berlin:Physica Verlag, pp. 243–248.
5. Silva, A. L., Bacelar-Nicolau, H., and Saporta, G. (2002). "Missing Data in Hierarchical Classification of Variables - a Simulation Study," in *Classification Clustering and Data Analysis*, eds. K. Jajuga and H.-H. Bock, Berlin:Springer, pp. 121-128.
6. Silva, A. L., Saporta, G., and Bacelar-Nicolau, H. (2002). "Dados Omissos em Classificacão Hierarquica de Variaveis e o Algoritmo Nipals," in *Proceedings of IX Jornadas de Classificação e Analise de Dados*, Lisbon:ESCS-IPL, pp.42–43.
7. Silva, A. L., Saporta, G., and Bacelar-Nicolau, H. (2003). "Classification Hierarchique Ascendante avec Imputation Multiple des Donnees Manquantes," in *Methodes et Perspectives en Classification (10emes Rencontre de la Societe Francophone de Classification)*, eds. Y. Dodge and G. Melfi, Neuchatel, pp. 59–62.
8. Tenenhaus, M. (1998). *La Regression PLS*, Editions Technip, Paris.
9. Vigneau, E., and Qannari, E. M. (2003). "Clustering of Variables Around Latent Components," *Communications in Statistics: Simulation and Computation*, **32**, 1131–1150.

The Treatment of Missing Values and its Effect on Classifier Accuracy

Edgar Acuña and Caroline Rodriguez

University of Puerto Rico at Mayaguez, Puerto Rico
edgar@cs.uprm.edu, caroline@math.uprm.edu

Abstract: The presence of missing values in a dataset can affect the performance of a classifier constructed using that dataset as a training sample. Several methods have been proposed to treat missing data and the one used most frequently deletes instances containing at least one missing value of a feature. In this paper we carry out experiments with twelve datasets to evaluate the effect on the misclassification error rate of four methods for dealing with missing values: the case deletion method, mean imputation, median imputation, and the KNN imputation procedure. The classifiers considered were the Linear Discriminant Analysis (LDA) and the KNN classifier. The first one is a parametric classifier whereas the second one is a nonparametric classifier.

1 Introduction

Missing data is a common problem in statistical analysis. Rates of less than 1% missing data are generally considered trivial, 1-5% are manageable. However, 5-15% requires sophisticated methods to handle, and more than 15% may severely impact any kind of interpretation. Several methods have been proposed in the literature to treat missing data. Many of these methods were developed for dealing with missing data in sample surveys (cf. Kalton and Kasprzyk, 1986; Mundfrom and Whitcomb, 1998), and have some drawbacks when they are applied to classification tasks. Chan and Dunn (1972) considered the treatment of missing values in supervised classification using the LDA classifier but only for two classes problems considering a simulated dataset from a multivariate normal model. Dixon (1979) introduced the KNN imputation technique for dealing with missing values in supervised classification. Tresp et al. (1995) also considered the missing value problem in a supervised learning context for neural networks. The interest in dealing with missing values has continued with the statistical applications to new areas such as data mining (Grzymala-Busse and Hu, 2000) and microarrays (Hastie et al., 1999;

Troyanskaya et al., 2001). These applications include supervised classification as well as unsupervised classification (clustering). Bello (1995) compared several imputation techniques in regression analysis, a area related to classification.

Little and Rubin (2002) divide methods for treating missing data into three categories: Case/Pairwise Deletion, Parameter Estimation, and Imputation. The first is easiest and most commonly applied. The second uses maximum likelihood procedures and variants of the Expectation-Maximization algorithm to handle parameter estimation in the presence of missing data. These methods are generally superior to case deletion methods, because they utilize all the observed data and especially good when the probability mechanism leading to missingness can be included in the model. However, they suffer from several limitations, including: a strict assumption of a model distribution for the variables, such as a multivariate normal model, which has a high sensitivity to outliers, and a high degree of complexity (slow computation). The third method replaces missing values with estimated ones based on information available in the data set. The objective is to employ known relationships that can be identified in the valid values of the data set to assist in estimating the missing values. There are many options varying from naive methods, like mean imputation, to some more robust methods based on relationships among attributes.

In this paper we compare four methods to treat missing values in supervised classification problems. We choose the case deletion technique (CD), the mean imputation (MI), the median imputation (MDI) and the k-nearest neighbor (KNN) imputation. The criteria to compare them are the effects on the misclassification rate in two classifiers: the Linear Discriminant Analysis (LDA) and the KNN classifier. The first is a parametric classifier and the second one is a nonparametric classifier. In Section 2 the four methods to treat missing values considered in this paper are described. In Section 3 we explain our experimental methodology and in Section 4 we present and discuss our results.

2 Four Methods for Missing Values

The following four methods are used in this paper to treat missing values in the supervised classification context. We also give a brief description of other methods not considered in this paper.

A. Case Deletion (CD). This method is also known as complete case analysis. It is available in all statistical packages and is the default method in many programs. This method consists of discarding all instances (cases) with missing values for at least one feature. A variation of this method consists of determining the extent of missing data on each instance and attribute, and deleting the instances and/or attributes with high levels of missing data. Before deleting any attribute, it is necessary to evaluate its relevance to the analysis. Unfortunately, relevant attributes should be kept even with a high degree of missing values. CD is less hazardous if it involves minimal loss of sample size (minimal missing data or a sufficiently large sample size) and there is no structure or pattern to the missing data. For other situations, where the sample size is insufficient or some structure exists in the missing data, CD has been shown to produce more biased estimates than alternative methods. CD should be applied only in cases in which data are missing completely at random (see Little and Rubin (2002)).

B. Mean Imputation (MI). This is one of the most frequently used methods. It consists of replacing the missing data for a given feature (attribute) by the mean of all known values of that attribute in the class where the instance with missing attribute belongs. Let us consider that the value x_{ij} of the k-th class, C_k, is missing then it will be replaced by

$$\hat{x}_{ij} = \sum_{i:x_{ij} \in C_k} \frac{x_{ij}}{n_k}, \tag{1}$$

where n_k represents the number of non-missing values in the j-th feature of the k-th class. In some studies the overall mean is used but we believe that this does not take in account the sample size of the class to which the instance with the missing values belongs. According to Little and Rubin (2002), among the drawbacks of mean imputation are (a) sample size is overestimated, (b) variance is underestimated, (c) correlation is negatively biased, and (d) the distribution of new values is an incorrect representation of the population values because the shape of the distribution is distorted by adding values equal to the mean. Replacing all missing records with a single value will deflate the variance and artificially inflate the significance of any statistical tests based on it. Surprisingly though, mean imputation has given good experimental results in data sets used for supervised classification purposes (Chan and Dunn, 1972; Mundfrom and Whitcomb, 1998).

C. Median Imputation (MDI). Since the mean is affected by the presence of outliers it seems natural to use the median instead just to assure robustness. In this case the missing values for a given feature are replaced by the median of all known values of that attribute in the class to which the instance with the missing feature belongs. This method is also a recommended choice when the distribution of the values of a given feature is skewed. Let us consider that the value x_{ij} of the k-th class, C_k, is missing. It will be replaced by

$$\hat{x}_{ij} = \text{median}_{\{i:x_{ij} \in C_k\}} \{x_{ij}\}. \tag{2}$$

In case of a missing value in a categorical feature we can use mode imputation instead of either mean or median imputation. These imputation methods are applied separately in each feature containing missing values. Notice that the correlation structure of the data is not being considered in the above methods. The existence of other features with similar information (high correlation), or similar predicting power, can make the missing data imputation useless, or even harmful.

D. KNN Imputation (KNNI). In this method the missing values of an instance are imputed by considering a given number of instances that are most similar to the instance of interest. The similarity of two instances is determined using a distance function. The algorithm is as follows:

---

(1) Divide the data set D into two parts. Let D_m be the set containing the instances in which at least one of the features is missing. The remaining instances will complete feature information form a set called D_c.
(2) For each vector x in D_m:
   a) Divide the instance vector into observed and missing parts as $x = [x_o; x_m]$.
   b) Calculate the distance between the x_o and all the instance vectors from the set D_c. Use only those features in the instance vectors from the complete set D_c, which are observed in the vector x.
   c) Use the K closest instances vectors (K-nearest neighbors) and perform a majority voting estimate of the missing values for categorical attributes. For continuous attributes replace the missing value using the mean value of the attribute in the k-nearest neighborhood. The median could be used instead of the median.

The advantages of KNN imputation are: (i) k-nearest neighbor can predict both qualitative attributes (the most frequent value among the k nearest neighbors) and quantitative attributes (the mean among the k nearest neighbors); (ii) it does not require one to create a predictive model for each attribute with missing data—actually, the k-nearest neighbor algorithm does not create explicit models; (iii) it can easily treat instances with multiple missing values; (iv) it takes in consideration the correlation structure of the data.

The disadvantages of KNN imputation are: (i) The choice of the distance function. It could be Euclidean, Manhattan, Mahalanobis, Pearson, etc. In this work we have considered the Euclidean distance. (ii) The KNN algorithm searches through all the dataset looking for the most similar instances. This is a very time consuming process and it can be very critical in data mining where large databases are analyzed. (iii) The choice of k, the number of neighbors. In similar fashion as it is done in Troyanskaya et al. (2001), we tried several numbers and decided to use k=10 based on the accuracy of the classifier after the imputation process. The choice of a small k produces a deterioration in the performance of the classifier after imputation due to overemphasis of a few dominant instances in the estimation process of the missing values. On the other hand, a neighborhood of large size would include instances that are significantly different from the instance containing missing values hurting their estimation process and therefore the classifier's performance declines. For small datasets k smaller than 10 can be used.

Other imputation methods are:

Hot deck Imputation. In this method, a missing attribute value is filled in with a value from an estimated distribution for the missing value from the current data. In Random Hot deck, a missing value (the recipient) of a attribute is replaced by a observed value (the donor) of the attribute chosen randomly. There are also cold deck imputation methods that are similar to hot deck but in this case the data source to choose the imputed value must be different from the current data source. For more details see Kalton and Kasprzyk (1986).

Imputation using a prediction model. These methods consist of creating a predictive model to estimate values that will substitute the missing data. The attribute with missing data is used as the response attribute, and the remaining attributes are used as input for the predictive model. The disadvantages of this approach are (i) the model estimated values are usually more well-behaved than the true values would be; (ii) if there are no relationships among attributes in the data set and the attribute with missing data, then the model will not be precise for estimating missing values; (iii) the computational cost is large since we have to build a many models to predict missing values.

Imputation using decision trees algorithms. All the decision tree classifiers handle missing values by using built-in approaches. For instance, CART replaces a missing value of a given attribute with the corresponding value of a surrogate attribute which has the highest correlation with the original attribute. C4.5 uses a probabilistic approach to handle missing data in both the training and the test samples.

Multiple imputation. In this method the missing values in a feature are filled in with values drawn randomly (with replacement) from a fitted distribution for that feature. Repeat this a number of times, say M=5 times. After that we can apply the classifier to each "complete" dataset and compute the misclassification error for each dataset by averaging the misclassification error rates to obtain a single estimate and also we can estimate the variance of the error rate. Details can be found in Little and Rubin (2002) and Shafer (1997).

3 Experimental Methodology

Our experiments were carried out using twelve datasets coming from the Machine Learning Database Repository at the University of California, Irvine. A summary of the characteristics of each dataset appears in Table 1. The number in parenthesis in the column *Features* indicates the number of relevant features for each dataset. The Missing Val. column contains the percentage of missing values with respect to the whole dataset and the Missing Inst. column contains the percentages of instances with at least one missing value. Considering these two values for *Hepatitis* we can conclude that its missing values are distributed in a large number of instances. The last two columns of Table 1 show the 10-fold cross-validation error rates for the the LDA and

KNN classifier, respectively. For the datasets with missing values these error rates correspond to the case deletion method to treat missing values.

Table 1. Information about the datasets used in this paper. Some features in the Ionosphere and Segment datasets were not considered in our experiment.

Dataset	n	Classes (no., size) (no., size)	Features	Missing Val.(%)	Missing Inst.(%)	LDA	KNN
Iris	150	3 (50,50,50)	4(3)	0	0	3.18	4.68
Hepatitis	155	2 (32,123)	19(10)	5.67	48.38	27.7	28.95
Sonar	208	2 (111,97)	60(37)	0	0	26.60	14.74
Heartc	303	2 (164,139)	13	0.15	1.98	16.51	19.42
Bupa	345	2 (145,200)	6(3)	0	0	35.04	36.46
Ionosphere	351	2 (225,126)	34(21)	0	0	16.59	13.23
Crx	690	2 (383,307)	15(9)	0.64	5.36	13.62	25.09
Breastw	699	2 (458,241)	9(5)	0.25	2.28	3.66	3.41
Diabetes	768	2 (500,268)	8(5)	0	0	24.59	27.37
Vehicle	846	4, all $\approx$ 200	18(10)	0	0	29.15	34.87
German	1000	2 (700,300)	20(13)	0	0	24.38	29.7
Segment	2310	7, all 330	19(11)	0	0	9.15	4.64

In the *Ionosphere* dataset we have discarded features 1 and 2 since feature 2 assumes the same value in both classes and feature 1 assumes only one value in one of the classes. For similar reasons in the *Segment* dataset we have not considered three features (3,4, and 5). Note that *Hepatitis* has a high percentage of instances containing missing values.

To evaluate more precisely the effect of missing values imputation on the accuracy of the classifier we worked only with the relevant variables in each dataset. This also sped up the imputation process. The relevant features were selected using the RELIEF, a filter method for feature selection in supervised classification, see Acuña et al. (2003) for more details. Batista et al. (2002) run a similar experiment but they choose only the three most important features and entered them one by one.

First we considered the four datasets having missing values. Each of them was passed through a cleaning process where features with more than 30% of missing values as well as instances with more than 50% of missing values were eliminated. We have written a program to perform this task that allows us to change these percentages as we want. This cleaning process is carried out in order to have minimize the number of imputations needed. After that is done we apply the four methods to treat missing values and once that is finished and we have a "complete" dataset we compute the 10-fold cross-validation estimates of the misclassification error for both the LDA and the KNN classifiers. The results are shown in Table 2.

Table 2. Cross-validation errors for the LDA and KNN classifiers using the four methods to deal with missing data.

Datasets	LDA				KNN			
	CD	MI	MDI	KNNI	CD	MI	MDI	KNNI
Hepatitis	27.7	31.50	32.07	30.83	28.95	38.32	37.67	39.23
*H*eartc	16.51	16.08	16.16	15.99	19.42	18.79	18.62	18.70
*C*rx	13.62	14.49	14.49	14.49	25.09	25.20	24.71	24.58
*B*reastw	3.66	3.72	3.66	3.96	3.41	3.84	3.88	3.61

Next, we considered the eight datasets without missing values and the "complete" versions of *Heartc*, *Breastw*, and *Crx*, obtained by case deletion. *Hepatitis* was not considered here because of its high percentage of instances containing missing values. In each of these 11 datasets we randomly insert a given percentage of missing values distributed proportionally according to the class size. We tried several percentages varying from 1% to 20%, but here, due to the lack of space, we only show the results for three of them. We recorded also also percentage of instances containing the missing values generated, but they are not shown in the table. After that we apply the four methods to treat missing values and compute 10-fold cross-validation estimates of the misclassification error rates for both the LDA and KNN classifiers. The results are shown in table 3.

4 Conclusions and Discussion

From Table 2 we can conclude that in datasets with a small number of instances containing missing values there is not much difference between case deletion and imputation methods for both types of classifiers. But this is not the case for datasets with a high percentage of instances with missing values, such as in *Hepatitis*.

From Tables 2 and 3 we can see that is not much difference between the results obtained with mean and median imputation. It is well known that most of datasets used here have features whose distributions contain outliers in both directions and their effects cancel out. Otherwise one could expect a better performance of the median imputation. From the same tables we can see that there is some difference between MI/MDI and KNN imputation only when a KNN classifier is used. However there is a noticeable difference between case deletion and all the imputation methods considered. Comparing the error rates from Tables 1 and 3 we can see that CD performs badly in *Sonar*, *Breast* and *German*, mostly due to the distribution of the missing values in a high percentage of instances. Overall KNN imputation seems to perform better than the other methods because it is most robust to bias when the percentage of missing values increases. In general, doing imputation does

Table 3. Cross-validation errors for LDA and KNN classifiers using the four missing data methods with missing rates shown in column MR.

Datasets	MR	LDA				KNN			
		CD	MI	MDI	KNNI	CD	MI	MDI	KNNI
Iris	1	2.89	3.82	3.72	3.64	4.82	4.81	4.70	4.86
	7	3.34	3.38	3.32	2.82	5.89	4.76	4.69	4.65
	13	3.82	2.97	3.16	3.04	4.28	2.28	2.65	3.44
Sonar	1	29.87	26.59	26.58	26.16	17.41	14.52	15.25	14.71
	3	31.63	25.48	25.91	26.14	24.06	11.50	12.24	12.99
	7	46.31	23.27	23.40	23.38	27.36	13.36	13.68	13.26
Heartc	5	12.96	14.84	14.11	15.66	16.44	18.25	18.32	18.53
	11	18.00	14.54	13.75	15.22	11.22	13.42	11.36	13.05
	21	11.75	12.94	10.64	13.64	17.12	12.41	10.23	12.59
Bupa	1	34.88	35.20	35.42	35.21	35.35	36.18	36.43	35.32
	3	36.50	36.23	36.66	35.70	35.98	37.22	37.02	36.37
	7	33.83	35.13	35.39	35.18	36.71	35.18	35.19	33.24
Ionosphere	1	15.57	16.04	16.16	16.17	14.63	12.52	12.44	12.87
	5	21.91	15.86	15.64	16.05	17.42	13.81	12.82	13.68
	9	27.87	15.28	15.13	15.83	18.97	13.81	12.82	13.68
Crx	3	15.05	13.18	13.16	13.35	24.60	24.93	25.39	25.65
	11	12.17	11.94	11.94	12.52	25.07	22.76	24.00	22.64
	21	16.44	10.82	10.71	10.71	34.70	18.97	18.24	23.97
Breastw	3	3.60	3.68	3.54	3.91	3.30	3.32	3.26	3.33
	11	4.68	3.46	3.59	3.78	3.34	2.82	2.82	2.86
	21	5.05	2.93	3.10	3.47	2.12	1.92	1.97	2.07
Diabetes	3	23.60	24.59	24.80	24.41	27.49	26.38	26.45	26.29
	9	24.09	24.09	24.24	24.42	25.35	25.82	24.56	26.05
	11	23.22	24.02	23.85	24.40	30.36	24.16	23.01	23.58
Vehicle	5	30.96	30.28	30.36	28.85	38.40	36.33	34.95	33.25
	13	30.91	34.49	34.81	28.81	40.30	33.78	32.83	32.41
	21	32.80	34.92	33.48	32.75	42.66	31.94	31.51	30.17
German	5	26.05	24.22	24.28	24.40	31.19	29.56	28.91	28.67
	13	26.00	23.88	22.70	23.96	35.92	28.03	28.93	27.61
	21	29.14	22.14	21.53	23.60	41.43	23.49	23.55	23.51
Segment	5	8.88	9.32	9.37	9.17	6.51	6.24	6.11	4.39
	13	8.29	9.35	9.44	8.84	9.41	7.04	6.60	5.31
	21	8.96	7.81	7.69	7.48	9.12	7.67	6.81	5.07

not seem to hurt too much the accuracy of the classifier, even if sometimes there is a high percentage of instances with missing values. This agrees with the conclusions obtained by Dixon (1979). We recommend that one can deal with datasets having up to 20% of missing values. For the CD method one can have up to 60% of the instances containing missing values and still have reasonable performance.

The R functions for all the procedures discussed in this paper are available in www.math.uprm.edu/~edgar, and were tested in a DELL workstation with 3GB of memory RAM and a dual processor PENTIUM Xeon.

5 Acknowledgment

This work was supported by grant N00014-00-1-0360 from ONR and by grant EIA 99-77071 from NSF

References

1. Acuña, E., Coaquira, F. and Gonzalez, M. (2003). "A Comparison of Feature Selection Procedures for Classifiers Based on Kernel Density Estimation," in *Proceedings of the International Conference on Computer, Communication and Control Technologies*, Orlando, FL:CCCT'03, Vol I, pp. 468–472.
2. Batista G. E. A. P. A., and Monard, M. C. (2002). "K-Nearest Neighbour as Imputation Method: Experimental Results," Technical Report 186, ICMC-USP.
3. Bello, A. L. (1995). "Imputation Techniques in Regression Analysis: Looking Closely at Their Implementation," *Computational Statistics and Data Analysis*, **20**, 45–57.
4. Chan, P., and Dunn, O. J. (1972). "The Treatment of Missing Values in Discriminant Analysis," *Journal of the American Statistical Association*, **69**, 473-477.
5. Dixon J. K. (1979). "Pattern Recognition with Partly Missing Data," *IEEE Transactions on Systems, Man, and Cybernetics*, SMC-9, **10**, 617–621.
6. Grzymala-Busse, J. W., and Hu, M. (2000). "A Comparison of Several Approaches to Missing Attribute Values in Data Mining," in *Rough Sets and Current Trends in Computing 2000*, pp. 340–347.
7. Hastie, T., Tibshirani, R., Sherlock, G., Eisen, M, Brown, P. and Bolstein, D. (1999). "Imputing Missing Data for Gene Expression Arrays," Techical Report, Division of Biostatistics, Stanford University.
8. Kalton, G., and Kasprzyk, D. (1986). "The Treatment of Missing Survey Data," *Survey Methodology*, **12**, 1–16.
9. Little, R. J., and Rubin, D. B. (2002). *Statistical Analysis with Missing Data*, second edn., John Wiley and Sons, New York.
10. Mundfrom, D. J., and Whitcomb, A. (1998). "Imputing Missing values: The Effect on the Accuracy of Classification," *Multiple Linear Regression Viewpoints*, **25**, 13–19.
11. Schafer, J. L. (1997). *Analysis of Incomplete Multivariate Data*, Chapman and Hall, London.
12. Tresp, V., Neuneier, R., and Ahmad, S. (1994). "Efficient Methods for Dealing with Missing Data in Supervised Learning," in *NIPS 1994*, eds. G. Tesauro, D. S. Touretzky, and T. K. Leen, Cambridge, MA:MIT Press, pp. 689–696.
13. Troyanskaya, O., Cantor, M., Sherlock, G., Brown, P. Hastie, T., Tibshirani, R., Bostein, D. and Altman, R. B. (2001). "Missing Value Estimation Methods for DNA Microarrays," *Bioinformatics*, **17**, 520–525.

Clustering with Missing Values: No Imputation Required

Kiri Wagstaff

Jet Propulsion Laboratory, California Institute of Technology, U.S.A.
kiri.wagstaff@jpl.nasa.gov

Abstract: Clustering algorithms can identify groups in large data sets, such as star catalogs and hyperspectral images. In general, clustering methods cannot analyze items that have missing data values. Common solutions either fill in the missing values (imputation) or ignore the missing data (marginalization). Imputed values are treated as being just as reliable as the observed data, but they are only as good as the assumptions used to create them. In contrast, we present a method for encoding partially observed features as a set of supplemental soft constraints and introduce the KSC algorithm, which incorporates constraints into the clustering process. In experiments on artificial data and data from the Sloan Digital Sky Survey, we show that soft constraints are an effective way to enable clustering with missing values.

1 Introduction

Clustering is a powerful analysis tool that divides a set of items into a number of distinct groups based on a problem-independent criterion, such as maximum likelihood (the EM algorithm) or minimum variance (the k-means algorithm). In astronomy, clustering has been used to organize star catalogs such as POSS-II (Yoo et al., 1996) and classify observations such as IRAS spectra (Goebel, 1989). Notably, the Autoclass algorithm identified a new subclass of stars based on the clustering results (Goebel, 1989). These methods can also provide data compression or summarization by quickly identifying the most representative items in a data set.

One challenge in astronomical data analysis is *data fusion*: how to combine information about the same objects from various sources, such as a visible-wavelength catalog and an infra-red catalog. A critical problem that arises is that items may have missing values. Ideally, each object in the sky should appear in both catalogs. However, it is more likely that some objects will not. The two instruments may not have covered precisely the same regions of the sky, or some objects may not emit at the wavelengths used by one of the catalogs. Missing values also occur due to observing conditions, instrument sensitivity limitations, and other real-world considerations.

Clustering algorithms generally have no internal way to handle missing values. Instead, a common solution is to fill in the missing values in a preprocessing step. However, the filled-in values are inherently less reliable than the observed data. We propose a new approach to clustering that divides the data features into *observed features*, which are known for all objects, and *constraining features*, which contain missing values. We generate a set of constraints based on the known values for the constraining features. A modified clustering algorithm, KSC (for "K-means with Soft Constraints"), combines this set of constraints with the regular observed features. In this paper, we discuss our formulation of the missing data problem, present the KSC algorithm, and evaluate it on artificial data as well as data from the Sloan Digital Sky Survey. We find that KSC can significantly outperform data imputation methods, without producing possibly misleading "fill" values in the data.

2 Background and Related Work

Green et al. (2001), among others, identified two alternatives to handling missing values: *data imputation*, where values are estimated to fill in missing values, and *marginalization*, where missing values are ignored. However, imputed data cannot and should not be considered as reliable as the actually observed data. Troyanskaya et al. (2001) stated this clearly when evaluating different imputation methods for biological data: "However, it is important to exercise caution when drawing critical biological conclusions from data that is partially imputed. [. . .] [E]stimated data should be flagged where possible [. . .] to avoid drawing unwarranted conclusions."

Despite this warning, data imputation remains common, with no mechanism for indicating that the imputed values are less reliable. One approach is to replace all missing values with the observed mean for that feature (also known as the "row average" method in DNA microarray analysis). Another method is to model the observed values and select one according to the true distribution (if it is known). A more sophisticated approach is to infer the value of the missing feature based on that item's observed features and its similarity to other (known) items in the data set (Troyanskaya et al., 2001). Ghahramani and Jordan (1994) presented a modified EM algorithm that can process data with missing values. This method simultaneously estimates the maximum likelihood model parameters, data cluster assignments, and values for the missing features. Each of these methods suffers from an inability to discount imputed values due to their lack of full reliability.

We therefore believe that marginalization, which does not create any new data values, is a better solution. Most previous work in marginalization has focused on supervised methods such as neural networks (Tresp et al., 1995) or Hidden Markov Models (Vizinho et al., 1999). In contrast, our approach handles missing values even we have no labeled training data. In previous work, we developed a variant of k-means that produces output guaranteed to satisfy a set of hard constraints (Wagstaff et al., 2001). Hard constraints dictate that certain pairs of items must or must not be grouped together. Building on this work, we present an algorithm that can incorporate soft constraints, which indicate how strongly a pair of items should or should not be grouped together. In the next section, we will show how this algorithm can achieve good performance when clustering data with missing values.

3 Clustering with Soft Constraints

Constraints can effectively enable a clustering algorithm to conform to background knowledge (Wagstaff and Cardie, 2000; Klein et al., 2002). Previous work has focused largely on the use of hard constraints that must be satisfied by the algorithm. However, in the presence of uncertain or approximate information, and especially for real-world problems, soft constraints are more appropriate.

3.1 Soft Constraints

In this work, we divide the feature set into F_o, the set of observed features, and F_m, the set of features with missing values. We also refer to F_m as the set of *constraining* features, because we use them to constrain the results of the clustering algorithm; they represent a source of additional information.

Following Wagstaff (2002), we represent a soft constraint between items d_i and d_j as a triple: $\langle d_i, d_j, s\rangle$. The strength, s, is proportional to distance in F_m. We create a constraint $\langle d_i, d_j, s\rangle$ between each pair of items d_i, d_j with values for F_m, where

$$s = -\sqrt{\sum_{f \in F_m} (d_i.f - d_j.f)^2} \tag{1}$$

We do not create constraints for items that have missing values. The value for s is negative because this value indicates the degree to which d_i and d_j should be separated. Next, we present an algorithm that can accommodate these constraints while clustering.

3.2 K-means Clustering with Soft Constraints

We have chosen k-means (Macqueen, 1967), one of the most common clustering algorithms in use, as our prototype for the development of a soft constrained clustering algorithm. The key idea is to cluster over F_o, with constraints based on F_m.

Table 1. KSC algorithm

KSC(k, D, SC, w)

(1) Let $C_1 \ldots C_k$ be the initial cluster centers.
(2) For each instance d in D, assign it to the cluster C such that:

$$C := \underset{C_i}{\operatorname{argmin}} \left((1-w)\frac{\operatorname{dist}(d, C_i)^2}{V_{max}} + w\frac{CV_d}{CV_{max}} \right) \tag{2}$$

where CV_d is the sum of (squared) violated constraints in SC that involve d.
(3) Update each cluster center C_i by averaging all of the points $d_j \in C_i$.
(4) Iterate between (2) and (3) until convergence.
(5) Return the partition $\{C_1 \ldots C_k\}$.

The k-means algorithm iteratively searches for a good division of n objects into k clusters. It seeks to minimize the total variance V of a partition, i.e., the sum of the (squared) distances from each item d to its assigned cluster C:

$$V = \sum_{d \in D} \operatorname{dist}(d, C)^2$$

Distance from an item to a cluster is computed as the distance from the item to the center of the cluster. When selecting the best host cluster for a given item d, the only component in this sum that changes is $\operatorname{dist}(d, C)^2$, so k-means can minimize variance by assigning d to the closest available cluster:

$$C = \underset{C_i}{\operatorname{argmin}} \operatorname{dist}(d, C_i)^2$$

When clustering with soft constraints, we modify the objective function to penalize for violated constraints. The KSC algorithm takes in the specified number of clusters k, the data set D (with F_o only), a (possibly empty) set of constraints SC, and a weighting factor w that indicates the relative importance of the constraints versus variance (see Table 1).

KSC uses a modified objective function f that combines normalized variance and constraint violation values. The normalization enables a straightforward specification of the relative importance of each source, via a weighting factor $w \in [0, 1]$.

$$f = (1-w)\frac{V}{V_{max}} + w\frac{CV}{CV_{max}} \tag{3}$$

Note that w is an overall weight while s is an individual statement about the relationship between two items. The quantity CV is sum of the squared strengths of violated constraints in SC. It is normalized by CV_{max}, the sum of all squared constraint strengths, whether they are violated or not. A negative constraint, which indicates that d_i and d_j should be in different clusters, is violated if they are placed into the same cluster. We also normalize the

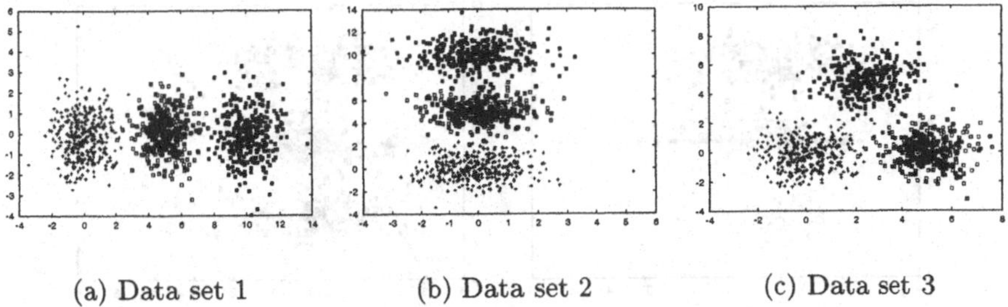

(a) Data set 1 (b) Data set 2 (c) Data set 3

Fig. 1. Three artificial data sets used to compare missing data methods.

variance of the partition by dividing by V_{max}, the largest possible variance given D. This is the variance obtained by assigning all items to a single cluster.

In deciding where to place item d, the only constraint violations that may change are ones that involve d. Therefore, KSC only considers constraints in which d participates and assigns items to clusters as shown in Equation 2.

4 Experimental Results

We have conducted experiments on artificial data as well as observational data from the Sloan Digital Sky Survey. As we will show, KSC in combination with constraints can often outperform typical data imputation methods. We will compare our approach to three common methods for handling missing data.

The first method, NOMISSING, does not impute data. Instead, it discards all of the features in F_m, relying only on the features in F_o. In doing so, it may discard useful information for the items that do possess values for F_m. Since our approach also bases its clustering only on features in F_o, any difference in performance will be due to the effect of including the soft constraints.

The second approach is MEANVALUE, which replaces each missing value with the mean of the observed values for that feature. The third approach is PROBDIST, which replaces missing values based on the observed distribution of values. For each item d with a missing value for feature f, we sample randomly from the observed values for f and select one to replace the missing value.

4.1 Partitioning Artificial Data

We created three artificial data sets (see Figure 1). In each case, the data set contains 1000 items in three classes that form Gaussian distributions. Data set 1 consists of three classes that are separable according to feature 1 (along the x-axis). Data set 2 consists of the same data mirrored so that the classes are separable according to feature 2. Data set 3 is data set 1 except with the rightmost class moved up and between the other two classes. In the final case, the three classes are not separable with either feature in isolation.

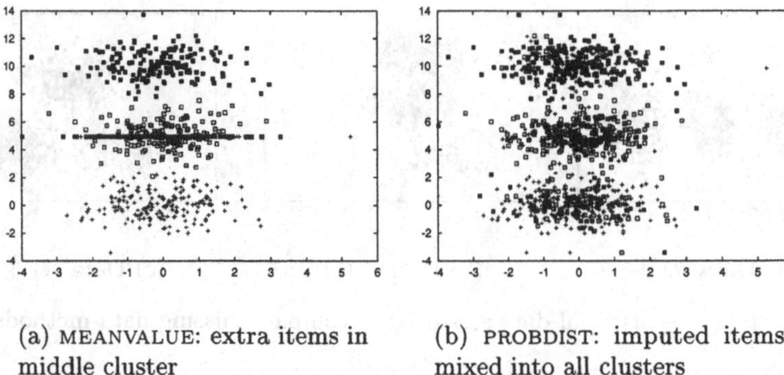

(a) MEANVALUE: extra items in middle cluster

(b) PROBDIST: imputed items mixed into all clusters

Fig. 2. Imputed data for data set 2 when 50% of feature 2's values are missing.

We have tested each method by generating variants of these data sets that contain increasing fractions of randomly missing values. For consistency, we only remove values in feature 2 (the y-axis). Figure 2 illustrates the problems associated with both imputation methods by showing the resulting data sets when 50% of the feature 2 values for items in data set 2 are removed, then imputed. MEANVALUE positions all of the imputed data in the middle cluster, while PROBDIST thoroughly mixes the data between clusters.

To create the soft constraints for KSC, we examine each pair of items d_i, d_j. If both have values for feature 2, we create a soft constraint between them proportional to their distance in feature 2 (cf. Equation 1):

$$s = -|d_i.f_2 - d_j.f_2| \tag{4}$$

The constraint is negative because it indicates how likely the two items are to be in different clusters. We then cluster using only feature 1, similar to NOMISSING, but with the additional constraint information.

We also need to select a value for w, the weight that is given to the constraint information. For data set 1, we know that feature 2 is not very useful for distinguishing the clusters, so we set $w = 0.01$. For data set 2, feature 2 is critical, so we set $w = 0.99$. For data set 3, where both features are important, we use the "equal weight" default value of $w = 0.5$. If the importance of F_m is unknown, it can be estimated by clustering with several different values for w on a small labeled subset of the data.

To evaluate performance, we compare the resulting partition (P_1) to the true partition (P_2) via the adjusted Rand index (Hubert and Arabie, 1985), averaged over ten trials. Let n_{ij} be the number of items that appear in cluster i in P_1 and in cluster j in P_2. Then R is the total agreement between P_1 and P_2, and we calculate

$$\text{Rand}(P_1, P_2) = \frac{R - E[R]}{M[R] - E[R]}, \quad R = \sum_{ij} \binom{n_{ij}}{2}$$

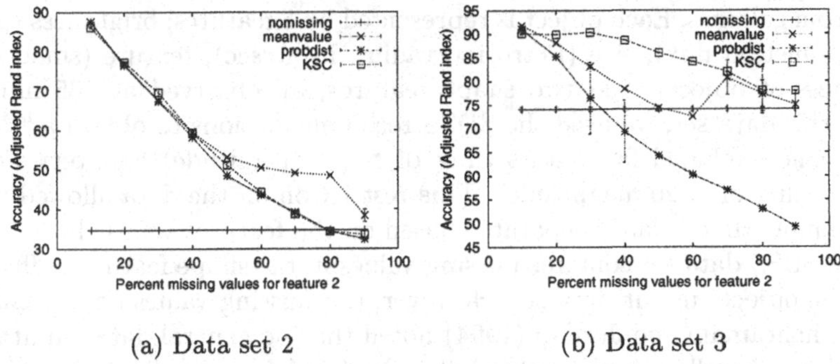

(a) Data set 2 (b) Data set 3

Fig. 3. Accuracy for all four methods on two artificial data sets ($k = 3$, 10 trials); bars indicate +/− one standard deviation.

where $E[R] = \left[\sum_i \binom{n_{i\cdot}}{2} \sum_j \binom{n_{\cdot j}}{2}\right] / \binom{n}{2}$ is the expected value of R and $M[R] = \frac{1}{2}\left[\sum_i \binom{n_{i\cdot}}{2} + \sum_j \binom{n_{\cdot j}}{2}\right]$ is the maximum possible value for R.

Because data set 1 is readily separable without any information from feature 2, we found that performance was identical for all methods at all fractions of missing values, at 98.8%. However, we observe dramatic differences for the other two data sets (see Figure 3). Performance for NOMISSING is independent of the fraction of missing values, because it only uses feature 1 to cluster the data. For data set 2, PROBDIST and KSC perform almost identically, though they make different kinds of errors. The output of PROBDIST assigns items with missing values arbitrarily to one of the three clusters. KSC's output comes to resemble that of NOMISSING when less constraint information is available (i.e., more values are missing). And MEANVALUE outperforms the other methods for missing fractions $\geq 50\%$, largely by placing the majority of the items all into the middle cluster. Although items from the top and bottom clusters are not correctly clustered, all of the items in the middle cluster are. This could be an artifact of using three clusters.

We find that KSC and MEANVALUE outperform PROBDIST for data set 3. In addition, KSC is much more robust to an increasing fraction of missing values. It is consistently the best performer for missing fractions greater than 10%. Overall, KSC performs as well or better than discarding or imputing data, without generating any potentially misleading data values. The exception to this trend is for data where the clusters are not separable in the observed features, when little information is available as constraints.

4.2 Separating Stars from Galaxies

In addition to our experiments with artificial data, we have also used KSC to analyze a portion of the SDSS star catalog. Our data set contains 977 objects:

354 stars and 623 galaxies. The goal is to produce a partition that separates stars from galaxies. Each object is represented by 5 features: brightness (point spread function flux), size (Petrosian radius, in arcsec), texture (small-scale roughness of object), and two shape features, all observed at 365 nm. To obtain this data set, we used the SDSS recommendations to obtain a "clean" sample and excluded faint stars (flux of $>$ 20 magnitude) and very bright galaxies (flux of $\leq$ 20 magnitude). This restriction on the data allowed us to get a sample that is fairly separable based on the features we used.

The SDSS data set contains missing values in the shape features, affecting 49 of the objects in our data set. However, the missing values only occur for stars. Ghahramani and Jordan (1994) noted that no general data imputation method can handle missing data that is confined to a single class, which is another reason to favor non-imputation methods. The fully observed features (F_o) are brightness, size, and texture. We created imputed versions of the data set for MEANVALUE and PROBDIST as described in the previous section. We created the set of soft constraints by generating, for each pair d_i, d_j that did have values for both features in F_m, a soft constraint according to Equation 1. The resulting set contained 873,920 constraints. Without any specific guidance as to the importance of F_m, we used a default value of $w = 0.5$.

However, in examining the output of each method we discovered that better performance could be obtained when clustering the data into *three* clusters, as shown in the following table. Three clusters allow finer divisions of the data, though splitting stars or galaxies across clusters is still penalized. This result suggests that there is a distinct star type that is easily confused with galaxies. The third cluster permitted these ambiguous items to be separated from the true star and galaxy clusters.

Method	NOMISSING	MEANVALUE	PROBDIST	KSC, $w = 0.5$
$k = 2$	80.6	70.6	70.6	68.3
$k = 3$	88.0	82.6	81.5	84.2

In both cases, NOMISSING achieved the best performance, suggesting that the shape features may not be useful in distinguishing stars from galaxies. To test this theory, we ran KSC with w values ranging from 0.1 to 0.9 (see Figure 4). We find that shape information *can* be useful, if properly weighted. For $w = 0.3, 0.4$, KSC outperforms NOMISSING, attaining a peak value of 90.4%. Otherwise, NOMISSING is the best method. There is no general rule for selecting a good w value, but existing knowledge about the domain can point to a value.

The large standard deviation for KSC is due to the occasional solution that does not satisfy very many constraints. For example, when $w = 0.4$, four of 50 trials converged to a solution that satisfied only 23% of the constraints (Rand 62%). The remaining trials satisfied about 46% of the constraints and achieved 90% performance. Thus, the constraint information, when satisfied, is very useful. Abd MEANVALUE and PROBDIST also have standard deviations of about 5.0 (not shown in Figure 4 for clarity).

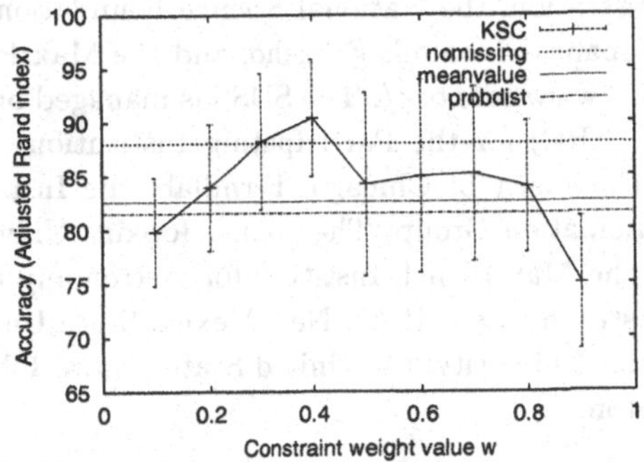

Fig. 4. Accuracy when clustering SDSS data with different weights for the constraints ($k = 3$, 50 trials); bars indicate $+/-$ one standard deviation for KSC.

5 Conclusions and Future Work

In this paper, we presented a new approach to the missing value problem for clustering algorithms. We have discussed, and demonstrated, the difficulties of data imputation methods that process imputed values as if they were as reliable as the actual observations. We presented a new approach that divides the data features into F_o, the observed features, and F_m, the features with missing values. We generate a set of soft constraints based on distances calculated on known values for F_m. A new algorithm, KSC, can apply these soft constraints. In experiments with artificial data and the SDSS star/galaxy catalog, we have shown that KSC can perform as well as or better than data imputation methods. In some cases, knowledge of the relative importance of the missing features is necessary.

In future work, we plan to compare KSC directly to the EM-based algorithm of Ghahramani and Jordan (1994). Although their goals were different (recovering missing data values vs. determining the correct partition), a comparison would provide further understanding of the applicability of KSC.

Another consideration is the complexity of the KSC approach. The number of constraints is $\mathcal{O}(n^2)$, where n is the number of items that possess values for features in F_m. Klein (2002) have suggested a technique for propagating hard constraints through the feature space, obtaining equivalent results with fewer explicit constraints. Although their work was restricted to hard constraints, we would like to explore options for extending their method to work with soft constraints as well.

Acknowledgments

This work was partially supported by NSF grant IIS-0325329. We wish to thank Victoria G. Laidler and Amy McGovern for their input on an early draft of this paper. Funding for the Sloan Digital Sky Survey (SDSS) has been provided by the Alfred P. Sloan Foundation, the Participating Institutions, the National Aeronautics and Space Administration, the National Science Foundation, the U.S. Department of Energy, the Japanese Monbukagakusho, and the Max Planck Society. The SDSS Web site is http://www.sdss.org/. The SDSS is managed by the Astrophysical Research Consortium (ARC) for the Participating Institutions. The Participating Institutions are The University of Chicago, Fermilab, the Institute for Advanced Study, the Japan Participation Group, The Johns Hopkins University, Los Alamos National Laboratory, the Max-Planck-Institute for Astronomy (MPIA), the Max-Planck-Institute for Astrophysics (MPA), New Mexico State University, University of Pittsburgh, Princeton University, the United States Naval Observatory, and the University of Washington.

References

1. Ghahramani, Z. and Jordan, M. I. (1994). "Learning from Incomplete Data," Tech. Report, Massachusetts Inst. of Technology Artificial Intelligence Lab.
2. Goebel, J., Volk, K., Walker, H., Gerbault, F., Cheeseman, P., Self, M., Stutz, J., and Taylor, W. (1989). "A Bayesian Classification of the IRAS LRS Atlas," *Astronomy and Astrophysics*, **222**, L5–L8.
3. Green, P. D., Barker, J., Cooke, M. P., and Josifovski, L. (2001). "Handling Missing and Unreliable Information in Speech Recognition," in *Proceedings of AISTATS 2001*, pp. 49-56.
4. Hubert, L. and Arabie, P. (1985). "Comparing Partitions," *Journal of Classification*, **2**, 193–218.
5. Klein, D., Kamvar, S. D., and Manning, C. D. (2002). "From Instance-Level Constraints to Space-Level Constraints: Making the Most of Prior Knowledge in Data Clustering," in *Proc. of the 19th Intl. Conf. on Machine Learning*, Morgan Kaufmann, pp. 307-313.
6. MacQueen, J. B. (1967). "Some Methods for Classification and Analysis of Multivariate Observations" in *Proceedings of the Fifth Berkeley Symposium on Math, Statistics, and Probability*, Berkeley:University of California Press, pp. 281-297.
7. Tresp, V., Neunier, R., and Ahmad, S. (1995). "Efficient Methods for Dealing with Missing Data in Supervised Learning," in *Advances in Neural Information Processing Systems 7*, pp. 689-696.
8. Troyanskaya, O., Cantor, M., Sherlock, G., Brown, P., Hastie, T., Tibshirani, R., Botstein, D., and Altman, R. B. (2001). "Missing Value Estimation Methods for DNA Microarrays," *Bioinformatics*, **17**, 520–525.
9. Vizinho, A., Green, P., Cooke, M., and Josifovski, L. (1999). "Missing Data Theory, Spectral Subtraction and Signal-to-Noise Estimation for Robust ASR: An Integrated Study," in *Proc. of Eurospeech '99*, pp. 2407–2410.
10. Wagstaff, K. (2002) *Intelligent Clustering with Instance-Level Constraints*, Ph.D. dissertation, Cornell University.
11. Wagstaff, K., Cardie, C., Rogers, S., and Schroedl, S. (2001). "Constrained k-Means Clustering with Background Knowledge," in *Proceedings of the 18th International Conference on Machine Learning*, San Mateo:Morgan Kaufmann, pp. 577–584.
12. Yoo, J., Gray, A., Roden, J., Fayyad, U., de Carvalho, R., and Djorgovski, S. (1996). "Analysis of Digital POSS-II Catalogs Using Hierarchical Unsupervised Learning Algorithms," in *Astronomical Data Analysis Software and Systems V*, vol. 101 of ASP Conference Series, pp. 41–44.